THE GREATEST BENEFIT
TO MANKIND

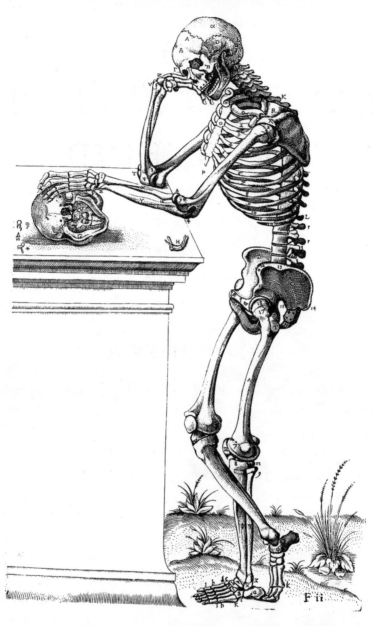

Renaissance anatomical illustrations often followed artistic conventions (situating the skeleton in a lifelike pose in a landscape) and played wittily on the tensions between life and death. The contemplation of the skull prefigures Hamlet's later meditation. Line drawing, Valverde de Hamusco, *Historia de la composicion del cuerco humano* (Rome: A. Salamanca & A. Lafreri, 1556).

THE
GREATEST BENEFIT
TO MANKIND

A Medical History of
Humanity from
Antiquity to the Present

ROY PORTER

HarperCollins*Publishers*

HarperCollins*Publishers*
77–85 Fulham Palace Road,
Hammersmith, London w6 8jb

Published by HarperCollins*Publishers* 1997
1 3 5 7 9 8 6 4 2

ISBN 0 00 215173 1

Set in Janson by Rowland Phototypesetting Limited
Bury St Edmunds, Suffolk

Printed and bound in Great Britain by
Caledonian International Book Manufacturing Ltd, Glasgow

All pictures courtesy of the Wellcome Institute Library,
London, except 'FDR photographed in his wheelchair at Warm Springs',
courtesy of the Franklin D. Roosevelt Library, Hyde Park,
New York; 'Brain in Skull', courtesy of GJLP/CNRI/Science Photo Library;
'A British hospital ward in the 1990s', courtesy of Emma Taylor,
St. George's Hospital Medical School.

TO

Mikuláš Teich,
true friend and scholar

Sick – Sick – Sick . . . O Sick – Sick – Spew

DAVID GARRICK, in a letter

I'm sick of gruel, and the dietetics,
I'm sick of pills, and sicker of emetics,
I'm sick of pulses, tardiness or quickness,
I'm sick of blood, its thinness or its thickness, –
In short, within a word, I'm sick of sickness!

THOMAS HOOD, 'Fragment', c. 1844

They are *shallow* animals, having always employed their minds about Body and Gut, they imagine that in the whole system of things there is nothing but Gut and Body.

SAMUEL TAYLOR COLERIDGE, on doctors (1796)

CONTENTS

FIGURES

ILLUSTRATIONS

An Apothecary with a Pestle and Mortar to Make up a Prescription by A. Park.
The interior of a pharmaceutical laboratory with people at work.
Philadelphia College of Pharmacy and Science.

Between pages 576 and 577

Portrait of René Théophile Hyacinthe Laennec
Portrait of Louis Pasteur by E. Pirou.
Portrait of William Gorgas.
Portrait of Joseph Lister.
Christiaan Barnard, photographed by B. Govender.
Mentally ill patients in the garden of an asylum by K. H. Merz.
Sigmund Freud, Carl Gustav Jung, Ernest Jones, Sandor Ferenczi, Abraham
Bill and G. Stanley Hall.
A male smallpox patient in sickness and in health.
A Fijian man with elephantiasis of the left leg and scrotum.
An Allegory of Malaria by Maurice Dudevant.
A white doctor vaccinating African girls all wearing European clothes at a
mission station by Meisenbach.
Portrait of Florence Nightingale.
A Nurse Checking on a Playful Child by J. E. Sutcliffe.
'A district health centre where crowds of local children are being vaccinated'
by E. Buckman.
Franklin D. Roosevelt.
The Hôtel Dieu.
Lister and his assistants in the Victoria Ward.
A British hospital ward in the 1990s photographed by Emma Taylor.
The bones of a hand, with a ring on one finger, viewed through X-ray.
Tomographic scan of a brain in a skull.

ACKNOWLEDGEMENTS

THE USUAL SUSPECTS will be heartily tired of hearing their praises sung yet again. As always, Frieda Houser has been a marvellous secretary, keeping everything on the road while I was deep in this book; Caroline Overy an infallible research assistant; Sheila Lawler and Jan Pinkerton indefatigable on the word-processor, and Andy Foley a wiz on the xerox machine. I have been so lucky having their help and friendship for so long. Thanks!

New to me have been the help and friendship I have received from Fontana Press. The series of which this book forms a part was first planned ten years ago, and since then Stuart Proffitt, Philip Gwyn Jones and Toby Mundy have been ever supportive, skilled equally in the use of sticks and carrots. Biddy Martin's copy editing uncovered ghastly errors and eliminated stylistic horrors, and Drusella Calvert compiled a truly thorough index.

Friends old and new have read this book at various stages and shared their thoughts, knowledge and criticisms with me. My thanks to Michael Neve, who always reads my manuscripts, and to Bill Bynum and Tilli Tansey for being patient with one who lacks a sound medico-scientific education; and to Hannah Augstein, Cristina Alvarez, Natsu Hattori, Paul Lerner, Eileen Magnello, Diana Manuel, Chandak Sengoopta, Sonu Shamdasani and Cassie Watson, all of whom have read the text, saved me from constellations of errors, shared insights and information, levelled cogent criticisms and helped to keep me going at the moments when all seemed sisyphean. Catherine Draycott and William Schupbach have been immensely helpful with the illustrations. My aim first and foremost is to tell a story that is clear, interesting and informative to students and general readers alike. My thanks to all who have helped the book in that direction.

I also wish to thank all the medical historians and other scholars whose papers I have heard, whose books I have read, and whose company

I have shared over the last twenty years. I have the deepest admiration for the expertise and the historical vision of scholars in this field. Panning from Stone Age to New Age, from Galen to Gallo, I cannot pretend personal knowledge on more than a few frames of the times and topics covered. As will be plain to see, I am everywhere profoundly dependent on the work of others. It would simply be distracting in a work like this to acknowledge all such debts one after another in thickets of footnotes. The Further Reading must serve not just by way of recommendation for what to read next but as a collective thank-you to all upon whose work I have freely and gratefully drawn.

I have written this book because when my students and people at large have asked me to recommend an up-to-date and readable single-volume history of medicine, I have felt at a loss to know what to suggest. Rather than bemoaning this fact, I thought I should have a shot at filling the gap. Writing it has made it clear why so few have attempted this foolhardy task.

The author and publishers are grateful to the following for permission to reproduce material: extracts from *The Illustrated History of Surgery* by Knut Haeger, courtesy of Harold Starke Publishers; extracts from *A History of Medicine* by Jean Starobinski, courtesy of Prentice Hall; extracts from *Hippocrates I–IV* and *The Complete Letters of Sigmund Freud to Wilhelm Fleiss, 1887–1904*, edited by Jeffrey Masson, courtesy of Harvard University Press; extracts from *The Odes of Pindar*, edited and translated by Richmond Lattimore, courtesy of Chicago University Press; extracts from *Medicine Out of Control: The Anatomy of Malignant Technology* by Richard Taylor, courtesy of Sun Books; extracts from *A History of Syphilis* by Claude Quétel, courtesy of Blackwell Publishers; extracts from *Doctor Dock. Teaching and Learning Medicine at the Turn of the Century* by Horace W. Davenport, courtesy of Rutgers University Press; an extract from Steven Sondheim's *West Side Story* courtesy of Boosey & Hawkes, Music Publishers Ltd. All reasonable efforts have been made by the author and the publisher to trace the copyright holders of the quotations contained in this publication. In the event that any of the untraceable copyright holders comes forward after the publication of this edition, the author and the publishers will endeavour to rectify the situation accordingly.

THE
GREATEST BENEFIT
TO MANKIND

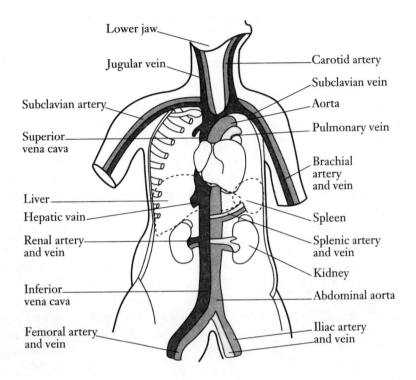

Lower jaw

Jugular vein

Subclavian artery

Superior
vena cava

Liver

Hepatic vain

Renal artery
and vein

Inferior
vena cava

Femoral artery
and vein

Carotid artery

Subclavian vein

Aorta

Pulmonary vein

Brachial
artery
and vein

Spleen

Splenic artery
and vein

Kidney

Abdominal aorta

Iliac artery
and vein

The main organs of the body

CHAPTER I

INTRODUCTION

THESE ARE STRANGE TIMES, when we are healthier than ever but more anxious about our health. According to all the standard benchmarks, we've never had it so healthy. Longevity in the West continues to rise – a typical British woman can now expect to live to seventy-nine, eight years more than just half a century ago, and over double the life expectation when Queen Victoria came to the throne in 1837. Break the figures down a bit and you find other encouraging signs even in the recent past; in 1950, the UK experienced 26,000 infant deaths; within half a century that had fallen by 80 per cent. Deaths in the UK from infectious diseases nearly halved between 1970 and 1992; between 1971 and 1991 stroke deaths dropped by 40 per cent and coronary heart disease fatalities by 19 per cent – and those are diseases widely perceived to be worsening.

The heartening list goes on and on (15,000 hip replacements in 1978, over double that number in 1993). In myriad ways, medicine continues to advance, new treatments appear, surgery works marvels, and (partly as a result) people live longer. Yet few people today feel confident, either about their personal health or about doctors, healthcare delivery and the medical profession in general. The media bombard us with medical news – breakthroughs in biotechnology and reproductive technology for instance. But the effect is to raise alarm more than our spirits.

The media specialize in scare-mongering but they also capture a public mood. There is a pervasive sense that our well-being is imperilled by 'threats' all around, from the air we breathe to the food in the shops. Why should we now be more agitated about pollution in our lungs than during the awful urban smogs of the 1950s, when tens of thousands died of winter bronchitis? Have we become health freaks or hypochondriacs luxuriating in health anxieties precisely because we are so healthy and long-lived that we have the leisure to enjoy the luxury of worrying?

These may be questions for a psychologist but, as this book aims to demonstrate, they are also matters of historical inquiry, examining the dialectics of medicine and mentalities. And to understand the dilemmas of our times, such facts and fears need to be put into context of time and place. We are today in the grip of opposing pressures. For one thing, there is the 'rising-expectations trap': we have convinced ourselves that we can and should be fitter, more youthful, sexier. In the long run, these are impossibly frustrating goals, because in the long run we're all dead (though of course some even have expectations of cheating death). Likewise, we are healthier than ever before, yet more distrustful of doctors and the powers of what may broadly be called the 'medical system'. Such scepticism follows from the fact that medical science seems to be fulfilling the wildest dreams of science fiction: the first cloning of a sheep was recently announced and it will apparently be feasible to clone a human being within a couple of years. In the same week, an English widow was given permission to try to become pregnant with her dead husband's sperm (but only so long as she did it in Belgium). These are amazing developments. We turn doctors into heroes, yet feel equivocal about them.

Such ambiguities are not new. When in 1858 a statue was erected in the recently built Trafalgar Square to Edward Jenner, the pioneer of smallpox vaccination, protests followed and it was rapidly removed: a country doctor amidst the generals and admirals was thought unseemly (it may seem that those responsible for causing deaths rather than saving lives are worthy of public honour). Even in Greek times opinions about medicine were mixed; the word *pharmakos* meant both remedy and poison – 'kill' and 'cure' were apparently indistinguishable. And as Jonathan Swift wryly reflected early in the eighteenth century, 'Apollo was held the god of physic and sender of diseases. Both were originally the same trade, and still continue.' That double idea – death and the doctors riding together – has loomed large in history. It is one of the threads we will follow in trying to assess the impact of medicine and responses to it – in trying to assess Samuel Johnson's accolade to the medical profession: 'the greatest benefit to mankind.'

'The art has three factors, the disease, the patient, the physician,' wrote Hippocrates, the legendary Greek physician who has often been called the father of medicine; and he thus suggested an agenda for history. This book will explore diseases, patients and physicians, and their inter-relations, concentrating on some more than others. It is, as its sub-title suggests, a *medical* history.

My focus could have been on disease and its bearing on human history. We have all been reminded of the devastating effects of pestilence by the AIDS epidemic. In terms of death toll, cultural shock and socio-economic destruction, the full impact of AIDS cannot yet be judged. Other 'hot viruses' may be coming into the arena of history which may prove even more calamitous. Historians at large, who until recently tended to chronicle world history in blithe ignorance of or indifference to disease, now recognize the difference made by plague, cholera and other pandemics. Over the last generation, distinguished practitioners have pioneered the study of 'plagues and peoples'; and I have tried to give due consideration to these epidemiological and demographic matters in the following chapters. But they are not my protagonists, rather the backdrop.

Equally this book might have focused upon everyday health, common health beliefs and routine health care in society at large. The social history of medicine now embraces 'people's history', and one of its most exciting developments has been the attention given to beliefs about the body, its status and stigmas, its race, class and gender representations. The production and reproduction, creation and recreation of images of Self and Other have formed the subject matter of distinguished books. Such historical sociologies or cultural anthropologies – regarding the body as a book to be decoded – reinforce our awareness of the importance, past and present, of familiar beliefs about health and its hazards, about taboo and transgression. When a body becomes a clue to meaning, popular ideas of health and sickness, life and death, must be of central historical importance. I have written, on my own and with others, numerous books exploring lay health cultures in the past, from a 'bottom-up', patients' point of view, and hope soon to publish a further work on the historical significance of the body.

This history, however, is different. It sets the history of *medical* thinking and *medical* practice at stage centre. It concentrates on medical ideas about disease, medical teachings about healthy and unhealthy bodies, and medical models of life and death. Seeking to avoid anachronism and judgmentalism, I devote prime attention to those people and professional groups who have been responsible for such beliefs and practices – that is healers understood in a broad sense. This book is principally about what those healers have done, individually and collectively, and the impact of their ideas and actions. While placing developments in a wider context, it surveys medical theory and practices.

This approach may sound old-fashioned, a resurrection of the Whiggish 'great docs' history which celebrated the triumphal progress of medicine from ignorance through error to science. But I come not to praise medicine – nor indeed to blame it. I do believe that medicine has played a major and growing role in human societies and for that reason its history needs to be explored so that its place and powers can be understood. I say here, and I will say many times again, that the prominence of medicine has lain only in small measure in its ability to make the sick well. This always was true, and remains so today.

I discuss disease from a global viewpoint; no other perspective makes sense. I also examine medicine the world over. Chapter 2 surveys the emergence of health practices and medical beliefs in some early societies; Chapter 3 discusses the rise of formal, written medicine in the Middle East and Egypt, and in Greece and Rome; Chapter 4 explores Islam; separate chapters discuss Indian and Chinese medicine; Chapter 8 takes in the Americas; Chapter 15 surveys medicine in more recent colonial contexts, and other chapters have discussions of disorders in the Third World, for instance deficiency diseases. The book is thus not narrowly or blindly ethnocentric.

Nevertheless, I devote most attention to what is called 'western' medicine, because western medicine has developed in ways which have made it uniquely powerful and led it to become uniquely global. Its ceaseless spread throughout the world owes much, doubtless, to western political and economic domination. But its dominance has increased because it is perceived, by societies and the sick, to 'work' uniquely well, at least for many major classes of disorders. (Parenthetically, it can be argued that western political and economic domination owes something to the path-breaking powers of quinine, antibiotics and the like.) To the world historian, western medicine is special. It is *conceivable* that in a hundred years time traditional Chinese medicine, shamanistic medicine or Ayurvedic medicine will have swept the globe; if that happens, my analysis will look peculiarly dated and daft. But there is no real indication of that happening, while there is every reason to expect the medicine of the future to be an outgrowth of present western medicine

– or at least a reaction against it. What began as the medicine of Europe is becoming the medicine of humanity. For that reason its history deserves particular attention.

Western medicine, I argue, has developed radically distinctive approaches to exploring the workings of the human body in sickness and in health. These have changed the ways our culture conceives of the body and of human life. To reduce complex matters to crass terms, most peoples and cultures the world over, throughout history, have construed life (birth and death, sickness and health) primarily in the context of an understanding of the relations of human beings to the wider cosmos: planets, stars, mountains, rivers, spirits and ancestors, gods and demons, the heavens and the underworld, and so forth. Some traditions, notably those reflected in Chinese and Indian learned medicine, while being concerned with the architecture of the cosmos, do not pay great attention to the supernatural. Modern western thinking, however, has become indifferent to all such elements. The West has evolved a culture preoccupied with the self, with the individual and his or her identity, and this quest has come to be equated with (or reduced to) the individual body and the embodied personality, expressed through body language. Hamlet wanted this too solid flesh to melt away. That – except in the context of slimming obsessions – is the last thing modern westerners want to happen to their flesh; they want it to last as long as possible.

Explanations of why and how these modern, secular western attitudes have come about need to take many elements into account. Their roots may be found in the philosophical and religious traditions they have grown out of. They have been stimulated by economic materialism, the preoccupation with worldly goods generated by the devouring, reckless energies of capitalism. But they are also intimately connected with the development of medicine – its promise, project and products.

Whereas most traditional healing systems have sought to understand the relations of the sick person to the wider cosmos and to make readjustments between individual and world, or society and world, the western medical tradition explains sickness principally in terms of the body itself – its own cosmos. Greek medicine dismissed supernatural powers, though not macrocosmic, environmental influences; and from the Renaissance the flourishing anatomical and physiological programmes created a new confidence among investigators that everything that needed to be known could essentially be discovered by probing more deeply and ever more minutely into the flesh, its systems, tissues, cells, its DNA.

This has proved an infinitely productive inquiry, generating first knowledge and then power, including on some occasions the power to conquer disease. The idea of probing into bodies, living and dead (and especially *human* bodies) with a view to improving medicine is more or less distinctive to the European medical tradition. For reasons technical, cultural, religious and personal, it was not done in China or India, Mesopotamia or pharaonic Egypt. Dissection and dissection-related experimentation were performed only on animals in classical Greece, and rarely. A medicine that seriously and systematically investigated the stuff of bodies came into being thereafter – in Alexandria, then in the work of Galen, then in late medieval Italy. The centrality of anatomy to medicine's project was proclaimed in the Renaissance and became the foundation stone for the later edifice of scientific medicine: physiological experimentation, pathology, microscopy, biochemistry and all the other later specialisms, to say nothing of invasive surgery.

This was not the only course that medicine could have taken; as is noted below, it was not the course other great world medical systems took, cultivating their own distinct clinical skills, diagnostic arts and therapeutic interventions. Nor did it enjoy universal approval: protests in Britain around 1800 about body-snatching and later antivivisectionist lobbies show how sceptical public opinion remained about the activities of anatomists and physicians, and suspicion has continued to run high. However, that was the direction western medicine followed, and, bolstered by science at large, it generated a powerful medicine, largely independent of its efficacy as a rational social approach to good health.

The emergence of this high-tech scientific medicine may be a prime example of what William Blake denounced as 'single vision', the kind of myopia which (literally and metaphorically) comes from looking doggedly down a microscope. Single vision has its limitations in explaining the human condition; this is why Coleridge called doctors '*shallow* animals', who 'imagine that in the whole system of things there is nothing but Gut and Body'. Hence the ability of medicine to understand and counter pathology has always engendered paradox. Medicine has offered the promise of 'the greatest benefit to mankind', but not always on terms palatable to and compatible with cherished ideals. Nor has it always delivered the goods. The particular powers of medicine, and the paradoxes its rationales generate, are what this book is about.

*   *   *

It may be useful to offer a brief resumé of the main themes of the book, by way of a sketch map for a long journey.

All societies possess medical beliefs: ideas of life and death, disease and cure, and systems of healing. Schematically speaking, the medical history of humanity may be seen as a series of stages. Belief systems the world over have attributed sickness to illwill, to malevolent spirits, sorcery, witchcraft and diabolical or divine intervention. Such ways of thinking still pervade the tribal communities of Africa, the Amazon basin and the Pacific; they were influential in Christian Europe till the 'age of reason', and retain a residual shadow presence. Christian Scientists and some other Christian sects continue to view sickness and recovery in providential and supernatural terms; healing shrines like Lourdes remain popular within the Roman Catholic church, and faith-healing retains a mass following among devotees of television evangelists in the United States.

In Europe from Graeco-Roman antiquity onwards, and also among the great Asian civilizations, the medical profession systematically replaced transcendental explanations by positing a natural basis for disease and healing. Among educated lay people and physicians alike, the body became viewed as integral to law-governed cosmic elements and regular processes. Greek medicine emphasized the microcosm/macrocosm relationship, the correlations between the healthy human body and the harmonies of nature. From Hippocrates in the fifth century BC through to Galen in the second century AD, 'humoral medicine' stressed the analogies between the four elements of external nature (fire, water, air and earth) and the four humours or bodily fluids (blood, phlegm, choler or yellow bile and black bile), whose balance determined health. The humours found expression in the temperaments and complexions that marked an individual. The task of hygiene was to maintain a balanced constitution, and the role of medicine was to restore the balance when disturbed. Parallels to these views appear in the classical Chinese and Indian medical traditions.

The medicine of antiquity, transmitted to Islam and then back to the medieval West and remaining powerful throughout the Renaissance, paid great attention to general health maintenance through regulation of diet, exercise, hygiene and lifestyle. In the absence of decisive anatomical and physiological expertise, and without a powerful arsenal of cures and surgical skills, the ability to diagnose and make prognoses was highly valued, and an intimate physician-patient relationship was fostered. The teachings of antiquity, which remained authoritative until the eighteenth century and still supply subterranean reservoirs of medical folklore, were more successful in assisting people to cope with chronic conditions and soothing lesser ailments than in conquering life-threatening infections which became endemic and epidemic in the civilized world: leprosy, plague, smallpox, measles, and, later, the 'filth diseases' (like typhus) associated with urban squalor.

This personal tradition of bedside medicine long remained popular in the West, as did its equivalents in Chinese and Ayurvedic medicine. But in Europe it was supplemented and challenged by the creation of a more 'scientific' medicine, grounded, for the first time, upon experimental anatomical and physiological investigation, epitomized from the fifteenth century by the dissection techniques which became central to medical education. Landmarks in this programme include the publication of *De humani corporis fabrica* (1543) by the Paduan professor, Andreas Vesalius, a momentous anatomical atlas and a work which challenged truths received since Galen; and William Harvey's *De motu cordis* (1628) which put physiological inquiry on the map by experiments demonstrating the circulation of the blood and the heart's role as a pump.

Post-Vesalian investigations dramatically advanced knowledge of the structures and functions of the living organism. Further inquiries brought the unravelling of the lymphatic system and the lacteals, and the eighteenth and nineteenth centuries yielded a finer grasp of the nervous system and the operations of the brain. With the aid of microscopes and the laboratory, nineteenth-century investigators explored the nature of body tissue and pioneered cell biology; pathological anatomy came of age. Parallel developments in organic chemistry led to an understanding of respiration, nutrition, the digestive system and deficiency diseases, and founded such specialities as endocrinology. The twentieth century became the age of genetics and molecular biology.

Nineteenth-century medical science made spectacular leaps forward in the understanding of infectious diseases. For many centuries, rival epidemiological theories had attributed fevers to miasmas (poisons in the air, exuded from rotting animal and vegetable material, the soil, and standing water) or to contagion (person-to-person contact). From the 1860s, the rise of bacteriology, associated especially with Louis Pasteur in France and Robert Koch in Germany, established the role of micro-organic pathogens. Almost for the first time in medicine, bacteriology led directly to dramatic new cures.

In the short run, the anatomically based scientific medicine which emerged from Renaissance universities and the Scientific Revolution contributed more to knowledge than to health. Drugs from both the Old and New Worlds, notably opium and Peruvian bark (quinine) became more widely available, and mineral and metal-based pharmaceutical preparations enjoyed a great if dubious vogue (e.g., mercury for syphilis). But the true pharmacological revolution began with the introduction of sulfa drugs and antibiotics in the twentieth century, and surgical success was limited before the introduction of anaesthetics and antiseptic operating-room conditions in the mid nineteenth century. Biomedical understanding long outstripped breakthroughs in curative medicine, and the retreat of the great lethal diseases (diphtheria, typhoid, tuberculosis and so forth) was due, in the first instance, more to urban improvements, superior nutrition and public health than to curative medicine. The one early striking instance of the conquest of disease – the introduction first of smallpox inoculation and then of vaccination – came not through 'science' but through embracing popular medical folklore.

From the Middle Ages, medical practitioners organized themselves professionally in a pyramid with physicians at the top and surgeons and apothecaries nearer the base, and with other healers marginalized or vilified as quacks. Practitioners' guilds, corporations and colleges received royal approval, and medicine was gradually incorporated into the public domain, particularly in German-speaking Europe where the notion of 'medical police' (health regulation and preventive public health) gained official backing in the eighteenth century. The state inevitably played the leading role in the growth of military and naval medicine, and later in tropical medicine. The hospital sphere, however, long remained largely the Church's responsibility, especially in Roman Catholic parts of Europe. Gradually the state took responsibility for the health of emergent industrial society, through public health regulation and custody of the insane in the nineteenth century, and later through national insurance and national health schemes. These latter developments met fierce opposition from a medical profession seeking to preserve its autonomy against encroaching state bureaucracies.

The latter half of the twentieth century has witnessed the continued phenomenal progress of capital-intensive and specialized scientific medicine: transplant surgery and biotechnology have captured the public imagination. Alongside, major chronic and psychosomatic disorders persist and worsen – jocularly expressed as the 'doing better but feeling worse' syndrome – and the basic health of the developing world is deteriorating. This situation exemplifies and perpetuates a key facet and paradox of the history of medicine: the unresolved disequilibrium between, on the one hand, the remarkable capacities of an increasingly powerful science-based biomedical tradition and, on the other, the wider and unfulfilled health requirements of economically impoverished, colonially vanquished and politically mismanaged societies. Medicine is an enormous achievement, but what it will achieve practically for humanity, and what those who hold the power will allow it to do, remain open questions.

The late E. P. Thompson (1924–1993) warned historians against what he called the enormous condescension of posterity. I have tried to understand the medical systems I discuss rather than passing judgment on them; I have tried to spell them out in as much detail as space has permitted, because engagement with detail is essential if the cognitive power of medicine is to be appreciated.

Eschewing anachronism, judgmentalism and history by hindsight does not mean denying that there are ways in which medical knowledge has progressed. Harvey's account of the cardiovascular system was more correct than Galen's; the emergence of endocrinology allowed the development in the 1920s of insulin treatments which saved the lives of diabetics. But one must not assume that diabetes then went away: no cure has been found for that still poorly understood disease, and it continues to spread as a consequence of western lifestyles. Indeed one could argue that the problem is now worse than when insulin treatment was discovered.

Avoiding condescension equally does not mean one must avoid 'winners' history. This book unashamedly gives more space to the Greeks than the Goths, more attention to Hippocrates than to Greek root-gatherers, and stresses strands of development leading from Greek medicine to the biomedicine now in the saddle. I do not think that 'winners' should automatically be privileged by historians (I have myself written and advocated writing medical history from the patients' view), but there is a good reason for bringing the winners to the foreground – not because they are 'best' or 'right' but because they are powerful. One can study winners without siding with them.

Writing this book has not only made me more aware than usual of my own ignorance; it has brought home the collective and largely irremediable ignorance of historians about the medical history of mankind. Perhaps the most celebrated physician ever is Hippocrates yet we know literally nothing about him. Neither do we know anything concrete about most of the medical encounters there have ever been. The historical record is like the night sky: we see a few stars and group them into mythic constellations. But what is chiefly visible is the darkness.

CHAPTER II

THE ROOTS OF MEDICINE

PEOPLES AND PLAGUES

IN THE BEGINNING WAS THE GOLDEN AGE. The climate was clement, nature freely bestowed her bounty upon mankind, no lethal predators lurked, the lion lay down with the lamb and peace reigned. In that blissful long-lost Arcadia, according to the Greek poet Hesiod writing around 700 BC, life was 'without evils, hard toil, and grievous disease'. All changed. Thereafter, wrote the poet, 'thousands of miseries roam among men, the land is full of evils and full is the sea. Of themselves, diseases come upon men, some by day and some by night, and they bring evils to the mortals.'

The Greeks explained the coming of pestilences and other troubles by the fable of Pandora's box. Something similar is offered by Judaeo-Christianity. Disguised in serpent's clothing, the Devil seduces Eve into tempting Adam to taste the forbidden fruit. By way of punishment for that primal disobedience, the pair are banished from Eden; Adam's sons are condemned to labour by the sweat of their brow, while the daughters of Eve must bring forth in pain; and disease and death, unknown in the paradise garden, become the iron law of the post-lapsarian world, thenceforth a vale of tears. As in the Pandora fable and scores of parallel legends the world over, the Fall as revealed in Genesis explains how suffering, disease and death become the human condition, as a consequence of original sin. The Bible closes with foreboding: 'And I looked, and behold a pale horse' prophesied the Book of Revelation: 'and his name that sat on him was Death, and Hell followed with him. And power was given unto them over the fourth part of the earth, to kill with sword, and with hunger, and with death, and with the beasts of the earth.'

Much later, the eighteenth-century physician George Cheyne drew attention to a further irony in the history of health. Medicine owed its foundation as a science to Hippocrates and his successors, and such founding fathers were surely to be praised. Yet why had medicine originated among the Greeks? It was because, the witty Scotsman explained, being the first civilized, intellectual people, with leisure to cultivate the life of the mind, they had frittered away the rude vitality of their warrior ancestors – the heroes of the *Iliad* – and so had been the first to *need* medical ministrations. This 'diseases of civilization' paradox had a fine future ahead of it, resonating throughout Nietzsche and Freud's *Civilization and its Discontents* (1930). Thus to many, from classical poets up to the prophets of modernity, disease has seemed the dark side of development, its Jekyll-and-Hyde double: progress brings pestilences, society sickness.

Stories such as these reveal the enigmatic play of peoples, plagues and physicians which is the thread of this book, scotching any innocent notion that the story of health and medicine is a pageant of progress. Pandora's box and similar just-so stories tell a further tale moreover, that plagues and pestilences are not acts of God or natural hazards; they are of mankind's own making. Disease is a social development no less than the medicine that combats it.

In the beginning ... Anthropologists now maintain that some five million years ago in Africa there occurred the branching of the primate line which led to the first ape men, the low-browed, big-jawed hominid Australopithecines. Within a mere three million years *Homo erectus* had emerged, our first entirely upright, large-brained ancestor, who learned how to make fire, use stone tools, and eventually developed speech. Almost certainly a carnivorous hunter, this palaeolithic pioneer fanned out a million years or so ago from Africa into Asia and Europe. Thereafter a direct line leads to *Homo sapiens* who emerged around 150,000 BC.

The life of early mankind was not exactly arcadian. Archaeology and palaeopathology give us glimpses of forebears who were often malformed, racked with arthritis and lamed by injuries – limbs broken in accidents and mending awry. Living in a dangerous, often harsh and always unpredictable environment, their lifespan was short. Nevertheless, prehistoric people escaped many of the miseries popularly associated with the 'fall'; it was later developments which exposed their descendants to the pathogens that brought infectious disease and have since done so much to shape human history.

The more humans swarmed over the globe, the more they were themselves colonized by creatures capable of doing harm, including parasites and pathogens. There have been parasitic helminths (worms), fleas, ticks and a host of arthropods, which are the bearers of 'arbo' (arthropod-borne) infections. There have also been the micro-organisms like bacteria, viruses and protozoans. Their very rapid reproduction rates within a host provoke severe illness but, as if by compensation, produce in survivors immunity against reinfection. All such disease threats have been and remain locked with humans in evolutionary struggles for the survival of the fittest, which have no master plot and grant mankind no privileges.

Despite carbon-14 and other sophisticated techniques used by palaeopathologists, we lack any semblance of a day-to-day health chart for early *Homo sapiens*. Theories and guesswork can be supported by reference to so-called 'primitive' peoples in the modern world, for instance Australian aborigines, the Hadza of Tanzania, or the !Kung San bush people of the Kalahari. Our early progenitors were hunters and gatherers. Pooling tools and food, they lived as nomadic opportunistic omnivores in scattered familial groups of perhaps thirty or forty. Infections like smallpox, measles and flu must have been virtually unknown, since the micro-organisms that cause contagious diseases require high population densities to provide reservoirs of susceptibles. And because of the need to search for food, these small bands did not stay put long enough to pollute water sources or accumulate the filth that attracts disease-spreading insects. Above all, isolated hunter-foragers did not tend cattle and the other tamed animals which have played such an ambiguous role in human history. While meat and milk, hides and horns made civilization possible, domesticated animals proved perennial and often catastrophic sources of illness, for infectious disease riddled beasts long before spreading to humans.

Our 'primitive' ancestors were thus practically free of the pestilences that ambushed their 'civilized' successors and have plagued us ever since. Yet they did not exactly enjoy a golden age, for, together with dangers, injuries and hardships, there were ailments to which they were susceptible. Soil-borne anaerobic bacteria penetrated through skin wounds to produce gangrene and botulism; anthrax and rabies were picked up from animal predators like wolves; infections were acquired through eating raw animal flesh, while game would have transmitted the microbes of relapsing fever (like typhus, a louse-borne disease), brucellosis and haemorrhagic fevers. Other threats came from organisms co-evolving with humans, including tapeworms and such bacteria as *Treponema*, the agent of syphilis, and the similar skin infection, yaws.

Hunter-gatherers being omnivores, they were probably not mal-nourished, at least not until rising populations had hunted to extinction most of the big game roaming the savannahs and prairies. Resources and population were broadly in balance. Relative freedom from disease encouraged numbers to rise, but all were prey to climate, especially during the Ice Age which set in from around 50,000 BC. Famine took its toll; lives would have been lost in hunting and skirmishing; childbirth was hazardous, fertility probably low, and infanticide may have been practised. All such factors kept numbers in check.

For tens of thousands of years there was ample territory for dispersal, as pressure on resources drove migration 'out of Africa' into all corners of the Old World, initially to the warm regions of Asia and southern Europe, but then farther north into less hospitable climes. These nomadic ways continued until the end of the last Ice Age (the Pleistocene) around 12,000–10,000 years ago brought the invention of agriculture.

Contrary to the Victorian assumption that farming arose out of mankind's inherent progressiveness, it is now believed that tilling the soil began because population pressure and the depletion of game sup-plies left no alternative: it was produce more or perish. By around 50,000 BC, mankind had spilled over from the Old World to New Guinea and Australasia, and by 10,000 BC (perhaps much earlier) to the Americas as well (during the last Ice Age the lowering of the oceans made it possible to cross by land bridge from Siberia to Alaska). But when the ice caps melted around ten thousand years ago and the seas rose once more, there were no longer huge tracts of land filled with game but empty of humans and so ripe for colonization. Mankind faced its first ecological crisis – its first survival test.

Necessity proved the mother of invention, and Stone Age stalkers, faced with famine – elk and gazelle had thinned out, leaving hogs, rabbits and rodents – were forced to grow their own food and settle in one place. Agriculture enhanced mankind's capacity to harness natural resources, selectively breeding wild grasses into domesticated varieties of grains, and bringing dogs, cattle, sheep, goats, pigs, horses and poultry under control. This change had the rapidity of a revolution: until around 10,000 years ago, almost all human groups were hunter-gatherers, but within a few thousand years cultivators and pastoralists predominated. The 'neolithic revolution' was truly epochal.

In the fertile crescent of the Middle East, wheat, barley, peas and lentils were cultivated, and sheep, pigs and goats herded; the neolithic peoples of south-east Asia exploited rice, sweet potatoes, ducks and chickens; in Mesoamerica, it was maize, beans, cassava, potatoes and guinea pigs. The land which a nomadic band would have stripped like locusts before moving on was transformed by new management techniques into a resource reservoir capable of supporting thousands, year in, year out. And once agriculture took root, with its systematic planting of grains and lentils and animal husbandry, numbers went on spiralling, since more could be fed. The labour-intensiveness of clearing woodland and scrub, weeding fields, harvesting crops and preparing food encouraged population growth and the formation of social hierarchies, towns, courts and kingdoms. But while agriculture rescued people from starvation, it unleashed a fresh danger: disease.

The agricultural revolution ensured human domination of planet earth: the wilderness was made fertile, the forests became fields, wild beasts were tamed or kept at bay; but pressure on resources presaged the disequilibrium between production and reproduction that provoked later Malthusian crises, as well as leading to ecological deterioration. As hunters and gatherers became shepherds and farmers, the seeds of disease were sown. Prolific pathogens once exclusive to animals were transferred to swineherds and goatherds, ploughmen and horsemen, initiating the ceaseless evolutionary adaptations which have led to a current situation in which humans share no fewer than sixty-five microorganic diseases with dogs (supposedly man's best friend), and only slightly fewer with cattle, sheep, goats, pigs, horses and poultry.

Many of the worst human diseases were created by proximity to animals. Cattle provided the pathogen pool with tuberculosis and viral poxes like smallpox. Pigs and ducks gave humans their influenzas, while horses brought rhinoviruses and hence the common cold. Measles, which still kills a million children a year, is the result of rinderpest (canine distemper) jumping between dogs or cattle and humans. Moreover, cats, dogs, ducks, hens, mice, rats and reptiles carry bacteria like *Salmonella*, leading to often fatal human infections; water polluted with animal faeces also spreads polio, cholera, typhoid, viral hepatitis, whooping cough and diphtheria.

Settlement helped disease to settle in, attracting disease-spreading

insects, while worms took up residence within the human body. Parasit-
ologists and palaeopathologists have shown how the parasitic round-
worm *Ascaris*, a nematode growing to over a foot long, evolved in
humans, probably from pig ascarids, producing diarrhoea and malnutrition. Other helminths or wormlike fellow-travellers became common
in the human gut, including the *Enterobius* (pinworm or threadworm),
the yards-long hookworm, and the filarial worms which cause elephantiasis and African river blindness. Diseases also established themselves
where agriculture depended upon irrigation – in Mesopotamia, Egypt,
India and around the Yellow (Huang) River in China. Paddyfields har-
bour parasites able to penetrate the skin and enter the bloodstream of
barefoot workers, including the forked-tailed blood fluke *Schistosoma*
which utilizes aquatic snails as a host and causes bilharzia or schistosomiasis (graphically known as 'big belly'), provoking mental and physical
deterioration through the chronic irritation caused by the worm. Investigation of Egyptian mummies has revealed calcified eggs in liver and
kidney tissues, proving the presence of schistosomiasis in ancient Egypt.
(Mummies tell us much more about the diseases from which Egyptians
suffered; these included gallstones, bladder and kidney stones, mastoiditis and numerous eye diseases, and many skeletons show evidence of
rheumatoid arthritis.) In short, permanent settlement afforded golden
opportunities for insects, vermin and parasites, while food stored in
granaries became infested with insects, bacteria, fungoid toxins and
rodent excrement. The scales of health tipped unfavourably, with infections worsening and human vitality declining.*

Moreover, though agriculture enabled more mouths to be fed, it
meant undue reliance on starchy cereal monocultures like maize, high

---

* Smallpox, the largest of all viruses, is the product of a long evolutionary adaptation
of cowpox to humans – something clearly perceived two hundred years ago by Edward
Jenner. His *An Inquiry into the Causes and Effects . . . of the Cow Pox* (1798) noted that:

> The deviation of man from the state in which he was originally placed by
> nature seems to have proved to him a prolific source of diseases. From the
> love of splendour, from the indulgence of luxury, and from his fondness for
> amusement he has familiarized himself with a great number of animals, which
> may not originally have been intended for his associates.

Jenner thus perceived the dangers animals posed to human health. Now, in the late
1990s, the transmission chain between the cattle disease, bovine spongiform
encephalopathy (BSE), and the human Creutzfeldt-Jakob Disease (CJD), is a hot
epidemiological and political issue in Europe.

in calories but low in proteins, vitamins and minerals; reduced nutritional levels allowed deficiency diseases like pellagra, marasmus, kwashiorkor and scurvy to make their entry onto the human stage. Stunted people are more vulnerable to infections, and it is a striking comment on 'progress' that neolithic skeletons are typically some inches shorter than their palaeolithic precursors.

MALARIA

Settlement also brought malaria. 'There is no doubt', judged the distinguished Australian immunologist, Macfarlane Burnet (1899–1985), 'that malaria has caused the greatest harm to the greatest number' – not through cataclysms, as with bubonic plague, but through its continual winnowing effect. First in sub-Saharan Africa and elsewhere since, conversion of forests into farmland has created environments tailormade for mosquitoes: warm waterholes, furrows and puddles ideal for rapid breeding. Malaria is worth pausing over, since it has coexisted with humans for thousands of years and remains out of control across much of the globe.

The symptoms of malarial fevers were familiar to the Greeks, but were not explained until the advent of tropical medicine around 1900. They are produced by the microscopic protozoan parasite *Plasmodium*, which lives within the body of an *Anopheles* mosquito, and is transmitted to humans through mosquito bites. The parasites move through the bloodstream to the liver, where they breed during an incubation stage of a couple of weeks. Returning to the blood, they attack red blood cells, which break down, leading to waves of violent chills and high fever.

Malarial parasites have distinct periodicities. *Plasmodium vivax*, the organism causing benign tertian malaria, once present in the English fenlands, has an incubation period of ten to seventeen days. The fever lasts from two to six hours, returning every third day (hence 'tertian'); marked by vomiting and diarrhoea, such attacks may recur for two months or longer. In time, as Greek doctors observed, the spleen enlarges, and the patient becomes anaemic and sometimes jaundiced. Quartan malaria, caused by *Plasmodium malariae*, is another mild variety.

Malignant tertian malaria, caused by *Plasmodium falciparum*, is the most lethal, producing at least 95 per cent of all malarial deaths. The incubation period is shorter but the fever more prolonged; it may be continuous, remittent or intermittent. *Plasmodium falciparum* proliferates fast, producing massive destruction of red blood cells and hence dangerous anaemia; the liver and spleen also become enlarged.

Malaria may sometimes appear as quotidian fever, with attacks lasting six to twelve hours – the result of multiple infection. Patients may also develop malarial cachexia, with yellowing of the skin and severe spleen and liver enlargement; autopsy shows both organs darkened with a black pigment derived from the haemoglobin of the destroyed red blood cells. What the ancients called melancholy may have been a \ malarial condition.

Malaria shadowed agricultural settlements. From Africa, it became established in the Near and Middle East and the Mediterranean littoral. The huge attention Graeco-Roman medicine paid to 'remittent fevers' shows how seriously the region was affected, and some historians maintain the disease played its part in the decline and fall of the Roman empire. Within living memory, malaria remained serious in the Roman Campagna and the Pontine marshes along Italy's west coast.

Coastal Africa was and remains heavily malarial, as are the Congo, the Niger and hundreds of other river basins. Indigenous West African populations developed a genetically controlled characteristic, the 'sicklecell', which conferred immunity against virulent *Plasmodium falciparum*. But, though protective, this starves its bearers, who are prone to debility and premature death: typical of such evolutionary trade-offs, gains and losses are finely balanced.

India was also ripe for malarial infection. Ayurvedic medical texts (see Chapter Six) confirm the antiquity of the disease in the subcontinent. China, too, became heavily infected, especially the coastal strip from Shanghai to Macao. And from the sixteenth century Europeans shipped it to Mesoamerica: vivax malaria went to the New World in the blood of the Spanish *conquistadores*, while falciparum malaria arrived with the African slaves whom the Europeans imported to replace the natives they and their pestilences had wiped out.

Malaria was just one health threat among many which set in with civilization as vermin learned to cohabit with humans, insects spread gastroenteric disorders, and contact with rodents led to human rickettsial (lice-, mite- and tick-borne) arbo diseases like typhus. Despite such infections encouraged by dense settlement and its waste and dirt, man's restless inventive energies ensured that communities, no matter how unhealthy, bred rising populations; and more humans spawned more diseases in upward spirals, temporarily and locally checked but never terminated. Around 10,000 BC, before agriculture, the globe's human population may have been around 5 million; by 500 BC it had probably leapt to 100 million; by the second century AD that may have doubled; the 1990 figure was some 5,292 million, with projections suggesting 12 billion by 2100.

Growing numbers led to meagre diets, the weak and poor inevitably bearing the brunt. But though humans were often malnourished, parasite-riddled and pestilence-smitten, they were not totally defenceless. Survivors of epidemics acquired some protection, and the mechanisms of evolution meant that these acquired sophisticated immune systems enabling them to coexist in a ceaseless war with their micro-organic assailants. Immunities passed from mothers across the placenta or through breast-feeding gave infants some defence against germ invasion. Tolerance was likewise developed towards parasitic worms, and certain groups developed genetic shields, as with the sickle-cell trait. Biological adaptation might thus take the edge off lethal afflictions.

THE ERA OF EPIDEMICS

Some diseases, however, were not so readily coped with: those caused by the zoonoses (animal diseases transmissible to man) which menaced once civilization developed. By 3000 BC cities like Babylon, with populations of scores of thousands, were rising in Mesopotamia and Egypt, in the Indus Valley and on the Yellow River, and later in Mesoamerica. In the Old World, such settlements often maintained huge cattle herds, from which lethal pathogens, including smallpox, spread to humans, while originally zoognostic conditions – diphtheria, influenza, chickenpox, mumps – and other illnesses also had a devastating impact. Unlike malaria, these needed no carriers; being directly contagious, they spread readily and rapidly.

The era of epidemics began. And though some immunity would develop amongst the afflicted populations, the incessant outreach of civilization meant that merchants, mariners and marauders would inevitably bridge pathogen pools, spilling diseases onto virgin susceptibles. One nation's familiar 'tamed' disease would be another's plague, as trade, travel and war detonated pathological explosions.

The immediate consequence of the invasion of a town by smallpox or another infection was a fulminating epidemic and subsequent decimation. Population recovery would then get under way, only for survivors' heirs to be blitzed by the same or a different pestilence, and yet another, in tide upon tide. Settlements big enough to host such contagions might shrink to become too tiny. With almost everybody slain or immune, the pestilences would withdraw, victims of their own success, moving on to storm other virgin populations, like raiders seeking fresh spoils. New diseases thus operated as brutal Malthusian checks, sometimes shaping the destinies of nations.

Cities assumed a decisive epidemiological role, being magnets for pathogens no less than people. Until the nineteenth century, towns were so insanitary that their populations never replaced themselves by reproduction, multiplying only thanks to the influx of rural surpluses who were tragically infection-prone. In this challenge and response process, sturdy urban survivors turned into an immunological elite – a virulently infectious swarm perilous to less seasoned incomers, confirming the notoriety of towns as death-traps.

The Old Testament records the epidemics the Lord hurled upon the Egypt of the pharaohs, and from Greek times historians noted their melancholy toll. The Peloponnesian War of 431 to 404 BC, the 'world war' between Athens and Sparta, spotlights the traffic in pestilence that came with civilization. Before that war the Greeks had suffered from malaria and probably tuberculosis, diphtheria and influenza, but they had been spared truly calamitous plagues. Reputedly beginning in Africa and spreading to Persia, an unknown epidemic hit Greece in 430 BC, and its impact on Athens was portrayed by Thucydides (460 – after 404 BC). Victims were poleaxed by headaches, coughing, vomiting, chest pains and convulsions. Their bodies became reddish or livid, with blisters and ulcers; the malady often descended into the bowels before death spared sufferers further misery. The Greek historian thought it killed a quarter of the Athenian troops, persisting on the mainland for a further four years and annihilating a similar proportion of the population.

What was it? Smallpox, plague, measles, typhus, ergotism and even syphilis have been proposed in a parlour game played by epidemiologists. Whatever it was, by killing or immunizing them, it destroyed the Greeks' ability to host it and, proving too virulent for its own good, the disease disappeared. With it passed the great age of Athens. Most early nations probably experienced such disasters, but Greece alone had a Thucydides to record it.

Epidemics worsened with the rise of Rome. With victories in Macedonia and Greece (146 BC), Persia (64 BC) and finally Egypt (30 BC), the Roman legions vanquished much of the known world, but deadly pathogens were thus given free passage around the empire, spreading to the Eternal City itself. The first serious outbreak, the so-called Antonine plague (probably smallpox which had smouldered in Africa or Asia before being brought back from the Near East by Roman troops) slew a quarter of the inhabitants in stricken areas between AD 165 and 180, some five million people in all. A second, between AD 211 and 266, reportedly destroyed some 5,000 a day in Rome at its height, while scourging the countryside as well. The virulence was immense because populations had no resistance. Smallpox and measles had joined the Mediterranean epidemiological melting-pot, alongside the endemic malaria.

Wherever it struck a virgin population, measles too proved lethal. There are some recent and well-documented instances of such strikes. In his *Observations Made During the Epidemic of Measles on the Faroe Islands in the Year 1846*, Peter Panum (1820–85) reported how measles had attacked about 6,100 out of 7,864 inhabitants on a remote island which had been completely free of the disease for sixty-five years. In the nineteenth century, high mortality was also reported in measles epidemics occurring in virgin soil populations ('island laboratories') in the Pacific Ocean: 40,000 deaths in a population of 150,000 in Hawaii in 1848, 20,000 (perhaps a quarter of the population) on Fiji in 1874.

Improving communications also widened disease basins in the Middle East, the Indian subcontinent, South Asia and the Far East. Take Japan: before AD 552, the archipelago had apparently escaped the epidemics blighting the Chinese mainland. In that year, Buddhist missionaries visited the Japanese court, and shortly afterwards smallpox broke out. In 585 there was a further eruption of either smallpox or measles. Following centuries brought waves of epidemics every three or four years, the most significant being smallpox, measles, influenza, mumps and dysentery.

This alteration of occasional epidemic diseases into endemic ones typical of childhood – it mirrors the domestication of animals – represents a crucial stage in disease ecology. Cities buffeted by lethal

epidemics which killed or immunized so many that the pathogens themselves disappeared for lack of hosts, eventually became big enough to
house sufficient non-immune individuals to retain the diseases permanently; for this an annual case total of something in the region of 5,000–
40,000 may be necessary. Measles, smallpox and chickenpox turned into
childhood ailments which affected the young less severely and conferred
immunity to future attacks.

The process marks an epidemiological watershed. Through such
evolutionary adaptations – epidemic diseases turning endemic –
expanding populations accommodated and surmounted certain once-
lethal pestilences. Yet they remained exposed to other dire infections,
against which humans were to continue immunologically defenceless,
because they were essentially diseases not of humans but of animals.
One such is bubonic plague, which has struck humans with appalling
ferocity whenever populations have been caught up in a disease net
involving rats, fleas and the plague bacillus (*Yersinia pestis*). Diseases like
plague, malaria, yellow fever, and others with animal reservoirs are
uniquely difficult to control.

PLAGUE

Bubonic plague is basically a rodent disease. It strikes humans when
infected fleas, failing to find a living rat once a rat host has been killed,
pick a human instead. When the flea bites its new host, the bacillus
enters the bloodstream. Filtered through the nearest lymph node, it
leads to the characteristic swelling (bubo) in the neck, groin or armpit.
Bubonic plague rapidly kills about two-thirds of those infected. There
are two other even more fatal forms: septicaemic and, deadliest of all,
pneumonic plague, which doesn't even need an insect vector, spreading
from person to person directly via the breath.

The first documented bubonic plague outbreak occurred, predictably enough, in the Roman empire. The plague of Justinian originated in Egypt in AD 540; two years later it devastated Constantinople,
going on to massacre up to a quarter of the eastern Mediterranean
population, before spreading to western Europe and ricocheting around
the Mediterranean for the next two centuries. Panic, disorder and
murder reigned in the streets of Constantinople, wrote the historian
Procopius: up to 10,000 people died each day, until there was no place

to put the corpses. When this bout of plague ended, 40 per cent of the city's population were dead.

It was a subsequent plague cycle, however, which made the greatest impact. Towards 1300 the Black Death began to rampage through Asia before sweeping westwards through the Middle East to North Africa and Europe. Between 1346 and 1350 Europe alone lost perhaps twenty million to the disease. And this pandemic was just the first wave of a bubonic pestilence that raged until about 1800 (see Chapter 5).

Trade, war and empire have always sped disease transmission between populations, a dramatic instance being offered by early modern Spain. The cosmopolitan Iberians became subjects of a natural Darwinian experiment, for their Atlantic and Mediterranean seaports served as clearing-houses for swarms of diseases converging from Africa, Asia and the Americas. Survival in this hazardous environment necessitated becoming hyper-immune, weathering a hail of childhood diseases – smallpox, measles, diphtheria and the like, gastrointestinal infections and other afflictions rare today in the West. The Spanish *conquistadores* who invaded the Americas were, by consequence, immunological supermen, infinitely more deadly than 'typhoid Mary'; disease gave them a fatal superiority over the defenceless native populations they invaded.

TYPHUS

Though the Black Death ebbed away from Europe, war and the movements of migrants ensured that epidemic disease did not go away, and Spain, as one of the great crossroads, formed a flashpoint of disease. Late in 1489, in its assault on Granada, Islam's last Iberian stronghold, Spain hired some mercenaries who had lately been in Cyprus fighting the Ottomans. Soon after their arrival, Spanish troops began to go down with a disease never before encountered and possessing the brute virulence typical of new infections: typhus. It had probably emerged in the Near East during the Crusades before entering Europe where Christian and Muslim armies clashed.

It began with headache, rash and high fever, swelling and darkening of the face; next came delirium and the stupor giving the disease its name – *typhos* is Greek for 'smoke'. Inflammation led to gangrene that rotted fingers and toes, causing a hideous stench. Spain lost 3,000 soldiers in the siege but six times as many to typhus.

Having smuggled itself into Spain, typhus filtered into France and beyond. In 1528, with the Valois (French) and Habsburg (Spanish) dynasties vying for European mastery, it struck the French army encircling Naples; half the 28,000 troops died within a month, and the siege collapsed. As a result, Emperor Charles V of Spain was left master of Italy, controlling Pope Clement VII – with important implications for Henry VIII's marital troubles and the Reformation in England.

With the Holy Roman Empire fighting the Turks in the Balkans, typhus gained a second bridgehead into Europe. In 1542, the disease killed 30,000 Christian soldiers on the eastern front; four years later, it struck the Ottomans, terminating their siege of Belgrade; while by 1566 the Emperor Maximilian II had so many typhus victims that he was driven to an armistice. His disbanded troops relayed the disease back to western Europe, and so to the New World, where it joined measles and smallpox in ravaging Mexico and Peru. Typhus subsequently smote Europe during the Thirty Years War (1618–48), and remained widespread, devastating armies as 'camp fever', dogging beggars (road fever), depleting jails (jail fever) and ships (ship fever).

It was typhus which joined General Winter to turn Napoleon's Russian invasion into a rout. The French crossed into Russia in June 1812. Sickness set in after the fall of Smolensk. Napoleon reached Moscow in September to find the city abandoned. During the next five weeks, the *grande armée* suffered a major typhus epidemic. By the time Moscow was evacuated, tens of thousands had fallen sick, and those unfit to travel were abandoned. Thirty thousand cases were left to die in Vilna alone, and only a trickle finally reached Warsaw. Of the 600,000 men in Napoleon's army, few returned, and typhus was a major reason.

Smallpox, plague and typhus indicate how war and conquest paved the way for the progress of pathogens. A later addition, at least as far as the West was concerned, was cholera, the most spectacular 'new' disease of the nineteenth century.

COLONIZATION AND INDUSTRIALIZATION

Together with civilization and commerce, colonization has contributed to the dissemination of infections. The Spanish conquest of America has already been mentioned; the nineteenth-century scramble for Africa also caused massive disturbance of indigenous populations and environmental disruption, unleashing terrible epidemics of sleeping sickness and other maladies. Europeans exported tuberculosis to the 'Dark Continent', especially once native labourers were jammed into mining compounds and the slums of Johannesburg. In the gold, diamond and copper producing regions of Africa, the operations of mining companies like De Beers and Union Minière de Haute Katanga brought family disruption and prostitution. Capitalism worsened the incidence of infectious and deficiency diseases for those induced or forced to abandon tribal ways and traditional economies – something which medical missionaries were pointing out from early in the twentieth century.

While in the period after Columbus's voyage, advances in agriculture, plant-breeding and crop exchange between the New and Old Worlds in some ways improved food supply, for those newly dependent upon a single staple crop the consequence could be one of the classic deficiency diseases: scurvy, beriberi or kwashiorkor (from a Ghanaian word meaning a disease suffered by a child displaced from the breast). Those heavily reliant on maize in Mesoamerica and later, after it was brought back by the *conquistadores*, in the Mediterranean, frequently fell victim to pellagra, caused by niacin deficiency and characterized by diarrhoea, dermatitis, dementia and death. Another product of vitamin B (thiamine) deficiency is beriberi, associated with Asian rice cultures.

The Third World, however, has had no monopoly on dearth and deficiency diseases. The subjugation of Ireland by the English, complete around 1700, left an impoverished native peasantry 'living in Filth and Nastiness upon Butter-milk and Potatoes, without a Shoe or stocking to their Feet', as Jonathan Swift observed. Peasants survived through cultivating the potato, a New World import and another instance of how the Old World banked upon gains from the New. A wonderful source of nutrition, rich in vitamins B_1, B_2 and C as well as a host of essential minerals, potatoes kept the poor alive and well-nourished, but when in 1727 the oat crop failed, the poor ate their winter potatoes early and then starved. The subsequent famine led Swift to make his ironic 'modest proposal' as to how to handle the island's surplus population better in future:

> a young healthy Child, well nursed is, at a Year old, a most delicious, nourishing and wholesome Food; whether Stewed, Roasted, Baked, or Boiled; and, I make no doubt, that it will equally serve in a Fricassee, or Ragout ... I grant this Food will be somewhat dear, and therefore very proper for Landlords.

With Ireland's population zooming, disaster was always a risk. From a base of two million potato-eating peasants in 1700, the nation multiplied to five million by 1800 and to close on nine million by 1845. The potato island had become one of the world's most densely populated places. When the oat and potato crops failed, starving peasants became prey to various disorders, notably typhus, predictably called 'Irish fever' by the landlords. During the Great Famine of 1845–7, typhus worked its way through the island; scurvy and dysentery also returned. Starving children aged so that they looked like old men. Around a million people may have died in the famine and in the next decades millions more emigrated. Only a small percentage of deaths were due directly to starvation; the overwhelming majority occurred from hunger-related disease: typhus, relapsing fevers and dysentery.

The staple crops introduced by peasant agriculture and commercial farming thus proved mixed blessings, enabling larger numbers to survive but often with their immunological stamina compromised. There may have been a similar trade-off respecting the impact of the Industrial Revolution, first in Europe, then globally. While facilitating population growth and greater (if unequally distributed) prosperity, industrialization spread insanitary living conditions, workplace illnesses and 'new diseases' like rickets. And even prosperity has had its price, as Cheyne suggested. Cancer, obesity, gallstones, coronary heart disease, hypertension, diabetes, emphysema, Alzheimer's disease and many other chronic and degenerative conditions have grown rapidly among today's wealthy nations. More are of course now living long enough to develop these conditions, but new lifestyles also play their part, with cigarettes, alcohol, fatty diets and narcotics, those hallmarks of life in the West, taking their toll. Up to one third of all premature deaths in the West are said to be tobacco-related; in this, as in so many other matters, parts of the Third World are catching up fast.

And all the time 'new' diseases still make their appearance, either as evolutionary mutations or as 'old' diseases flushed out of their local environments (their very own Pandora's box) and loosed upon the wider world as a result of environmental disturbance and economic change. The spread of AIDS, Ebola, Lassa and Marburg fevers may all be the result of the impact of the West on the 'developing' world – legacies of colonialism.

Not long ago medicine's triumph over disease was taken for granted. At the close of the Second World War a sequence of books appeared in Britain under the masthead of 'The Conquest Series'. These included

The Conquest of Disease, *The Conquest of Pain*, *The Conquest of Tuberculosis*, *The Conquest of Cancer*, *The Conquest of the Unknown* and *The Conquest of Brain Mysteries*, and they celebrated 'the many wonders of contemporary medical science today'. And this was before the further 'wonder' advances introduced after 1950, from tranquillizers to transplant surgery. A signal event was the world-wide eradication of smallpox in 1977.

In spite of such advances, expectations of a conclusive victory over disease should always have seemed naive since that would fly in the face of a key axiom of Darwinian biology: ceaseless evolutionary adaptation. And that is something disease accomplishes far better than humans, since it possesses the initiative. In such circumstances it is hardly surprising that medicine has proved feeble against AIDS, because the human immunodeficiency virus (HIV) mutates rapidly, frustrating the development of vaccines and antiviral drugs.

The systematic impoverishment of much of the Third World, the disruption following the collapse of communism, and the rebirth of an underclass in the First World resulting from the free-market economic policies dominant since the 1980s, have all assisted the resurgence of disease. In March 1997 the chairman of the British Medical Association warned that Britain was slipping back into the nineteenth century in terms of public health. Despite dazzling medical advances, world health prospects at the close of the twentieth century seem much gloomier than half a century ago.

The symbiosis of disease with society, the dialectic of challenge and adaptation, success and failure, sets the scene for the following discussion of medicine. From around 2000 BC, medical ideas and remedies were written down. That act of recording did not merely make early healing accessible to us; it transformed medicine itself. But there is more to medicine than the written record, and the remainder of this chapter addresses wider aspects of healing – customary beliefs about illness and the body, the self and society – and glances at medical beliefs and practices before and beyond the literate tradition.

MAKING SENSE OF SICKNESS

Though prehistoric hunting and gathering groups largely escaped epidemics, individuals got sick. Comparison with similar groups today, for instance the Kalahari bush people, suggests they would have managed their health collectively, without experts. A case of illness or debility directly affected the well-being of the band: a sick or lame person is a serious handicap to a group on the move; hence healing rituals or treatment would be a public matter rather than (as Western medicine has come to see them) private.

Anthropologists sometimes posit two contrasting 'sick roles': one in which the sick person is treated as a child, fed and protected during illness or incapacity; the other in which the sufferer either leaves the group or is abandoned or, as with lepers in medieval Europe, ritually expelled, becoming culturally 'dead' before they are biologically dead. Hunter-gatherer bands were more likely to abandon their sick than to succour them.

With population rise, agriculture, and the emergence of epidemics, new medical beliefs and practices arose, reflecting growing economic, political and social complexities. Communities developed hierarchical systems, identified by wealth, power and prestige. With an emergent division of labour, medical expertise became the *métier* of particular individuals. Although the family remained the first line of defence against illness, it was bolstered by medicine men, diviners, witch-smellers and shamans, and in due course by herbalists, birth-attendants, bone-setters, barber-surgeons and healer-priests. When that first happened we cannot be sure. Cave paintings found in France, some 17,000 years old, contain images of men masked in animal heads, performing ritual dances; these may be the oldest surviving images of medicine-men.

Highly distinctive was the shaman. On first encountering such folk healers, westerners denounced them as impostors. In 1763 the Scottish surgeon John Bell (1691–1780) described the 'charming sessions' he witnessed in southern Siberia:

> [the shaman] turned and distorted his body into many different postures, till, at last, he wrought himself up to such a degree of fury that he foamed at the mouth, and his eyes looked red and staring. He now started up on his legs, and fell a dancing, like one distracted, till he trod out the fire with his bare feet.
>
> These unnatural motions were, by the vulgar, attributed to the operations of a divinity . . . He now performed several legerdemain tricks; such as stabbing himself with a knife, and bringing it up at his mouth, running himself through with a sword and many others too trifling to mention.

This Calvinist Scot was not going to be taken in by Asiatic savages: 'nothing is more evident than that these shamans are a parcel of jugglers, who impose on the ignorant and credulous vulgar.' Such a reaction is arrogantly ethnocentric: although shamans perform magical acts, including deliberate deceptions, they are neither fakes nor mad. Common in native American culture as well as Asia, the shaman combined the roles of healer, sorcerer, seer, educator and priest, and was believed to possess god-given powers to heal the sick and to ensure fertility, a good harvest or a successful hunt. His main healing techniques have been categorized as contagious magic (destruction of enemies, through such means as the use of effigies) and direct magic, involving rituals to prevent disease, fetishes, amulets (to protect against black magic), and talismans (for good luck).

In 1912 Sir Baldwin Spencer (1860–1929) and F. J. Gillen (1856–1912) described the practices of the aborigine medicine-man in Central Australia:

> In ordinary cases the patient lies down, while the medicine man bends over him and sucks vigorously at the part of the body affected, spitting out every now and then pieces of wood, bone or stone, the presence of which is believed to be causing the injury and pain. This suction is one of the most characteristic features of native medical treatment, as pain in any part of the body is always attributed to the presence of some foreign body that must be removed.

Stone-sucking is a symbolic act. As the foreign body had been introduced into the body of the sick man by a magical route, it had to be removed in like manner. For the medicine-man, the foreign body in his mouth attracts the foreign body in the patient.

As such specialist healers emerged, and as labour power grew more valuable in structured agricultural and commercial societies, the appropriate 'sick role' shifted from abandonment to one modelled on child care. The exhausting physical labour required of farm workers encouraged medicines that would give strength; hence, together with drugs to relieve fevers, dysentery and pain, demand grew for stimulants and tonics such as tobacco, coca, opium and alcohol.

In hierarchical societies like Assyria or the Egypt of the pharaohs, with their military–political elites, illness became unequally distributed and thus the subject of moral, religious and political teachings and judgments. Its meanings needed to be explained. Social stratification meanwhile offered fresh scope for enterprising healers; demand for medicines grew; social development created new forms of healing as well as of faith, ritual and worship; sickness needed to be rationalized and theorized. In short, with settlement and literacy, conditions were ripe for the development of medicine as a belief-system and an occupation.

Like earthquakes, floods, droughts and other natural disasters, illness colours experiences, outlooks and feelings. It produces pain, suffering and fear, threatens the individual and the community, and raises the spectre of that mystery of mysteries – death. Small wonder impassioned and contested responses to sickness have emerged: notions of blame and shame, appeasement and propitiation, and teachings about care and therapeutics. Since sickness raises profound anxieties, medicine develops alongside religion, magic and social ritual. Nor is this true only of 'primitive' societies; from Job to the novels of Thomas Mann, the experience of sickness, ageing and death shapes the sense of the self and the human condition at large. AIDS has reminded us (were we in danger of forgetting) of the poignancy of sickness in the heyday of life.

Different sorts of sickness beliefs took shape. Medical ethnologists commonly suggest a basic divide: natural causation theories, which view illness as a result of ordinary activities that have gone wrong – for example, the effects of climate, hunger, fatigue, accidents, wounds or parasites; and personal or supernatural causation beliefs, which regard illness as harm wreaked by a human or superhuman agency. Typically, the latter is deliberately inflicted (as by a sorcerer) through magical devices, words or rituals; but it may be unintentional, arising out of an innate capacity for evil, such as that possessed by witches. Pollution from an 'unclean' person may thus produce illness – commonly a corpse or a menstruating woman. Early beliefs ascribed special prominence to social or supernatural causes; illness was thus *injury*, and was linked with aggression.

This book focuses mostly upon the naturalistic notions of disease developed by and since the Greeks, but mention should be made of the supernatural ideas prominent in non-literate societies and present elsewhere. Such ideas are often subdivided by scholars into three categories: *mystical*, in which illness is the automatic consequence of an act or experience; *animistic*, in which the illness-causing agent is a personal

supernatural being; and *magical*, where a malicious human being uses
secret means to make someone sick. The distribution of these beliefs
varies. Africa abounds in theories of mystical retribution, in which
broken taboos are to blame; ancestors are commonly blamed for sickness. Witchcraft, the evil eye and divine retribution are frequently used
to explain illness in India, as they were in educated Europe up to the
seventeenth century, and in peasant parts beyond that time.

Animistic or volitional illness theories take various forms. Some
blame objects for illness – articles which are taboo, polluting or dangerous, like the planets within astrology. Other beliefs blame people –
sorcerers or witches. Sorcerers are commonly thought to have shot some
illness-causing object into the victim, thus enabling healers to 'extract'
it via spectacular rituals. The search for a witch may involve divination
or public witch-hunts, with cathartic consequences for the community
and calamity for the scapegoat, who may be punished or killed. Under
such conditions, illness plays a key part in a community's collective life,
liable to disrupt it and lead to persecutions, in which witchfinders and
medicine men assume a key role.

There are also systems that hinge on spirits – and the recovery of
lost souls. The spirits of the dead, or nature spirits like wood demons,
are believed to attack the sick; or the patient's own soul may go missing.
By contrast to witchcraft, these notions of indirect causation allow for
more nuanced explanations of the social troubles believed to cause illness; there need be no single scapegoat, and purification may be more
general. Shamanistic healers will use their familiarity with worlds
beyond to grasp through divination the invisible causes behind illness.
Some groups use divining apparatus – shells, bones or entrails; a question
will be put to an oracle and its answer interpreted. Other techniques
draw on possession or trance to fathom the cause of sickness.

Responses to sickness may take many forms. They may simply
involve the sick person hiding away on his own, debasing himself with
dirt and awaiting his fate. More active therapies embrace two main
techniques – herbs and rituals. Medicines are either tonics to strengthen
the patient or 'poisons' to drive off the aggressor. Choice of the right
herbal remedy depends on the symbolic properties of the plant and on
its empirical effects. Some are chosen for their material properties,
others for their colour, shape or resonances within broader webs of
symbolic meaning. But if herbs may be symbolic, they may also be
effective; after much pooh-poohing of 'primitive medicine', pharmacol-

ogists studying ethnobotany now acknowledge that such lore provided healers with effective analgesics, anaesthetics, emetics, purgatives, diuretics, narcotics, cathartics, febrifuges, contraceptives and abortifacients. From the herbs traditionally in use, modern medicine has derived such substances as salicylic acid, ipecac, quinine, cocaine, colchicine, ephedrine, digitalis, ergot, and other drugs besides.

Medicines are not necessarily taken only by the patient, for therapy is communal and in traditional healing it is the community that is being put to rights, the patient being simply the stand-in. Certain healing rituals are *rites de passage*, with phases of casting out and reincorporation; others are dramas; and often the patient is being freed from unseen forces (exorcism). Some rituals wash a person clean; others use smoke to drive harm out. A related approach, *Dreckapotheke*, involves dosing the patient with disgusting decoctions or fumigations featuring excrement, noxious insects, and so forth, which drive the demons away.

A great variety of healing methods employ roots and leaves in elaborate magical rituals, and all communities practise surgery of some sort. Many tribes have used skin scarifications as a form of protection. Other kinds of body decoration, clitoridectomies and circumcision are common (circumcision was performed in Egypt from around 2000 BC). To combat bleeding, traditional surgeons used tourniquets or cauterization, or packed the wound with absorbent materials and bandaged it. The Masai in East Africa amputate fractured limbs, but medical amputation has been rare. There is archaeological evidence, however, from as far apart as France, South America and the Pacific that as early as 5000 BC trephining was performed, which involved cutting a small hole in the skull. Flint cutting tools were used to scrape away portions of the cranium, presumably to deliver sufferers from some devil tormenting the soul. Much skill was required and callous formations on the edges of the bony hole show that many of the patients survived.

BODY LORE

Illness is thus not just biological but social, and concepts of the body and its sicknesses draw upon powerful dichotomies: nature and culture, the sacred and the profane, the raw and the cooked. Body concepts incorporate beliefs about the body politic at large; communities with rigid caste and rank systems thus tend to prescribe rigid rules about

bodily comportment. What is considered normal health and what constitutes sickness or impairment are negotiable, and the conventions vary
from community to community and within subdivisions of societies,
dependent upon class, gender and other factors. Maladies carry different
moral charges. 'Sick roles' may range from utter stigmatization
(common with leprosy, because it is so disfiguring) to the notion that
the sick person is special or semi-sacred (the holy fool or the divine
epileptic). An ailment can be a *rite de passage*, a childhood illness an
essential preliminary to entry into adulthood.

Death affords a good instance of the scope for different interpretations in the light of different criteria. The nature of 'physical' death is
highly negotiable; in recent times western tests have shifted from cess-
ation of spontaneous breathing to 'brain death'. This involves more
than the matter of a truer definition: it corresponds with western values
(which prize the brain) and squares with the capacities of hospital technology. Some cultures think of death as a sudden happening, others
regard dying as a process advancing from the moment of birth and
continuing beyond the grave. Bodies are thus languages as well as envel-
opes of flesh; and sick bodies have eloquent messages for society.

It became common wisdom in the West from around 1800 that the
medicine of orientals and 'savages' was mere mumbo-jumbo, and had
to be superseded. Medical missions moved into the colonies alongside
their religious brethren, followed in due course by the massive health
programmes of the modern international aid organizations. By all such
means Europeans and Americans sought to stamp out indigenous practices and beliefs, from the African witchdoctors and spirit mediums to
the *vaidyas* and *hakims* of Hindu and Islamic medicine in Asia. Native
practices were grounded in superstition and were perilous to boot; colonial authorities moved in to prohibit practices and cults which they saw
as medically, religiously or politically objectionable, thereby becoming
arbiters of 'good' and 'bad' medicine. Western medicine grew aggressive, convinced of its unique scientific basis and superior therapeutic
powers.

This paralleled prejudices developing towards folk or religious
medicine within Europe itself. The sixteenth-century French physician
Laurent Joubert (1529–83) wrote a huge tome exposing 'common
fallacies'. *Erreurs populaires* [1578] systematically denounced the
'vulgar errors' and erroneous sayings of popular medicine regarding
pregnancy, childbirth, lying-in, infant care, children's diseases and so

forth, insisting that 'such errors can be most harmful to man's health and even his life'. 'Sometimes babies, boys as well as girls, are born with red marks on their faces, necks, shoulders or other parts of the body,' Joubert noted. 'It is said that this is because they were conceived while their mother had her period ... But I believe that it is impossible that a woman should conceive during her menstrual flow.' Another superstition was that whatever was imprinted upon the imagination of the mother at the time of conception would leave a mark on the body of her baby.

Elite medicine sought to discredit health folklore, but popular medicine has by no means always been misguided or erroneous. Recent pharmacological investigations have demonstrated the efficacy of many traditional·cures. It is now known, for instance, that numerous herbal decoctions – involving rue, savin, wormwood, pennyroyal and juniper – traditionally used by women to regulate fertility have some efficacy. Today's 'green pharmacy' aims at the recovery of ancient popular medical lore, putting it to the scientific test.

Once popular medicine had effectively been defeated and no longer posed a threat, scholarly interest in it grew, and great collections of 'medical folklore' and 'medical magic', stressing their quaintness, were published in the nineteenth century. But it is a gross mistake to view folk medicine as a sack of bizarre beliefs and weird and wonderful remedies. Popular medicine is based upon coherent conceptions of the body and of nature, rooted in rural society. Different body parts are generally represented as linked to the cosmos; health is conceived as a state of precarious equilibrium among components in a fluid system of relations; and healing mainly consists of re-establishing this balance when lost. Such medical beliefs depend on notions of opposites and similars. For example, to stop a headache judged to emanate from excessive heat, cold baths to the feet might be recommended; or to cure sciatica, an incision to the ear might be made on the side opposite to the pain.

Traditional medicine views the body as the centre or the epitome of the universe, with manifold sympathies linking mankind and the natural environment. Analogy and signatures are recurrent organizing principles in popular medicine. By their properties (colour, form, smell, heat, humidity, and so on) the elements of nature signal their meaningful associations with the human body, well and sick. For instance, in most traditional medicine systems, red is used to cure disorders connected with blood; geranium or oil of St John's wort are used against cuts. Yellow plants such as saffron crocus (*Crocus sativus*) were chosen for jaundice, or the white spots on the leaves of lungwort (*Pulmonaria officinalis*) showed that the plant was good for lung disease, and so on. Sometimes it was argued that remedies had been put in places convenient for people to use. So, in England, the bark of the white willow (*Salix alba*) was valued for agues, because the tree grows in moist or wet soil, where agues chiefly abound, as the Revd Edmund Stone, of Chipping Norton in Oxfordshire, observed in his report to the Royal Society of London in 1763:

> the general maxim, that many natural maladies carry their cures along with them, or that their remedies lie not far from their causes, was so very apposite to this particular case, that I could not help applying it; and that this might be the intention of Providence here, I must own had some little weight with me.

Maintaining health required understanding one's body. This was both a simple matter (pain was directly experienced) and appallingly difficult, for the body's interior was hidden. Unable to peer inside, popular wisdom relied upon analogy, drawing inferences from the natural world. Domestic life gave clues for body processes – food simmering on the hob became a natural symbol for its processing in the stomach – while magic, folksong and fable explained how conception and birth, growth, decay and death mirrored the seedtime and the harvest. The landscape contained natural signs: thus peasant women made fertility shrines out of springs. To fathom abnormalities and heal ailments, countryfolk drew upon the suggestive qualities of strange creatures like toads and snakes (their distinctive habits like hibernation or shedding skins implied a special command over life and death), and also the evocative profiles of landscape features like valleys and caves, while the phases of the moon so obviously correlated with the menstrual cycle.

Nature prompted the idea that the healthy body had to flow. In an agrarian society preoccupied with the weather and with the changes of the seasons, the systems operating beneath the skin were intuitively understood as fluid: digestion, fertilization, growth, expulsion. Not structures but processes counted. In vernacular and learned medicine alike, maladies were thought to migrate round the body, probing weak spots and, like marauding bands, most perilous when they targeted central zones. Therapeutics, it was argued, should counter-attack by

forcing or luring ailments to the extremities, like the feet, where they
might be expelled as blood, pus or scabs. In such a way of seeing, a
gouty foot might even be a sign of *health*, since the big toe typically
afflicted was an extremity far distant from the vital organs: a foe in the
toe was trouble made to keep its distance.

In traditional medicine, as I have said, health is a state of precarious
balance – being threatened, toppled and restored – between the body,
the universe and society. More important than curing is the aim of
preventing imbalance from occurring in the first place. Equilibrium is
to be achieved by avoiding excess and pursuing moderation. Prevention
lies in living in accord with nature, in harmony with the seasons and
elements and the supernatural powers that haunt the landscape: purge
the body in spring to clean it of corrupt humours, in summer avoid
activities or foods which are too heating. Another preventative is good
diet – an idea encapsulated in the later advice, 'an apple a day keeps
the doctor away'. Foods should be consumed which give strength and
assimilate natural products which, resembling the body, are beneficial
to it, such as wine and red meat: 'meat makes flesh and wine makes
blood', runs a French proverb. The idea that life is in the blood is an
old one. 'Epileptic patients are in the habit of drinking the blood even
of gladiators,' noted the Roman author Pliny (AD *c.* 23–79): 'these
persons, forsooth, consider it a most effectual cure for their disease, to
quaff the warm, breathing, blood from man himself, and, as they apply
their mouth to the wound, to draw forth his very life.'

Clear-cut distinctions have frequently been drawn between 'science'
and 'superstition' but, as historians of popular culture today insist, in
societies with both a popular and an elite tradition (high and low, or
learned and oral cultures), there has always been complex two-way cultural traffic in knowledge, or more properly a continuum. While often
aloof and dismissive, professional medicine has borrowed extensively
from the folk tradition.

Take, for instance, smallpox inoculation. There had long been some
folk awareness in Europe of the immunizing properties of a dose of
smallpox, but it was not until around 1700 that this knowledge was
turned to use. The first account of artificial inoculation was published
in the *Philosophical Transactions* of the Royal Society of London in
1714, and widespread publicity was achieved thanks to the observations
of Lady Mary Wortley Montagu (1689–1762), wife of the British
consul in Constantinople, that Turkish peasant women routinely

performed inoculations. One English country doctor who practised inoculation was Edward Jenner. In his native Gloucestershire it was also known in the farming community that there was a disease of cattle – cowpox – which was occasionally contracted by human beings, particularly dairy-maids who milked the cows. This led Jenner to the idea behind vaccination; elite medicine clearly had much to learn from folk tradition.

We must thus avoid taking for granted the antagonistic presence of two distinct traditions: the scientific and the superstitious, the right and the wrong. In all complex societies there have been various ways of thinking about the body, health and disease. In early modern Europe there was nothing mutually exclusive about different types of therapeutics or styles of healing. The English parson–physician, Richard Napier (1559–1634), was a graduate of Oxford University and a learned scholar. Yet he was also an exponent of religious healing: he would pray for the recovery of his patients, and to protect them 'against evil spirits, fairies, witcheries' he would also give them protective sigils and amulets to wear, as well as purges. And when the diarist Samuel Pepys (1633–1703), who later became president of the Royal Society of London, surveyed his health and found himself in exceptionally good condition, he was unsure of the cause. On 31 December 1664, he balanced his books for the year:

> So ends the old year, I bless God with great joy to me; not only from my having made so good a year of profit, as having spent £420. and laid up £540 and upward.
> But I bless God, I never have been in so good plight as to my health in so very cold weather as this is, nor indeed in any hot weather these ten years, as I am at this day and have been these four or five months. But I am at a great loss to know whether it be my Hare's fote, or taking every morning a pill of Turpentine, or my having left off the wearing of a gowne.

As this suggests, for Pepys as for others, religion, magic and medicine coalesced for therapeutic ends. Bread baked on Good Friday would never go mouldy; if stored, it would treat all manner of disease; rings made out of silver collected at the Eucharist would cure convulsions; the sacrament of confirmation would ward off sickness. Such beliefs had been encouraged within the proliferating healing rites of medieval Catholicism. In Protestant countries, with the anathematizing of pilgrimages, relics, holy waters, invocation of saints and the like at the Reformation, similar rituals continued, though essentially without express ecclesiastical authorization.

Medical magic was accepted by the unlettered and the elite alike until at least the seventeenth century, and was thought to operate in many ways. Disease could be transferred, transplanted or transformed. A sick person should boil eggs in his own urine and then bury them; as the ants ate them, the disease would also be eaten up. To heal a swollen neck, one was to draw a snake along it, put the snake in a tightly corked bottle and bury it; as the snake decayed, the swelling would go. Similarly, whooping cough sufferers should stand on the beach at high tide; when the tide went out, it carried the cough with it. Warts might be treated by touching them with a pebble; the pebbles were placed in a bag which was 'lost' as the sufferer went to church. Whoever found the bag acquired the warts too.

It was also widely believed that disease could be transferred to the dead. The sick person should clutch a limb of someone awaiting burial; the disease would then leave his or her body and enter the corpse. This mode of magic explains why mothers crowded around a scaffold, struggling to get their sickly infants into contact with an executed felon's body.

The doctrine of signatures linking humans and nature, microcosm and macrocosm, was of course interwoven with astrology – a learned science as well as a popular belief. Understanding of the heavens was seen as providing the key to the particular properties of herbs and minerals. Plants governed by Venus, herbalists explained, were aids to fertility and childbirth; those under Mars provided strength, and the moon played a crucial part.

Above all, magic functioned with religion in popular healing. Christianity endorsed an articulate symbolic cosmology which asserted the supreme potency of non-material forces. Roman Catholicism etched onto believers' minds the notion of miracle cures and the healing powers of sacraments, relics, Latin incantations, invocation of saints and holy waters. Popular therapeutic magic and religious healing could be interchangeable. Rejecting Catholic 'superstition', Protestants fought such 'contamination' of religion with magic; but the Reformation's iconoclasm towards magic within the Church encouraged it to flourish in a kind of 'black market' outside. Modernizing forces – literacy, the availability of commercial medicines, the rise of the medical profession –

gradually peripheralized such beliefs. But the finger of God might continue to be seen in visitations of illness and injury. 'Last Wednesday night while carrying a bucket of water from the well,' noted the Revd Francis Kilvert (1840–79) in his journal on 26 December 1874, 'Hannah Williams slipped upon the icy path and fell heavily upon her back. We fear her spine was injured for though she suffers acute pain in her legs she cannot move them. The poor wild beautiful girl is stopped in her wildness at last, and perhaps by the finger of God.'

·What must be stressed is the ceaseless dialectic of popular and educated medicine, and everything between. Superficially at least, the distinctive medical systems seem to have nothing in common but animosity. The medical missionary and explorer, David Livingstone (1813–73), recorded an exchange between representatives of quite different medical systems:

> MEDICAL DOCTOR: Hail, friend! How very many medicines you have about you this morning! Why, you have every medicine in the country here.
> RAIN DOCTOR: Very true, my friend; and I ought; for the whole country needs the rain which I am making.
> M.D: So you really believe that you can command the clouds? I think that can be done by God alone.
> R.D: We both believe the very same thing. It is God that makes the rain, but I pray to him by means of these medicines, and, the rain coming, of course it is then mine.

As the Rain Doctor recognized, they had more in common than met the eye. And the similarities yet differences between diverse medical systems and practices have always been evident to the sick themselves. In modern Taiwan, for instance, the sick use modern western doctors for certain ailments, traditional Chinese medicine for others, Japanese medicine and local herbal medicine and healers.

This sense of difference in commonness should help focus our attention to what is special to modern western scientific medicine: it is one healing system among many, yet it has, formally at least, in large measure broken with the traditional wisdom of the body. Herein lie its strengths and weaknesses. A distinguished historian of medicine, Jean Starobinski, writes,

> The historian who hopes to make sense out of the development of medicine cannot simply list the discoveries in the field, adding

them up as if one grew spontaneously out of the other. These conquests have been made possible only by a never-ending struggle against entrenched error, and by an unflagging recognition that the accepted methods and philosophical principles underlying basic research must be constantly revised. . . . Disease is as old as life, but the science of medicine is still young.

Contained within those remarks are the ideology of western medicine and some genuine historical insights. The following pages explore these ambiguities.

CHAPTER III

ANTIQUITY

AT THE END OF THE LAST ICE AGE about ten thousand years ago, a revolution began which decisively changed the symbiosis of society and disease. As we saw in the previous chapter, communities learned to master animals, to herd them for food, yoke them for traction, and spur them to war. Familiarity with soils, seeds and seasons made it possible to harvest crops regularly. Settlements grew, and with them arts and crafts. Story-telling and public memory were cultivated and the gods propitiated through priestly rituals. With the Bronze Age (from about 4000 BC), metal-working was improved, the wheel exploited, the reckoning of time and space rationalized and the calendar invented. Learning was encouraged, cities administered, tributes extracted, treasure hoarded, laws promulgated, empires enlarged. All such developments – the ABC of civilization – brought new approaches to healing and, for the first time, the writing down of medical practice. Medicine entered history.

MESOPOTAMIA

By around 3000 BC the warm and fertile region in the Middle East watered by the Tigris and the Euphrates was cradling some of the world's first great civilizations: Ur on the Euphrates, founded by the Sumerians, a hundred miles upriver from the Persian Gulf; Babylon, farther up the Euphrates; Assyria, centred on Assur, and later Nineveh on the Tigris, near Mosul in modern Iraq. Assyria destroyed Babylon and Nineveh reached its height under its kings Sennacherib (r. 705– 681 BC) and Assurbanipal (r. 668–627 BC); its fall to the Persians in 608 BC is celebrated in the Bible.

44

All these Mesopotamian ('land between the rivers') kingdoms have left magnificent remains, archaeological and written, which permit reconstruction of their dynasties and deities, and the agrarian and bureaucratic infrastructures that sustained them. Their healing practices remain cloudy, but among the 30,000 or so surviving clay tablets covered with cuneiform writing there are about a thousand from the library of Assurbanipal on medicine, containing diagnoses and prognostications, remedies and their ingredients. These date from the seventh century BC, though the Sumerian/Assyrian healing traditions they record go back much further.

The chief text, called 'The Treatise of Medical Diagnosis and Prognosis', comprises some three thousand entries on forty tablets. It is basically a list of ailments, and some are identifiable today: 'the patient coughs continually. What he coughs up is thick and frequently bloody. His breathing sounds like a flute. His hand is cold, his feet are warm. He sweats easily, and his heart activity is disturbed' – this sounds like tuberculosis. Eye disorders are prominent, and mention of 'stinking disease' and distended bellies suggests the vitamin-deficiency diseases symptomatic of the new grain-growing economies.

The framework for disease interpretation was largely omen-based, using divination based on inspection of the livers of sacrificed animals (hepatoscopy), because the liver was regarded as the seat of life. Prognostication may also have involved techniques like observing a flickering flame. Medical practice mixed religious rites and empirical treatments. Mention is made of three types of healers, presumably cooperating with one another: a seer (bârû), specializing in divination; a priest (âshipu), who performed incantations and exorcisms; and a physician (âsû), who employed drugs and did bandaging and surgery. An official head physician presided, and court doctors were expected to take an oath of office and allegiance.

The sixth king of the first dynasty of Babylon, Hammurabi (1728–1686 BC) was a mighty ruler who made Babylon feared. Alongside the mathematical treatises, dictionaries, astrological, magical writings and other forms of learning that gave lustre to his reign, his greatest work was a legal code, whose 282 laws deal with the regulation of society, family life and occupations. The Code of Hammurabi, engraved on a two-metre-high stele found in 1901 at Susa in Iran and preserved in the Louvre, includes medical instructions for physicians. Its rules set out fees for treatment, with a sliding scale adjusting rewards according to the patient's rank (nobleman, commoner or slave), together with terrifying draconian fines for incompetence or failure. 'If a physician has performed a major operation on a lord with a bronze lancet and has saved the lord's life . . . he shall receive ten shekels of silver' (more than a craftsman's annual pay); but if he caused the death of such a notable, his hand would be chopped off. A doctor causing the death of a slave would have to replace him.

The Mesopotamian peoples saw the hand of the gods in everything: disease was caused by spirit invasion, sorcery, malice or the breaking of taboos; sickness was both judgment and punishment. An Assyrian text of around 650 BC describes epileptic symptoms within a demonological framework:

> If at the time of his possession, while he is sitting down, his left eye moves to the side, a lip puckers, saliva flows from his mouth, and his hand, leg and trunk on the left side jerk like a slaughtered sheep, it is *migtu*. If at the time of possession his mind is awake, the demon can be driven out; if at the time of his possession his mind is not so aware, the demon cannot be driven out.

Headaches, neck pain, intestinal ailments and impotence were read as omens, and remedies involved identifying the demons responsible and expelling them by spells or incantation, though when maladies were the work of a god they might be a portent of death. Sicknesses were also ascribed to cold, dust and dryness, putrefaction, malnutrition, venereal infection and other natural causes.

Physical symptoms might be treated with empirical remedies. The Babylonians drew on an extensive *materia medica* – some 120 mineral drugs and twice that number of vegetable items are listed in the tablets. Alongside various fats, oils, honey, wax and milk, active ingredients included mustard, oleander and hellebore; colocynth, senna and castor oil were used as laxatives; while wound dressings were compounded with dried wine dregs, salt, oil, beer, juniper, mud or fat, blended with alkali and herbs. They had discovered distillation, and made essence of cedar and other volatile oils. Use of dog dung seems to smack of Dreckapothecary treatments, faecal ingredients designed to drive off demons.

Such empirical remedies accompanied a prognostic bent reflecting Babylonian preoccupations with astrology, the casting of horoscopes and soothsaying through examination of animal entrails (haruspicy). Viewing disease as largely supernatural, Mesopotamian medicine might be regarded as sorcery systematized. Parallels to this are offered by Egyptian medicine, which developed at the same time and presents comparable healing practices involving prayers, magic, spells and sacrifices, together with practical drug treatments and surgery.

EGYPT

Egypt rose under the pharaohs in the third millennium BC; the great pyramids in the Valley of the Kings, dating from around 2000 BC, show a powerful regime possessed of stupendous ambition and technological virtuosity. The earliest written evidence of their medicine appears in papyri of the second millennium BC, but such records encode far older traditions. Among the medical texts, the most important, discovered in the nineteenth century, are the Edwin Smith and the Georg Ebers papyri.

Sometimes called a book of wounds, the Edwin Smith papyrus (c. 1600 BC, found near Luxor and named after an American Egyptologist) gives a head-to-foot inventory of forty-eight case reports, including various injuries and wounds, their prognosis and treatment. 'If you examine a man having a dislocation of his mandible, should you find his mouth open, and his mouth cannot close, you should put your two thumbs upon the end of the two rami of the mandible inside his mouth and your fingers under his chin and you should cause them to fall back so that they rest in their places.' The surgical conditions treated were wounds, fractures and abscesses; circumcision was also performed. Broken bones were set in ox-bone splints, supported by resin-soaked bandages. The papyrus refers to a raft of dressings, adhesive plasters, braces, plugs, cleansers and cauteries.

The Smith papyrus shows there was an empirical component to ancient Egyptian medicine alongside its magico-religious bent. In a similar style, the London papyrus (c. 1350 BC) describes maternal care, and the Kahun papyrus (c. 1850 BC) deals with animal medicine and gynaecology, including methods for detecting pregnancy and for contraception, for which pessaries were recommended made of pulverized crocodile dung and herbs now impossible to identify, mixed with honey. Their contraceptive measures, evidently aimed at blocking the passage of semen, may have worked, since the Egyptians seem to have been able to regulate family size without recourse to infanticide.

The Ebers papyrus (*c.* 1550 BC), deriving from Thebes, is, however, the principal medical document – indeed the oldest surviving medical book. Over twenty metres long, it deals with scores of diseases and proposes remedies including spells and incantations. This and other sources show the prominence of magic. Amulets were recommended, and treatments typically involved chants and supplications to the appropriate deities, the most popular being the falcon-headed sun god Ra; Thoth, the ibis-headed god of wisdom (later associated with the Greek Hermes or the Roman Mercury); and Isis and her son Horus, the god of health, whose eye formed the motif for a popular charm.

The Ebers papyrus covers 15 diseases of the abdomen, 29 of the eyes, and 18 of the skin, and lists no fewer than 21 cough treatments. About 700 drugs and 800 formulae are referred to, mainly herbs but also mineral and animal remedies. To cure night-blindness fried ox liver was to be taken – possibly a tried-and-tested procedure, as liver is rich in vitamin A, lack of which causes the illness. Eye disorders were common, and there were numerous cures:

> To drive away inflammation of the eyes, grind the stems of the juniper of Byblos, steep them in water, apply to the eyes of the sick person and he will be quickly cured. To cure granulations of the eye prepare a remedy of cyllyrium, verdigris, onions, blue vitriol, powdered wood, mix and apply to the eyes.

For stomach ailments a decoction of cumin, goose-fat and milk was recommended, but other remedies sound more exotic, including a drink prepared from black ass testicles, or a mixture of vulva and penis extracts and a black lizard, designed to cure baldness. Also good for hair growth was a compound of hippopotamus, lion, crocodile, goose, snake and ibex fat.

Egyptian medicine credited many vegetables and fruits with healing properties, and used tree resins, including myrrh, frankincense and manna. As in Mesopotamia, plant extracts – notably senna, colocynth and castor oil – were employed as purgatives. Recipes include ox spleen, pig's brain, honey-sweetened tortoise gall and various animal fats. Antimony, copper and other minerals were recommended as astringents or disinfectants. Containing ingredients from leeks to lapis lazuli – including garlic, onion, tamarisk, cereals, spices, condiments, resins, gums, dates, hellebore, opium and cannabis – compound drugs were administered in the form of pills, ointments, poultices, fumigations, inhalations, gargles and suppositories; they might even be blown into the urethra through a tube.

Archaeological evidence and papyri afford glimpses of Egyptian medical practice, at least among the elite. Part was hierarchically organized and under state control; physicians were appointed to superintend public works, the army, burial grounds and the pharaoh's palace. Court physicians formed the apex of the medical pyramid. Just as the gods governed different body parts, physicians (*swnu*) specialized in particular diseases or body organs; in the fifth century BC the Greek Herodotus observed that in Egypt 'one physician is confined to the study and management of one disease . . . some attend to the disorders of the eyes, others to those of the head, some take care of the teeth, others are conversant with all diseases of the bowels.'

As in Mesopotamia, the *swnu* formed one of three divisions of healers. The others were priests of Sekhmet, and sorcerers. Healers whose names have come down include Iri, Keeper of the Royal Rectum, presumably the pharaoh's enema expert. (Enemas had a divine origin, being invented by ibis-headed Thoth; they were widely used, because Egyptian health lore feared putrefaction in the guts and bowels.) There was also Peseshet, head female physician or overseer, proof of the existence, as in Mesopotamia, of female healers; and the celebrated Imhotep ('he who cometh in peace') chief vizier to Pharaoh Zozer (*fl.* 27 cent. BC), high priest at Heliopolis, renowned as an astrologer, priest, sage and pyramid designer (the Step Pyramid of Sakkarah), but above all as a physician.

Imhotep became a figure akin to the Greek god Asclepius (Aesculapius in Latin). His 'sayings' were later recorded and preserved among the classics of Egyptian wisdom, and within a few generations he was being deified. There is, however, little evidence of his cult for another millennium, and only around 300 BC did it blossom. As with Asclepius, Imhotep became associated with healing shrines and temple sleep (incubation cures). Patients would sleep overnight in the inner precincts where they would be visited in their dreams by a god, or an emissary like a snake, and their illness or infertility remedied.

The Egyptians believed well-being was endangered by earthly and supernatural forces alike, in particular evil spirits stealing into the body through the orifices and consuming the victim's vital substance. Health was associated with correct living, being at peace with the gods, spirits and the dead; illness was a matter of imbalance which could be restored to equilibrium by supplication, spells and rituals. Thus, someone struck blind might invoke a god: 'Ptah, the lord of Truth, has turned his justice against me; he has rightly chastised me. Have pity on me, deign to regard me with merciful countenance.' Handling burns, a magician would swab the wound with the milk of a mother of a baby boy, while appealing to Isis by repeating the words the goddess had supposedly used to rescue her son Horus from being burned: 'There is water in my mouth and a Nile between my legs; I come to quench the fire.'

Surgery was limited to repairing injuries and bone fractures; sutures and cautery were used, and wound dressings to promote healing, which combined honey with grease or resin; but no surgical instruments survive. Anatomical knowledge remained limited to bones and major organs. As mummification suggests, the Egyptians did not share the taboos that have so widely forbidden tampering with corpses, but embalmers formed a separate guild and were of low caste; moreover, since mummification aimed to preserve the body intact, embalmers did not open cadavers up; they eviscerated and extracted the organs through small incisions. The brain was removed through the nose by hooks, though the heart was left in place, being the seat of the soul.

According to Egyptian medical theory, humans were born healthy, but were susceptible to disorders caused not only by demons but by intestinal putrefaction. Life lay in breath, and a speculative heart-centred physiology pictured a mesh of vessels carrying blood, urine, air, semen, tears and solid wastes to all bodily parts. This vascular network was likened to the Nile and its canals and, as with that water-system, the point was to keep it free of obstruction. Rotting food and faeces clogging the system were considered perilous, hence the need to prevent pus formation and to cleanse the innards with laxatives. Herodotus noted that three days each month were set aside for evacuating the body with emetics and enemas.

As with Mesopotamia, Egypt's imposing political regime made for an organized medical practice. It is, however, with Greek civilization that evidence of recognizable medical discourse first appears.

GREECE

By 1000 BC the communities later collectively known as the Greeks were emerging around the Aegean sea, in Ionia (the western seaboard of Asia Minor or Turkey), the Greek mainland (the Peloponnese), and the intervening islands. How much medical knowledge they took from Egypt remains controversial. On Crete, midway between Africa and the Greek mainland, the remarkable Minoan civilization had developed after 2000 BC, with its dazzling pottery and frescos found at Knossos and other palaces; and the Greeks of the Mycenean period (*c.* 1200 BC) were in close touch with Egypt, certainly getting drugs from there. But the contrasts between old Egyptian and new Greek medicine are striking.

Little is known of Greek medicine before the appearance of written texts in the fifth century BC. Archaic Greece undeniably possessed folk healers, including priest healers employing divination and drugs. From early times (Olympic games are recorded from as early as 776 BC), the love of athletics gave rise to instructors in exercise, bathing, massage, gymnastics and diet. Throughout Greek civilization, as with the Roman later, ideals of manliness required keeping one's physique in peak condition; admiration for the lithe, fit, attractive warrior shines through classical art and myths. Dancing, martial arts and working out in the gymnasium with the help of trainers – men-only practices, women being excluded from public life – were regarded as essential for the well-being of the body. The archaic warrior developed into the beauty-loving citizen of the *polis* (city state), with his ideal of a cultivated mind in a disciplined body. Athenian sculpture and painting revered the human form, proudly displaying its naked magnificence and finding in its geometrical forms echoes of the fundamental harmonies of nature. A tradition was thus begun that would climax in the Renaissance image of 'Vitruvian Man', the representation of the naked male figure inscribed at the centre of the cosmos.

Glimpses of early Greek medicine are offered by the Homeric epics, dating from before 600 BC but incorporating older narratives. Painstaking scholars have counted some 147 cases of battle wounds in the *Iliad* (that is, 106 spear thrusts, 17 sword slashes, 12 arrow shots and 12 sling shots). Among survivors of arrow wounds was King Menelaus of Sparta, whose physician extracted the arrow, sucked out the blood and applied a salve. As with other medical interventions in Homer, this shows no Egyptian influence, supporting the idea that, even if Greek practice owed much to Egypt, it rapidly went its own way. Certainly Greek medicine as known from written sources is highly distinctive, for from the beginning Greek medical texts were essentially secular.

Admittedly Greek society at large drew heavily upon sacred healing. In Homer, Apollo appears as the 'god of healing' – now the spreader of plague, now the avenger. In the *Iliad* deities visited plagues upon humans, and Greek myths abound in injuries inflicted by the gods, for instance Prometheus having his liver torn out by an eagle. Various gods and heroes were identified with health and disease, the chief being Asclepius, who even had the power to raise the dead. A heroic warrior and blameless physician, Asclepius was the son of Apollo, sired upon a mortal mother. Taught herbal remedies by Chiron the centaur, he generously used them to heal humans. Incensed at being cheated of death, Hades (Roman: Pluto), the ruler of the underworld, appealed to the supreme god, Zeus, who obligingly dispatched Asclepius with a thunderbolt (though he was later elevated to the ranks of the gods).

A different version appears in Homer, who portrayed Asclepius as a tribal chief and a skilled wound healer, whose sons became physicians and were called Asclepiads, from whom all Asclepian practitioners descended. As the tutelary god of medicine, Asclepius is usually portrayed with a beard, staff and snake (the origin of the caduceus sign of the modern physician, with its two snakes intertwined, double-helix like, on a winged staff; the shedding of the snakes' skin symbolized the renewal of life). The god was often shown accompanied by his daughters, Hygeia (health or hygiene) and Panacea (cure-all).

Asclepius eventually became a cult figure and the physicians' patron. Pindar wrote:

> They came to him with ulcers the flesh had grown, or their
> Limbs mangled with the grey bronze, or bruised
> With the stone flung from afar,
> Or the body stormed with summer fever, or chill, and he
> Released each man and led him
> From his individual grief.

During the third century the cult of Asclepius spread, and by 200 BC every large town in Greece had a temple to the god. The best known of these Asclepieions were on the island of Cos, Hippocrates' birthplace, and at Epidaurus, thirty miles from Athens, but at least 200 other sites have been uncovered; they played a role similar to medieval healing shrines or to Lourdes today. The major shrines sported splendid temples and their cures were celebrated in memorial inscriptions. Pilgrims stayed the night in special incubation chambers where, before an image of Asclepius, they hoped through 'temple sleep' to receive a vision in a dream. The god would either perform the cure himself, or would give the patient a dream to be deciphered by the priest. The restored patient usually raised in the precinct a memorial of this marvel: 'Hermodikes of Lampsakos was paralysed in body. In his sleep he was healed by the god.' Physicians rarely acted as dream interpreters, but around the temples religious and secular healing rubbed shoulders.

The Greeks also went in for other religious healing, involving exorcists, diviners, shamans and priests. Certain diseases, notably epilepsy, were ascribed to celestial wrath: the *Iliad* opens with a plague sent by Apollo, and relief from the appalling great plague of Athens (430–427 BC) was sought through invoking the gods.

For all that, Hippocratic medicine, the foundation of Greek written medicine, explicitly grounds the art upon a quite different basis: a healing system independent of the supernatural and built upon natural philosophy. The author of the Hippocratic text, *On the Sacred Disease* (*c.* 410 BC), utterly rejected the received idea of a divine origin for epilepsy. He sarcastically paraded the different gods supposed to produce epileptic seizures: if the convulsive patient behaved in a goatlike way, or ground his teeth, the cause allegedly lay in Hera, the mother of the gods; Hecate, the goddess of sorcery, was to blame if the sufferer experienced nightmares and delirium; and so forth. But what evidence was there for any of these fantasies? 'Men regard its nature and cause as divine from ignorance and wonder', insisted the author, 'and this notion is kept up by their inability to comprehend it.' How foolish! For if a condition 'is reckoned divine because it is wonderful, instead of one there would be many diseases which would be sacred'. Nowhere in the Hippocratic writings is there any hint of disease being caused or cured by the gods.

This scoffing at the 'sacred disease' chimed with an elitist ideal of professional identity. Staking their claims in the medical market-place of the polis, Hippocratic doctors scolded traditional healers. Those pretenders 'who first referred this disease to the gods', the author complained, were like conjurors and charlatans. Elevating themselves above such dabblers in divination, the Hippocratics posited a *natural* theory of disease aetiology. *On the Sacred Disease* plucked disease from the heavens and brought it down to earth. The true doctor would no longer be an intermediary with the gods but the bedside friend of the sick.

This separation of medicine from religion points to another distinctive feature of Greek healing: its openness, a quality characteristic of Greek intellectual activity at large, which it owed to political diversity and cultural pluralism. In the constellation of city states dotting the mainland and the Aegean islands, healing was practised in the public sphere, and interacted with other mental pursuits. There was no imperial Hammurabic Code and, unlike Egypt, no state medical bureaucracy; nor were there examinations or professional qualifications. Those calling themselves doctors (*iatroi*) had to compete with bone-setters, exorcists, root-cutters, incantatory priests, gymnasts and showmen, exposed to the quips of playwrights and the criticism of philosophers. Medicine was open to all (as later in Rome, slaves sometimes practised medicine).

Doctrinally, too, there was great multiplicity, in complete contrast to what is known of Babylonian or Egyptian medicine, which have left no trace of controversy, being essentially lists of instructions. Greek medical writers loved speculation and argument, doubtless angling for public attention. Trading facts and chopping logic, physicians jousted to unsaddle their rivals.

The ultimate challenge was to fathom the order of the universe, and because this included the human body viewed as a microcosm of the grand order of nature (macrocosm), such metaphysical speculations had direct medical implications. The earliest Ionian philosophers hoped to identify a single elemental substance, but Parmenides of Elea in southern Italy criticized such monocausal theories. A shaman-like figure, Parmenides (*c.* 515–450 BC) maintained that the key question concerned not material essence but the processes governing change and stability within a regular universe.

Various solutions to the riddle of the cosmos followed. For the geometer Pythagoras (*c.* 530 BC), living at Croton in Sicily, the key lay in number and harmony – and the dynamic balance of contraries, based on the opposition of odd and even. For Heraclitus (*c.* 540–475 BC) the true constant was change itself, in a macrocosm composed of fire and water; for Democritus (*c.* 460 BC), the essence was a flux of atoms in a void.

Others, like the Sicilian Empedocles (*fl.* mid-5th century BC), regarded nature as composed of a small number of basic elements (earth, air, fire, and water) combining into temporarily stable mixtures. Building on Parmenides, Empedocles seems to have been the first to advance some of the key physiological doctrines in Greek medicine. These involve the concept of innate heat as the source of living processes, including digestion; the cooling function of breathing; and the notion that the liver makes the blood that nourishes the tissues.

His contemporary, Alcmaeon of Croton (*fl.* 470 BC), believed that the brain, not the heart, was the chief organ of sensation. This had a real observational basis: examination of the eyeball led him to discern the optic nerve leading into the skull. He gave similar explanations for the sensations of hearing and smelling, because the ear and nostrils suggested passages leading to the brain.

Discounting the role of demons in disease, Alcmaeon treated health in a rather Pythagorean way as the dance of primary pairs of bodily powers – hot and cold, sweet and sour, wet and dry. Seated in the blood, marrow or brain, illness could arise from an external cause or an internal imbalance, caused by too much or too little nutriment. Similar views can be found in several texts in the Hippocratic Corpus (440–340 BC), though no direct influence can be proved. Indeed, all these early writers are obscure, for their opinions survive only through later commentators and critics, such as Plato, who used them for their own polemical purposes.

What is clear is that in classical Greece *philosophical* speculations about nature became enmeshed in dialogue with *medical* beliefs about sickness and health; dialogue and debate were integral to Greek intellectual life. Unlike healing in the Near East, elite Greek medicine was not a closed priestly system: it was open to varied influences and accessible to outsiders, guaranteeing its flexibility and vitality.

This openness followed from the fact that Greek civilization developed in multiple centres from Asia Minor to Sicily, and no single sect of doctors possessed a state or professional monopoly. Athens was the first city to support a fair number of full-time healers making a livelihood out of fees, and, according to his younger contemporary Plato (427–347 BC), the great Hippocrates taught all who were prepared to pay.

HIPPOCRATES

All we know about Hippocrates (*c.* 460–377 BC) is legend. Early hagiographers say he was born on the island of Cos and that he lived a long and virtuous life. The sixty or so works comprising the Corpus were penned by him only in the sense that the *Iliad* is ascribed to Homer. They derive from a variety of hands, and, as with the books of the Bible, they became jumbled up, fragmented and then pasted together again in antiquity. What is now called the Corpus was gathered around 250 BC in the library at Alexandria, though further 'Hippocratic' texts were added later still. Scholarly ink galore has been spilt as to which were authentic and which spurious; the controversy is futile.

The Corpus is highly varied. Some works like *The Art* are philosophical, others are teaching texts; some, like the *Epidemics*, read like case notes. What unites them is the conviction that, as with everything else, health and disease are capable of explanation by reasoning about nature, independently of supernatural interference. Man is governed by the same physical laws as the cosmos, hence medicine must be an understanding, empirical and rational, of the workings of the body in its natural environment. Appeal to reason, rather than to rules or to supernatural forces, gives Hippocratic medicine its distinctiveness. It was also to win a name for being patient-centred rather than disease-oriented, and for being concerned more with observation and experience than with abstractions.

Hippocratic medicine did not offer all the answers. The workings of the body and the springs of disease remained thorny issues dividing physicians. This was partly because knowledge was limited. Hippocratic doctors had a sound grasp of surface anatomy, but first-hand knowledge of the innards and living processes depended heavily on wound observation and animal dissection, for in the classical period the dignity the human body enjoyed forbade dissection.

Analogy might help – hens' eggs offered models for human foetal development, and the digestion of food could be compared to cooking over a fire – but even animal experiments were rare, and the body's hidden workings had to be deduced largely from what went in and what came out. With internal physiology hidden, disease might be conjecturally explained: *On the Sacred Disease* argued that epilepsy, as natural as any other disease, was caused by phlegm blocking the airways, which then convulsed the body as it struggled to free itself.

The cardinal concept in the Hippocratic Corpus was that health was equilibrium and illness an upset, an explanation probably owing much to pre-Socratic attempts to understand the stability yet changeability of nature. *On Regimen* pictured the body as being in perpetual flux: health was a matter of keeping it within bounds. More commonly, notably in *On the Nature of Man*, the body was viewed as stable until illness subverted it. Imbalance would produce illness if it resulted in undue concentration of fluid in a particular body zone. Thus a flow (defluxion) of humours to the feet would produce gout, or catarrh (defluxion of phlegm from the head to the lungs) would be the cause of coughing. It was the healer's job to apply his skill to preserving balance or, if illness befell, to restoring it.

What was being kept in balance or upset were bodily fluids or *chymoi*, translated as 'humours'. Sap in plants and blood in animals were the fount of life. Other and perhaps less salutary bodily fluids became visible only in case of illness – for example, the mucus of a cold or the runny faeces of dysentery. Two fluids were particularly associated with illness: bile and phlegm, though naturally present in the body, seemed to flow immoderately in sickness. Winter colds were due to phlegm, summer diarrhoea and vomiting to bile, and mania resulted from bile boiling in the brain. *Airs, Waters, Places* also attributed national characteristics to bile and phlegm: the pasty, phlegmatic peoples of the North were contrasted with the swarthy, hot, dry, bilious Africans. Both were judged inferior to the harmonious Greeks in their ideally equable climate.

Bile and phlegm were visible mainly when exuded in sickness, so it made sense to regard them as harmful. But what of other fluids? Since Homeric times, blood had been associated with life, yet even blood was expelled naturally from the body, as in menstruation or nose-bleeds. Such natural evacuation suggested the practice of blood-letting, devised by the Hippocratics, systematized by Galen, and serving for centuries as a therapeutic mainstay.

The last of the humours, black bile (melancholy), entered disease theory late, but in *On the Nature of Man* it assumed the status of an essential, if mainly harmful, humour. Visible in vomit and excreta, it was perhaps thought of as contributing to the dark hue of dried blood. Indeed, the idea of four humours may have been suggested by observation of clotted blood: the darkest part corresponded to black bile, the serum above the clot was yellow bile, the light matter at the top was phlegm. Black bile completed a coherent, symmetrical grid in binary oppositions, and the four humours – blood, yellow bile, black bile and phlegm – proved wonderfully versatile as an explanatory system. They could be correlated to the four primary qualities – hot, dry, cold and wet; to the four seasons, to the four ages of man (infancy, youth, adulthood and old age), to the four elements (air, fire, earth and water), and the four temperaments. They thus afforded a neat schema with vast explanatory potential. On the assumption, for example, that blood predominated in spring and among the young, precautions against excess

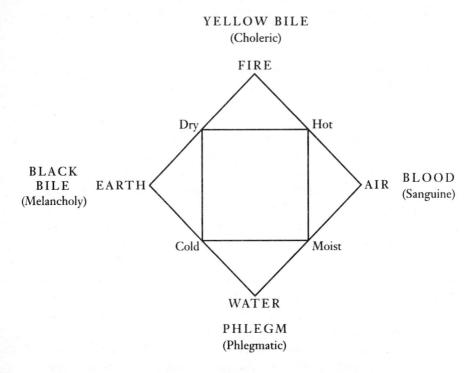

The four humours and four elements

could be taken, either by eliminating blood-rich foods, like red meat, or by blood-letting (phlebotomy) to purge excess. The scheme (which finds parallels in Chinese and Indian medicine) could be made to fit with observations, and afforded rationales for disease explanation and treatment within a causal framework.

The Hippocratics specialized in medicine by the bedside, prizing trust-based clinical relations:

> Make frequent visits; be especially careful in your examinations, counteracting the things wherein you have been deceived at the changes. Thus you will know the case more easily, and at the same time you will also be more at your ease. For instability is characteristic of the humours, and so they may also be easily altered by nature and by chance.
>
> ... Keep a watch also on the faults of the patients, which often make them lie about the taking of things prescribed. For through

non compliance!

not taking disagreeable drinks, purgative or other, they sometimes die. What they have done never results in a confession, but the blame is thrown upon the physician.

Their therapeutic stance was 'expectant': they waited and watched their patients, talking, winning trust and giving a helping hand to the 'healing power of nature' (*vis medicatrix naturae*) emphasized in the text *On Ancient Medicine*. Believing that 'our natures are the physicians of our diseases', they scorned heroic interventions and left risky procedures to others. The *Oath* forbade cutting, even for the stone, and other texts reserved surgery for those used to handling war wounds. That was a sensible division of labour, but surgery was also regarded as an inferior trade, the work of the hand rather than the head – a fact reflected in its name: 'surgery' derives from the Latin *chirurgia*, which comes from the Greek *cheiros* (hand) and *ergon* (work). Surgery was handiwork.

The Hippocratic doctor might disown the knife, but he prided himself on his knowledge of surgical matters – indeed the Corpus contains much now regarded as such, including a treatise *On Head Injuries*. Hippocratic advice proved highly influential: wounds should be kept dry, but suppuration was deemed essential to healing; the pus supposedly derived from vitiated blood which needed to be expelled from the body: pus was thus a desirable evacuation. Fractures were to be reduced and immobilized with splints and bandages. For bladder stones, catheterization was advocated, never lithotomy – such operations were left to 'such as are craftsmen therein'; and, as a last resort in case of gangrene, amputation might be performed (vascular ligature was unknown).

Hippocratic surgical texts were thus conservative in outlook, encouraging a tradition in which doctors sought to treat complaints first through management, occasionally through drugs and finally, if need be, by surgical intervention. Hippocrates and Galen alike were dubious about surgery for cancer.

Drug therapy too was cautious. The preferred Hippocratic treatment lay in dietary regulation. Unlike sheep and goats, humans could not eat rough food; good diet was crucial to health and so, as the saying went, the first cook was the first physician. But diet meant more than food and drink – *diatetica* (dietetics), the cornerstone of the healing art, involved an entire lifestyle. Ancient authors linked this therapy to athletic training, and to the well-regulated life as urged by philosophers. *On Regimen* gave advice on taking exercise, so important to the culture of free-born Greeks, and also on sex, bathing and sleep. In winter, for instance, 'sexual intercourse should be more frequent . . . and for older men more than for the younger'.

Hippocratic healing was patient-oriented, focusing on 'dis-ease' rather than diseases understood as ontological entities. But observation identified certain illness patterns. To the Hippocratics the paradigm acute disease was fever, and its model seems to have been malaria, the seasonal onset and regular course of which allowed it to be documented and explained in terms of humours and times of the year. Though ignorant of the role played by mosquitoes, Hippocratic physicians had a shrewd grasp of the connexions between fever and weather, season and locality. *Airs, Waters, Places* observed that if the rains occurred normally in autumn and winter, the year would be healthy, but if they were delayed until spring, many fever cases would occur during the summer, 'for whenever the great heat comes on suddenly while the earth is soaked by reason of the spring rains . . . the fevers that attack are of the acutest type.'

Hippocratic physicians posited a broad correlation between humours and times of the year. In each season, one humour was thought to predominate. Bodily phlegm increased during the winter because, being cold and wet, it was akin to the chilly and rainy weather of a Mediterranean winter; colds, bronchitis and pneumonia were then more prevalent. When spring came, blood increased in quantity, and diseases would follow from a plethora of blood, including spring fever outbreaks (primarily benign tertian malaria), dysentery and nose-bleeds. By summer, the weather was hotter and drier, yellow bile (hot and dry) increased, and so the diseases resulting from yellow bile would multiply, that is severe fevers (falciparum malaria). With the cooler weather at the end of summer, fevers waned, but many would display the consequences of repeated fever attacks, their skins showing a dirty yellowish tinge and their spleens enlarged. The autumnal decline of fevers indicated to the Hippocratic physician that yellow bile had diminished while black bile was increasing. Seemingly the most problematic humour, black bile makes good sense in the light of awareness of the effects of malarial fevers. Philiscus, whose evidently malarial condition was described in *Epidemics I*, suffered from black urine and his 'spleen stuck out'; the spleen was considered the seat of black bile. Faced with fevers, Hippocratic doctors predictably did not attempt anything heroic. Valuing regimen and diet, they gave barley water, hydromel (honey and water) or oxymel (honey and vinegar) – a 'low' diet with adequate fluids.

The doctor should therefore observe sickness, attending the patient and identifying symptom clusters and their rhythms. *Airs, Waters, Places* took it as axiomatic that understanding of locales would enable the healer on arrival in a faraway town to grasp the local diseases, so that he could 'achieve the greatest triumphs in the practice of his art', something important in a competitive market.

The art of diagnosis involved creating a profile of the patient's way of life, habitation, work and dietary habits. This was achieved partly by asking questions, and partly by the use of trained senses:

> When you examine the patient, inquire into all particulars; first how the head is . . . then examine if the hypochondrium and sides be free of pain, for . . . if there be pain in the side, and along with the pain either cough, tormina or bellyache, the bowels should be opened with clysters . . . The Physician should ascertain whether the patient be apt to faint when he is raised up, and whether his breathing is free.

Hippocratics prided themselves on their clinical acuity, being quick to pick up telltale symptoms, as with the *facies hippocratica*, the facial look of the dying: 'a protrusive nose, hollow eyes, sunken temples, cold ears that are drawn in with the lobes turned outward, the forehead's skin rough and tense like parchment, and the whole face greenish or black or blue-grey or leaden'. Experience was condensed into aphorisms; for instance, 'when sleep puts an end to delirium, it is a good sign.'

Hippocratic doctors cultivated diagnostic skills, but the technique they really prized was *prognosis* – a secular version of the prognostications of earlier medicine:

> It appears to me a most excellent thing for the physician to cultivate Prognosis; for by foreseeing and foretelling, in the presence of the sick, the present, the past, and the future, and explaining the omissions which patients have been guilty of, he will be the more readily believed to be acquainted with the circumstances of the sick; so that men will have confidence to intrust themselves to such a physician.

This skill had a social function: prognostic flair created a favourable impression, setting the gifted healer above quacks and diviners. To be able to tell a patient's medical history and prospects displayed acuity.

And by declaring, if need be, that death was impending, a healer escaped blame for apparent failure.

Hippocratics made no pretence to miracle cures, but they did undertake that they would first and foremost do no harm (*primum non nocere*) and presented themselves as the friends of the sick. This philanthropic disposition attested the physician's love of his art – above fame and fortune – and reassured anxious patients and their relatives. Such concerns are addressed in the Hippocratic Oath (see box, overleaf).

For all its later prominence, little is known about the Oath's origins, though it dates from between the fifth and third centuries BC. It certainly did not set general standards of conduct, for the sanctity it accords to human life is anomalous to classical moral thought and practice, abortion and infanticide being familiar practices, condoned by Plato and Aristotle. The fact that it prohibits prescribing a 'destructive pessary' suggests a Pythagorean influence, with their belief in the transmigration of souls.

The Oath foreshadowed the western paradigm of a profession (one who *professes* an oath) as a morally self-regulating discipline among those sharing craft knowledge and committed to serving others. But it was equally an agreement between apprentice and teacher. As it makes clear, Hippocratic medicine was a male monopoly, although male physicians might cooperate with midwives and nurses.

Hippocratic medicine had its weaknesses – it knew little of the inner workings of the body – but its striking innovation lay in perceiving sickness as a disturbance in the health of the individual, who would then be accorded devoted personal attention. 'Life is short, the art long, opportunity fleeting, experience fallacious, judgment difficult,' proclaims the first of the Hippocratic aphorisms, outlining the arduous but honourable labour of the physician.

The significance of Hippocratic medicine was twofold: it carved out a lofty role for the selfless physician which would serve as a lasting model for professional identity and conduct, and it taught that understanding of sickness required understanding of nature.

MEDICINE AND PHILOSOPHY

With Greek philosophers praising health as one of the greatest blessings of life, medicine became implicated in wider debates about human nature and the status of the body. The earliest writer to mention

THE OATH

I swear by Apollo the healer, by Aesculapius, by Health and all the powers of healing, and call to witness all the gods and goddesses that I may keep this Oath and Promise to the best of my ability and judgment.

I will pay the same respect to my master in the Science as to my parents and share my life with him and pay all my debts to him. I will regard his sons as my brothers and teach them the Science, if they desire to learn it, without fee or contract. I will hand on precepts, lectures and all other learning to my sons, to those of my master and to those pupils duly apprenticed and sworn, and to none other.

I will use my power to help the sick to the best of my ability and judgment; I will abstain from harming or wronging any man by it.

I will not give a fatal draught to anyone if I am asked, nor will I suggest any such thing. Neither will I give a woman means to procure an abortion.

I will be chaste and religious in my life and in my practice.

I will not cut, even for the stone, but I will leave such procedures to the practitioners of that craft.

Whenever I go into a house, I will go to help the sick and never with the intention of doing harm or injury. I will not abuse my position to indulge in sexual contacts with the bodies of women or of men, whether they be freemen or slaves.

Whatever I see or hear, professionally or privately, which ought not to be divulged, I will keep secret and tell no one.

If, therefore, I observe this Oath and do not violate it, may I prosper both in my life and in my profession, earning good repute among all men for all time. If I transgress and forswear this Oath, may my lot be otherwise.

Hippocrates and his theories, Plato (427–437 BC) developed a series of analogies to divide human nature into three functions – reason, spirit, and appetites – located respectively within the brain, the heart and the liver, and all potentially in conflict. Only in the philosopher would reason, aided by spirit, triumph over sordid desires. The *Republic*'s distinctions between reason and appetite, mind and body, was of utmost philosophical and psychological significance. Plato's place in later medical thinking, however, rests on the *Timaeus* (*c.* 375 BC). This pictured the body as built up from transcendental geometrical shapes. The human frame was constructed by the Creator with specific purposes in mind; hence medicine had a discernible teleology. Somatic in orientation, the *Timaeus* taught that morality was not simply a matter of education; behaviour might also be determined by organic constituents, by excesses or deficiencies in the spinal marrow which affected the sensations of pleasure and pain; madness might thus have a physiological cause, to be treated by medical means. Because the mind was influenced by the body, the doctor had a part to play in teaching virtue. Advancing a physiology compatible with Hippocratic medicine, the *Timaeus* became a highly influential text, linking medicine and philosophy, health and politics.

'The soul and body being two, they have two arts corresponding to them,' Plato stated, making similar links in the *Gorgias*: 'there is the art of politics attending on the soul; and another art attending on the body, of which I know no single name, but which may be described as having two divisions, one of them gymnastic, and the other medicine.' Thanks to Plato, western thinking could consider medicine as having its share in understanding human nature. Greek thinking thus emphasized the common ground between what would later become the separate disciplines of philosophy, medicine and ethics. Health depended upon temperance and wisdom, or proper self-control. Achieved through moderation in eating, drinking, sex and exercise, bodily health became the template for healthy thinking (*sōphrosynē*, soundness of mind). To later Stoic philosophers likewise, the wisdom of the sage required the attainment of true health; for their part Epicureans stressed the supreme desirability of freedom from pain.

Plato's pupil Aristotle also put forward hugely influential views on the constitution of life. A doctor's son from Stagira in Thrace, Aristotle (384–322 BC) went to Athens to study with Plato, later becoming tutor to Alexander the Great (356–323 BC). His towering role in theorizing about metaphysics and cosmology, ethics, politics, poetics and thinking itself involved many achievements: the creation of a scientific method; the pursuit of teleological ways of thinking; and the impetus he gave to biological research. Questioning Plato's transcendental ideas, Aristotle called for the systematic observation of nature. Whereas Plato distrusted sense experience, his pupil launched a programme of empirical investigation into the natural world – into zoology, botany and meteorology. Nature did nothing in vain, so body parts had to be explained in respect of their purpose (teleology). Aristotle discussed such final causes in terms of a wider fourfold theory of causation. For nearly two thousand years, Aristotelian methodology provided the framework for scientific investigation.

Later hailed by Dante as the 'master of the men who know', Aristotle was the first who systematically used dissection findings (animal not human) as a grounding for his biomedical theories. What he recorded occasionally puzzled his successors. In his description of the heart, he refers to 'three chambers' connected to the lung; later investigators were baffled which animals he was referring to. While revealing the veins as a connected system of vessels extending from the heart throughout the whole body, he did not distinguish between veins and arteries, applying the same term to both.

Observing the embryo developing within eggs, Aristotle perceived the beating heart as the first sign of life, concluding that it must be the prime mover of life and coeval with the whole body. The blood contained within the heart and blood vessels became correspondingly decisive. Blood was the nutrient the vessels absorbed from the intestines: 'this explains why the blood diminishes in quantity when no food is taken, and increases when much is consumed.'

The idea of a nervous system paralleling the veins and arteries was as yet unformulated, so it is not surprising that Aristotle did not locate the seat of the soul, the source of movement and sensation, within the brain, but in the heart, stressing its physiological primacy within the human body. It was also the source of innate heat; pulsation was the result of a sort of boiling movement (ebullition) in the blood, causing it to press against the heart walls and pour out into the blood vessels. The heart's heat dilated the lungs, fresh air rushed in, cooled the blood, and, warmed by the blood's heat, was then expired. The brain had a part to play in these vital processes. Being naturally cold, it served as a refrigerator, helping to cool the blood's innate heat. It also brought on sleep. Its function was that of a regulator, adjusting the organism as a whole.

The discussions of psychology in Aristotle's *On the Soul, On Sleep and Waking, On Sensation* and *On Memory* long intrigued doctors and philosophers alike; and two thousand years later his teleological doctrines shaped the physiology of William Harvey (See Chapter Nine).

In the shorter term his anatomy was taken up and revised by the next generation, particularly by Diocles of Carystos (*fl.* 320 BC), and two doctors working in Alexandria, Herophilus and his contemporary Erasistratus.

ALEXANDRIAN MEDICINE

Aristotle's royal pupil, Alexander, routed all his rivals, lamented there were no more worlds to conquer, and expired in 323 BC, supposedly exclaiming, 'I die by the help of too many physicians.' His destruction of the Persian Emperor Darius III had brought Egypt within the hellenistic sphere of influence, and after Alexander's death science gained a prominent place at the court of King Ptolemy, who ruled from 323 to 282 BC and established his capital at Alexandria, at the mouth of the Nile.

King Ptolemy's main cultural creations, the Alexandrian Library and the Museum (sanctuary of the Muses) installed Greek learning in a new Egyptian environment: Archimedes, Euclid and the astronomer Ptolemy were later to teach there. The library became a wonder of the scholarly world, eventually containing, it was said, 700,000 manuscripts, and its facilities included an observatory, zoological gardens, lecture halls and rooms for research.*

Thanks to Alexander's conquests, the hellenistic world stretched from the Persian Gulf to Sicily, with Greek becoming the *lingua franca* of the elite. One consequence was a remarkable increase of new information on animals, plants, minerals and drugs. Alexandria also attracted medical talent, notably Herophilus of Chalcedon (*c.* 330–260 BC) and his contemporary, Erasistratus of Chios (*c.* 330–255 BC). Their writings having been lost, we know about them only through later physicians. Cornelius Celsus (*fl.* AD 60) reported that they dissected, or at least experimented upon, living humans, which is not inconceivable, for

---

* The life of learning could be precarious, as is clear from the fate of even the great Alexandrian library. Part was wrecked in 48 BC during riots sparked by Julius Caesar's arrival; later Christian leaders encouraged the destruction of the Temple of Muses and other pagan idols. And, so legend has it, in AD 395 the last scholar at the museum, the female mathematician Hypatia, was hauled out of the museum by Christian fanatics and beaten to death. The Muslim conquest of the city in the seventh century resulted in the final destruction of the library.

Greeks may have used their privileged status in Alexandria to experiment on their inferiors, especially condemned criminals.

Herophilus was apparently a student of Praxagoras of Cos (*fl.* 340 BC), who had improved Aristotelian anatomy by distinguishing arteries from veins. Praxagorus saw the arteries as air tubes, similar to the trachea and bronchi, conducting the breath of life (*pneuma*) from the lungs to the left side of the heart and thence through the aorta and other arteries to the whole body. The arteries stemmed from the heart; the veins, by contrast, Praxagoras believed, arose from the liver, their function being to carry the blood, created from digested food, to the rest of the body. The combining of blood and pneuma generated innate heat.

Herophilus practised medicine in Alexandria under the first two Ptolemies, apparently dissecting human cadavers in public. He wrote at least eleven treatises. Three were on anatomy: it was he who discovered and named the prostate and the duodenum (from the Greek for twelve fingers, the length of gut he found). He also wrote on the pulse as a diagnostic guide, on therapeutics, ophthalmology, dietetics and midwifery, and a polemic 'Against Common Notions'.

Continuing Praxagoras' differentiation between veins and arteries, Herophilus pointed out that the coats of the arteries were much thicker than those of the veins. Unlike Praxagoras, however, he held that the arteries were filled not with air but with blood. His most striking dissection feat was the delineation of the nerves. Demonstrating their source in the brain enabled him to conclude that they played the part preceding thinkers had ascribed to the arteries: transmitting motor impulses from the soul (intelligence centre) to the extremities. Rebutting Aristotle, he thus established the importance of the brain, distinguishing the cerebrum from the cerebellum and displaying the nerve paths from the brain and spinal cord. His description of the *rete mirabile*, the network of arteries at the base of the brain, shows he dissected animals as well as human corpses, since it does not exist in humans.

Herophilus also devoted attention to the liver and to 'veins' ending in glandular bodies which, he believed, nourished the intestines but did not pass to the liver. These 'veins' must have been the lacteals or chyle-vessels, whose function was explained by Aselli some two thousand years later. Praxagoras' interest in the pulse was taken up by Herophilus. Identifying pulsation as derived from the heart, he developed a speculative classification of different classes of pulse, on the basis of magnitude, strength, rate and rhythm, and is reputed to have tried to calculate pulse by means of a portable water clock.

Erasistratus is far more nebulous and controversial. He supposedly studied medicine in Athens before settling in Alexandria, where he experimented on living animals and perhaps humans. His main discoveries concerned the brain which, like Herophilus but unlike Aristotle, he regarded as the seat of intelligence. He too distinguished the cerebrum from the cerebellum, described the cerebral ventricles within the brain, and distinguished between motor and sensory nerves. Nerves were hollow tubes containing pneuma ('spirit' or air), which transmitted sensation, enabling muscles to produce motion.

In a tradition going back to Alcmaeon, he also believed that pneuma alone – not blood – was contained in the arteries: it was taken in through the lungs, piped to the heart (which he compared to a blacksmith's bellows) and then pumped out to fill the arteries. Blood by contrast was formed in the liver and carried by the veins. Why then was it blood that spurted from a cut artery? It was drawn in, Erasistratus reasoned, because nature abhorred a vacuum.

Erasistratus has been portrayed as an early mechanist, because of his model of bodily processes: digestion for instance involved the stomach grinding food. Yet this may be a caricature created by Galen for polemical purposes. Even Galen applauded his remarkable investigations of brain anatomy, while being scathing about his other views, particularly the idea that the arteries contained air alone. Erasistratus was clearly a radical; for want of evidence, he is also a riddle.

In the following centuries medicine, like philosophy, split into sects: Hippocratics, Herophileans and Erasistrateans were later challenged by the Pneumatists, who regarded *pneuma* as a fifth element which flowed through the arteries, sustaining vitality. All such sects were later given the label of 'rationalist', to signal their antagonism to the Empirics, a band of physicians led by Heraclides of Tarentum (*fl.* 80 BC), who spurned medicine based on speculation about hidden disease causes in favour of one grounded on experience. What mattered, Empirics claimed, was not cause but cure, and so they collected case histories and remedies. Knowledge, they held, could be better gained at the bedside than by dissection; what counted was which drugs worked. Hence theory must bow to experience – a claim later opponents, principally Galen, rejected as shallow.

MEDICINE IN THE ROMAN ERA

Greek medicine spread throughout the Mediterranean, not least to Italy, where the southern cities shared Greek culture – doctors at Elea, Tarentum and Metapontum were like their colleagues in Athens or Alexandria. Rome was different. No-nonsense Roman tradition held that one was better off without doctors. Romans had no need of professional physicians, insisted authors like Cato (234–149 BC), for they were hale and hearty, unlike the effete Greeks. 'Beware of doctors', he cried; they would bring death by medicine. 'It is our duty, my young friends', reflected Cicero (106–43 BC), 'to resist old age; to compensate for its defects by a watchful care; to fight against it as we would fight against disease; to adopt a regimen of health; to practise moderate exercise; and to take just enough food and drink to restore our strength and not to overburden it.'

Romans enjoyed bad-mouthing Greek physicians: according to Pliny (AD c. 23–79), who deplored the recent influx of 'luxury' and worthless Greek physicians, an inscription, echoing Alexander, was now sprouting up on monuments in Rome: 'It was the crowd of physicians that killed me.'*

Romans liked to think healing should take place in the family, under the care of the paterfamilias, who would dispense herbs and charms. Cato, who dosed his family on cabbage soup, derided Greek physicians as the antithesis of Roman virtue: they were frauds who cheated patients and 'have sworn to kill all barbarians with their drugs'. Prejudices such as these may explain the tardy emergence of native Italian physicians.

The contrast drawn by Cato and Pliny between homespun healing and hellenistic speculation was xenophobic prejudice. The real difference was not between Greece and Rome, but between rustic medicine and that of the big city. Greek medicine arrived with city life as Rome was hellenized. For long professional doctors (*medici*) in Italy were immigrants; the first noted Roman practitioner, Asclepiades (c. 120–30 BC),

---

* Pliny compiled a *Natural History*, completed AD 77, a compendium of all natural learning. Books 12–19 deal with botany and 20–27 with *materia medica* from botanical sources, followed by five books (28–32) on animal *materia medica*. His remedies proved of great influence, being quarried by Isidore of Seville and subsequent medieval encyclopaedists.

was a native of Bithynia in Asia Minor. Modified by his pupil, Themison of Tralles (*fl.* 70 BC), his doctrines gave rise to the Methodist sect. Its physiology was based not upon the Hippocratic four humours but upon corpuscular theory. In the body the proper arrangement of atoms and their intermediate pores produced health; any obstruction or undue looseness led to disease, so health was the balance between tension and relaxation. This atomist physiology enabled the doctor to reduce diagnosis to the 'common conditions' – the constricted, the lax and the mixed – deducible from visible symptoms. Hence the Asclepiadean or Methodist doctor did not need intimate familiarity with the life history of his patients: plain symptoms were sufficient. Cure was by opposites, enlarging narrow pores and reducing large ones, for which Asclepiades promoted massage, exercise and cold-water bathing. His slogan *cito, tute et jucunde* – swiftly, safely, sweetly – is reflected in his rejection of heroic bleeding, his preference for gentle medicines, his prescription of wine and his stress on convalescence. Self-styled Asclepiadeans flourished for three centuries, though their rejection of philosophical reasoning riled Galen, who sneered at their pre-packed therapies.

More light on the infiltration of Greek medicine into Rome is offered by the physician Scribonius Largus (*c.* AD 1–50). Born in Sicily, he probably learned his craft from hellenistic practitioners on the island, and in AD 43 he accompanied the Emperor Claudius on his campaign to subdue Britain. His sole surviving medical text is a Latin handbook of drug recipes, the *Compositiones*. It contains 271 recipes for conditions from headache to gout, all claimed of proven value. In his preface, Scribonius set out his views on medical ethics, becoming our earliest witness to the use of the Hippocratic oath. How widespread was his endorsement of a professional ethic is unclear, for no other ancient writer made such an open commitment.

The early empire brought the first surviving survey of medicine in Latin. An encyclopaedic compilation, Celsus' *Artes* [The Sciences] originally contained at least twenty-one books, of which only the eight devoted to medicine survive in full. No professional physician but a wealthy estate owner who presumably treated his family and friends, Celsus (*fl.* AD *c.* 30) was acquainted with both theory and treatments, writing in an elegant Latin which won him the title of the Cicero of the physicians.

The eight books are introduced by a long preface tracing the story of medicine from the time of the Trojan war, and lamenting the rise of clashing sects: Dogmatists, who stressed the need to seek out unseen causes; Empirics, whose emphasis was on experience; and Methodists, wedded to 'common conditions'. Medicine, in Celsus' view, required not just experience but reason.

Celsus' first book is on the preservation of health and on diet; Book 2 deals with signs the doctor should watch for, and remedies; Book 3 concerns diseases of the whole body – fevers, jaundice and so on; Book 4 lists the diseases of individual body parts in the top-to-toe order which was to become customary; and the lengthy Book 5 falls into two parts, a description of various drugs, and treatments for bites and ulcers. Book 6 handles treatments of diseases of the parts of the body, again from top to bottom. Subsequent books deal with surgery, opening with a brief history of the art, and moving on to a list of surgical conditions occurring anywhere in the body, before examining surgical techniques for individual parts, again from head to heel. The final book deals with fractures, ruptures and luxations, including such ambitious operations as removal of bone splinters from the skull. After surgery the physician must be alert to the four cardinal signs of inflammation – *calor, rubor, dolor* and *tumor* (heat, redness, pain and swelling). As the first major medical author writing in Latin and offering a summary of the whole of medicine in a single work, Celsus exercised a powerful influence.

The medical colossus of the Roman era is Galen (AD 129–c. 216), but he had significant contemporaries who stand in his shadow, in part because he belittled them, in part because their works, unlike his, survive only in fragments. One was Aretaeus of Cappadocia (*fl.* AD 140) who proclaimed his loyalties by writing in Greek and frequently alluding to Hippocrates. His work, known in Latin as *De causis et signis acutorum et diuturnorum morborum* [Acute and Chronic Diseases] provides the best disease descriptions of any surviving ancient author. A 'rationalist', he inclined to the pneumatic school, believing that in the universe and in man alike, pneuma (spirit) bound everything together, and any change in it led to illness.

Aretaeus made disease the hub of his inquiries, recording nothing about his patients – or himself for that matter. He gave fine descriptions, among other things, of dropsy and diabetes, mental disorders and epilepsy. Diabetes represented 'a liquefaction of the flesh and bones into urine', so much so that 'the kidneys and bladder do not cease emitting urine'. His description of tetanus gives evidence of his clinical experience:

Tetanus consists of extremely painful spasms, which are a peril to life and very difficult to relieve. The attack begins in the jaw muscles and tendons, but spreads to the whole body, because all bodily parts suffer in sympathy with the one first affected.

There are three types of spasms. Either the body is stretched, or it is bent either backward or forward. With stretching the disease is called *tetanus*: the subject is so rigid that he cannot turn or bend. The spasms are named according to the tension and the position of the forward and backward arching. When the posterior nerves are affected and the patient arches backward, we call the condition *opisthotonus*; when the anterior nerves are affected and the arching is forward, the condition is called *emprosthotonus*.

Another doctor then active was Soranus, practising in Ephesus AD *c.* 100. His *Gynaecology*, the largest early treatment of that subject, should be understood in the context of traditional Hippocratic thinking on the diseases of women, which presumably reflected prevailing male prejudices. Children born at seven months were said, implausibly, to have a greater chance of surviving than those born at eight; the 'wandering womb' was blamed for hysteria-like illnesses; and the female constitution was an imperfect version of the male. Soranus, however, was sceptical of many of these traditions, and dismissive of the 'wandering womb'. His *Gynaecology*, which enjoyed wide circulation, is divided into four sections. The first, dealing with conception and pregnancy, also discusses virginity and the right age for intercourse (not before menarche, at about fourteen). Advice was given on contraception, though Soranus disapproved of abortion by mechanical means. The next section treats labour, recommending the sitting position and the Roman birthing-chair. In case of difficult labour, he taught 'podalic version' – easing a hand into the uterus and pulling down one of the baby's legs, so that it would be born feet-first. The third part examines women's maladies, including uterine fluxes and womb-caused diseases, and the final section is concerned with problems in the birth itself: how to remove the placenta after birth and tie the umbilical cord.

Another physician associated with Ephesus was Rufus (AD 70–120), who learnt anatomy in Alexandria and spent some time in Rome. He wrote commentaries on several Hippocratic writings, accepting the doctrine of the four humours and of cure by opposites. His writings were praised by Galen. Galen's sun, however, outshone his ideas, as it did everyone else's.

GALEN

Galen's dominion over medicine for more than a millennium was partly the consequence of his prolific pen. More of his opus survives than of any other ancient writer: some 350 authentic titles ranging from the soul to bloodletting polemics – about as much as all other Greek medical writings together. He had vast erudition and a matching ego.

Born in AD 129 in Pergamon (now Bergama, Turkey), one of the fairest cities in the Greek-speaking empire, Galen was the son of a wealthy architect, Nicon, and a shrewish woman ('My mother . . . used to bite her serving maids, and was perpetually shouting at my father'). He enjoyed a long, lavish, liberal education; when he was sixteen, his father was visited in a dream by Asclepius, after which the son was piously steered towards medicine. He studied with Alexandrian teachers and travelled in Egypt, learning about drugs from India and Africa. Returning home in 157, he was appointed physician to the gladiators, a job which enlarged his anatomical and surgical expertise, since wounds afforded windows onto the body. But Pergamon was provincial, and in 162 he left for Rome, where public debates against Methodists and high-profile public anatomical displays spread his fame. One of his party tricks, revealing his genius for self-advertisement as well as experiment, was to sever the nerves in the neck of a pig. As these were severed, one by one, the pig continued to squeal; but when Galen cut one of the laryngeal nerves the squealing stopped, impressing the crowd. Leading senators and dignitaries began to employ him, and from AD 169 Galen was in imperial service, first with the emperor's son, Commodus, and later a succession of emperors. He liked reminding readers that his patients were of the highest rank. 'Something really amazing happened when the emperor [Marcus Aurelius] himself was my patient', he wrote:

> Just when the lamps were lit, a messenger came and brought me to the Emperor as he had bidden. Three doctors had watched over him since dawn, and two of them felt his pulse, and all three thought that a fever attack was coming. I stood alongside, but said nothing. The Emperor looked first at me and asked why I did not feel his pulse as the other two had. I answered: 'These two colleagues of mine have already done so and, as they have followed

you on the journey, they presumably know what your normal pulse is, so they can judge its present state better.'

When I said this, he bade me, too, to feel his pulse. My impression was that – considering his age and body constitution – the pulse was far from indicating a fever attack, but that his stomach was stuffed with the food he had eaten, and that the food had become a slimy excrement. The Emperor praised my diagnosis and said, three times in a row: 'That is it. It is just as you say. I have eaten too much cold food.'

He then asked what measures should be taken. I replied what I knew of a similar case, saying: 'If you were any plain citizen of this country, I would as usual prescribe wine with a little pepper. But to a royal patient as in this case, doctors usually recommend milder treatment. It is enough for a woollen cover to be put on your stomach, impregnated with warm spiced salve.'

Expert in one-upmanship, Galen couched an inflated sense of his importance in terms of the dignity of medicine, scolding colleagues as dimwits. He was invariably right; there is no denying that he was an erudite man and an accomplished philosopher, particularly in constructing an image of the organism as a teleological unity open to reasoning. For him, anatomy proved the truth of Plato's tripartite soul, with its seats in the brain, heart and liver; and Aristotelian physics with its elements and qualities explained the body system.

Philosophy should promote medicine, Galen taught, though the physician must master philosophy – logic (the discipline of thinking), physics (the science of nature), and ethics (the science of action). Philosophy and medicine were thus counterparts: the best doctor was also a philosopher, while the unphilosophical healer (the Empiric) was like an architect without a plan. A good physician would practise for the love of mankind, while accepting his due rewards in fame and fortune.

The patient's trust was essential in the healing process. It could be won by a punctilious bedside manner, by meticulous explanation, and by mastery of prognosis, an art demanding experience, observation and logic. Galen brought psychosomatic conditions to light, including uneasiness amongst defendants in court cases or those whose pulses raced through guilty passions.

Galen prided himself on being more than a fine clinician; he was a medical scientist. He performed dissections, mainly of apes, sheep, pigs and goats and even of an elephant's heart, but not of humans. He knew much skeletal anatomy, but, dissection being out of the question, little internal human anatomy. Two mistakes were particularly critical for the future. Dissections of calves revealed a network of nerves and vessels, the *rete mirabile* at the base of the brain, earlier found by Herophilus, which he assumed also existed in humans. This, he said, was the site where the vital spirits in the arteries turned into animal spirits. He also misleadingly described the liver (which he believed to be the source of the veins) as grasping the stomach with its lobes as if by fingers, an image derived from dissection of pigs or apes. Forced to apply animal findings to humans, his human womb also had cotyledons like a dog's. Such mistakes aside, his explanations of anatomical phenomena in terms of the teleology of a divinely ordered universe were internally coherent and provided a rational basis for further investigation.

Gross anatomy and experiments offered paths to understanding, but Galen did not restrict himself to sensory perceptions. By combining his observations with Platonic speculations about the macrocosm at large, he formulated models of concealed bodily structures. Each part functioned only when its basic elements were properly adapted, and any change would result in functional failure or disease. The unknown was thereby explained in terms of a structural/functional physiology. His systematizing zeal was both a boon and a bane.

Galen presented his work as 'perfecting' Hippocrates' legacy, and this gives his *oeuvre* a remarkable unity, fusing the clinical and the theoretical. Take his writings on fever: fever might result from either an excess of yellow bile, black bile or phlegm (a condition he called *cacochymia*), or from an excess of blood (*plethora*). Surplus humours might accumulate in some bodily part where they would cause putrefaction and excessive heat or fever. To remove such superfluities and restore humoral balance, he advocated energetic blood-letting. The physician should let blood from a patient not only when he was ill but prophylactically, whenever a fever was on the cards. Indications were given of when and how much blood to draw, depending on the patient's age and constitution, the season of the year, the weather and the place. Instead of the earlier Hippocratic treatment of fevers by starvation, Galen urged venesection (letting blood from the veins) to cool the body.

He justified blood-letting in terms of his elaborate pulse lore. Written in the early 170s, his sixteen books on the pulse were divided into four treatises, each four books long. The first, *On the Differences between Pulses*, displayed his learning, logic and linguistic skills. In the next four books *On the Diagnosis of Pulses*, he explained how to take the pulse and interpret it, raising key questions. How was it possible to tell whether a pulse was 'full', 'rapid' or 'rhythmical'? Such questions he resolved partly from experience and partly by reference to earlier authorities.

On the Causes of Pulsation addressed anatomy. Although Galen was convinced, *pace* Erasistratus, that arteries contained blood from the heart, his idea of pulsation was quite different from ours. The heart and the artery contracted simultaneously and arterial expansion and contraction were separate, active movements. In contraction, super-fluities were expelled; in expansion, atmospheric air was taken in to cool things down and, by mixing with blood in the heart, to generate vital spirits (pneuma). It was this vital spirit which was mainly responsible for creating the pulsative power within the coats of the artery.

Blood, Galen taught, was made in the liver, incorporating ingested foods in the form of chyle; it then moved to the extremities carrying natural spirits which supported the vegetative functions of growth and nutrition. This dark venous blood, passing from the liver to the right ventricle of the heart, divided into two streams. One passed to the lungs via the pulmonary artery; the other crossed the heart through 'interseptal pores' into the left ventricle, where it mixed with *pneuma* (air), became heated, moved thence from the left ventricle to the aorta, and finally to the periphery. His belief that the veins originated in the blood-making liver, carrying nutrition to the parts whenever needed, while the arteries originated in the heart, was one of the errors in his model of the circulatory system which, after dominating medicine for well over a millennium, was challenged by Renaissance anatomy.

From a clinical standpoint, Galen was principally concerned to teach the doctor to read the various pulse phenomena. This he provided in the final part, *On Prognosis from the Pulse*, where he adopted a double strategy. The first two books described the complaints a specific pulse type might betray: for example, the 'double-hammer pulse' was a fre-quent sign of heart weakness. The last books detailed the sort of pulse found in specific disorders: for example, in hectic fevers the pulse increased in frequency and rapidity.

Whatever the disorder – even blood loss – Galen judged bleeding proper. All depended on knowing where and when to do it, and how much blood to take. For severe conditions he recommended phlebotomy twice a day; the first should be stopped before the patient fainted, but the second time the physician could bleed as far as unconsciousness.

Convinced that nature prevented disease by discharging excess blood, he pointed out that menstruation spared women many diseases – gout, epilepsy, apoplexy – to which males were prone. The quantities of blood he removed were large, and would often, to our thinking, have been harmful. His teachings on plethora and venesection remained influential until the nineteenth century.

Galen took clinical Hippocratic medicine and set it within a wider anatomo-physiological framework. In broad terms this built on the Platonic doctrine of a threefold division of the soul, which distinguished vital functions into processes governed by vegetative, animal, and rational 'souls' or 'spirits'. Animal life was possible only because of the existence of pneuma. Within the human body, *pneuma* (air), the life breath of the cosmos, was modified by the three principal organs, the liver, heart and brain, and distributed by three types of vessels: veins, arteries and nerves. Pneuma, modified by the liver, became the nutritive soul or natural spirits which supported the vegetative functions of growth and nutrition; this nutritive soul was distributed by the veins. The heart and arteries were responsible for the maintenance and distribution of innate heat and pneuma or vital spirits to vivify the parts of the body. The third alteration, occurring in the brain, ennobled vital spirits into animal spirits, distributed through the nerves (which Galen thought of as empty ducts) to sustain sensation and movement.

For Galen, anatomy, logic and experience fitted together. Not least because he had an explanation for everything, Galenic medicine proved monumental, as he intended it should:

> I have done as much for medicine as Trajan did for the Roman Empire when he built bridges and roads through Italy. It is I, and I alone, who have revealed the true path of medicine. It must be admitted that Hippocrates already staked out this path . . . he prepared the way, but I have made it passable.

MEDICINE IN THE AGE OF GALEN

Personal in Greece, medicine remained personal in Rome. No medical degrees were conferred or qualifications required. In the absence of colleges and universities, the private, face-to-face nature of medical instruction encouraged fluidity and diversity; students attached themselves to an individual teacher, sitting at his feet and accompanying him on his rounds. Medical authors frequently engaged in pugnacious polemics, contributing to the proliferation of rival schools.

Many different sorts of medical care were available. Self-help was universal; Celsus' *On Medicine* was written for a non-professional readership willing to wield the scalpel as well as the plough and sword. Some healers in Italy were slaves or ex-slaves; others, especially in Asia Minor, hailed from medical dynasties or, like Galen, from prosperous backgrounds. In large cities there were swarms of healers, reputable and dubious, including body-builders, schoolteachers, 'wise women', root-gatherers and hucksters. Women were not confined to treating female troubles, and both Soranus and Galen expressed respect for good midwives and nurses; one of Herophilus' pupils, according to legend, was the Athenian Agnodice, who, distressed by the anguish of women who would rather die than be examined by a man, cross-dressed so as to study and practise medicine. She became a heroine among those rallying support for female medical education in the nineteenth century.

The affluent sick could receive treatment in a doctor's house, while the poor might hobble to a shrine. In big households there were slave physicians caring for their sick fellows in *valetudinaria* (hospitals). And in the Roman army, buildings were set aside for treating the sick and wounded. A standard military hospital plan evolved, with individual cells off a long corridor, a large top-lit hall, latrines and baths. A good example has been excavated at Inchtuthil in Scotland. In Rome itself, civil engineering and public works helped to maintain health. Fourteen great aqueducts (some still in use today) brought millions of gallons of fresh water to the capital; public lavatories were installed; dwellings were provided with plumbed sanitation; and civic officials oversaw the water and sewage systems and the public granaries. Vitruvius' *On Architecture* (c. 27 BC) set out sanitary ideals for towns, stressing the need for good water supplies.

With the exception of the great plague of Athens in 430 BC, the diseases of the Greek world seem to have been local. This pattern changed with the Roman empire, however, once smallpox, brought back from Mesopotamia by the legions, ravaged the entire Mediterranean. This Antonine plague was the most lethal disease invasion in antiquity.

Disease explanations changed little. Public authorities still ascribed famines and pestilences to the gods, and during the Antonine plague processions were staged, with sacrifices to city-protecting deities. Latter-day Hippocratics continued to emphasize individual susceptibility and bad air (*miasma*), and stressed dietetics. Galen reiterated a personal, constitutional medicine and said nothing on contagion. Astrology had its devotees, though Galen rejected divination while making use of dream prognostication. What truth there was in astrology and bird divination was explained naturalistically: the flight of birds indicated changes in the weather. He similarly rationalized the use of amulets.

Therapeutics, too, changed little, and the old predilections for diet over drugs and drugs over surgery continued. The range of drugs reaching great cities increased, leading to more complex compounds. For example, theriac, originally prescribed as a snakebite antidote and used as a general tonic, grew extremely elaborate. In the version associated with Mithridates VI, King of Pontus (132–63 BC), it had forty-one ingredients, but Galen's recipe had swollen to seventy-one ingredients, including vipers' flesh, ground-up lizard and other animal ingredients. Princes had an interest in such remedies, since they lived in fear of poisoning. Mithridates swallowed antidotes to make himself immune to all known poisons; when his son staged a coup, he sensibly had his father stabbed.

Antiquity produced two writers who put the study of *materia medica* on a systematic basis. Theophrastus (*c.* 371–*c.* 287 BC), a pupil of Aristotle, took over as head of the Peripatetic school of Athens. His two treatises on plants deal respectively with their description (the *De historia plantarum* [Investigations into Plants]) and their aetiology (the *Causis plantarum* [Explanations of Plants]). Using as his model Aristotle's writings on the animal kingdom, he laid the groundwork for botany.

The *Investigations* classifies plants into trees, shrubs and herbs. Some 550 species and varieties are described, with habitats ranging from the Atlantic to India (his Indian material being gathered by members of Alexander's expedition in the 320s BC). The second treatise on botany in seven books is intended to account for the common characteristics of plants. His rediscovery in the Renaissance led to the revival of medical botany and botanical gardens.

The other notable writer was Dioscorides (*c.* AD 40–*c.* 90), a Greek surgeon to Nero's army. His *De materia medica* (written in Greek, but known by its Latin title) is in five books. Book I deals with aromatics like saffron, oils, salves, shrubs and trees; Book II with animals, cereals, and herbs; Book III with roots, juices, herbs and seeds; Book IV with other roots and herbs; and Book V with wines and minerals, including salts of lead and copper. Providing detailed descriptions based largely on external appearance, Dioscorides aimed to enable the doctor to choose the right plant, listed by its pharmacological properties. He noted the various plant names, their uses in treatments, techniques of harvesting, modes of storage and possible adulterants. From an early date, these verbal descriptions were supplemented by drawings. Many of his remedies were common herbs and spices: cinnamon and cassia for instance were said to be valuable for internal inflammations, snake bites, runny nose and menstrual disorders; others were bizarre, like bed bugs mashed with meat and beans for malarial fevers. Some herbs had many properties. The bramble ('batos', *Rubus fruticosus*), according to an early translation,

> binds and drys; it dyes ye hair. But the decoction of the tops of it being drank stops ye belly, & restrains ye flux of women, & is convenient for ye biting of ye Prester. And the leaves being chewed do strengthen ye gums, and heal ye Apthae. And ye leaves being applied, do restrain ye Herpetas, & heal ye running ulcers which are in ye head, & ye falling down of the eyes.

Galen described 473 drugs of vegetable, animal and mineral origin as well as a large number of compound drugs. Together with theriac, he recommended two remedies that became universally celebrated, *hiera picra* and *terra sigillata*. His *hiera picra* formula called for aloes, spices and herbs; the compound was made into an electuary. Its 'signal Virtues' according to William Salmon, a seventeenth-century commentator, were that it was 'a good thing to loosen the body . . . It heats . . . drys . . . opens obstruction, and urges thick Phlegmatick humours.' *Terra sigillata* (sealed earth) was a greasy clay, containing silica, alumina, chalk, magnesia and oxide of iron, found on the Greek islands of Lemnos, Melos, and Samos. It was formed into large tablet-like units upon which the seal of the place of origin was impressed. It was meant to be drying and binding, and useful against poisons.

INSANITY

Throughout antiquity, one disorder provoked divergent responses, paving the way for lasting controversy. Madness was, of course, well known within the general culture. Herodotus described the mad destructive King Cambyses of Persia mocking religion – who but a madman would dishonour the gods? The deranged Ajax slaughtered sheep in the belief that they were enemy soldiers, a scene presaging Don Quixote's tilting at windmills. Violence, grief, blood-lust and cannibalism were commonly taken as signs of insanity.

Graeco-Roman law sought to prevent the mad from destroying life, limb and property, and made provision for guardians for the insane. Insanity was a family responsibility and there were no lunatic asylums. The seriously disturbed were restrained at home, while others were allowed to wander, though, as evil spirits (*keres*) might fly out of them to possess other people, the crazed were feared and shunned.

Madness found medical explanations. In the Hippocratic tradition the most common labels for such conditions were mania and melancholia, the former characterized by excitement, the latter by depression. Both were marked by delusions, and, like all other maladies, were understood humorally, usually in terms of choler and black bile. In *On the Sacred Disease*, which claimed madness as well as epilepsy for medicine, the Hippocratic author stated that 'those maddened through bile are noisy, evil-doers and restless, always doing something inopportune . . . But if terrors and fears attack, they are due to a change in the brain.'

Hippocratic medicine thus did not envisage an independent discipline of psychiatry, but it did accept certain psychological elements. In one case, a woman with symptoms of depression and incoherent speech was explained as suffering from 'grief', while another, 'after a grief', would 'fumble, pluck, scratch, pick hairs, weep and then laugh, but . . . not speak'. Melancholy madness caused by black bile was occasionally seen as the spark of genius, originating the notion of melancholy as a disease of superior wits which achieved its most erudite treatment in Robert Burton's *Anatomy of Melancholy* (1621). Plato could similarly represent madness as a transcendental divine fire with the power to inspire, a view influential in the Renaissance and the Romantic movement.

Galen held that mania was a disease of yellow bile or the vital spirits in the heart. A cooling regimen was indicated, for mania was a 'hot' disease. Soranus devoted chapters to mania and melancholia, describing symptoms in detail and discussing aetiology. Among the causes of mania were 'continual sleeplessness, excesses of venery, anger, grief, anxiety, or superstitious fear, a shock or blow, intense straining of the senses and the mind in study, business, or other ambitious pursuits'. Something which could later be interpreted as hysteria – a disorder marked by palpitations, migratory pain, breathing difficulties and the *globus hystericus* – might be attributed to a wandering uterus. By way of cure for many female psychological disorders, doctors recommended marriage.

The consolidation of Greek and Roman medicine over the course of some seven hundred years laid solid foundations for learned medicine, including the naturalistic notion of disease as part of cosmic order, and the idea of the human body as regulated by a constitution, intelligible to experience and reason. It created the ideal of the union of science, philosophy and practical medicine in the learned physician, who would be the personal attendant of the patient rather than a medicine-man interceding with the gods or a functionary working for the state.

For the next thousand years and more, medical knowledge would change little. This was partly the consequence of the break-up of the Mediterranean civilizations, but also because of the solidity of these foundations. Galen's enduring reputation was the epitome of these beliefs: he unified theory and practice, discourse and the doctor, but his death brought that tradition to a halt.

CHAPTER IV

MEDICINE AND FAITH

THE PASSAGE FROM THE GLORIOUS DAYS of Rome to the Middle Ages was often violent, especially in the West, with wave after wave of barbarian onslaughts from the East. These culminated in the sack of the Eternal City by Alaric's Goths in AD 410, which effectively put an end to the western empire and frayed the thread of learned medicine.

Fortified from AD 324 by its new capital, Constantinople (later Byzantium, modern Istanbul) on the Bosphorus, the eastern empire remained a bastion of imperial strength and a treasury of hellenistic learning and culture. From 364, the empire formally split, the two halves being ruled by separate emperors, and by the close of the sixth century the West had splintered further into fragmented kingdoms ruled by descendants of the invading Goths and Vandals. Its economy was feebler than that of the East, its cities declined or collapsed altogether – Londinium (London), once boasting a population of 30,000, became a ghost town – and civic institutions dwindled. In such circumstances, it was inevitable that eastern and western medicine would go separate ways.

CHRISTIANITY

Throughout the Mediterranean the mental climate began to shift from 313 with the Emperor Constantine's establishment of Christianity as one of the official imperial faiths; from the early fifth century it was the sole official religion. Thereafter, by contrast with the naturalistic bent of Hippocratic and Galenic medicine, healing became more spiced with religion, for the rising Church taught there was a supernatural plan and purpose to everything (every human had a soul to be saved) and Christian doctrines, rituals and sacraments covered every stage through which believers passed from womb to tomb, and beyond.

Religion, of course, shared common ground with medicine. Etymologically, the words 'holiness' and 'healing' stem from a single root, conveying the idea of wholeness. But early Christianity also made demarcations between the body and the soul, implying the subordination of medicine to religion, and of doctor to priest, the one attending merely to the cure of bodies, the other to the cure of souls. The boundaries between temporal and eternal were of course endlessly blurred, and physic and faith, while generally complementary and enjoying a fairly peaceful coexistence, sometimes tangled in border disputes.

Christian outlooks on the body and sickness drew on various traditions. The faith absorbed aspects of eastern asceticism, which prized the soul or spirit above the flesh, and Jewish healing traditions were also influential. Early Judea had its distinctive healers, not least King Solomon (r. 970–931 BC), who was credited not only with wisdom but with magical and medical powers. Hebrew ideas on healing expressed in the Old Testament (compiled between the eighth and the third centuries BC), and the Talmud (between 70 BC and the second century AD), shared with Egypt and Mesopotamia a religious orientation: disease signified the wrath of God. 'It shall come to pass', it was recorded in Deuteronomy,

> if thou wilt not hearken unto the voice of the LORD thy God ... the LORD shall make the pestilence cleave unto thee, until he have consumed thee from off the land; whither thou goest to possess it.
>
> The LORD shall smite thee with a consumption, and with a fever, and with an inflammation, and with an extreme burning, and with the sword, and with blasting, and with mildew; and they shall pursue thee until thou perish.

Certain maladies were associated with the Almighty's punishments for sin, including *Zara'ath*, which has usually been translated as leprosy, though this identification is medically dubious. 'When a man shall have in the skin of his flesh a rising [a swelling], a scab, or bright spot, and it be in the skin of his flesh like the plague [the spots] of leprosy,' states the Book of Leviticus, then he shall be brought unto Aaron the priest, or unto one of his sons the priests; and the priest shall look on the plague in the skin of the flesh: and when the hair in the plague is turned white, and the plague in sight be deeper than the skin of his flesh it is a plague of leprosy: and the priest shall look on him, and pronounce him unclean.

Such polluting diseases were curable by the Lord alone, and this encouraged certain Jews to reject human medicine in favour of divine, citing the fate of King Asa (c. 914–874 BC), who 'sought not the Lord, but his physicians', and whose foot sores consequently worsened and he died. Jewish sacred writings have no place for the professional physician as such, nor even for priestly healers; Jahweh alone is the healer. Naaman the leper was instructed by the prophet Elisha to wash himself seven times in the River Jordan, so as to be cleansed; the only surgical operation mentioned in the Old Testament is the religious rite of circumcision.

Suffering could be a godsend and a trial. 'Blessed is the man whom God correcteth,' declared Job, singled out by the Lord to undergo great suffering, 'therefore despise not thou the chastening of the Almighty: For he makes sore, and bindeth up: he woundeth, and his hands make whole.' For devout Jews, the pagan assumption that a healthy body was a great blessing could seem trifling.

Nevertheless, the Hebrews did develop teachings about the body and its well-being. Blood was probably viewed as the vehicle for the soul (one rationale for kosher meat, from which the blood is drained, and also for the refusal of blood transfusions by Jehovah's Witnesses), but life lay in the breath. Believing physical cleanliness bespoke spiritual purity, rules were formulated for personal hygiene, social gatherings and sexual intercourse, and prohibitions were issued against eating unclean animals. Though some modern Jewish apologists argue that the dietary bans on pork and shellfish in Leviticus arose from awareness that these foods could pass on diseases such as trichinosis, the fact is that Jewish dietary rituals (kosher food) were principally expressions of precepts about pollution and purification. Nevertheless, cleanliness rites indirectly spurred public health: no well was to be dug near burial or waste ground, water should be boiled before drinking, and waste had to be burned or buried beyond encampments. Judaism also taught the obligation of caring for co-religionists, and by AD 400 Jewish communities were instructed to possess a healer.

Christians often expressed disdain for Jews as the people of the law, exalting by contrast their faith of the spirit; and this difference is discernible in their distinctive approaches to health. But one must not oversimplify: the New Testament presents many models of healing, secular and sacred alike. 'Costly physicians' were condemned, but Luke the Evangelist was himself a physician. In the parable of the good Samaritan, the use of wine as a disinfectant reflects Greek wound treatment, whereas in the Acts of the Apostles healing is portrayed as a matter of faith, involving prayer and the laying-on of hands. When Jesus met a man born blind, he asked who had sinned; and he told the man who suffered from a palsy that his sins were forgiven. Sin was thus assumed to be perhaps a cause of sickness, or at least sin and sickness were similar states; in either case spiritual healing might be requisite. 'Is any sick among you?', asked the Apostle James. 'Let him call for the elders of the church, and let them pray over him, anointing him with oil in the name of the Lord; and the prayer of faith shall save the sick, and the Lord shall raise him up.'

Early Christianity exhibits a medley of attitudes towards healing, shaping fluid relations between medicine and the Church. Many old healing practices were dressed up in new Christian garbs; Christian shrines were raised upon the ruins of pagan temples, and the leading healing saints, Cosmas and Damian, were in some respects revampings of the heathen Castor and Pollux.

Christian theology embraced but modified the radical dualism of some Levantine religious and philosophical sects which elevated the immaterial soul while disparaging the mortal body, commonly viewed as the soul's prison house. Christianity taught that the spirit was eternal; the flesh was weak, corruptible and fallen. Adam and Eve's disobedience in Eden had brought disease and death into the world and made nakedness a source of shame. The Desert Fathers and saintly hermits pursued ascetic practices designed to deaden desire and restore the spiritual powers enjoyed by Adam in Eden.

Such beliefs challenged the classical, Athenian man-centred and *polis*-oriented ideals of balance and beauty, looking to mortification of the flesh as the release of the spirit. A glorification of suffering associated with release from the throbbing flesh remained a powerful force within Christianity, especially Catholicism. Thérèse Martin, later canonized as Saint Thérèse of Lisieux, died of tuberculosis in 1897, barely out of her teens. 'God has deigned to make me pass through many types of trials,' she affirmed in her diary, 'I am truly happy to suffer.'

Yet Christianity also taught that man had been created in God's image in a paradise garden of physical bliss in which disease and death had no part; and it proclaimed the raising up of the bodies of the faithful at the Last Judgment, as prefigured by Christ's own resurrection. Orthodoxy anathematized the manichean heresy that viewed the flesh as the Devil's domain. The human body belonged not to man or Satan but to God, and had to be properly looked after – hence the suicide taboo.

While suffering and disease could appear as chastisement of the wicked or a trial of those the Lord loved, the Church also developed a healing mission. Was not Luke 'the beloved physician'? And did not Christ, though he told physicians to heal themselves, give proofs of his own divine powers by acts of healing? Some thirty-five such miracles are recorded in the Bible, and the apostles subsequently exercised healing as 'a gift of the spirit'. From the start, Christianity won converts among those desperate to be cured; and, like a self-fulfilling prophecy, healing miracles proliferated, often wrought by holy relics like drops of the Virgin's milk. Sober ecclesiastics condemned this vulgar zeal for healing marvels, presenting Christ as the physician of the soul. Whereas members of his congregation brought infants for baptism hoping the holy water would heal leprosy or blindness, St Augustine (354–430) viewed cures by holy oil, relics or baptism not as a routine health service but as providences. Overall, Church fathers steered a middle course, accepting a role, but a subordinate one, for secular medicine.

Christianity made its mark through action. Jewish traditions of help and hospitality were extended, and Christ's instruction to his disciples to care for the sick and needy assumed institutional form through the appointment of deacons charged with distributing alms. By 250 the Church in Rome had developed an elaborate charitable outreach, with wealthy converts providing food and shelter for the poor. After Constantine's official recognition of Christianity, alms found expression in bricks and mortar. Leontius, bishop of Antioch from 344 to 358, set up hostels in his see; around 360, Bishop Eustathius of Sebasteia built a poorhouse; and St Basil erected outside the walls of Caesarea 'almost a new city' for the sick, poor and leprous.

Similar institutions sprang up somewhat later in the Latin West. A hospital was founded in 390 by Fabiola (d. 399), an affluent Christian convert, who, after two wretched marriages, dedicated her life to charity

among Rome's sick poor. 'She assembled all the sick from the streets
and highways', wrote her teacher, St Jerome,

> and personally tended the unhappy and impoverished victims of
> hunger and disease. I have often seen her washing wounds which
> others – even men – could hardly bear to look at . . . She founded
> a hospital and gathered there the sufferers from the streets, and
> gave them all the attention of a nurse. Need I describe the many
> woes which can befall a human being: the cut-off noses, lost eyes,
> mangled feet, leprous arms, swollen bellies, withered thighs, the
> ailing flesh that is filled up by hungry worms? How often she
> carried home, on her own shoulders, the dirty and poor who were
> plagued by epilepsy! How she washed the pus from sores which
> others could not even behold!

Greek and Roman paganism had acknowledged no such duties.

In the East, hospitals (in Greek *nosokomeia*, places to care for the
sick) became large and complex. By the mid sixth century Jerusalem
had one with 200 beds, and St Sampson's in Constantinople was bigger
still, with surgical operations being performed and a wing for eye disorders. Edessa had a women's hospital, and major hospitals at Antioch
and Constantinople were divided into male and female wards. By 650,
the Pantokrator in Constantinople had a hierarchy of physicians and
even teaching facilities, a home for the elderly and, beyond the walls,
a leper house. To care for lepers and thus expose oneself to infection was
a mark of holiness. Christianity planted the hospital: the well-endowed
establishments of the Levant and the scattered houses of the West
shared a common religious ethos of charity.

THE LEGACY OF GALEN

During a long fallow time of the intellect, some authors passed on the
baton of medical learning. Oribasius (325–97), physician to Julian the
Apostate, came from a wealthy family in Pergamon in Asia Minor
(Galen's hometown) and studied medicine at Alexandria. Three of his
works became influential. The earliest comprised excerpts from the
best medical authorities. Its four books described hygiene and diet; the
properties of simple drugs and indications for use, and the body – its
maladies and treatments from top to toe. What remains of it reveals
broad reading and his respect for Galen and Rufus of Ephesus. He also

wrote a shorter practical medical compendium for the traveller, and an even briefer summary. He was worried about the state of medicine, bemoaning (in a familiar way) the proliferation of quacks and the want of practical handbooks. Oribasius played an important role as mediator and synthesizer: he preserved excerpts from many authors otherwise lost, created a pattern for later digests, and shaped the package of Galenism that dominated later centuries. Having simplified, synthesized and publicized the master's writings, his work was rehashed by others in the same mould – Aetius, Alexander of Tralles and Paul of Aegina – before being further systematized by the Arabs.

In North Africa, Caelius Aurelianus (*c.* 420) produced a large Latin nosographical handbook, *De morbis acutis et chronicis* [On Acute and Chronic Diseases]. A follower of the Methodist sect, he subscribed to the doctrine of stricture and laxity among atoms and pores: diseases were due either to excessive tension or relaxation. Fragments survive of a medical catechism, of parts of his Latin translation of Soranus' *Gynaecology*, and of the eight books on *Acute and Chronic Diseases*.

The Greek physician Alexander of Tralles (sixth century) was best known for his *Libri duodecim* [Twelve Books on Medicine], popular in Latin, Greek and Arabic. After travelling in Greece, Italy, Spain and Gaul, he settled in Rome. He was the first European to champion the eastern laxative, rhubarb, later so prized, but was also keen on more exotic remedies, for example live beetles. Henbane, he taught, was effective only if held between the left thumb and index finger while the moon was in Pisces or Aquarius; and he advised epileptics to 'take a nail of a wrecked ship, make it into a bracelet and set therein the bone of a stag's heart taken from its body whilst alive; put it on the left arm; you will be astonished at the result.' Over the next centuries, the rational medicine of antiquity went through a long process of being diluted, or rather spiced up, with more magic ingredients and more exotic recipes.

Slightly later, Paul of Aegina (*fl.* 640) studied and practised medicine in Alexandria. A Galenist, he wrote on gynaecology and poisons, but his only extant work is his medical encyclopaedia, *Epitome medicae libri septem* [Seven Books of Medicine]. It opens with pregnancy, the diseases of childhood and of old age, and then passes to diet and regimen. Illness is dealt with in Book II. Maladies affecting specific parts are next treated from top to toe. For mental illness he recommends gentle treatments, including music, but also alludes to satanic possession. Book IV is concerned with skin diseases, beginning with scabies and elephantiasis (presumably a form of leprosy) and progressing to herpes, oedemas, cancers and ulcers. Discussion of conditions caused by noxious body humours is followed in Book V by a survey of external agents, principally poisons, with a brief appendix on impostors. Book VI deals with surgery, including an account of tracheotomy, and a final long book is taken up with drugs, including the use of colchicum for gout. As a practical introduction, his *Epitome* was esteemed by Islamic physicians.

Such writers as Oribasius and Paul of Aegina saw it as their job to stitch extracts from earlier writers into a compendium of teachings and remedies. Their encyclopaedias spread Galen's influence far and wide; they also reveal emergent tensions between theory and practice. Galen's insistence on the need for a doctor to understand philosophy was interpreted as a call for logic and book-learning. This encouraged a drift towards treating medicine in terms of set texts. Though Galen had laid down no canon, by AD 500 in Alexandria there was not only a syllabus of Hippocratic texts (those which Galen had followed) but an embryonic Galenic canon, which became known as the sixteen books, taught with commentaries and studied in a set order, beginning with *On Sects* and the *Art of Medicine*. Alexandrian scholars also summarized the sixteen books for ease of memory, thus imparting to Galenism a more dogmatic air. Just as Christ's teachings were theologized by the Church, classical medicine was being given its own orthodoxy. Medicine was becoming a matter of great texts.

While a scholarly tradition maintained itself in the eastern Roman empire, promoting a somewhat stilted Galenism, learned medicine was languishing in the West, where erudite doctors almost disappeared. Schools dwindled and Latin became confined to the Church. Cassiodorus (*c.* 540–*c.* 583) advised his monks at Vivarium in southern Italy to tend the sick and trust in God, while recommending a few practical medical texts: 'read above all the translations of the *Herbarium* of Dioscorides, which describes with surprising exactness the herbs of the field,' together with some Latin Hippocrates, Galen's *Method of Healing*, Caelius Aurelianus' *On Medicine*, and a handful of others. But that amounted to a sparse diet, and such texts were largely practical. The *Lorch Book of Medicine*, written about 795 in a Benedictine abbey in Germany, similarly contains brief introductory texts on anatomy, the humours and prognostics, and ends with recipes and dietary advice. The range of learned medicine was shrinking.

Knowledge was also transmitted in the West through encyclopaedias like the *Etymologiae* of Isidore, archbishop of Seville (*c.* 560–636), a medieval bestseller. Writing amid the turmoil in Spain – Goths ruled the country while Arian heretics (those who denied that Jesus was divine in the same way as God the Father) were bickering with the pope – the young Isidore felt called upon to shore up classical culture. His *Etymologiae* (the name reflects his passionate interest in the origins of words) takes in theology as well as history, grammar, mathematics, law and virtually all other learning. The fourth book concerns medicine, drawing on late-classical compendia, including the works of Caelius Aurelianus.

Isidore served up a beginner's guide to Greek science, philosophy and medicine. The physical world was explained in terms of the four qualities (hot, cold, wet, dry), and the four elements (earth, air, fire, and water). The body operated on a similar plan, ruled by the four humours (blood, choler, phlegm, melancholy). Disease in the microcosm was caused by humoral imbalance, and treatment had to restore that equilibrium allopathically by diet, regimen or drugs. The medical sections of his encyclopaedia abstracted learned medicine, but his very title highlighted the new focus of study: words not bodies. Semantics was the key to a cosmos created by the Divine Logos, an orientation symptomatic of the cloistering of learning in the Latin West during those times of which little evidence survives: the 'Dark Ages'.

The Venerable Bede (*c.* 672–735) was the English Isidore, a man aware of the need to meld healing and holiness. Although their Northumberland lay on the outer rim of the civilized world, Bede and his monks possessed many medical writings. Indeed, England was unique in producing a medical literature in a non-Latin tongue, Anglo-Saxon. Knowledge of plant remedies was extensive, and the English healer (*laece* or leech) used chants and charms, predicated on the belief that certain diseases and bad luck were caused by darts shot by elves, while others involved a 'great worm', a term applied to snakes, insects, and dragons. Bald and Cild's do-it-yourself *Leechbook* (AD 900) mirrors medical tracts common elsewhere in western Europe, simplifying Latin recipes by removing the more exotic ingredients and interweaving local remedies. Disease could be cured by prayers or by invoking saints' names, by exorcism, or by transferring it to animals, plants or the soil. Christian amulets were prescribed, together with number magic (the Anglo-Saxons favoured nines). For paralysis, 'scarify the neck after the setting of the sun and silently pour the blood into running water. After that, spit three times, then say: "Have thou this unheal and depart with it".'

Anglo-Saxon medicine conveys the spirit of early medieval Europe. A basis of classical therapeutics endured, explained by a sprinkling of Greek theory. The emphasis, however, had shifted to practicalities: recipes, meteorological and astrological advice, tips for uroscopy and bleeding, all indicative of an unstable society where books and learning had grown precious. The torch of medicine had meanwhile moved from Galen's Rome to the east.

ISLAM

The eastern Mediterranean experienced turmoil of its own. Prolonged warfare between the Byzantine (Roman) and Persian empires caused chaos; within Byzantium, ethnic tensions between Greeks, Semites, Persians, Armenians and Slavs were exacerbated by vitriolic doctrinal splits amongst Christian sects. The heroic military efforts of Justinian (r. 524–65) to recover the western Roman Empire and his ruinous building ambitions caused further upheaval. The appearance of bubonic plague in 541 heralded two hundred years of devastating outbreaks. The Greek heritage grew less assured. Learned medicine continued in large cities, especially Alexandria, but most doctors were increasingly working in isolation, and religion assumed a dominant role in everyday life. The scene was set for Islam.

Muhammad (570–632) was a member of the tribe of Quraysh who ruled Mecca. He began life as a poor orphan but rose to become a wealthy merchant. When he was about forty, he received a call, and the Qur'an (Koran) was revealed to him in visions. He gradually assumed the mantle of the last of the prophets in a long line beginning with Adam and Noah. In 622 an assassination plot against the Muslims in Mecca led him to flee to Medina where he commanded a growing following.

By the time of his death, practically all of Arabia had been won over for Islam, and a century later his adherents had conquered half of Byzantine Asia, all of Persia, Egypt, the Maghreb (North Africa) and Spain, where Cordova became capital of the western caliphate, the Baghdad of the West, the source of Hispano–Arabian culture, together with Seville and Toledo, which peaked in the twelfth century, and later still Granada. Unlike Christianity, Islam was not a proselytizing faith which saw itself as superseding earlier faiths, and the Qur'an granted Christians and Jews special status as 'People of the Book' (*ahl al-Kitab*), adherents of the other scripture-based faiths. Before the papacy launched the Crusades, Christians, Jews, Muslims and others rubbed along well together. What brought some unity to the Arab empire was not religion but a common language.

The pre-Islamic Near and Middle East possessed a popular medicine akin to that of the Mediterranean. *Materia medica* included plants and herbs familiar to Greek medicine, though certain remedies were distinct. Truffle juice was applied to eye disorders, clarified butter was used against fever, dates were prescribed for children's maladies, while camel's urine toned up the system. Cupping, cautery and leeches were employed for blood-letting; wounds were disinfected with alkali-rich saltwort, and ashes were applied to stanch bleeding. Knowledge of internal organs was meagre, and surgery was basic.

Interwoven with these practices were animist beliefs. Ill health was widely attributed to spirits. To restore well-being, the sick had to outwit them or recruit the protection of superior magical powers. The forces responsible for ill health were the *jinn* and the evil eye (*al-'ayn*), a glance believed to harm those upon whom it fell. The *jinn* (plural: *jinni*, whence genie) was a lesser spirit interfering with human beings; one could see, bargain with and even kill *jinni*, and they could bring good luck as well as bad. Healthwise, however, their activity was harmful, and they were held particularly to blame for fevers, madness and children's diseases.

Avoidance of sickness thus demanded practical and magical precautions to ward off evil spirits. There were incantations against ailments like leg ulcers and night-blindness, and charms guaranteed a safe delivery for pregnant women. Popular observances countered unwelcome visitations from spirits: thus a boy suffering from a blistered lip would beg for food and then toss any offerings to the dogs; as the blister had originally been attracted by his eating food, it would be drawn to the scraps and so transferred to the dogs. Practical medicine was everyone's business, but those who, like bleeders and cuppers, possessed particular skills were paid for their services, while the magical side of traditional medicine was performed by diviners, seers and charmers.

Initially the rise of Islam posed no threat to this traditional lore. The Qur'an has almost nothing to say about medicine, apart from advice to the faithful to wash for prayer and praise for the healing powers of honey. Scripture accepted the *jinn*, and Islam raised no objection to the indigenous medicine of conquered provinces; formal learning, including medicine, continued in the (Christian) Jacobite and Nestorian monasteries of Syria and Mesopotamia.

The seventh and eighth centuries, however, brought the transformation of Islam from a simple monotheistic creed to a formal faith, laying down theological orthodoxy. Popular medicine became mired in controversy because of its animistic bent, and many traditional practices were condemned. Conflict was sharpened by the fact that, in the centuries after the Prophet's death (632), discussion of issues tended to be dominated by claims that Muhammad or his companions must have pronounced on the matter. Such pious dicta grew into a distinct corpus called *hadith*, the sayings of the Prophet. Old-style healers also began to claim Muhammad's support: traditions alleged to be from the Prophet told, for example, that 'the evil eye is real'; that there was medicinal power in his saliva; and that the water of the well of Zamzam in Mecca had healing properties. Being God's word, the Qur'an too must have great powers. Hence, to assist a woman in labour, certain verses should be written on a slate, cleaned off, and the water given her to drink. The parallels with Christian healing are plain.

As Islam developed, traditional medicine was called into question. One major dilemma was plague. Early views had attributed epidemics to the *jinn*. This explanation was displaced by beliefs setting pestilence within the monotheistic framework of an Allah who was the ordainer of all things (including disease), yet was just and merciful. Though with the growth of Islam, many folkloric practices were attacked, medicine itself was not called into question, since Islam taught that 'God sends down no malady without also sending down with it a cure.'

It is often held that a distinctive Arab–Islamic medicine dates from the time of the Prophet and stems from a hospital (*bimaristan*: Persian for house for the sick) and academy at Jundishapur, near Susa in southern Persia. Jundishapur was certainly a meeting-place for Arab, Greek, Syriac and Jewish intellectuals, but there is no evidence that any *medical* academy existed there. Only in the early ninth century did Arab–Islamic learned medicine take shape. The first phase of this revival lay in a major translation movement, arising during the reign of Harun al-Rashid (r. 786–809) and gaining impetus in the caliphate of his son, al-Ma'mum (r. 813–33). It was stimulated by a socioeconomic atmosphere favourable to the pursuit of scholarship, a perceived need among both Muslims and Christians for access in Arabic to ancient medicine, and the ready availability of the relevant texts.

Crucial in this 'age of translations' was the establishment in Baghdad, capital of the Islamic empire under the Abbasid caliphs, of the Bayt al-Hikma (832), a centre where scholars assembled texts and translated into Arabic a broad range of non-Islamic works. The initial translation work was dominated by Christians, thanks to their skills in Greek and Syriac. The main figure was Hunayn ibn Ishaq (d. 873), later known in the West as Johannitius, a Nestorian Christian from the southern Iraqi town of al-Hira. Hunayn, who travelled to the Byzantine empire in search of Galenic treatises and was said to wander the streets of Baghdad reciting Homer in Greek, was amazingly prolific. With his pupils, he translated 129 works of Galen into Arabic (and others into Syriac), providing the Arabic world with more Galenic texts than survive today in Greek.

Encouraged by official patronage, the translation drive proceeded rapidly. Hundreds of Greek texts were rendered into accurate and elegant Arabic; works in Syriac and Sanskrit were also translated, reflecting the cosmopolitanism of ninth-century Baghdad. The impact was enormous, not least in view of the hundreds of ancient texts saved in Arabic for posterity. The favoured author was Galen, and he thereby became the father figure for Arabic medicine. Even the Hippocratic Corpus was known primarily through his commentaries.

Continuing into the early eleventh century, the translation movement revived learned medicine, made Arabic a tongue for original scholarship, and gave Islamic culture access to a galaxy of learning. The early translators also launched an original medical literature of their own. Hunayn authored essays on ophthalmology, known as his *Kitab al-'ashr maqalat fi l-'ayn* [Book of the Ten Treatises on the Eye]. His *Medical Questions and Answers*, a student text book, adopted the threefold scheme of discussing first the natural organisation of the body, then neutral factors, and finally unnatural (or contra-natural) disease – a handling reproduced by all Arabic writers in the Galenic tradition. By the late ninth century medical men had access to a stock of ancient texts in superior Arabic translations and an expanding corpus of original scholarship glossing Greek works.

This in turn created a need for fresh syntheses, leading to the supreme achievement of Arab–Islamic medicine, the medical compendia. The first was the *Firdaws al-hikma* [Paradise of Wisdom] by 'Ali ibn Rabban al-Tabari (*c.* 850), in which the author, an Islamic convert, sought to collect a *summa* of medical erudition worthy for presentation

to the Caliph al-Mutawakkil. His sources were Arabic and Persian translations of ancient classics, and his citations included not only Hippocrates, Galen and Dioscorides but Persian and Indian writers (this Indian
element was soon, however, eclipsed by the Greek tradition).

Persia produced one of the greatest Muslim physicians and philosophers, Muhammad ibn Zakariya al-Razi, known in the West as Rhazes
(865–925), author of some 200 treatises. In his youth (anecdotes tell
us) al-Razi studied and practised medicine at the *bimaristan* of Baghdad.
He later returned to Rayy, near Teheran, as head of its hospital, at the
invitation of Persia's ruler, Mansur ibn Ishaq; al-Razi dedicated to him
Al-Kitab al-mansuri fi'l-tibb [The Mansurian Book of Medicine], a
manual in ten books. The first six ran through such concerns as anatomy,
physiology and *materia medica*, while the last four dealt with clinical
matters: diagnosis, therapy, surgery and pathology, discussing diseases
from head to foot. His separate work, *al-Tibb al-ruhani* [Spiritual Physic]
handled diseases of the soul within a discussion of philosophy. Having
won fame in Rayy, al-Razi went to Baghdad to take charge of its new
al-Mu'tadidi Hospital. He spent his declining years in Rayy suffering
from glaucoma, before becoming blind.

Al-Razi developed a medical philosophy. In the first chapter ('On
the Excellence and Praise of Reason') of *al-Tibb al-ruhani*, he asserted
that reason (*al-'aql*) was the ultimate authority which 'should govern,
and not be governed; should control, and not be controlled; should
lead, and not be led'. He condemned slavish authority, devoting a large
book, *Fi'l-Shukuk 'ala Jalinus* [Doubts about Galen], to criticism of
precepts in Galen, beginning with *al-Burhan* [Demonstration], and ending with his large work, *Fi'l-Nabd* [On the Pulse]. In his introduction
to *Fi'l-Shukuk*, he nevertheless declared himself Galen's disciple; but
since the art of healing was a form of philosophy, it could neither
renounce criticism nor benefit from worshipping the dead. Extolling
the progress of scientific knowledge, he wrote in *Fi Mihnat al-tabib* [On
Examining Physicians and on Appointing Them] that 'he who studies
the works of the Ancients, gains the experience of their labour as if he
himself had lived thousands of years spent on investigation.' Nevertheless 'all that is written in books is worth much less than the experience
of a wise doctor.'

Al-Razi's best-known work, *al-Hawi fi'l-tibb* [*Continens*, or Comprehensive Book of Medicine], was a commonplace book of detailed notes
and transcribed bits of texts, beginning with diseases of the head and

working down. Devoted to specific subjects, these files were gradually
filled with jottings; the result was a kind of filing system, organized by
subject though lacking overall form. Al-Razi incorporated case histories
from earlier sources, notably Galen, but he also registered his own
cases, recording the patient's name, age, sex and occupation. Clinical
observations of his own illnesses are also preserved: notes on how he
had treated throat inflammation by gargling with strong vinegar; elsewhere he wrote about his swollen right testicle (emetics helped recovery). From these notes, al-Razi took the material for books such as
al-Qulani [Cholic] and *al-Jadari wa'l-hasba* [Smallpox and Measles].
Hitherto all exanthemata (infections causing rashes) had tended to be
lumped together; al-Razi was the first to distinguish them as separate
diseases: 'The physical signs of measles are nearly the same as those of
smallpox, but nausea and inflammation are more severe, though the
pains in the back are less. The rash of measles usually appears at once,
but the rash of smallpox spot after spot.' It is intriguing to find measles
regarded as the more severe.

     Al-Razi had many asides on medical practice: noblemen, he judged,
echoing Galen, were entitled to special consideration in prescribing; for
them unpleasant tasting drugs should be made palatable. But he did not
neglect the poor, for whom he wrote his *Man la yahduruh al-tabib* [Who
has no Physician to Attend Him]. *Khawass al-ashya'* [Properties of
Things] included the role of alchemy in medicine and the secret recipes
and remedies of nature. Experience must be the touchstone of truth:

> since many wicked people tell lies with regard to such properties,
> and we do not possess decisive means to distinguish the truth of
> rightful men from the false testimony of liars – save only actual
> experience – it will be useful not to leave these claims scattered
> but to collect and write them all. We shall not accept any property
> as authentic unless it has been examined and tried.

Al-Razi won renown, and his medical works later enjoyed ascendancy
in the Latin West. In 1279 *al-Hawi fi'l-tibb* was Latinized under the
title of *Continens* by the Sicilian Jew Faraj ibn Salim (Farragut), and
printed five times between 1488 and 1542. His *al-Mansuri fi'l-tibb*
[*Liber ad Almansorem*] and his *al-Tibb al-muluki* [*Liber regius*] were also
popular. His work was in turn mentioned by Abu Rayhan ibn Ahmad
al-Biruni (Al-Biruni, 973–c. 1050), who wrote on a variety of subjects:
astronomy and astrology, mathematics, geography, history, philosophy

and religion, mechanics, mineralogy and medicine. As well as editing al-Razi, he translated much of Galen's otherwise lost *Commentary on the Hippocratic Oath*.

The Arabic medical compendium culminated in two works of the tenth and eleventh centuries. 'Ali ibn al'-Abbas al-Majusi (Haly Abbas, d. late tenth century) was a native of al-Ahwaz in southern Persia, but little is known about his life. Following al-Razi's example, he divided his *Kamil al-sina'a al-tibbiya* [The Complete Medical Art] into two sections, on theoretical and on practical medicine, each including ten treatises on specialized topics, and his introduction surveyed the development of medicine up to his own times. Well-organized, practical, and devoting greater attention than al-Razi to anatomy and surgery, it secured al-Majusi's medical reputation, winning a place second only to Ibn Sina's *Qanun*.

The talents of Abu Ali al-Husayn ibn 'Abdallah ibn Sina (Avicenna, 980–1037) were evident from early youth. A Persian tax-collector's son, he could, it is piously recorded, recite the *Qur'an* at the age of ten and was practising medicine by sixteen. If somewhat mythologized, Ibn Sina represents the pinnacle of the Galenic ideal of the philosopher– physician in Islam: he was the first scholar to create a complete philosophical synthesis in Arabic.

In a wandering life driven by burning intellectual curiosity, Ibn Sina held positions as a jurist, a teacher of philosophy, an administrator, and as physician to various courts. His autobiography boasts that his writing was done on horseback during military campaigns, in hiding, in prison and even after drinking bouts. The outcome was two hundred and seventy titles which include two monumental encyclopaedias, one on science (*Kitab al-Shifa*) and one on medicine (*Kitab al-Qanun*).

The *Kitab al-Qanun* [Canon, or The Medical Code] arranges in its million words the whole of medical science: the legacies of Hippocrates, Galen, Dioscorides and the late Alexandrian physicians, enriched by the works of Arab predecessors. It consists of five books arranged by subject, with subdivisions and summaries. Book I deals with general principles, starting with the theory of the elements, humours and temperaments and moving on to anatomy, physiology, hygiene, aetiology, symptoms and treatment of diseases. Book II is on *materia medica*, describing the physical properties of simple drugs, and how to collect and preserve them (a separate section lists 760 drugs alphabetically). Book III deals with specific diseases, classified from head to heel, together with the aetiology, symptoms, diagnosis, prognosis and treatment of each. Anatomy is also discussed. Book IV is concerned with diseases, such as fevers, affecting the whole body; it also covers ulcers, abscesses, swellings, pustules, fractures and injuries, as well as poisons, and there is even a section on anorexia and obesity. Book V describes compound drugs – theriacs, electuaries, emetics, pessaries, liniments, and so on – together with their medicinal uses.

In addition to the *Canon*, Ibn Sina wrote about forty works on medical subjects. The best known is *Urjuza fi'l-tibb* [A Medical Poem], a summary of the principles of medicine in verse as a mnemonic aid to students. But it was the *Qanun* that became the authoritative text on medicine for centuries, both in Islam, where it remains influential, and in Latin Christendom, earning him such titles as the 'Galen of Islam'. His pre-eminent standing in the Latin West is symbolized by Dante's ennobling him between Hippocrates and Galen.

Critics have alleged that al-Razi's and Ibn Sina's work stifled independent thought. Certainly the *Canon* was taught and annotated, but some of the commentaries were highly critical, notably that of the Andalusian physician, Ibn Rushd (Averroës, 1126–98). Criticism of its anatomy section also gave rise to the description by Ibn al-Nafis (d. 1288) of the pulmonary (lesser) circulation, nearly three hundred years before Servetus and Realdo Colombo (see below).

All these great compendia originated in Persia, but texts were also produced elsewhere, including the work of Abu'l-Qasim Khalaf ibn Abbas al-Zahrawi (Albucasis, 936–1013). Born in Cordova, al-Zahrawi was author of a medical compendium entitled *Al-Tasrif li-man 'ajaza 'an al-ta'lif* [The Recourse of Him Who Cannot Compose (a Medical Work of His Own)]. Some 1500 pages in length, and divided into thirty treatises, it offers information on topics elsewhere neglected, including surgery, midwifery and child-rearing, and detailed accounts of bleeding, cupping and cautery. Treatise 30, the most celebrated, deals with surgery, describing operations for the stone, cauterization of wounds, sutures, obstetrical and dental procedures, setting fractures and dislocations, procedures for opening abscesses and eye surgery, to say nothing of 200 illustrations of medical and dental instruments, many of which he designed himself. This surgical treatise won enormous acclaim in the Latin West.

Albucasis gave a definitive account of cautery, which was central to Arabic surgical practice, being used to open abscesses, burn skin tumours and haemorrhoids, cleanse wounds, and stanch blood flow. Like blood-letting, it was also performed in the treatment of internal diseases, and Albucasis advised the cauterizing iron for almost every ailment, including epilepsy, stroke and melancholy. Apart from him, it is unlikely that the Arabic surgical authors ever practised surgery themselves.

Also Spanish-born was Abu-l-Walid Muhammad ibn Ahmad ibn Muhammad ibn Rushd (d. 1198), latinized as Averroës. Physician, philosopher and jurist, Ibn Rushd is known in the West for his classic commentaries on Aristotle. Coming from a long line of lawyers, he served as a judge in Cordova and Seville and also as physician to the ruling Almohad family – though he later came under attack for his views, leading to exile and the burning of his philosophical works. His major medical text is the encyclopaedic *al-Kulliyat* [The Book of General Principles], written between 1153 and 1169. Consisting of seven books dealing with anatomy, health, pathology, symptoms, dietetics and drugs, hygiene and therapeutics, it was conceived as a companion to *al-Taisir*, written by his colleague, Ibn Zuhr (Avenzoar, *c.* 1091–1162), which dealt with specific diseases. Together they constituted a comprehensive medical treatise, becoming familiar in the West through their Hebrew and Latin translations [*Colliget*], and printed together in Venice in 1482. On physiological issues he preferred Aristotelian explanations over Galen's, but he was not a slavish follower, and both the *Colliget* and the *Commentaries* show independent thinking.

Rabbi Moshe ben Maimun (1135–1204: Moses Maimonides or Abu 'Imran ibn 'Ubdaidalla Musa ibn Maimun) was another scholar who testifies to the intellectual pre-eminence of Spain at this time. The ascendancy of a fanatic Muslim ruling group forced the Jewish Maimonides, like Averroës, to flee Cordova in 1148, and he spent the next ten years in exile. In 1158, he settled in Fez, but moved on a few years later to Cairo where he stayed until his death. His medical practice earned him celebrity; in 1174 he was appointed court physician to Saladin, sultan of Egypt and Syria, and he became the head of the Jewish community in Egypt.

Paralleling the Islamic intellectuals of his day, Maimonides was a polymath, combining philosophy, logic, theology, astronomy and medicine. Apart from his major fourteen-volume religious work, the *Mishneh Torah*, which is in Hebrew, his books were written in Arabic. His ten medical works, all surviving, mostly in Arabic but some only in Hebrew translation, include the *Extracts from Galen*, a collection of Galen's writings, and a *Commentary on the Hippocratic Aphorisms*. His *Medical Aphorisms* is of particular interest because of its criticism of Galen for preferring Aristotelian over biblical cosmology. He emphasized the duties of physicians: 'may I never see in the patient anything but a fellow creature in pain.'

There are various treatises on individual topics (on haemorrhoids, asthma, poisons and their antidotes, and so forth), but Maimonides' most famous medical book was his *Regimen of Health* – short, much reproduced, often translated, and full of solid advice:

> How can a person heal his intestines if they are slightly constipated?
> If he is a young boy, he should eat salty foods, cooked and spiced
> with olive oil, fish brine and salt, without bread, every morning;
> or he should drink the liquid of boiled spinach or cabbage in olive
> oil and fish brine and salt. If he is an old man, he should drink honey
> mixed with warm water in the morning and wait approximately four
> hours, and then he should eat his meal. He should do this for one
> day or three or four days if it is necessary, until his intestines soften.

While not adding anything original to Graeco–Arabic medicine, Maimonides' considerable literary output earned him respect, and, like other contemporaries, he was widely cited by leading European authorities such as Henri de Mondeville, Arnald of Villanova and Guy de Chauliac.

An original aspect of Arab–Islamic medicine was its contribution to pharmacology. The lands overrun by Arab warriors yielded an abundance of plants, animals and minerals; hence, whereas Dioscorides' *materia medica* had included less than a thousand plants, animals and minerals, that of Ibn al-Baytar (d. 1248) astonishingly listed over 3000 items, including 800 botanical drugs, 145 mineral drugs, and 130 animal drugs. The medical formulary of al-Kindi (Yaqub ibn-Ishaq al-Kindi, *c.* 800–870) served as a source for Arabic treatises on pharmacology, botany, zoology and mineralogy. His writings contained many Persian, Indian or Oriental drugs unknown to the Greeks, including camphor, cassia, senna, nutmegs and mace, tamarind and manna.

In the eleventh century, al-Biruni described more than a thousand simples in his *Kitab al-Saydanah fi al Tibb* [Book of Pharmacy in the Healing Art]. The *Minhaj al-Dukkan wa Dustur al-'yan* [Handbook for the Apothecary Shop], written in Cairo in 1259 by the Jewish pharmacist Abu al-Muna Kohen al-'Attar, was much more than a mere formulary of the *materia medica*. Intended to provide instruction for his son, it included drug synonyms, recipes for syrups, remedies to aid digestion, fumigations and liniments and pharmaceutical weights – and also covered the duties and shop practices of the pharmacist.

The word 'drug' is of Arabic origin, as are alcohol (it then referred to a sulphurous powder), alkali, syrup, sugar, jujube and spinach; and many new drugs were introduced by the Arabs – benzoin, camphor, myrrh, musk, laudanum, naphtha, senna and alcohol. From the time of the 'father' of Arabic alchemy, Jabir ibn Hayyan (Jebir or Geber), who lived in the tenth century, they developed the alchemical techniques of crystallization, filtration, distillation and sublimation, alongside investigations into the properties of things contained in a 'secrets of nature' tradition paralleling that in the West. They created the first pharmacies, which also served as rendezvous for the exchange and discussion of information.

Overall, the value of Arab contributions to medicine lies not in their novelty but in the thoroughness with which they preserved and systematized existing knowledge. Great effort was devoted to its dissemination and medical texts were repeatedly copied. Over 5000 medical manuscripts in Arabic, Turkish, and Persian survive in libraries in Turkey alone, with more than fifty copies of Ibn Sina's *Qanun*, and still more transcripts of the many later commentaries on it. And though the era of the great Arabic medical compendia ended with the *Qanun*, such works long continued as foci of scholarly attention, commentaries in turn becoming the bases for super-commentaries, such as that of 'Ala' al-Din ibn al-Nafis (1200–88).

Growing up in Damascus, Ibn al-Nafis studied at the famous Nuri hospital there. As with so many Arabic physicians, his interests were wide: medicine, logic, grammar and theology; he also wrote numerous commentaries on Hippocrates and Ibn Sina. His *Mujiz al-Qanun*, an epitome of Ibn Sina's *Canon*, was vastly popular, but the work for which he is best known today is the commentary on the anatomy of Ibn Sina, the *Sharh Tashrih al-Qanun*, since one passage contains the first description of the pulmonary circuit.

Contrary to the Galenic description of the passage of blood from the right ventricle directly through 'invisible pores' to the left ventricle, Ibn al-Nafis states that no blood could pass through the interventricular septum, 'the substance of the heart there being impermeable . . . therefore, the blood must pass only through the lungs'. He thus proposed for the first time the pulmonary circuit of the blood:

This is the right cavity of the two cavities of the heart. When the blood in this cavity has become thin, it must be transferred into the left cavity, where the pneuma is generated. But there is no passage between these two cavities; the substance of the heart there seems impermeable. It neither contains a visible passage, as some people have thought, nor does it contain an invisible passage which would permit the passage of blood, as Galen thought. . . . It must, therefore, be that when the blood has become thin, it is passed into the arterial vein [pulmonary artery] to the lung, in order to be dispersed inside the substance of the lung, and to mix with the air. The finest parts of the lung are then strained, passing into the venous artery [pulmonary vein] reaching the left of the two cavities of the heart.

His description, however, seems to have fallen into obscurity. A similar description of the pulmonary circuit appeared in 1553 by the Spaniard Michael Servetus, and then in 1559 by the Italian, Realdo Colombo, but there is no evidence that either had access to his work.

HEALTH CARE

What of health care in general in Islam? Damascus and Cairo were no dirtier or cleaner than Naples, Paris, or any other pre-modern cities. Livestock was kept at home, waste left in the streets, and epidemics wrought havoc. Medieval sources frequently refer to 'pestilence', sometimes smallpox, though the greatest scourge was bubonic plague, which devastated the region in wave after wave between 541 and 749, returning as the Black Death in 1347–9. Cairo, the world's second largest city with half a million people, lost half its population.

To serve the sick, a range of medical practitioners and services was on offer. The formative period was marked by the predominance of Christian doctors, with lesser numbers of Jews and pagans. Many physicians had several occupations, and sidelines in trade were common. Healing remained more flexible and unregulated than in Christendom: there were no licensing requirements, no fixed curricula or sites for learning medicine, and no laws defining the profession. Islamic society tolerated a spectrum of practitioners and remedies, partly because popular lore was upheld by custom and the approval of the Prophet. In any case, learned medicine was often unavailable in the countryside, and within the cities it was beyond most people's pockets.

There were various ways to prepare for a medical career. Some doctors were self-taught, like Ibn Sina. Others underwent formal study under a teacher. Muslims sometimes taught in mosques, and hospitals were natural places for instruction, since patients were to hand and many hospitals had libraries. Teaching methods and curricula varied according to the master, though instruction often focused on the key Galenic works. Mathematics and logic were also studied, and the novice had an array of manuals, later supplemented by the cribs generated around Ibn Sina's *Qanun*. Textual mastery was paramount; texts were usually read aloud and committed to heart, and classwork meant sitting with a mentor who posed questions and glossed obscurities. Anatomy was not taught in a hands-on manner, since dissection was abhorrent to Muslim sensibilities: the dead were believed to feel pain, and dissection was desecration. Clinical experience was obtained in hospitals: physicians used patients to illustrate maladies and problems to students who trailed them on their rounds. Pupils probably shouldered certain basic duties, such as venesection.

Physicians had certain public duties to fulfil, some quite bureaucratic. Doctors were frequently called upon to make official statements – for example, when a leper was seeking public assistance. Jewish physicians were often leaders of their communities, and Muslims found themselves in administrative positions such as army physician or hospital medical superintendent.

The hospital, though not part of a wider 'health policy', was a centre of Islamic medical practice. These institutions (the greatest were in Baghdad, Damascus, Cairo and Cordova) were initially inspired by the precedent of sick-relief services offered at Christian monasteries, although the Islamic hospital became a more elaborate medical institution. The first was apparently founded in Baghdad around 805 on the initiative of Harun al-Rashid, and this was followed by others. The movement spread to Persia, and by the twelfth century a hospital graced every large Islamic town; thirty-four have been identified in Muslim cities from Spain to Moghul India. One of the best known was built in Cairo in 1283 by al-Mansur Qalawun, who dedicated it to all who needed care – rich and poor, old and young, male and female, of all faiths. It had special wards for physical and mental diseases, a surgery, pharmacy, dispensary, library and lecture rooms, and a chapel for Christians as well as a mosque; it was still in use when Napoleon invaded Egypt.

Separate hospitals for the insane were also set up. The Qur'an required humane care of the mad, and the first institutions created primarily for mental cases appeared in Muslim lands. Called *maristans*, these had a good reputation, and European travellers marvelled at the humanity shown to the insane. The Islamic tradition had some impact, the first European mental hospitals being built in former Muslim Spain, beginning with Granada in 1365.

Nevertheless, the role of hospitals in medieval Islam should not be exaggerated. They were a drop in the ocean for the vast size of the populations they had to serve, and their true function lay in highlighting ideals of compassion and bringing together the activities of the medical profession.

With Cordova falling to the Christians in 1236 and Baghdad sacked by the Mongols in 1258, Arab civilization was beginning to decline after 1300. The Ottoman Turks who dominated the Levant in the succeeding centuries did not inspire new intellectual glories. Nevertheless, the medical system described flourished in the Muslim world until the nineteenth century, when it gradually receded before the tide of modern western medicine. It continues in India and Pakistan as Yunani medicine.

CHAPTER V

THE MEDIEVAL WEST

BARBARIAN INVASIONS, the collapse of the western Roman empire, and the rise of warrior fiefdoms spelt catastrophe for civilization and its amenities – including the teaching and practice of learned medicine. City life collapsed in Europe into a landscape dominated by castles and cathedrals, with literate men and women confined to monastic cloisters. The medical thread was, however, unbroken, even if it frayed and threatened to snap. Through what are known as the Dark Ages medical manuscripts were at least preserved, copied and studied within the sanctuaries provided by abbeys and cathedral schools. The medicine they kept alive was, however, but a shadow of its brilliance in Galen's day: a basic survival kit when book-learning itself was under threat.

The revival of formal medicine took place centuries later in the backward West than in the Islamic world – not until around 1100, emerging first in Salerno in southern Italy, thirty miles south of Naples and seventy miles from the glorious Benedictine monastery of Monte Cassino. And it had to be imported and replanted.

THE WEST COMES TO LIFE AGAIN

The Salerno medical school was supposedly founded by four scholars – a Latin teacher, a Jew, an Arab and a Greek who had brought to the West the writings of Hippocrates. This legend carries a figurative truth. Sited in mid-Mediterranean and protected by the modernizing Norman dukes of Sicily, Salerno lay at a crossroads – cultural, economic and ethnic. In 1063, Alphanus (d. 1085), a Benedictine monk of Monte Cassino who had become archbishop of Salerno, travelled to Constantinople where he became acquainted with Greek medical texts. His

Premnon Physicon introduced into the Latin-speaking world a Christianized Galenism, while his writings on the humours and the pulse reflected Byzantine medicine. Together Alphanus's works amount to a more philosophical approach to medicine than that hitherto available in the West, hellenizing it and enabling the physician to set himself above the workaday healer.

Later Salernitan teaching texts continued the latinization of Greek writings, and Salerno channelled Arabic medicine into the West, under the stimulus of Constantinus Africanus (*c.* 1020–87). A native of Carthage (in modern Tunisia) who became a monk of Monte Cassino, Constantine relayed texts of Arabic and Greek medicine, the most important of his translations being the *Pantegni* [The Whole Art] of Haly Abbas (d. 994). Many Greek texts which had been translated into Arabic were now latinized by Constantine, notably Galen's *Method of Healing*, his commentaries on Hippocrates' *Aphorisms*, his *Regimen in Acute Diseases*, *Prognostic* and the *Art of Medicine*. Constantine also made a version of Hunayn's (Johannitius') *Medical Questions*, known as the *Liber Ysagogarum* [Isagogue or Introduction]. By the mid-twelfth century these texts were seeping beyond Italy.

Constantine's translations were crucial, providing as they did the means whereby Latin Christendom gained access to the tradition of Hippocratic learning rationalized by Galen and digested by the Arabs. For the first time since the sixth century, Latin speakers could share in contemporary medical thinking. Providing a framework for medical teaching on diagnosis and therapy, the *Liber Ysagogarum* became a foundation text in the medical schools which sprang up in Italy and France, forming the basis of the *Articella* (see below).

The *Liber Ysagogarum* also broadened and gave greater prominence to the Galenic idea of the 'six non-naturals' – food and drink, environment, sleep, exercise, evacuations (including sexual) and state of mind; by regulating these, natural body balance could be preserved in the medical analogue to monastic rule. Stressing regimen, the non-naturals set the mould for medieval therapeutics, particularly in popular health books emanating from Salerno. The *Regimen sanitatis salernitanum* [Salernitan Regime of Health], a book of verses probably compiled in the thirteenth century and sometimes credited to Arnald of Villanova (1240–1311), supplied tips for healthy living from youth to old age, highlighting hygiene, exercise, diet and temperance. The first of the home health manuals, its enduring popularity is shown by the number of later printed editions: some 240 versions in Latin and other European languages, as well as Hebrew and Persian. And no wonder, since it was simple and even entertaining in its advocacy, alongside Galenic venesection, of Drs Quiet, Diet and Merryman.*

Salernitan translations and teachings created a new canon of medical authority known as the *Articella* [Little Art of Medicine], which included the *Liber Ysagogarum* and Hippocrates' *Aphorisms* and *Prognostic*, supplemented by Galen's *Tegni* and the Hippocratic *On Regimen in Acute Diseases* in a translation by Gerard of Cremona (*fl.* 1150–87). Rapidly becoming canonical, the *Articella* or *Ars medicinae* marked a turning point in the revival of medicine in the West. It combined translations from Greek and Arabic; it was concerned with theory, providing a basis of philosophical knowledge organized around key themes; its discussions set medicine within a wider conception of nature; and its Aristotelian orientation appealed to university scholastics. Not least, the *Articella* gave medicine a distinctly Galenic complexion. Pre-Salernitan compendia had included texts drawn from the Methodist as well as the Hippocratic tradition; Galen had not eclipsed all others. But the *Articella* texts were wholly Galenic: a proper doctor could thenceforth be defined as a man who knew his Galen.

Learned medicine continued to develop, thanks to the rise of universities (discussed below) and further access to scholarship via translation. The business of Latin translation proceeded through several stages. The first, the Salernitan, involved both Greek and Arabic texts. From the 1140s, there was a great outpouring of Latin translations from Arabic made in Muslim Spain, sometimes by way of Hebrew intermediaries. This development, which included philosophical texts, especially Aristotle, as well as medical, was led by Gerard of Cremona. Settling in Toledo, he translated an incredible quantity of material from Arabic – twenty-four works on medicine alone, including the *Qanun* of Avicenna, the *Liber Almansorius* of Rhazes (al-Razi), the last part of Albucasis' *De cirurgia*, the *Ars parva* and other works of Galen, and the *Commentary*

---

* Take for instance this section in the English translation by Sir John Harington (1561–1612) (who was, incidentally, the inventor of the water-closet):

> Although you may drink often while you dine,
> Yet after dinner touch not once the cup, . . .
> To close your stomach well, this order suits,
> Cheese after flesh, Nuts after fish or fruits.

on Galen's Art of Medicine by Haly Rodoan (Ali-ibn Ridwan). The *Qanun* or *Canon of Medicine* became the cornerstone of the medical curriculum at the University of Montpellier, remaining a textbook there until 1650! These translations created a richer terminology for learned medicine in Latin and provided Galenic medicine with a logical backbone. Medicine could now speak the language of scholasticism.

A century later there came a further burst of translations, mainly in Spain and Italy, latinizing other major works of Arabic science. These included the *Continens* [All-Embracing Book] of al-Razi (trans. 1282); and the *Colliget* [The Book of Universals] of Ibn Rushd, translated in Padua in 1283. The key figure in this drive was Arnald of Villanova. After studying medicine at Montpellier, he became a teacher and a polymath. Not only a translator of medical works, he was physician to the popes and the Aragonese royal family in Spain; later in life, he pored over theology, propounding heterodox ideas – his astrological computations predicted the world would end in 1378. As a theoretician, Arnaud aspired to rationalize Galenic medical theory with mathematical precision, by drawing on Arabic writers, notably al-Kindi and Averroës.

His Italian contemporary Pietro d'Abano (1257–*c.* 1315) made versions directly from Greek manuscripts he had carried back from Constantinople, including the beginning of a translation of Galen's *On the Use of the Parts of the Body*. Niccolò da Reggio (*fl.* 1315–48) translated over fifty Galenic writings, many for the first time, including the entire text of that work. There was also translation from Latin into the vernacular, in growing demand when town life was reviving and courts and burghers were hungry for knowledge. The *Surgery* of John of Arderne (*c.* 1307–70), discussed below, exists in both Latin and English versions, and Bartholomew the Englishman's (d. 1260) *De proprietatibus rerum* (1246) [On the Properties of Things] also enjoyed wide circulation in both tongues. Parts of the *Articella* were made available in French and English, and even in Welsh and Gaelic. For a couple of centuries, the translation movement had no less momentous consequences in Europe than in Islam, bolstering the prestige of antiquity and canonizing a Galenic medicine set in an arabized Aristotelian framework. Medical knowledge was buttressed not just by its classical heritage but by its place within the divine scheme of Christianity.

RELIGION

Medicine and religion intersected at many points. Conventional histories of medicine still retail the view that the Church arrested medical
progress, for instance, by supposedly banning dissection. Some ecclesiastics did indeed disparage medicine – St Bernard of Clairvaux (1090–
1153) asserted that 'to consult physicians and take medicines befits not
religion and is contrary to purity' – and it was a popular gibe that *ubi
tre physici, dui athei* (where there are three doctors, there are two atheists);
but in general such judgments miss the mark. Medieval hospitals have
been criticized for their religious ethos, but without the Christian virtue
of charity would such hospitals have existed at all?

The Church's position was clear: the divine was above the temporal.
Sometimes the Lord's will was to punish sinners with plagues; sometimes
it was man's duty to preserve life and health, for the glory of God and the
salvation of souls. But the body was to be subordinated to the soul, and
healing, like every other temporal activity, had to be under ecclesiastical
regulation. Thus in the case of the dying, it was more important that they
should be blessed by a priest than bled by a doctor. Concern for salvation
occasionally led to suspicions being voiced against Jewish doctors: the
Lateran Council of 1215 forbade practitioners not approved by the
Church from attending the sick, but this applied only on paper, for
the highly valued Jewish doctors were everywhere, especially in Spain.

Monks and clerics, for long the only body of learned men, commonly practised medicine, while in the northern European universities
medical students often entered minor holy orders. Petrus Hispanus
(Peter of Spain *c.* 1210–77), whose *Thesaurus pauperum* [Treasury of
the Poor] was popular despite its recommendation of pig shit to stanch
nosebleeds, even became Pope in 1276 as John XXI. (He died a year
later when the roof of a palace he had built collapsed; one trusts he was
a better doctor than architect.) Various ecclesiastical regulations were
passed covering medicine; the aim was not to curb it but to uphold the
Church's dignity and prevent clerics developing lucrative sidelines which
would seduce them from holy poverty and divine service. Thus when
the Lateran Council of 1215 forbade clerics in higher orders from
shedding blood, this was not (as often interpreted) an attack on surgery:
it aimed, not unlike the Hippocratic oath, to detach the clergy from a

manual and bloody craft. Clerics could continue to practise healing but not for gain. Nor did the Church authorities prohibit dissection: in 1482 Pope Sixtus IV informed the University of Tübingen that, provided the body came from an executed criminal and was finally given a Christian burial, there was no objection to human anatomy.

The Benedictine rule states that 'the care of the sick is to be placed above and before every other duty, as if indeed Christ were being directly served by waiting on them'; hence it is no surprise that monasteries became key medical centres, more important than universities prior to 1300. As well as offering shelter for pilgrims, most had an infirmary (*infirmarium*) for sick monks. Separate hospital facilities were founded for the general public.

Healing shrines flourished, and scores of saints were invoked – rather as in Egyptian medicine, each organ of the body and each complaint acquired a particular saint. Supplanting the pagan Asclepius, Damian and Cosmas became the patron saints of medicine. Brothers living in Cilicia (Asia Minor) around the close of the third century, they became celebrated for their healing powers. Their martyrdom under Diocletian is stirring stuff: despite being burnt, stoned, crucified and sawn in half, they survived, perishing only after decapitation. The pair appear in the heraldry of barber-surgeon companies, and churches were dedicated to them, often claiming to house their remains in fine reliquaries. Their chief medical miracle credits them with the first transplant: they amputated a (white) man's gangrenous leg and grafted in its place that of a dead Moor. In many paintings depicting this scene, the patient, with one leg white and one leg black, lies supine as the spectators stare awestruck upon the miracle.

In addition to this pair, St Luke or St Michael might be called upon for all manner of illnesses, but other saints were specialists: St Anthony was invoked for erysipelas (St Anthony's fire); St Artemis for genital afflictions, St Sebastian for pestilence. St Christopher dealt with epilepsy, St Roch protected against plague buboes (he had visited many sufferers on missions of mercy, fell sick himself, then was healed by an angel); St Blaise was good for goitre and other throat complaints, St Lawrence for backache, St Bernardine for the lungs, St Vitus for chorea (St Vitus's dance) and St Fiacre for sore arses. St Apollonia became the patron saint of toothache because all her teeth had been knocked out during her martyrdom, while St Margaret of Antioch was the patron of women in labour. Out walking, she had encountered a dragon, which swallowed her whole. In its stomach, she piously made the sign of the cross; this materialized into a real cross, growing until the dragon burst open, thus delivering the saint.

Healing shrines developed a great range of relics, pious images and souvenirs. Some, like Bury St Edmunds or Rocquemadour in the south of France, attracted pilgrims by the thousand. The blood of St Thomas à Becket cured blindness, insanity, leprosy and deafness – and ensured Canterbury's popularity. In Catholic Europe, many medieval shrines continue to this day.

Certain diseases, for instance the much-feared epilepsy, assumed supernatural connotations and cures; Hippocrates would have turned in his grave! Treatments for the falling sickness involved a mishmash of folklore, humoral medicine, sorcery, pagan beliefs and pious healing. John of Gaddesden (1280–1349), physician to Edward II and compiler of the encyclopaedic *Rosa anglica medicinae* [The English Rose of Medicine], recommended reciting the gospel over an epileptic patient while bedecking him with peony and chrysanthemum amulets or the hair of a white dog. The folk conviction that mistletoe cured the falling sickness was given a sacred rationalization: keeping watch over his father's flocks, the young King David saw a woman collapse in a fit. When he prayed for a remedy, an angel appeared to him, announcing, 'Whoever wears the oak mistletoe in a finger ring on the right hand, so that the mistletoe touches the hand, will never again be bothered by the falling sickness.'

Mistletoe was also used in other ways against epilepsy. In central Europe, the stalk was hung round children's necks to prevent seizures, while in Scandinavia countryfolk carried a knife with a handle cut from oak mistletoe. In the mid seventeenth century, the leading experimentalist and founder-member of the Royal Society, Robert Boyle, was still endorsing pulverized mistletoe: 'as much as can be held on a sixpence coin, early in the morning, in black cherry juice, during several days around the full moon'. The pious Boyle believed in religious cures, but sought their scientific basis.

HOSPITALS

Medieval hospitals were religious foundations through and through. Those planted in the West had originally been small and mainly for pilgrims; their late medieval successors were often more impressive.

St Leonard's in York had 225 sick and poor in 1287; still larger were the civic hospitals of Milan, Siena and Paris. In Florence alone, a city of some 30,000 inhabitants, there were over thirty foundations by the fifteenth century. Some had only ten beds, others hundreds. In England hospitals and almshouses totalled almost five hundred by 1400, though few were of any size or significance. London's St Bartholomew's dates from 1123 and St Thomas's from around 1215. At Bury St Edmunds six hospitals were endowed between 1150 and 1260 to cater for lepers, pilgrims, the infirm and the aged.

Small hospitals were essentially hostels or hospices lacking resident medical assistance, but physicians were in attendance by 1231 at the Paris Hôtel Dieu, next to Notre Dame, and Sta Maria Nuova in Florence was gradually medicalized: from twelve beds in 1288 for 'the sick and the poor', this 'first hospital among Christians', as one Florentine patriot called it, expanded by 1500 to a medical staff of ten doctors, a pharmacist and several assistants, including female surgeons. Although catering largely for the indigent, it had eight private rooms 'reserved for the sick of the higher classes'. Within hospital walls the Christian ethos was all-pervasive.

In hospital expansion the Crusades played their part, since crusading orders such as the Knights of St John of Jerusalem (later the Knights of Malta), the Knights Templar, and the Teutonic Knights built hospitals throughout the Mediterranean and German-speaking lands. By the fourteenth century non-military brotherhoods, such as the Order of the Holy Spirit, were also running infirmaries from Alsace to Poland, while the Order of St John of God appeared in Spain in the sixteenth century, building insane asylums and putting up about 200 hospitals in the New World.

LEARNED MEDICINE

The great age of hospital building from around 1200 coincided with the flourishing of universities in Italy, Spain, France and England, sustained by the new wealth and confidence of the High Middle Ages. Paris was founded in 1110; Bologna in 1158; Oxford in 1167, Montpellier in 1181, Cambridge in 1209, Padua in 1222 and Naples in 1224. The universities extended the work of Salerno in medical education. By the 1230s Montpellier was drawing medical students from afar; there, as in

Paris, Bologna, Oxford and other centres, medical teaching initially developed informally, but teachers later banded themselves into an official faculty.

There were some differences between the clerically dominated universities of the north like Paris, Cologne and Oxford, where the theology faculty was supreme, and the more secular ones of Montpellier and Italy, where arts and law faculties led; but all had much in common. The Bachelor of Medicine (MB) took around seven years of study, including a preliminary Arts training; a medical doctorate (MD) was awarded after around ten years' study. Hence there were hardly swarms of medical students: Bologna granted 65 degrees in medicine and only one in surgery between 1419 and 1434; Turin a mere 13 between 1426 and 1462. The single big school and true centre of excellence was Padua, where medical students comprised one tenth of the student population. Its medical faculty was unusually large, numbering 16 in 1436 – Oxford had only a single MD teaching.

Following the model established in universities at large, medical education was based on set books, usually parts of the *Articella* and Avicenna's *Canon*, expounded in lectures. It was also heavily influenced by the new Aristotelianism associated with Thomas Aquinas (1226–74) and Albertus Magnus (1200–80). A Dominican monk who taught at the new university of Cologne, Albert was wrongly credited with many medicinal recipes and occult treatises, as well as with the *De secretis mulierum* [On the Secrets of Women], all of which blocked his canonization until 1931.

After perhaps seven years' study beyond the Arts degree, doctoral graduation rested on having attended the requisite lectures, disputations and oral examinations and – at some universities, including Bologna and Paris – on having worked under a physician (such clinical experience had to be acquired extra-murally). From about 1300 at Bologna and a generation later at Montpellier, university requirements further demanded that students attend a dissection, to supplement traditional anatomical lessons on dead animals. The academic justification of a medical education lay in the acquisition of rational knowledge (*scientia*) within a natural philosophical framework. Medical professors aimed to prove that their discipline formed a noble chapel of the temple of science and philosophy; the learned physician who knew the reasons for things would not be mistaken for the hireling with a knack for healing.

Renaissance humanists and subsequent historians have sneered at medieval academic medicine for its Galenolatry and its abstract disputation topics ('Can sleep be harmful?'). But formulaic teaching was unavoidable in an age when books were few. And if much of the knowledge seems rather formal, this is because the student had to understand the medieval forerunner of what is now prized as 'basic science': the theory of the physical world and its laws and purposes. Grasp of universal truths was needed to comprehend individual cases, and the ability to reason and cite chapter and verse raised the true physician above the empiric.

Graduates got the pick of the patients; princes and patricians in Italy, France and Spain welcomed cultured doctors who could explain the whys and wherefores. The duties of physicians in the service of King Edward III of England were clearly laid down:

> And muche he should talke with the steward, chamberlayn, assewer, and the maister cooke, to devyse by counsayle what metes and drinkes is best according with the Kinge.... Also hym ought to espie if any of this courte be infected with leperiz or pestylence, and to warn the soveraynes of hym, till he be purged clene, to keepe hym oute of courte.

The learned physician claimed, in the Hippocratic manner, to prevent disorders or restore health by dietetics and drugs. For that he would need to form a diagnosis. Feeling the pulse and scrutinizing urine (uroscopy) were routine, and the doctor's *consilium* (advice) would be a personal prognosis based on a patient's history. Drug prescriptions were also personalized, involving compound mixtures (polypharmacy), often called 'Galenicals'.

Highly prized was medical mathematics, which sought to achieve an understanding of the significance for health of the motions of the heavens, in a tradition going back to the Hippocratic *Epidemics* and embracing subsequent developments in Ptolemaic astronomy and astrology. Following Galen, disease was enumerated as involving sequences of 'critical days' when an illness would reach crisis point and then either subside or prove fatal. The physician on Chaucer's Canterbury pilgrimage was proud of his astrological learning:

> With us ther was a DOCTOUR OF PHISYK,
> In al this world ne was ther noon him lyk
> To speke of phisik and of surgerye;
> For he was grounded in astronomye.

He kepte his pacient a full greet del
In houres, by his magik naturel.
Wel coude he fortunen the ascendent
Of his images for his pacient.
He knew the case of everich maladye,
Were it of hoot or cold, or moiste, or drye,
And where engendred, and of what humour;
He was a verrey parfit practisour.

Medical astrology might require arcane and labyrinthine calculations, but there were handy charts to illustrate planetary influences over the organs of the body and their maladies. Princely courts often housed a physician-astrologer, though it could prove a risky trade: the physician John of Toledo (d. 1275) was accused of dabbling in necromancy, and thrown into prison.

Zodiacs and nativities were also used to ascertain the right time for blood-letting. Recommended in spring and the beginning of September, its benefits, according to the *Salernitan Rule of Health*, included sound sleep, toning up the spirits, calmness, and better sight and hearing. Bleeding was left mainly to surgeons and barber-surgeons, who also cupped, pulled teeth, leeched, gave enemas, curetted fistulas, applied ointments, drained running sores, sutured wounds, removed superficial tumours and stopped haemorrhaging. Descriptions of trusses and eye-glasses began to appear in the thirteenth century.

Dietetics, by contrast, was the main therapeutic recourse of the physician regulating lifestyle in accordance with the six non-naturals. Spurred by the revival of international commerce, pharmacy also developed, especially in Venice, where drugs imported from the East were traded in large stores (*apothecai*), which came to mean a druggist's shop.

Relations between physicians and surgeons were not always plain-sailing, especially with eminent surgeons like Henri de Mondeville, Guy de Chauliac and John of Arderne (*c.* 1307–70) laying claim to learning as well as a good eye, a steady hand and a sharp blade. According to de Mondeville, 'it is impossible to be a good surgeon if one is not familiar with the foundations and general rules of medicine [and] it is impossible for anyone to be a good physician who is absolutely ignorant of the art of surgery.'

Among the famous early surgical writers was Lanfranc of Milan (*c.* 1250–1306). Italian by birth, he settled in Paris where he wrote his

Chirurgia magna, an expansion of his more popular *Chirurgia parva*. They were both translated into French, Italian, Spanish, German, English, Dutch and Hebrew. The *Grand Surgery* is divided into sections on general principles, and on anatomy, embryology, ulcers, fistulas, fractures and luxations, baldness and skin diseases, phlebotomy and scarification, cautery and diseases of various organs. There is also a lengthy section on herbs and pharmacy. Lanfranc was valued by his distinguished successors, de Mondeville and de Chauliac.

Henri de Mondeville (*c.* 1260–*c.* 1320) was born in Normandy, studying at Montpellier, Paris and Bologna. Travelling widely, he spent some time as a military surgeon to the French royal family, and lectured in surgery and anatomy at Montpellier and Paris. He planned his *Cyrurgia* (begun in 1306 but never completed) along traditional lines, opening with anatomy and moving on to wounds. Attention was paid to the contentious topic of wound treatment. Mondeville advocated simple bathing of wounds and immediate closure, followed by dry dressings with minimal loss of flesh or skin. His preference was for dry healing without pus formation, a view contradicting Hippocratic wisdom but already advocated by Hugo of Lucca (*c.* 1160–1257) and his disciple, Theoderic (1205–96), who had boldly maintained in his *Chirurgia* (1267) that 'it is not necessary that pus be formed in wounds'.

This new approach met opposition from supporters of conventional wound salves: plasters and powders designed to promote suppuration; since Greek times it had been taught that certain types of pus (known as 'laudable pus') were beneficial, conveying poisoned blood out of the body. The Salernitan school had thus recommended keeping wounds open to allow for suppuration and healing *per intentio secundam* (by second intention), from the base of the wound up.

The most prominent surgeon of the next generation was Guy de Chauliac (1298–1368), educated at Montpellier and Bologna. His great work, the *Chirurgia magna*, was fully comprehensive, covering anatomy, inflammation, wounds, ulcers, fractures, dislocations and miscellaneous diseases belonging to surgery. An astonishing exercise in surgical erudition, it contains no fewer than 3299 references to other works, including 890 quotations from Galen. This parade of sources was calculated, since Chauliac was concerned to show surgery to be a learned art:

> The conditions necessary for the surgeon are four: first, he should
> be learned, second, he should be expert: third, he must be ingeni-

ous, and fourth, he should be able to adapt himself. It is required for the first that the surgeon should know not only the principles of surgery, but also those of medicine in theory and practice.

Chauliac's *Chirurgia* was translated into several languages. In the *pus bonum et laudibile* debate, he did not exactly take sides, though he appears to have been hostile to traditional wound salves, judging they did more harm than good. The work also contains fascinating details about his own times, including first-hand reports of the Black Death, descriptions of surgical instruments and operations, and his often damning judgments on his contemporaries. Like most medieval practitioners, he offered a pot-pourri of Hippocratic treatments and ones of a magico-religious flavour. Epileptics, for instance, were to write in their own blood on a piece of parchment the names of the Three Wise Men, and to recite three Pater Nosters and three Ave Marias daily for three months.

The most distinguished English surgeon was John of Arderne, who served under John of Gaunt in the Hundred Years War and produced a *Treatment of Anal Fistulas*. For this operation, his technique was to place the patient in the lithotomy position. Four ligatures were taken up through the fistula, and their ends, drawn down through the anus, were knotted to stop the bleeding. Next, he pushed one grooved instrument through the fistula into the rectum, where it made contact with another. He then made a bold cut with his scalpel to remove the whole intervening segment, and stopped the bleeding between the ligatures with a hot sponge. The wound was cared for by cleaning and the patient was given daily enemas.

MEDICINE AND THE PEOPLE

From the twelfth century, Europe blossomed: population rose, trade boomed, and courts and cities acquired a new sophistication. Such circumstances helped medicine. While learned physicians were at the top of the tree, they constituted only a small fraction of all those offering medical services, and larger towns attracted a diversity of healers. Around 1400 Florence boasted not only graduates of Padua and Bologna, but bone-setters from Rome and families specializing in eye-diseases, hernia and the stone. Herbalists, midwives and pedlars of folk remedies thrived, and parish priests plied pious cures.

With numbers rising, medicine needed to organize itself. This happened first in urban Italy, where medical guilds assumed responsibilities for apprenticeship, examination of candidates, location of pharmacists and supervision of drugs, food and herbs. As early as 1236 Florentine physicians and pharmacists grouped into a single guild, recognized as one of the city's seven major crafts.

Medical organization took various forms. In southern Europe there was no great gulf between surgeon and physician: surgery was a desirable skill for a physician to acquire. In Frederick II's regulations for the Kingdom of Sicily (c. 1231), a licence to practice medicine could be gained only after five years of study which included surgery, and in Italy the chance to learn surgery at university helped to prevent professional rancour between the two branches. Elsewhere the gap widened, however, for beyond Italy surgery was excluded from the academic curriculum. In northern Europe surgical training and practice were organized on a guild basis, through apprenticeship, and so were regarded by physicians as *infra dig*.

In Paris, the surgeons' organization began in 1210 when the College of St Cosme (Côme or Cosmas) was established. Its members were divided into the long- and the short-robed, only the former being entitled to operate. Training was mainly practical and the college granted three degrees: a bachelor's, a licence and a master's. A three-cornered tussle developed between physicians of the faculty, the surgeons of the college, and the barbers, who did bleeding and the like. The introduction of anatomy added to the confusion, for dissections were under the direction of a physician but the knife-work was performed by a surgeon. Not till 1516 was the conflict resolved, with the surgeons ceding precedence to the physicians, for both could unite in antipathy towards the 'ignorant' barbers. In the German states and England, the barber-surgeon became typical, but in Italy, Spain and southern France, that hybrid occupation never gained prominence.

In London, the Fellowship of Surgeons came into being in 1368–9, and a Company of Barbers was chartered in 1376. The tiny band of university-trained physicians did not organize themselves until 1423, when a group led by the cleric and court physician, Gilbert Kymer (c. 1385–1463) petitioned for a joint college 'for the better education and control of physicians and surgeons practising in the city'. Not until the founding of the College of Physicians of London in 1518 could the physicians regulate metropolitan practice. Though intra-professional conflicts flared, they were not universal. In small cities like Bristol or

Norwich, physicians, surgeons and barbers found strength in unity. And, in any event, professional tussles in the late medieval centuries reflect the surging number of healers and their dawning sense of civic standing.

This proliferation provoked attempts by princes and city authorities at regulation and 'protection'. In the Kingdom of Sicily the royal physician took charge of licensing, while in the 1340s the Aragonese King Peter licensed Jewish practitioners who had been denied medical degrees from Christian universities. Church authorities often licensed midwives, on the grounds that their morals needed to be impeccable.

Urban expansion also explains the emergence, initially in northern Italy, of community-employed public physicians. The earliest known public contracts for such *medici condotti* were at Reggio in 1211 and in neighbouring Bologna in 1214, where the appointee was to treat soldiers as well as citizens. Contracts typically imposed a residence requirement, balanced the doctor's private and public duties, and set scales of fees. Especially in time of plague, the civic doctor was to assist at inquests and trials, to attend hospitals, and to tend injuries resulting from judicial torture.

This system spread. By 1300, public physicians were found in all the large towns of northern Italy; a century later the office was almost universal in northern and central Italy and in the Venetian territories in Dalmatia and Greece, and it had also been adopted in major centres in Provence, Aragon and Valencia. By 1500 civic doctors were being appointed in northern France, Flanders and many German cities, though Britain lagged behind.

Meanwhile rising urban populations contributed to overcrowding and worsening sanitary problems, due to the contamination of drinking water and food, waste accumulation and the keeping of livestock. Water began to be piped into towns, and by 1300 Bruges had built a municipal water system. Many towns paved their main thoroughfares; every large house in Paris was required to have a chamber draining into the sewers, and Milan passed ordinances for cesspools and sewers. Some German cities prohibited pig-pens facing onto the street; municipal slaughterhouses were established, and cities also tried to monitor food markets and curb river pollution. For example, tanners were not allowed to wash their skins or dyers to dump their waste in public waters. Nonetheless filth began to pose mounting threats. Plague struck in the fourteenth century (see below) and typhus from the close of the fifteenth.

LEPROSY

Certain diseases loomed large both in reality and in the public imagination, notably leprosy, now called Hansen's disease after Armauer Hansen (1841–1912), the discoverer of the bacillus *Mycobacterium leprae*. Its physical symptoms – scaly flesh, mutilated fingers and toes and bone degeneration, in short 'uncleanliness' – made it seem a living death and led to deeply punitive attitudes. The disease has a puzzling history. From as early as 2400 BC Egyptian sources contain references to a skin condition interpreted as leprosy, and 900 years later, the Ebers papyrus mentions a leprous disease seemingly confirmed by Egyptian skeleton evidence. True leprosy probably existed in the Levant from biblical times, but the term was also used for various dermatological conditions producing disfiguring ulcers and sores.

Leprosy became highly stigmatized. Authorized by ancient Levitical decrees, leper laws were strict in medieval Europe. They were forbidden all normal social contacts and became targets of shocking rites of exclusion. They could not marry, they were forced to dress distinctively and to sound a bell warning of their approach. According to the liturgical handbook, the Sarum Use, in thirteenth-century England,

> I forbid you ever to enter churches, or go into a market, or a mill, or a bakehouse, or into any assemblies of people.
> I forbid you ever to wash your hands or even any of your belongings in spring or stream of water of any kind . . .
> I forbid you ever henceforth to go out without your leper's dress, that you may be recognized by others . . .
> I forbid you to have intercourse with any woman except your wife . . .
> I forbid you to touch infants or young folk, whosoever they may be, or to give them or to others any of your possessions.
> I forbid you henceforth to eat or drink in any company except that of lepers . . .

They were segregated in special houses outside towns, lazarettos, following the injunction in Leviticus that the 'unclean' should dwell beyond the camp. There was also a leper mass, conducted with the victim in attendance, declaring the sufferer to be 'dead among the living', and the 1179 Lateran Council ordered them cast out from society, with their own burial places. The only consolation the Church gave was to interpret the leper's suffering as a purgatory on earth, destined to bring swifter reward in heaven. God, proclaimed de Chauliac, loved the leper; after all, did not the Bible (Matthew 8:3) show Jesus extending his hand, saying 'be thou clean'?

Leprosy provided a prism for Christian thinking about disease. No less a religious than a medical diagnosis, it was associated with sin, particularly lust, reflecting the assumption that it was spread by sex. In *The Testament of Cresseid* by Robert Henryson (*fl.* 1470–1500), the heroine is punished by God with leprosy for her lust and pride. Lepers were thus scapegoated with Jews and heretics in what historians have called a 'persecuting society'.

From the eleventh century there was a rapid surge in the number of hospitals built to house lepers. By 1226 there may have been around 2,000 in France alone, and in England about 130. By 1225 there were a staggering 19,000 leprosaria in Europe, offering shelter while enforcing isolation. Yet by 1350 leprosy was in decline. The epidemiology of that watershed is much disputed: some have speculated that the Black Death killed so many that the disease died out, others that it might be connected with the rise of tuberculosis, which has a similar but more aggressive pathogen; the TB bacillus could have elbowed out the leprosy. But though the disease waned, its menace remained, becoming a paradigm for later diseases of exclusion, and for persecution generally. Leprosaria were used for the poor and those suspected of carrying infectious diseases. Some became hospitals: on the then outskirts of Paris, the Hôpital des Petites Maisons, near the monastery of St Germain des Prés, founded as a leprosarium, was used for the mentally disordered and for indigent syphilitics. St Giles-in-the-Fields, then just outside London, was a lazaretto and later a hospital, as were the hospitals for incurables built outside Nuremberg.

PLAGUE

The Black Death is the most catastrophic epidemic ever to have struck Europe, killing perhaps twenty million people in three years. Absent from Europe for eight hundred years since the plague of Justinian, it was endemic for the next three centuries. The Great Pestilence of 1347–51 probably originated in China; in 1346 it migrated from beyond

Tashkent in central Asia to the Black Sea, where it broke out among the Tatars fighting Italian merchants in the Crimea. A chronicler tells how the Christians took refuge in the citadel at Kaffa (Feodosia), where they were besieged. Plague forced the Tatars to raise the siege, but before withdrawing they invented biological warfare by catapulting corpses of plague victims over the citadel walls, causing the disease to flare among the Christians. When they in turn escaped, it travelled with them into the Mediterranean, breaking out in Messina and Genoa and raging through the rest of Europe. According to Fra Michele di Piazze,

> In the first days of October 1347, twelve Genoese galleys fleeing before the wrath of our Lord over their wicked deeds, entered the port of Messina. The sailors brought in their bones a disease so violent that whoever spoke a word to them was infected and could in no way save himself from death ... Those to whom the disease was transmitted by infection of the breath were stricken with pains all over the body and felt a terrible lassitude. There then appeared, on a thigh or an arm, a pustule like a lentil. From this the infection penetrated the body and violent bloody vomiting began. It lasted for a period of three days and there was no way of preventing its ending in death.

Within a couple of years, plague killed around a quarter of Europe's population – and far more in some towns; the largest number of fatalities caused by a single epidemic disaster in the history of Europe. This provoked a lasting demographic crisis. Thousands of villages were abandoned, and by 1427 Florence's population had plummeted by 60 per cent from over 100,000 to about 38,000. A Europe which had been relatively epidemic-free turned into a crucible of pestilences, spawning the obsessions haunting late medieval imaginations: death, decay and the Devil, the *danse macabre* and the Gothic symbols of the skull and crossbones, the Grim Reaper and the Horsemen of the Apocalypse.

Boccaccio (1313–75) gave the most graphic account of plague in the *Decameron*, a collection of tales related by a group of young men and women who had fled Florence to escape it (the regular advice was 'flee early, flee far, return late'). Noting that most of the afflicted died within three days, he recorded:

> Such was the cruelty of heaven and to a great degree of man that between March [1348] and the following July it is estimated that more than 100,000 human beings lost their lives within the walls

of Florence, what with the ravages attendant on the plague and the barbarity of the survivors towards the sick.

So virulent was the plague, 'that the sick communicated it to the healthy who came near them, just as a fire catches anything dry or oily near it' (a sign that ordinary people regarded it as contagious). 'How many valiant men, how many fair ladies, breakfasted with their kinsfolk and that same night supped with their ancestors in the other world.'

Social breakdown followed. In Siena, wrote one survivor,

> Father abandoned child, wife husband, one brother another ...
> none could be found to bury the dead for money or friendship ...
> they died by the hundreds, both day and night, and all were thrown
> in ditches and covered with earth. And as soon as those ditches
> were filled, more were dug. And I, Agnolo di Tura ... buried my
> five children with my own hands.

Though epidemiological controversies have raged, the Black Death was almost certainly bubonic plague, caused by transmission of the bacillus *Yersinia pestis* from rats to humans via fleas (notably *Xenopsylla cheopis*). When the bacillus enters the body through the bite of an infected flea (it can disgorge up to 24,000 in one bite), the disease follows the pattern called bubonic. After a six-day incubation, victims suffer chest pains, coughing, vomiting of blood, breathing troubles, high fever and dark skin blotches caused by internal bleeding (hence the name Black Death), as well as hard, painful egg-sized swellings (buboes) in the lymph nodes in the armpit, groin, neck and behind the ears. Restlessness, delirium, and finally coma and death generally follow. Not all the features familiar in contemporary Asia match those recounted in medieval chronicles. The swift onset suggests that some direct human-to-human transmission also took place, perhaps in the form of pneumonic plague, spread by droplet infection.

Many explanations were inevitably offered: God in His wisdom had sent plague to punish mankind for its sins; it might be the result of planetary conjunctions; amongst the 'natural causes', alterations in the environment could cause a 'pestilential atmosphere' resulting from effluvia, vapours from stagnant pools, dungheaps, decaying corpses, the breath of sufferers themselves – or poisoning of the air by 'enemies' such as Jews. Laymen like Boccaccio referred to contagion, but most medical theorists, loyal to their Greek learning, stood by constitutional factors: if the body was robust, illness should not result; if not, one would sicken and die.

Responses depended upon which theory was accepted. If the plague was truly God-sent, only prayer and fasting could be effective. This encouraged flagellant bands to trudge from town to town, whipping each other, hoping by their lashings and denunciations of Jews and sinners to propitiate divine wrath; which in turn sparked persecution of Jews, who were accused of poisoning the wells. In Basel, Jews were penned up in a wooden building and burnt alive; 2000 were said to have been slaughtered in Strasbourg and 12,000 in Mainz; while in July 1349 the flagellants led the burghers of Frankfurt into the Jewish quarter for a wholesale massacre. But, however pious, the flagellants themselves posed a serious threat to public order by creating panic and challenging authority, leading Pope Clement VI to prohibit them.

Seeking to protect themselves with long leather gowns, gauntlets, and masks with snouts stuffed with aromatic herbs, physicians put the accent on individual treatment, on the assumption that plague involved atmospheric putrefaction. They recommended sniffing amber-scented nosegays and pomanders and administering strong-smelling herbs – aloes, dittany, myrrh and pimpernel, all supposed to have cleansing properties, to say nothing of those princes of pharmacy, mithridatium and theriac. Fires should be lit and rooms fumigated with aromatic wood or vinegar. Writing in 1401, the Florentine doctor Lapo Mazzei (1350–1412) suggested 'it would help you to drink, a quarter of an hour before dinner, a full half-glass of good red wine, neither too dry nor too sweet.'

Faced with plague, physicians had no power to effect public-health measures; that was the magistrate's business. In Venice a committee of three nobles laid down burial regulations, banning the sick from entering the city and jailing intruders. In Milan, the council sealed in the occupants of affected houses and left them to die (perhaps this draconian measure worked: Milan had only a 15 per cent death rate). In Florence a committee of eight was given dictatorial powers, though ordinances requiring the killing of dogs and cats ironically removed the very animals that might have contained the rats. At that time, however, no one had any reason to suspect rats.

Secular and religious strategies were sometimes at odds. In 1469, despite the risks of congregating in large numbers, the civic authorities in Brescia allowed the Corpus Christi procession to go ahead because deliverance, hoped the pious, would come through divine intervention. By contrast, in time of plague the Venice Health Board banned preaching, processions and feast-day assemblies. Churches were locked, and in 1523 and 1529 even the shrine of St Roch, a popular intercessor against plague, was shut.

Certain routines became standard. The committees appointed to co-ordinate public health measures began to remove the sick to leper houses beyond city limits (hence 'lazaretto' came to mean a plague hospital), while also establishing a system of exclusion, banning persons or goods from entering or leaving. Such measures were adopted throughout Italy. In 1377 Ragusa (Dubrovnik, Croatia) instituted a regular thirty-day isolation period on a nearby island for all arriving from plague-infected areas; in 1397 this was increased to forty, thus becoming a true quarantine (*quarantenaria*, forty days). Marseilles took similar action in 1383; Venice imposed quarantine measures in 1423; in 1464 Pisa followed and Genoa three years later.

Before the fifteenth century such health boards, composed of nobles and officials, were *ad hoc* creations. In Milan, however, a permanent magistracy 'for the preservation of health' was established around 1410, with (by 1450) a staff of a physician, surgeon, notary and barber, two horsemen, three footmen and, sensibly, two grave-diggers. Doctors acted not as full members of such boards but as advisers. Other Italian cities followed; in 1486, Venice appointed a permanent Commission of Public Health, consisting of three noblemen; Florence set up a similar commission of five in 1527, and Lucca one of three in 1549. Bills of Mortality were initiated in Milan, listing names and causes of death. Health Boards extended quarantines and the closing of borders, and health passes were introduced. In this respect, north European towns lagged behind Italy by more than a century.

The regulation of markets, streets, hospitals and cemeteries, the control of beggars, prostitutes and Jews – in short, public health measures – fell under the health boards. Resentment was expressed about their cost and powers, especially since economic disaster was almost inevitable once plague had been declared official, with commerce and travel suspended and markets closed.

Obliquely, therefore, medical practitioners became more involved in public administration. Midwives, too, performed policing functions. Laws required them to report illegitimate births, and to press unmarried mothers for the names of the father, so as to secure financial support for the babies. The oaths sworn by English midwives seeking a bishop's licence included promises to extract the truth about paternity and to refuse requests for secret births.

MADNESS

Alongside leprosy and plague, another condition of public concern was insanity. Madness remained particularly disputed. On Galen's authority, medical writers distinguished four main categories: frenzy, mania, melancholy and fatuity, each the result of a particular humoral imbalance. Folklore believed the moon caused lunacy; theology saw it as a consequence of diabolical possession or sorcery. Some viewed it as divinely inspired, perhaps involving the gift of tongues; others praised the innocence of the village idiot; while troubadours might sing of tragic love-madness.

Nor was there agreement over remedies. Some advocated drugs and bleeding to sedate the demented and evacuate peccant humours. Shock treatment might be tried, such as hurling a maniac into a river. For demoniacal possession, there was exorcism, while certain saints had the power to cure madness. Three shrines enjoyed a special reputation: St Mathurin at Larchant and St Acairius at Haspres (both in northern France), and St Dymphna at Geel in Flanders. A hospice built there to house the mentally ill proved too small and many were lodged in village households. From this a special 'family colony' developed, in which the mentally ill were tended by the villagers. The Geel community still exists.

Public attitudes towards the insane were mixed. German municipalities sometimes expelled idiots or insane persons, whipping them out of town – though the celebrated 'ship of fools' is not a reality but a literary conceit, symbolizing humanity's follies. The insane were cared for in monasteries; various towns had madmen's towers (*Narrentürme*); in Paris, special cells were set aside at the Hôtel Dieu; and the Teutonic Knights' hospital at Elbing had a madhouse (*Tollhaus*). Specialized hospitals began to appear, notably under the influence of Islam in Spain: Granada (1365), Valencia (1407), Zaragoza (1425), Seville (1436), Barcelona (1481) and Toledo (1483). The priory of St Mary of Bethlehem in London, founded in 1247, was by 1403 housing six men 'deprived of reason'; it developed into the notorious Bedlam. Such moves towards incarceration were counterbalanced by the image of the mad person as a holy fool, while in the 'feast of fools' medieval society came to terms with mental alienation through the carnival notion of the world turned upside down – madness as dionysian release.

The insane also became linked to witchcraft, with demonic possession serving as an explanation for deranged behaviour. Haunted by plague and heresy, the late medieval church warned against the Devil and his minions; women were considered particularly susceptible to Satan; and during the next 300 years the witch-craze seized Europe, leading to the execution, often after judicial torture, of upwards of 50,000 victims, mainly women (the figure of nine million burnings, often cited in feminist writings, is pure fantasy).

An individual of whom much is known is the English mystic, Margery Kempe (b. 1393). A wealthy woman who owned a brewery in King's Lynn, she fell victim to puerperal insanity and began to behave oddly. Undertaking pilgrimages to Jerusalem, Rome and Spain, she described her spiritual experiences. *The Book of Margery Kempe* (c. 1423), perhaps the very first English autobiography, reveals the contested borderland between illness and religious experience. To some of her companions she was a sick woman, indeed a confounded nuisance with her non-stop wailings; to others, she was the mouthpiece of God – or was possessed by the Devil. 'Many said', she wrote,

> there was never saint in heaven that cried as she did, and from that they concluded she had a devil within her which caused that crying. And this they said openly, amid much more evil talk. She took everything patiently for our Lord's love, for she knew very well that the Jews said much worse of His own person than people did of her, and therefore she took it the more meekly.

WOMEN

Margery Kempe's difficulties derived in part from perceptions of her gender; certain disorders were associated with women and their reproductive systems. Giving birth is depicted in medieval texts as an all-female business, the mother being supported by relatives, neighbours and a midwife. Midwives rose in status, as some town councils paid them to act in an official capacity in cases involving female illness, obstetrics and infant care. They were called upon to test for virginity or sterility, and to certify infant deaths.

A few obstetrical texts were directed to female readers, and male writers discussed gynaecological problems and prescribed remedies for female sexual disorders, advising not least on contraception. The *Treasury of the Poor*, ascribed to Peter of Spain (later Pope John XXI), gave over a hundred prescriptions concerning fertility, aphrodisiacs and contraceptives, presumably derived from popular tradition. Medical attitudes towards sex were far from puritanical, for sexual release was regarded as requisite for humoral balance, and female orgasm was widely believed essential for conception.

Female healers abounded, sometimes learning their craft from a male member of the family, and a few women wrote medical texts. Hildegard of Bingen (1098–1179), who had been put in a convent at the age of eight and began having religious visions soon after, practised medicine in her role as abbess of Rupertsberg. Her main work was the *Liber simplicis medicinae* (*c.* 1150–60) [Book of Simple Medicine], on the curative powers of herbs, stones and animals; she also wrote on the natural causes of diseases. These texts summarize traditional lore concerning the medical uses of animals, vegetables and minerals, advising treatments on the principle of opposites, while for terrible diseases like leprosy she commended exotic remedies involving unicorn liver and lion heart. Herbs were God's gifts; either they would cure or the patients 'will die for God did not will that they should be healed'.

Another acclaimed woman healer is more enigmatic. Obstetrical writings and other treatises of women's disorders are attributed to a certain Trotula, said to be a female member of the medical school of Salerno during the twelfth century; but 'Trotula', anglicized as 'Dame Trot', was more likely a male writing in drag. Texts called *The English Trotula* long circulated, containing advice on conception, pregnancy and childbirth and motherhood (nursing mothers should avoid highly salted or spiced food).

A few female healers were accepted into the Florentine practitioners' guild, and English records show women called 'leech' or '*medica*'; at St Leonard's Hospital, York, a Sister Ann was described in 1276 as a *medica*. But women were excluded in the later Middle Ages, marginalized by professional conflicts and guild restrictive practices. In 1421, the English physician Gilbert Kymer and his cronies petitioned Parliament to ban women from practising. The limitation of medical and surgical practice to those who had received a university training or were enrolled in a guild tended to confine women to nursing, midwifery and home physic.

Control of midwifery became more common from the fifteenth century. The Papal Bull of 1484 denouncing witchcraft drew attention to alleged attacks by sorceresses on virility and fertility; in their viciously misogynistic *Malleus maleficarum* (1486) [Hammer of Witches], the Dominicans Henricus Institoris (Heinrich Krämer, *fl.* 1470–1501) and Jacob Sprenger (*fl.* 1468–94) accused midwives of murdering babies in the womb, roasting them at sabbaths or offering them to the Devil. There is little evidence, however, that female healers were charged with witchcraft.

Medieval authors on sex and childbirth (or 'generation' as the subject was known) drew on a variety of traditions: Aristotle, Galen, Soranus and the Bible. The standard view was that men and women shared a common physiology, but in perfect and flawed versions. Female generative organs were like those of men, but inverted and inferior – the vagina was an inverted penis which had never fully developed. Thus, the female form was a faulty version of the male, weaker, because menstruation and tearfulness displayed a watery, oozing physicality; female flesh was moister and flabbier, men were more muscular. A woman's body was deficient in the vital heat which allowed the male to refine into semen the surplus blood which women shed in menstruation; likewise, women produced milk instead of semen. Women were leaky vessels (menstruating, crying, lactating), and menstruation was polluting.

De secretis mulierum [On Women's Secrets] spelt out the harmful effects of menstruation:

> women are so full of venom in their time of menstruation that they poison animals by their glance; they infect children in the cradle; they spot the cleanest mirror; and whenever men have sexual intercourse with them, they are made leprous and sometimes cancerous.

The womb was an unstable organ, making women less balanced than men. Social consequences followed from these physiological teachings. According to the instigator of the Reformation, Martin Luther (1483–1546),

> Men have broad and large chests, and small narrow hips, and more understanding than women, who have but small and narrow breasts,

and broad hips, to the end they should remain at home, sit still, keep house, and bear and bring up children.

Controversies flared among doctors, philosophers and theologians over the gendering and engendering of the body. The roles of the male and female in fecundation were disputed, as Aristotle's distinction between superior male 'form' and inferior female 'matter' (seed and seedbed), clashed with the Galenic theory of the confluence of male and female semen to make a baby. Such niceties could have weighty implications: how, for example, had the Virgin Mary conceived Christ – was it from menstrual blood, or was such blood a waste product? Contrasting explanations could also be given regarding the means and the moment of the soul's entering the foetus.

In the later Middle Ages, medical and Christian views cross-fertilized at many points as the body assumed heightened significance in the humanistic theology of the times. While some, like the early Church Fathers, still viewed it as the prison of the spirit, new emphasis came to be placed on the soul's incarnation in the flesh, the doctrine of immanentism. In the consecration of the host in the eucharist, the bread was transubstantiated into Christ's body, turning miraculously to flesh. There was similar stress on bodily resurrection at the Last Judgment. In Catholic rituals, a saint's power was associated with relics of the body: a hallowed bone, tooth or toenail protecting against evil; hence the booming relics business.

BODIES

Theological concerns loomed large in readings of the body, yet medicine too was concerned with the implications of the theory of embodiment and the soul. Scholastic medicine subscribed to the Chain of Being or Scale of Nature, with man as the midpoint between angels and brutes, distinguished from the beasts by possession of a rational soul. One consequence of this doctrine was that, considered in a purely physical light, the human body could be described in the same terms as that of a pig or a monkey. Belief in such a continuum of creation explains why the earliest medieval anatomies, conducted at Salerno and Bologna, could be performed on animals: the human soul was unique, so similarities between human and animal cadavers were not theologically worrying.

The first recorded public human dissection was conducted in Bologna around 1315 by Mondino de' Luzzi (*c.* 1270–1326). Born into a medical family, Mondino graduated at Bologna, and rose to a chair of medicine there. His fame rests on his *Anatomia mundini* (*c.* 1316), which became the standard text on the subject. Built on personal experience of human dissection, the *Anatomia* was a brief, practical guide, treating the parts of the body in the order in which they would be handled in dissection, beginning with the abdominal cavity, the most perishable part. Relying on Galen and the Arabs, the *Anatomia* perpetuated old errors derived from animal dissections, such as the five-lobed liver and the three-ventricled heart. Mondino's achievement derived from his intuition that the developing university-based education of his day required an introductory anatomy manual. The first printed version appeared in 1478, followed by at least forty editions – a clear recognition of how central anatomy was becoming to medical expertise.

Hitherto anatomy had played little part in medical education; it had no place in the *Articella* or the medical school of Salerno, though pigs had been dissected there. But from Mondino's time learned physicians began to enunciate the view that medicine should be anatomy-based. Thereafter academic physicians gloried in public displays of human dissection and anatomy theatres were built. Dissection was justified largely in terms of natural philosophy and piety (the body demonstrated the wisdom of the Creator); the surgical benefits were rarely mentioned – clear evidence of the professional function of physicians' anatomical knowledge.

Various factors contributed to the rise of human anatomy, among them Galen's prestige (after all Galen had prided himself upon his dissecting abilities). Tampering with human remains was far from unknown in medieval Christendom. The wish to bring dead crusaders back from the Holy Land for burial had led to the custom of boiling up bodies to leave only the bones, and to the preservation of the heart of the deceased. Though this practice was condemned by Boniface VIII in 1300, the papal ban proved ineffective. From around 1250, autopsies also became regular in Italian, French and German towns, with surgeons called in to investigate homicide and establish cause of death. The step from a coroner's postmortem to dissection was small.

Public dissection was spectacle, instruction and edification all in one. The corpse would be that of an executed criminal, presupposing municipal cooperation. It was sometimes staged in a church, usually in winter, since cold slowed putrefaction. Mondino's order of dissection of the three main bodily cavities – first the lower abdomen, then the thorax and the skull – was designed with decay in mind. In illustrations of dissections, a physician resplendent in academic robes sits on a throne, intoning from a Galenic anatomical text, while a surgeon slits the cadaver with his knife, and a teaching assistant points out notable features. Whether or not dissections were actually conducted in this way, what is conveyed is the ritual of the performance: religious, civic, and university authorities agreed that the occasion must be accorded due gravity.

Book-driven anatomy – a demonstration of what was already known, within the explanatory framework of learned medicine – served many purposes, providing guidance to the student, who would not have been able to see much for himself. From Bologna, human dissection spread; the next key centre was Padua, which was popular with foreign students. In Spain, the first public dissection took place at Lerida in 1391; Vienna held its first in 1404. In England and Germany anatomy teaching with a human corpse did not become routine before 1550.

Anatomy had an impact upon medical illustrations – a subject bedevilled by modern prejudices about 'realism', for medievals who drew 'childish' images of the bones and arteries have been adversely contrasted with the new 'scientific' artists of the Renaissance (notably Leonardo da Vinci), admired for their realistic anatomical drawings. But the comparison is misleading. For one thing, Leonardo at times followed tradition rather than his eye, adopting, for instance, the standard five-lobed liver. For another, it is wrong to think that the apparent crudity of medieval images reveals ineptitude. Late medieval illustrations were not meant to depict minute documentary detail; they were diagrammatic teaching aids, schematically representing general truths – mnemonic rather than photographic.

The most common type of medieval medical illustration was the 'Zodiac man': a male figure marked up with blood-letting points or with the zodiac signs (Taurus controlled and cured diseases of the neck and throat, Scorpio the genitals, Capricorn the knees, Pisces the feet, and so forth). The right way and place to let blood was gauged by study of the constellations and the moon. There was also the group known as the 'five-picture series', standing for the five systems: arteries, veins, bones, nerves and muscles. Squatting figures with legs astride were occasionally used to show diseases, wounds and the influence of the stars and planets on body parts. There were also charts explaining how to examine urine. The success of such images is evident: they survived into the age of print, wound-men in particular continuing to crop up in surgery texts.

The late Middle Ages wear a gloom-laden appearance: painters gave Death a mocking grin and portrayed him accosting peasants, merchants and princes. Perhaps for this reason, and because it was roundly disparaged by Renaissance humanists, medieval medicine has never enjoyed a good press. Proud of recovering Hippocrates and Galen in the original Greek, humanists chid and despised their muddle-headed predecessors.

We should not blindly accept these judgments. Much was afoot before 1500: in particular the fifteenth century brought a rise in practical medicine, associated with the books of *practica* and case-histories (*consilia*) produced by Italian professors. Bedside consultations, autopsies and the spread of dissection gave Italian medical training an increasingly hands-on emphasis. It is ironic that from the 1490s the medical humanists reverted to theory, to philology and medicine's 'sacred' books, notably through the Galen revival.

The later Middle Ages also consolidated the role of medicine in European society, with new institutions and regulations. At the time when the Salerno school was founded, physicians were to be found only in monasteries and palaces; five hundred years later they had infiltrated society (remember the physician on Chaucer's pilgrimage) and were facing competition from other practitioners like barber-surgeons, professional bickering being but one sign of this growing medical presence. Other domains of life were falling under medical control: health officials directed urban hygiene and combated plague. From birth to death – and even beyond, if one had the misfortune to be cut up for a public anatomy display – medicine gained a hold that it had previously lacked or lost.

CHAPTER VI

INDIAN MEDICINE

EACH AREA OF THE GLOBE has created a medicine of its own. The neolithic revolution in India and China produced civilizations comparable in complexity and achievements to the developments discussed in the Middle East, the Levant and the eastern Mediterranean, like these, founded upon an agrarian economy sustaining, and sustained by, political overlords and large urban settlements. In the great Asiatic empires social hierarchy and the consequent division of labour facilitated the emergence of specialist healers, together with priests, wise men and bureaucrats.

The consolidation of writing encouraged learned traditions which helped to give permanence to particular corpuses of medical (as well as religious and philosophical) erudition. As with the writings of Hippocrates and Galen in the West, the result tended to be a glorification of tradition, and the associated belief that a fixed, permanent and perfect medicine had, in a quasi-divine manner, been handed down from some far-distant origin. It was the duty of successors to uphold such a tradition, protecting and purifying it against the threat of corruption. Such values imparted into Asian medical systems a great durability; they certainly gave no encouragement to innovation. Indian and Chinese medicine alike proved tenacious and encouraged myths of an essential unchangingness – though this was actually belied by developments. The consequence was that both traditional Indian and traditional Chinese medicine continued in place; yet both experienced in due course a tense and ambiguous encounter with western 'scientific medicine', which left them compelled to take aspects of it on board.

EARLY INDIA

As in many other parts of the world, the first settled agricultural communities in India appeared at the end of the last Ice Age about ten
thousand years ago; around 3000 BC, as archaeology reveals, developments took place around the Indus river leading to elaborate civilization.
Excavations of the imposing Indus cities of Harappa, Mohenjo-daro and
Lothal have revealed what must have been a complex urban social order,
with well-defined social and occupational hierarchies. As well as priests,
healers must have existed: perhaps the function was twinned. Remains
of great public water tanks in these cities suggest communal bathing
and hence cleansing rites, perhaps linking ritual to hygiene.

Around 1500 BC, this Indus civilization seems to have fallen into
decay; the explanation for this may lie in climatic and environmental
changes affecting the water courses. Meanwhile, the Indo-European
peoples were migrating into south Asia, and their civilization achieved
a position of dominance in the subcontinent. Brotherhoods of hereditary
priests (*brahmana*) grew powerful, becoming the masters and guardians
of Sanskrit religious teachings called *veda* (the knowledge). Though
there is no distinctive 'Vedic medicine', such religious writings shed
some indirect light on contemporary beliefs about health and healing.

It seems that a magico-religious outlook on illnesses and treatments
became established which broadly parallels Mesopotamian or Egyptian
practices. Distinctive healing powers were associated with particular
deities, it being believed that diseases could be produced by wicked
spirits or by happenstance. The deities who brought disease visitations
were to be propitiated by rites involving *mantra* (incantations), supplications and expiation. Herbs were valued for their therapeutic powers,
while injuries and broken bones were attributed to everyday causes; but
some diseases – conditions like *yaksma* (perhaps consumption) and *tak-
man* (fevers associated with the monsoon season) – were judged to be
signs of demonic and magical interventions. Beliefs about the body and
its workings came from various sources. Vedic rites involved the use of
animal and human sacrifice, and the ceremonial texts contain some
listings of anatomical parts. Some basic forms of surgery were also
recorded, cauterization being employed to stanch wounds, and reeds
were used as catheters to relieve the retention of urine. Vedic writings

speak of the value of water, whether to be bathed in, drunk or ritually applied.

From perhaps 1000 BC, Veda constituted the main faith of north India. Other groups also were appearing, seemingly dedicated to making religion a more spiritual matter and placing emphasis upon the need to lead a life of moral uprightness. Alongside many individual ascetics, the chief and best known of such groups was the Buddhist community, founded by Gautama Sakyamuni (the Buddha, 563–483 BC). Others included those subsequently called the Jains. These gatherings gave rise to new medical practices.

The monastic rule which governed the lives of Buddhist monks, dedicated to acquiring the 'peace of mind brought about by the abandonment of desire', declared that among their meagre belongings should be included five elementary medicines: fresh butter, clarified butter (*ghee*), oil, honey and molasses. This list expanded in time to embrace a large pharmacopoeia and divers foodstuffs. Archaeological evidence from the fourth century AD shows that some Buddhist monasteries included a sick-room, which may have developed into a more distinct hospital, at around the same time as the emergence of hospitals in the Christian West. Initially, the monks' healing activities were for fellow brethren, but, as in the West, the monasteries also served the lay community.

In contrast to the earlier Vedic medicine, which is not at all similar to Ayurveda, there are striking resemblances between these Buddhist texts and later Ayurvedic texts on medicinal herbs and on specific treatments. In terms of origins and influences, the Ayurvedic texts are themselves misleading, since they claim a derivation from the Vedic tradition. The reality is that, while the situation is complex and controversial, they probably developed out of the newer ascetic milieu. Best scholarly opinion today holds that the ascetic communities of the fourth century BC onwards, particularly the Buddhist community, played a vital part in the evolution of Ayurveda.

AYURVEDIC MEDICINE

The archetypal system of Indian medicine is called *Ayurveda* – the knowledge (Sanskrit: *veda*) needed for longevity (*ayus*). Ayurvedic teachings amount to a code of life and consist of practical advice concerning all aspects of life, from washing to diet, from exercise to regimen, within a wider Hindu religious philosophy of rebirth, renunciation, and the maintenance of the balance of the soul. Their theoretical foundation lies in the notion of three basic bodily humours (*dosas*) – wind, bile, and phlegm – which reflect the macrocosmic forces of wind, sun and moon. There are also seven fundamental bodily constituents: chyle, blood, flesh, fat, bone, marrow and semen. The Ayurvedic pharmacopoeia is mainly herbal, prescribing an assortment of therapies including oint-ments, enemas, douches, massage, sweating and surgery. Though met-allic compounds came into medical use from around AD 1000, these remained marginal; opium too was brought in, apparently from Islamic sources, to relieve dysentery. For achieving health, the canonical texts stress temperance in all matters – food, sleep, exercise, sex and medicines themselves. The healthy life is to be consonant with the harmonies of the universe and true religious teachings.

Written in Sanskrit, the earliest surviving Ayurveda texts date from the early centuries of the Christian era; traditional claims among prac-titioners that Ayurveda dates back thousands of years are pious. Of the various Sanskrit writings that expound the Ayurveda, the earliest are the *Caraka Samhita* [Caraka's Compendium] and the *Susruta Samhita* [Susruta's Compendium], supposedly the work of the sages Caraka and Susruta. Very substantial in bulk, they form the cornerstone of Ayur-veda. A third early text, the *Bhela Samhita*, survives only in a single damaged manuscript.

The *Caraka Samhita* tradition is connected with north-western India, and in particular the ancient university of Taksasila; the *Susruta Samhita* was supposedly composed in Benares on the River Ganges. Their original composition date is a matter of speculation: earlier ver-sions may derive from as far back as the time of the Buddha (early fourth century BC). Caraka may date to around AD 100; Susruta to the fourth century. The Sanskrit texts which became canonical represent the works in the form they had attained around AD 1000.

There are other subsequent prominent Brahminic texts. These include the *Astangahrdaya Samhita* of Vagbhata (AD *c.* 600), which includes midwifery, the *Rugviniscaya* of Madhavakara (AD *c.* 700), the *Sarngadhara Samhita* of Sarngadhara (*c.* fourteenth century AD), and the *Bhavaprakasa* of Bhavamisra (sixteenth century). Madhavakara's work broke new ground through rearranging medical topics according to pathological categories, thereby establishing the model of thematic grouping followed by almost all later works. Sarngadhara was the first Sanskrit author to introduce new foreign elements, including opium and metallic compounds, into the *materia medica*, and the use of pulse lore in diagnosis and prognosis.

The *Caraka Samhita* and the *Susruta Samhita* stem from a common intellectual tradition. The *Caraka Samhita* is marked by long reflective and philosophical passages, including discussions of causality and so forth. The *Susruta Samhita* for its part contains extensive descriptions of sophisticated surgical techniques: eye operations, plastic surgery, etc., which do not appear in the *Caraka Samhita* at all or only in less detail. Both are huge compendia of medical teachings on subjects such as a balanced diet; the powers of plants and vegetables; the causes and symptoms of various maladies; epidemic diseases; the right techniques for examining patients; the parts of the body; conception, pregnancy and the way to take care of foetuses; diagnosis and prognosis; stimulants and aphrodisiacs; the nature and treatment of fever, heated blood, swellings, urinary and skin disorders, consumption, insanity, epilepsy, dropsy, piles, asthma, coughs and hiccups and scores of other conditions; cupping, blood-letting, the use of leeches, and many other treatments; the right use of alcohol; the properties of vegetables, nuts, and other *materia medica*; the use of enemas – and all alongside incantations, omens and fears of sorcery.

The medicines described in the *Caraka Samhita* and the *Susruta Samhita* comprise a rich menu of animal, vegetable, and mineral substances. For dealing with the 200 diseases and 150 other conditions mentioned, the *Caraka Samhita* refers to 177 materials of animal derivation, including snake dung, the milk, flesh, fat, blood, dung, or urine of such animals as the horse, goat, elephant, camel, cow and sheep, the eggs of the sparrow, pea-hen and crocodile, beeswax and honey, and various soups; 341 items of vegetable origin (seeds, flowers, fruit, tree-bark and leaves), and 64 substances of mineral origin (assorted gems, gold, silver, copper, salt, clay, tin, lead and sulphur). The use of dung and urine are standard; since the cow is a holy animal to orthodox Hindus, all its products are purifying. Cow dung was judged to possess disinfectant properties and was prescribed for external use, including fumigation; urine was to be applied externally in many recipes.

The *Caraka Samhita* praises the virtuous healer: 'Everyone admires a twice-born [brahmin] physician who is courteous, wise, self-disciplined, and a master of his subject. He is like a guru, a master of life itself.' Quacks, by contrast, are roundly condemned: 'As soon as they hear someone is ill, they descend on him and in his hearing speak loudly of their medical expertise.' In respect of the true physician, the *Caraka Samhita* tenders an Oath of Initiation, comparable to the Hippocratic Oath. A pupil in Ayurvedic medicine had to vow to be celibate, to speak the truth, to adhere to a vegetarian diet, to be free of envy, and never to carry weapons. He was to obey his master and pledge himself to the relief of his patients, never abandoning or taking sexual advantage of them. He was not to treat enemies of the king or wicked people, and had to desist from treating women unattended by their husbands or guardians. The student had to visit the patient's home properly chaperoned, and respect the confidentiality of all privileged information pertaining to the patient and his or her household.

The diagnostic and therapeutic aspects of Ayurveda depended on knowledge of the canonical Sanskrit texts. The good physician (*vaidya*) memorized material consisting largely of verses which specified the correlations between the three humours (wind, bile and phlegm), and the various symptoms, complaints and treatments. He conducted an examination of his patient which took into account the symptoms, in the process recalling verses applicable to the patient's condition. These would trigger remembrance of further verses containing the same combinations of humoral references, all of which would lead to a prognosis and a proposed therapy.

The Ayurvedic schemes of substances, qualities and actions offered the *vaidya* an effective combination of solid learned structure and freedom to act. The practice of Ayurveda depended heavily upon oral traditions, passed down from master to pupil, in which a huge magazine of memorized textual material was recreated to fit particular circumstances, while remaining faithful to the fundamental meaning of the text. (The role of precedent within English Common Law offers a parallel.)

The *Susruta Samhita* is distinctive for its wide-ranging section on surgery, which describes how a surgeon should be trained and the various operations he should perform. There are, among other things, descriptions of cutting for stone, couching for cataract, the way to extract arrowheads and splinters, suturing, and the examination of human corpses as part of the study of anatomy. The text maintains that surgery is the oldest and most useful of the eight branches of medical knowledge, and elaborate surgical techniques are described. However, there is little evidence to confirm that these practices persisted. A description of the couching operation for cataract exists in the ninth-century *Kalyanaka-raka* by Ugraditya, and texts based on the *Susruta Samhita* copy out the sections on surgery with other material. But medical texts give no evidence of any continuous development of surgical thinking; no ancient or even medieval surgical instruments survive; nor is surgery described in literary or other sources. A parallel may be found in the apparent fate of surgery within the Islamic tradition.

One possible explanation for this apparent waning of surgery is that, as the caste system grew more rigid, taboos concerning physical contact became stronger and, a little like Hippocratic doctors, *vaidyas* may have shunned therapies which involved applying the knife to the body, transferring their attention to less intrusive approaches, including examination of the pulse and the tongue. Whatever the reasons, the early sophistication of surgical knowledge seems to have been an isolated phenomenon in the development of the Indian medical tradition.

There is, however, one well-documented historical event which suggests that surgery akin to the *Susruta Samhita* remained widely known. In March 1793, an operation was undertaken in Poona of significance for the later course of plastic surgery. A Maratha named Cowasjee, a bullock driver with the English army, having been captured by Tipu Sultan's forces, had his nose and one hand cut off – a customary punishment for adultery. He turned to a man of the brickmakers' caste to have his face repaired. Thomas Cruso (d. 1802) and James Trindlay, surgeons in the Bombay Presidency, witnessed this operation, publishing in 1794 an account of what they had seen, with an engraving of the patient and diagrams of the skin-graft procedure. The obscure brickmaker, reported the English surgeons, had performed a superb skin-graft and nose reconstruction using a technique superior to anything they had ever seen. It was taken up in Europe and became known as the 'Hindu method'.

This may seem to be proof of the persistence of Susruta's surgery during the course of well over a thousand years, but there are puzzling elements to the tale – notably the fact that rhinoplasty of this kind is not delineated in any detail in the *Susruta Samhita*. Furthermore, as a member of the brickmakers' caste, the surgeon who performed the Poona operation was not himself a *vaidya*. He probably knew no Sanskrit: his skill lay in his hands, not in his head. It is conceivable that this represents a survival of a procedure from Susruta's time, but if so it seems to have been passed down independently of the practice of educated physicians. There is no evidence from other written sources of the practice of such operations in the intervening period.

A similar puzzle is posed by smallpox. Before the nineteenth century, inoculation was popular knowledge and widely used for protection against the disease, with the expectation that a mild episode would follow. After the graft the patient was kept quarantined in a controlled environment. A detailed account by an English surgeon, dating from 1767, describes the practice and states that it was widespread in Bengal. No trace of inoculation appears, however, in any Sanskrit medical text. The disease was undeniably identified in Ayurvedic writings, where it is called the 'lentil' disease, but again the link between theory and practice is tenuous. It seems that techniques recorded in texts, though still related in the learned tradition, fell into disuse, while new developments were widely practised without being inscribed in approved medical learning.

In this light it is easy to fall into the trap of assuming that the Ayurvedic tradition was static and 'timeless' – that later texts did no more than to elaborate a coherent and comprehensive set of teachings set out, once and for all, in the *Caraka Samhita* and the *Susruta Samhita*. This supposition is given some support by the fact that these two texts do present themselves as unchanging bodies of knowledge; moreover, it is in line with native and foreign stereotypes of India as the fountainhead of eternal truths. But while the canonical texts present the appearance of homogeneity, research into the development of Sanskrit Ayurvedic literature has revealed that numerous authors dissented from orthodox viewpoints. In the course of time new diseases were reported and identified. From the sixteenth century syphilis (known as 'foreigners' disease' in Sanskrit) was described in texts (mercury, brought to India by Islamic physicians, was used to treat it); and from the eighteenth century writings embraced disease descriptions evidently borrowed from western medicine.

There were also innovations in diagnostics. Close attention to urine, and techniques for its inspection, stem from the eleventh century. Before the thirteenth century there is no mention of pulse examination in Sanskrit texts, but it subsequently developed into a key diagnostic method. A technique called 'examination of the eight bases' (*astasthanapariksa*) – the routine diagnostic method for examining the patient's pulse, urine, faeces, tongue, eyes, general appearance, voice and skin – emerged in the sixteenth century. Novel prognostic techniques also came into use. For example, from about the same time, a procedure was taught whereby a bead of oil was dropped on the surface of a patient's urine. The remaining span of his life was read from the way the oil spread.

In therapy, a discernible shift lay in the rise of standardized compound medicines (*yoga*). Consisting of a large number of ingredients, *yoga* is regularly described in terms of its specific effectiveness against a particular ailment; this brings into question the conventional western view that Ayurvedic medicine was invariably holistic.

Though Ayurveda is the most familiar tradition of indigenous Indian medicine, others have flourished in the subcontinent, notably the Siddha system of the Tamils and the Yunani medicine of Islam. Other assorted therapies are also visible, from folk medicine and shamanism to faith-healing and astrology.

In south India, the form of medicine evolved in the Tamil-speaking areas was dissimilar in certain aspects to Ayurveda. Known as Siddha medicine (Tamil: *cittar*), this was basically an esoteric magical and alchemical system, presumably heavily influenced by tantric ideas. It was characterized by a greater use of metals, in particular mercury, than in Ayurveda, and prized a substance called *muppu*, credited with possessing great powers for physical and spiritual transformation. Pulse taking was highly valued for diagnosis. The semi-legendary founders of Siddha medicine include Bogar, who is said to have journeyed to China, teaching and learning alchemical lore, and Ramadevar, who supposedly travelled to Mecca, teaching the Arabs the arts of alchemy.

From earliest times, Ayurvedic medicine handled and treated a range of children's maladies, blaming them on the evil influence of celestial demons (*graha*, seizer), believed to attack children. The Sanskrit term *graha* was subsequently used to mean 'planet', and although *grahas* are clearly described as celestial beings in the *Susruta Samhita*, later rites for planetary propitiation are targeted at the same types of influence. Indian astrology and religious ordinances contain texts for placating heavenly bodies, as well as astrological prognostications regarding such matters as pregnancy and the sex of unborn children, dream interpretation, sickness and death. According to an early and significant legal work, 'one desirous of prosperity, of removing evil or calamities, of rainfall [for farming], long life, bodily health and one desirous of performing magic rites against enemies and others should perform sacrifice to planets.'

A work exemplifying the close relationship between medicine and astrology as therapeutic systems is the *Virasimhavaloka* by Virasimpa, written in AD 1383, probably in Gwalior. It deals with diseases from three points of view: astrology, religion, and medicine. The body parts are matched to the constellations and planets in an intricate scheme of influences and associations, and it is the astrologer's task to read this pattern of symbols to understand the patient's problem before advising remedies such as charms, expiations, prayers and herbs.

The Bower manuscript, one of the oldest surviving Indian works, contains a text on divination by dice. It reveals the outlook of a fifth-century healer interested in the therapeutic powers of garlic, in elixirs for eternal life, in the treatment of eye diseases, herbal medicines, butter decoctions, aphrodisiacs, oils, the care of children, and spells against snake-bites, as well as divination.

NEW ARRIVALS

Islam brought new medical practices to India, having a major impact after the eleventh-century Turco-Afghan invasions of Gujarat, and becoming entrenched especially around Lahore, Agra, Lucknow and Delhi. These were known as Yunani Tibb – *Yunani* (or *unani*) being an Indian representation of the word 'Ionian'. Yunani medicine derives in large part from Galenic medicine as interpreted in Ibn Sina's *Al-Qanun fi'l-tibb* [Canon], and continues to flourish in India today. It is practised by *hakims* (physicians) in rural areas especially and is advocated among those who wish to embrace a distinctively Islamic medicine.

Yunani medicine and Ayurveda have interacted to some degree, especially in *materia medica*. Though the primary languages of Yunani medicine are Persian and Arabic, there are also certain Sanskrit texts. Yunani postulates four basic humours, as distinct from Ayurveda's three, and it has more of an orientation towards treatments in hospitals. The major difference between them is their clientèle. Broadly, Yunani physicians treat Muslim patients, and Ayurvedic physicians treat Hindus.

In the first half of the sixteenth century Portuguese settlers came to Goa. The first medical book printed in India was the *Coloquios dos Simples, e Drogas he Cousas Mediçinais da India* (1563) [Colloquies on the Medical Simples and Drugs of India] by Garcia d'Orta (1490–1570). D'Orta had gathered his material from local physicians, and the signs are that there was a free exchange of medical ideas at that time between the Portuguese and the Indians. Relationships however declined, and after 1600 the Portuguese introduced restrictions which in effect banned Hindu physicians in Goa.

Dutch East India Company officials showed great interest in the natural history and medicines of the Malabar coast where they traded and settled. Heinrich van Rheede (1637–91), the Dutch governor, published between 1686 and 1703 a work containing nearly 800 plates of Indian plants. Paul Herman's (1646–95) herbarium and *Museum Zeylanicum* provided major sources for Linnaeus's *Flora Zeylanica* (1747).

The British arrived around 1600. Facing unfamiliar and severe health problems, East India Company traders were keen to learn from the local *vaidyas* and *hakims*, and Indian doctors were curious about British surgery, since the art had lapsed among *vaidyas*. It was observed by Sir William Sleeman (1788–1856) that 'the educated class, as indeed all classes, say that they do not want our physicians, but stand much in need of our surgeons.'

British physicians were initially prompted to adopt Indian methods by the problems involved in shipping medical stores from Europe. In time, however, they grew increasingly critical of the crudeness of indigenous drugs and contemptuous of what they saw as the shortcomings of Indian medicine. With characteristic ethnocentricity, East India Company attitudes towards Indian medicine hardened. When medical colleges had been founded in Bengal and elsewhere under the British Raj, the study of Ayurveda was given a semblance of support alongside British medicine; but with changes in educational policy after 1835 and the suppression of Ayurvedic teaching in state-funded medical colleges, British support for Ayurvedic training ceased. Ayurvedic physicians continued to practise, although their training was reduced to the traditional family apprenticeship system.

In the twentieth century, with the rise of the Indian independence movement, indigenous traditions received active encouragement from nationalists. In recent decades there have been divided loyalties: since independence in 1947, the Indian government has oscillated between commitment to western medicine in the name of progress, and acceptance of the fact that Ayurvedic medicine is widely practised, especially in the countryside, and commands sturdy loyalties. Many Indian physicians have a strong incentive to devote themselves to western medicine – it is a passport to practise throughout the world.

In 1970, the Indian Parliament passed the Indian Medicine Central Council Act, setting up a central council for Ayurveda. Since then government-accredited colleges and universities have provided professional training and qualifications. This training, however, includes some basic education in western methods, family planning and public health. In 1983, there were approximately one hundred officially approved Ayurvedic training colleges, many attached to universities. But although the number of Ayurvedic and Yunani colleges and dispensaries has multiplied since independence, government funding has been minimal. Popular perception is said to be that the students in the indigenous medical schools failed to gain admission to modern western medical or professional universities.

The traditions combine and are rarely exclusive. Private Ayurvedic practitioners make use of modern western treatments, often on the wishes of their patients: western-style injections are widely regarded as a powerful, almost magical cure. In a small 1970s study of fifty-nine indigenous practitioners in Punjab and Mysore, researchers found that the vast majority of drugs being used were antibiotics and similar western medicines. The idea that Ayurvedic physicians deal purely in herbs, roots, and therapeutic massage is a nostalgic myth. Today in India, the patient may take any of many available paths towards greater health. There exist side by side physicians of cosmopolitan medicine, Ayurveda, and Yunani, as well as others such as homoeopaths, naturopaths, traditional bone-setters, yoga teachers and faith-healers.

The trend, however, is towards the greater assimilation of western medicine, especially among the wealthy and cosmopolitan. It is noteworthy that Ayurvedic medicine has not yet achieved the vogue in the West acquired by Indian philosophy and (thanks to fascination with acupuncture and the yin-yang system) by Chinese medicine.

CHAPTER VII

CHINESE MEDICINE

AS WITH AYURVEDIC MEDICINE in the Indian subcontinent, traditional Chinese medicine has often been commended as ancient and timeless. Its champions (and occasionally its detractors) assert that Chinese medicine is essentially unchanged since the composition over two thousand years ago of the *Yellow Emperor's Inner Canon of Medicine* (so called because it includes a dialogue between the 'yellow emperor' Huang-ti and his chief minister, Ch'i Po).

This characterization – rather like the claim that, by contrast with western biomedicine, it is mild, draws only upon 'natural' substances and is holistic – is to some extent the expression of deep-seated preferences. Even so, the long history of Chinese medicine, and its ingrained attitudes towards knowledge and the human body, provide some grounds for the contrast. The upholding of traditional values and texts has counted for much and, unlike the West, novelty has never been greatly valued in the Chinese medical tradition, or for that matter in Chinese intellectual and cultural life in general.

Chinese medicine is certainly distinctive yet not totally different from other medical traditions, and that is partly because it is not wholly indigenous. Over the centuries, it absorbed many outside influences, from India, Tibet, central and south-east Asia. Since around 1850, it has been forced to come to terms with medicine from the West. It is thought that blood-letting and the needling techniques from which acupuncture developed may have originated in central Asian shamanic curing. Buddhism brought from India beliefs concerning the soul and salvation which endorsed care for the ill and debilitated: the needy could find help in monastic hospitals or secure charitable treatment at dispensaries.

Indian medical theories are not easily reconciled with Chinese models, however, though some scholars have held that the influence of Ayurvedic or even Galenic classifications may be found in the use of such categories as 'hot' and 'cold' in Chinese *materia medica*. (Such elements are more plausibly viewed as transcultural rather than as direct borrowings.) Buddhist charms were incorporated into classical Chinese therapy, and during the medieval period cataract operations were performed which probably derived from India. Certain of the key drugs in the *materia medica* were introduced or imported from abroad – ginseng from Korea, musk from Tibet, camphor, cardamom and cloves from south-east Asia, aniseed, saffron, frankincense and myrrh from Persia and Arabia.

Chinese medicine thus assimilated elements from elsewhere; and as the Chinese tongue, Chinese Buddhism and Confucian philosophy were embraced by elites in various parts of east Asia, so too was Chinese medicine. It was probably introduced to Korea with Buddhism before the sixth century AD, and Buddhist priests conveyed it from there to Japan. (Chinese medicine is known as *hanui* in Korea, and as *kanpo* in Japan.) From the sixteenth century, it was taken by migrants to Taiwan, the Philippines and much of south-east Asia, and from the nineteenth century to the Americas and other continents. In such areas, it flourishes today alongside western medicine. Certain aspects, notably moxibustion and its needling techniques, became reasonably familiar in the West from the seventeenth century, but they made few inroads into western medicine, though by the early nineteenth century acupuncture began to enjoy a vogue, especially in France. Only time will tell whether the current popularity of acupuncture and Chinese medical philosophies will be lasting.

CHINESE HEALING

Medical learning was pursued, taught, developed and practised by educated males, who mainly treated clients from the middle and higher strata of urban society. The great mass of peasants and other poor people had recourse to folk or religious healers.

The main source for our knowledge of the history of classical Chinese medicine lies in a corpus of texts: these include works on medical theory; on the classification, diagnosis, and treatment of diseases (including compilations of particular physicians' case histories); and on drug use and prescriptions. Some ten thousand such specialized medical works exist.

The earliest surviving texts date back about twenty-two centuries, and include even older materials. This is an outcome of political and dynastic circumstances. China became politically unified in 221 BC, and the first emperors of the Han dynasty (206 BC–AD 220) set about laying down political, philosophical and cosmological orthodoxy. This period brought the emergence of the medical canon which constitutes the theoretical basis for the 'high classical tradition' of medicine, which set the reference frame for subsequent thinking and debate. A unified empire created and demanded a unified body; the healthy state presupposed thinking about the healthy body.

The core works in this tradition are the *Inner Canon*, the *Divine Husbandman's Materia Medica*, the *Canon of Problems* and the *Treatise on Cold-Damage Disorders*. The former two works are scriptural in status, considered as comprising the wisdom and teachings of legendary sages. A learned physician would be expected to be completely familiar with these works. The two latter works were fundamental classics, which a physician would equally be expected to know by heart, but they were regarded as human knowledge acquired through experience, not divine revelation; such knowledge could be queried, revised and even overridden.

The divisions of the *Inner Canon* spell out teachings on core subjects: the physiological constitution of the body, including the circulation of *qi*; health and the onset and progression of disease; and therapy through needling (blood-letting or acupuncture). The *Canon of Problems* addresses eighty-one 'difficult issues' from the *Inner Canon*, relating mostly to diagnosis and needling treatment. Its significance as an adjunct to the *Inner Canon* was unquestioned until the Song dynasty (960–1279), but thereafter, where conflicts were remarked between the two works, medical authors simply assumed that the writer of the *Canon of Problems* had failed to grasp the definitive teachings of the *Inner Canon*.

The *Treatise on Cold-Damage Disorders* deals with the diagnosis and remedy of diseases caused by external cold factors (*shanghan bing*): what western medicine would call acute infectious fevers. Diagnosis is in line with what is known as the Six Warps theory, and treatment is not by needling but by medications. Particulars are given for 113 prescriptions, many still in use.

In the twelfth century Chinese physicians began to refine *shanghan* (cold-factor) theory into a doctrine of heat-factor disorders (*wenre bing*), thereby distinguishing between disorders said to have distinct aetiologies. This tendency gathered momentum during the seventeenth century, when there was a wave of serious epidemics. Dissatisfaction with the shortcomings of cold-damage theory led to a series of works on heat-factor disorders, chief of which was the *Wenre lun* of Ye Tianshi (*c.* 1740), which unfolded the 'triple burners' (*san jiao*) system to classify these.

The *Divine Husbandman's Materia Medica* contains a description of the properties and virtues of over three hundred vegetable, animal and mineral drugs, ordered into three classes: upper, middle and lower. The upper class of drugs was gentle and cumulative in action, fostering health and longevity; the more robust lower class was to be used in response to the actual onset of disease. The longevity-oriented classification was abandoned in later *materia medica* for systems more directly based on the curative qualities of drugs, categorized according to a system of correspondences between *yin yang* and *wu xing* (the 'five phases'). Thousands of listings of *materia medica* were produced over the centuries, the main being the late sixteenth-century *Bencao gangmu*.

THE TRADITION

Why did these ancient texts become so authoritative as the core of Chinese medicine? Were Chinese physicians concerned principally with theory and indifferent to empirical evidence and the teachings of experience? Was Chinese medicine essentially philosophically oriented? Some have seen it that way. Other histories of Chinese medicine of a Whiggish nature have been produced, seeking to show how a progressive winnowing took place of the grains of science from the husks of superstition. It has been claimed that Chinese physicians evolved theories (such as the heart as a pump) which match the evolutionary development of scientific medicine, but critics, by contrast, have dismissed Chinese medicine as an inchoate muddle of speculation.

It is important to remember that traditional Chinese medicine is a classical scheme of knowledge. The role of such basic concepts as *yin yang* and *wu xing* remained definitive, even if their meanings were susceptible to being modified. Canonical works were considered as the cardinal guides to comprehending the human body (microcosm) and its relations to the macrocosm. In the Chinese, as in other text-based traditions, there was a scholarly predisposition towards ironing out doctrinal differences by means of a quest for higher unity. Doctrines were built upon the belief that the human body represents a microcosm of the natural and social worlds. Bodily processes follow patterns comparable to those governing the workings of nature. To explain health and disorder, the *Inner Canon* thus standardly invokes the foursome of Heaven, Earth, Man and Society:

> A human body is the counterpart of a state.... The spirit [the body's governing vitalities, *shen*] is like the monarch; the blood *xue* is like the ministers; the *qi* is like the people. Thus we know that one who keeps his own body in order can keep a state in order. Loving care for one's people is what makes it possible for a state to be secure; nurturing one's *qi* is what makes it possible to keep the body intact.

Health depends on the preservation of harmony within the body, and harmony between the body, the environment and the larger order of things. Healing is a question of knowing how harmony can be restored; and the task of the physician is as much philosophical as technical.

Classical Chinese medical theory concentrates on the body viewed as a natural entity influenced by a terrestrial environment. Sickness can be brought on by some internal upset or by such external factors as cold, damp or contagion. In popular thinking, however, the factors responsible for illness were largely social or supernatural: sickness was often seen as punishment for causing offence to one's ancestors. Pestilence and plague might result from wrongdoing or from a ruler's wicked deeds – or from ancestral curses.

Before the Han dynasty which began in 206 BC, individual sickness had often been attributed to evil spirits or evil 'wind', which possessed the soul: cures were by exorcism or drugs and charms and talismans were used to ward off attacks. Children's anchoring to their souls was feeble, so they were particularly vulnerable. To this day, a major class of children's maladies is termed 'fright'. Although the emphasis on supernaturally caused disorders waned, most medical works recognized their existence.

From the earliest systematic formulations of cosmological principles around 200 BC, illness processes were regarded by physicians as determined by certain principles (one may compare Hippocratic thinking in

Greece). Chinese natural philosophy deals in relations, processes and cycles of transformation. The principal stuff of the natural world is *qi* (*ch'i*), variously translated as 'air', 'vapours' or 'energy' (and perhaps to be compared with the *pneuma* or *spiritus* of Greek medicine). In natural philosophy, *qi* stimulates a process of transformation, or is the medium through which such a process takes place. It permeates the cosmos; life comes from a build-up of *qi*, and death from its dissipation; in respect of living beings the word may be understood as 'vital energies'. A person must nurture the *qi* which regulates bodily functions, so as to preserve good health. But it can also be disruptive – 'pathogenic' *qi* triggers illness.

A concept fundamental for understanding the distribution of *qi* is the pairing of *yin yang*. To *yin* are ascribed qualities that westerners have sometimes viewed as the polar opposites of *yang*: female-male, dark-light, cold-hot, and so on. But these concepts are not static opposites; they are always relational. In any one phenomenon *yin* and *yang* are interrelated and subject to cyclical change. *Yin yang* gives structure to the patterning of space and time. *Yang* is more exterior, *yin* more interior. As pathogenic *qi* penetrates the outer *yang qi*, which constitutes the body's defences, it gains access to the inner regions of *yin qi*, which supplies the body with nourishment and growth; and thereby becomes more perilous. Like all natural processes, a malady will go through active *yang* phases and latent *yin* phases: after a *yang* sickness peaks, it moves into a *yin* phase for which distinctive treatment is required. *Yin yang* relations are elemental, complex, and have to be understood at many different levels. In health and in sickness, the body is in constant need of fresh assessment.

The term *wu xing* (five phases) was formerly translated as 'five elements' but it does not match the Greek notion of elements; 'phases' better conveys the dynamic quality. The five phases are wood, fire, earth, metal and water. Each is characterized by action or interaction; in a physiological context, wood denotes a growth phase and branching development; fire a phase of rapid upward dispersal, and so forth. Each is manifested in a characteristic colour, flavour, emotion, physiological system, bodily secretion, etc. The theory of how these phases interrelate is known as 'systematic correspondence'. The five phases spontaneously engender one another in the sequence mentioned (the order of 'mutual production'), and a cycle of 'mutual restraint' also occurs: wood, earth, water, fire, metal.

Overall, the body is a microcosm whose processes, normal and abnormal, are understood to be configured by the universal characteristics of *qi*, *yin yang*, and the five phases. It is contained and separated from the outer environment by a skin which is not impermeable but marked by pores which external pathogens can penetrate.

Within the body, *qi* has two components – these are often referred to as vital substances but they are processual rather than material. The *yang* element, likewise called *qi*, represents the capacity for action and transformation; the *yin* component, called *xue* (literally 'blood'), represents the capacity for circulation, nourishment and growth. Another vital substance, usually translated as 'essence' (*jing*), includes the nourishment obtained from food and the reproductive powers and substances (including semen) necessary for procreation. The vital substances circulate through the body in regular cycles along the circulation tracts (*jing luo* or *jing mai*). These passages include the anatomically identifiable blood vessels but also the invisible pathways along which *qi* in its various embodiments circulates. The circulation tracts connect the visceral systems.

Before the theory of systematic correspondence was fully elaborated, the conception of tracts and viscera was closer to western anatomy. Early texts identify tracts with blood vessels; others sketch the location of the viscera. Chinese physicians were not interested in the model of the body as a machine, however, nor was exact anatomical knowledge of the organs necessary as medical theory shifted from matter to processes.

Classical medical theory involves five *yin* visceral systems (the cardiac, hepatic, splenetic, pulmonary and renal), and six *yang* systems: gall-bladder, stomach, large intestine, small intestine, urinary bladder and the *san jiao* (triple burner). The *yin* systems create, transform, govern, and accumulate *qi*, *xue* and *jing*; the *yang* systems receive and process food to generate *qi*, *xue* and *jing* and get rid of the waste. Despite the superficial correspondence between most of these systems and western anatomical organs like the heart, lungs and liver, the primary focus is on functions and their interrelations; the triple burner, which evolved late in Chinese medicine, does not correspond to any anatomical entity, yet possesses a well-defined range of functions. The relations between the visceral systems, and the ways in which malfunctioning in one affects the others, are to be grasped in terms of the theory of systematic correspondence. Because the relationships between the viscera and the associated senses, organs, emotions and secretions are seen as systemic, there can be no such thing in Chinese medical thought as a Cartesian mind/ body dualism.

When *qi* is circulating correctly through the body, harmony and balance prevail, external threats are kept at bay, and the individual enjoys good health. This harmony is maintained through temperate behaviour. There are many ways for an individual to generate *qi*: through diet, exercise, preventative acupuncture or moxibustion, meditation or sexual techniques. Such methods not only enhance health but extend longevity – some texts decreed a lifespan of over a hundred years to be the norm to aim for – while others, in Taoist fashion, even aspire to immortality.

Disorder (*bing*) results from an imbalance of *yin* and *yang*, causing disturbance of *qi* circulation, which then impairs the normal transformative functions of the vital fluids and the visceral systems. Obstruction, accumulation or depletion of *qi* or *xue* in one of the visceral systems will modify its function and dispersion through the organism in a pattern dictated by phase dynamics and modified by the sufferer's constitution. If caught in the early *yang* phases, the imbalance can be treated and health restored. Once it reaches the life-threatening *yin* phases, the damage may be irreversible – indeed, a physician would be entitled to refuse to take on the case.

A disorder is produced by the irruption of an external pathogen or by internally generated imbalance. 'Excesses' are the main problem, but moderation precludes both excess and abstinence – gynaecological disorders are characteristic of widows deprived of sex, and lack of appropriate emotion can be as harmful as its excess. External pathogens (noxious *qi*) include heat, cold, damp, ingestion of poisonous substances, fright (in the case of children), or sexual intercourse with ghosts. The particular configuration of a disorder is shaped not only by the pathogen but by the constitution of the sufferer, which influences its phase dynamics. The range of disorders caused by one particular type of pathogen (cold-damage disorders, for example) thus follows a general pattern, but has a wide array of conceivable variations. Handbooks of diagnosis and treatment frequently classified them for convenience's sake by symptoms rather than causes, but they could not be cured unless their fundamental causes were grasped.

Classical Chinese medicine has what might be called a humoral or a constitutional approach to disease – 'biomedical' concepts of disease are largely absent. In the seventeenth century, however, a wave of epidemics led physicians to postulate the existence of certain types of pathogenic *qi*, which entered the body through the nose and mouth, and which, in the case of tuberculosis or smallpox, could be communicated by contact. This was a new concept, closer to the western one of infectious diseases, but was employed for a limited category of disorders only.

PRACTICE

A physician, when consulted by a patient, had to identify the disorder and its development before considering treatments. Very often, its root cause would be obscured by a plethora of complex symptoms. It was also crucial to know the background and constitution of the patient, which would influence the course of the illness and indicate the likely response to treatment.

The practitioner would reduce symptoms to a manageable set of dynamic characteristics: the fundamental cause, how the *qi* was affected, which visceral systems were impaired. The most popular system for determining the type of manifestation was the 'Eight Rubrics', first outlined in the *Inner Canon*, which loops four sets of polar opposites: inner-outer, cold-hot, depletion-repletion, and *yin-yang*. Another system is the Six Warps, first developed in the *Treatise on Cold-Damage Disorders*, which classifies manifestations according to the degree of penetration of the pathogenic *qi*. From the seventeenth and eighteenth centuries, this procedure was developed by heat-factor disorder theorists into a four-level classification based on the location of symptoms among the triple burners (*san jiao*).

The earliest medical texts emphasize pulse-taking as well as observation of physical and emotional signs. The pulse provided information about the circulation of *qi*, thus indicating the basic imbalances in the body and how the visceral systems were affected. It was elaborated into a complex art, the radial pulse of the wrist being palpated at three different depths at each of three locations, and classified according to strength, duration, resonance, texture, rhythm, and so forth. According to the twelve-volume *Mei Ching* (AD 280) [Book of the Pulse]:

> The human body is likened to a chord instrument, of which the different pulses are the chords. The harmony or discord of the organism can be recognized by examining the pulse, which is thus fundamental for all medicine.

Consideration also had to be given to the patient's complexion, breathing, emotional state, temperature, pain, sensory or motor problems, eating and digestive patterns. Deep-lying visceral effects were discernible in well-defined ways. Ailments of the hepatic system were manifested in the state of the eyes and were associated with anger; kidney disorders affected the bones and ears as well as sexual capacities, and elicited feelings of fear. Emotional or intellectual disorders were construed as symptoms of wider constitutional conditions rather than as 'psychiatric' diseases.

The physician took the case history from the patient and his or her family, and was interested not only in behaviour patterns that might be the immediate causes, (exhaustion, exposure to cold, melancholy, over-eating, etc.), but in validating cyclical patterns in the symptoms (insomnia, pain or fever, appetite loss, complications in childbearing). Diagnosis became more elaborated over the centuries, a systemization based on tongue examination, for example, appearing in the nineteenth century. The twentieth century has brought the incorporation of temperature measurement, blood count and blood-sugar levels. Nevertheless, the fundamentals of the 'Four Methods of Examination' remain interrogation, ocular inspection, auditory and olfactory examination, and pulse-taking. Therapy combines two aspects: it eliminates the pathogenic *qi* and counters its effects, while building up the orthogenic *qi* which constitutes the body's defences.

For almost all diseases a package of therapies was offered. The dangerous symptoms of an acute disorder, such as coma or elevated fever, had to be treated at once, before the underlying imbalance could be approached, but choice of treatment would always take those troubles into account. For instance, although certain *yin* drugs were highly efficacious in reducing acute fever, if it were a symptom of a *yang* depletion, *yin* drugs would aggravate the trouble. The physician adjusted the therapy step by step as the malady was gradually brought under control.

Almost all illnesses were understood as 'internal' – even skin problems or injuries. Problems of the eyes had to be cured through treatment of the hepatic system, and a disorder of the visceral system could be relieved only by restoring the *yin* and *yang* balance, not by directly attacking the diseased organ. 'External medicine' was of secondary importance. Apart from a short period predating the theory of systematic correspondence, surgery was not included in mainstream medicine.

Drugs form by far the most important therapy in traditional

medicine, and their action was classified in various ways. Some drugs replenished depleted *qi* or blood, others dispersed pathogenic *qi*, acted as sudorifics or as purgatives, expelled cold or reduced heat. Most prescriptions (*fang*) included a combination of drugs in specified proportions: perhaps a strong dose of a powerful 'principal' drug to break up thickened blood, smaller quantities of a 'leading' drug to direct the principal agent to the affected visceral system, one 'auxiliary' drug to complement the principal drug, and another auxiliary to prevent undesirable side-effects.

There are thousands of well-known *fang* which have been in use for centuries. Some medicines were pills or powders made up by the physician or the pharmacist; others were taken as syrups, decoctions or infusions. Some could be purchased readymade as patent medicines; others were secret, handed down within a family. Also important were acupuncture and moxibustion.

ACUPUNCTURE AND MOXIBUSTION

Acupuncture involves inserting fine metal needles one-half to several inches in length into the skin. The needles, which in some cases are driven in with great force and in others inserted gently, are set at different depths, and the point of insertion is of particular importance. The oldest existing catalogue of insertion points, the section called *Ling shu* in the *Inner Canon*, dates from about 100 BC, but the points are named in an earlier collection. There were 365 in the second century; the number grew.

Once inserted, the needles are twirled and vibrated. The physiology of acupuncture rests on the Taoist doctrine that the life force *qi*, or energy, circulates through all the body's organs. The acupuncture points are located on fourteen invisible lines or meridians running the length of the body, and points on those meridians 'control' certain physical conditions. All disease is the result of imbalance in the energy flow in the body. Pain or disease is the manifestation of imbalance, and acupuncture needles introduce a restorative and balancing *qi*.

Moxibustion is a technique involving the burning of small pellets of dried wormwood at points on the skin (a practice in some ways analogous to cupping in the West). Both acupuncture and moxibustion were believed to produce stimulation of key nodal points along the *qi* circulation tracts; they unblocked obstructed *qi*, redirected it to depleted viscera and so restored regular circulation.

Propriety dictated that the physical contact between physicians and genteel patients be kept to a minimum, especially with females who might remain concealed behind a screen and communicate with the physician only via a husband or a maidservant. While drug therapy was the most common treatment prescribed, there were acupuncture specialists who did not prescribe drugs; and many lay people performed acupuncture or moxibustion within the family. Massage was not performed by physicians; for that there were lower-class experts, as also for childbirth.

THE HEALERS

Classical Chinese medical cosmology was secular and naturalistic, even if the mass of the people saw illness as caused by malevolent ghosts, angry ancestors, insulted gods, karma and sin. The medical corpus depicted two kinds of healer. One was the so-called 'Confucian physician' (*ruyi*), a gentleman scholar of good family who studied the medical arts in a spirit of benevolence. This philosophical healer acquired acumen first through studying texts, then by personal experience. The second respectable practitioner was the 'hereditary physician' (*shiyi*). He came from a line of doctors, so his training included apprenticeship as well as book-learning. Such families often rose to fame by specializing in a certain disorder or holding some secret prescription. Some had the status of regular family doctors, receiving an annual retainer from well-to-do clients. They were expected to treat poor patients gratis.

These two categories of healer did not make up a profession in the modern western sense. The nearest to professional physicians were those who took medical examinations instituted by the state before serving as state medical officers. But their rank was not high, and they seldom shone in the medical pantheon. The medical corpus also refers to an array of quacks, 'vulgar doctors', itinerants, priests, shamans, acupuncturists, masseurs and old women. These healers had no prestige – they were not scholars or philosophers or gentlemen. Women healers were generally depicted as illiterate, ignorant and unscrupulous but, despite male reservations about their integrity, large numbers of midwives and wet-nurses served the health-care needs of gentlewomen. The Korean state introduced formal medical training for women in the fourteenth century, though it was of low status.

Case histories show that the sick were likely to seek help from a variety of healers, many of them religious. Religious healing still retains its importance throughout east Asia, and has even shown a resurgence in the People's Republic of China. The earliest hospices and charitable medical services in China were established by Buddhist monasteries in the early centuries AD. Confucians also took health services seriously; they believed in a link between the health of the body politic and the health of the people at large, care for the well-being of one's inferiors showed one's fitness to rule.

When Buddhist monasteries were nationalized during the Tang dynasty in the ninth century, imperial authorities assumed responsibility for their infirmaries. State initiatives continued throughout the Song and Yuan dynasties, when the government also sponsored the compilation of *materia medica* and established charity pharmacies and clinics. The decline of government medical services during the late Ming Dynasty (*c.* 1500–1644) was attended by a rise in private medical charities.

MODERN DEVELOPMENTS

Until the nineteenth century, Chinese medicine more or less matched its European counterpart in efficacy and prestige. The emperors allowed restricted access to westerners, but few Chinese physicians had any knowledge of European medicine.

Japanese scholars, however, had access through westerners permitted to live in the port of Nagasaki, and from the eighteenth century 'Dutch scholarship' (*rangaku*) flourished. Japanese *rangaku* physicians became interested in anatomy and surgery, and introduced Jennerian vaccination in 1824. Its success helped to undermine the authority of *kanpo*, and schools of western medicine appeared. But international politics more than scientific efficacy effected this change. By 1850, both Japan and China were forcibly confronted with the terrifying strength of the western powers and a medicine confident of its scientific superiority.

The Japanese Meiji government resolved to adopt the German system of medical training in 1869, sent many students to Germany for this purpose and restricted the practice of *kanpo*. A state system of western medical education and services was established, and by 1900 there were three imperial and eleven other state colleges of western medicine in Japan. By 1912 these institutions had trained 14,552 physicians – around two thirds of all those in practice. Similar policies were established when the Japanese annexed Taiwan (1895) and Korea (1910). Chinese medicine has made a comeback in modern Japan, together with other cultural revivals. It remains separate and largely private, although it has become professionalized, and standardized training, including basic anatomy and physiology, is offered in private medical colleges and hospitals. Both Japan and Korea include Chinese medical prescriptions and treatments in their insurance systems.

The Chinese became familiar with western medicine through missionaries, who arrived after the treaties of 1860. Many reformers thought Chinese medicine partly responsible for the country's defeats, but others preferred to reform and modernize rather than abandon it. In any case, the weak regime of the late Qing was in no position to effect Meiji-style reforms. The chief impulse for change came not from the state but from the detested foreigners, in particular the Chinese Medical Missionary Association, founded in 1886, which, together with the Rockefeller-funded Chinese Medical Commission, tried to regularize medical education and services by establishing union medical colleges in Peking (Beijing) and other major cities between 1903 and 1912. But by 1913 there were only 500 Chinese medical students receiving training in all mission services throughout China.

Republican China (1911–49) developed ambitious plans to establish a modern state medical system. In 1926, about one hundred cities had western-style medical practitioners or hospitals, and in 1928 the nationalist government used them as nuclei for health institutions, organizing medical education, health centres and hospitals from the capital right down to village paramedics. Peasant health care was a high priority: village health workers were given a few weeks' intensive training in elementary hygiene, diagnosis and treatment of standard minor illnesses, immunization against smallpox, typhoid and diphtheria, and referral of serious illnesses to higher authorities. The system drew upon western medicine; although Chinese medicine was not banned, it suffered from the competition.

After 1948, the nationalist health-care structure was taken over almost unchanged by the new communist regime, though Chinese medicine was integrated into the system. Science was touted as the key to the future, but nationalistic sentiment reinforced by anti-bourgeois ideology gave Chinese medicine a new symbolic authority, leading to professional parity with western medicine. Top physicians are required to have a basic training in western-style as well as traditional medicine. Indeed, in the late 1950s, when China was desperately short of skilled practitioners, up to 2000 doctors at a time were withdrawn from regular practice for three years' study of traditional medicine, and the government devoted much of its health budget to providing hospitals, clinics and medical schools for Chinese medicine. The 'barefoot doctors' of the 1960s and 1970s included among their skills simple acupuncture and a knowledge of Chinese *materia medica*.

The balance between western and Chinese medicine has fluctuated, and the notion of a 'syncretic medicine', combining the best of the two types became popular. Attempts have been made to establish an experimental, scientific basis for Chinese medicine, setting it up as a rival to biomedicine. There has been a switch from functionalism to materialism in medical concepts, accompanied by a tendency to reduce Chinese technical terms to their biomedical equivalents. However *xue* in classical medicine includes a whole range of meanings, only one of which more or less corresponds to the biomedical concept of 'blood'. While most contemporary practitioners recognize this distinction, there is a tendency to use the meanings interchangeably. Materialism provides a way of elucidating Chinese medical theory and therapeutics in western scientific terms, applying the methods of the experimental laboratory: the location of the acupuncture tracts has been explored, and explanations of the effects of acupuncture anaesthesia given in terms of endorphins; the pharmacological effects of Chinese drugs have also been tested.

The classical concept of knowledge continues to shape the thinking of contemporary practitioners of Chinese medicine: neither in Beijing, Tokyo, nor Seoul can a physician be trained without becoming acquainted with the works of the *Canon*. But classical Chinese is no longer an essential linguistic element of medical education. Physicians may become acquainted with the classical works and the traditions of exegesis through excerpts or quotations in modern textbooks. In the People's Republic and Taiwan, the emphasis on practice means that many doctors receive only a superficial training in the theoretical rationale underlying therapy. Chinese medical practitioners used to reinforce their prestige by their skills with the book; now they assume the trappings of western medicine: even traditional physicians carry stethoscopes.

From the wider perspective there is a key difference between the eastern and western medical traditions. Both initially shared common assumptions about the balanced and natural operations of the healthy body and these were inscribed in hallowed texts. Western medicine alone radically broke with this. An entirely new medicine grew up in the West – scientific medicine – building upon the new sorts of knowledge, programme and power that followed from anatomy and the investigations of the body it opened.

To this day the relations between the western and the eastern traditions remain unresolved. Early western physicians dabbled in moxibustion. But in 1794 European surgeons visiting China on an embassy led by Lord Macartney were openly contemptuous of traditional Chinese medicine for its ignorance of anatomy and hence of medicine's 'scientific' basis. And though acupuncture had small pockets of followers in nineteenth-century France and Britain it has been only in the last generation that the claims of Chinese medicine have found widespread acceptance in the West. This is due partly to a new multiculturalism and partly to rejection in some quarters of high-tech values; but it also results from 'scientific' explanations of acupuncture anaesthesia in terms of endorphins and other neurotransmitters. Whether East and West will ever meet, medically, remains unclear.

CHAPTER VIII

RENAISSANCE

THE OLD WORLD AND THE NEW

THE MOST MOMENTOUS EVENT FOR HUMAN HEALTH was Columbus's landfall in 1492 on Hispaniola (now the Dominican Republic and Haiti). The Europeans' discovery of America forged contact between two human populations isolated from each other for thousands of years, and the biological consequences were devastating, unleashing the worst health disaster there has ever been, and precipitating the conquest of the New World by the Old World's diseases.

The forebears of the 'Indians' Columbus encountered in his attempt to find a short-cut to the 'Indies' or China were hunter-gatherers. Before or around 10,000 BC such people had crossed the Bering Straits from Asia to Alaska via a land bridge created by the fall in sea levels during the last Ice Age. They were relatively disease-free; lacking domesticated animals, they had no walking disease-carriers except themselves, and on their travels they encountered no other humans.

The melting of the great North American glaciers isolated that continent while opening it up to the newcomers, who spread south. In time the Maya, Aztec and Inca to the south and the Mississippian peoples of North America settled into sedentary agriculture, cultivating maize and beans, cassava and potatoes, and in some cases building complex civilizations centred on vast cities – which spawned all the familiar health problems. Tuberculosis developed, as did pinta and other treponemal infections, including non-venereal syphilis, various disorders caused by intestinal parasites, and Chagas' disease. With agriculture came the nutritional maladies typical of monocultures.

The Amerindian peoples developed their own forms of medicine, with priests, shamans and sorcerers conducting healing rituals. Supernatural powers were believed to inflict pestilence to punish misdeeds, and in Mexico and Peru disease was connected with witchcraft and the malevolent shades of dead animals, demons and deities. Native Americans acquired knowledge of the healing properties of various vegetable products: Peruvian Indians chewed coca leaves against hunger and fatigue, while cacao (cocoa) was the Aztecs' most important tonic and medicinal beverage, powdered and boiled in water with honey, vanilla and pepper. The Incas had herbs for headaches and other pains; and they used scopolamine, a poison from the datura plant, as an anaesthetic. Broken bones were treated with fat from the ñandu, an ostrich-like bird, and llama kidney juice was dropped into aching ears.

North American Indian tribes had a less extensive *materia medica*. They used sassafras, holly, sunflower seeds and infusions of flaxseed, inhaled the smoke from burning twigs to treat chest conditions, and used decoctions of mushrooms and peyote as hallucinogens. A Spanish explorer, Cabeza de Vaca, travelling in the 1520s through what is now Texas, observed the healing practices of the native Indians: 'their method of cure is to blow on the sick, the breath and the laying-on of hands supposedly casting out the infirmity.' He had no doubt what to think of that: 'We scoffed at their cures.'

The New World peoples were not living in a golden age, but they had been spared Eurasian afflictions. Thus they were vulnerable virgin soil, entirely without resistance to epidemics imported by the *conquistadores*. This was not the first time Spanish conquest had brought diseases to a virgin population. In the fifteenth century, the Iberian conquest of the Canary islands had meant total devastation of the native inhabitants, the Guanches, whose immune systems were helpless against European infections. Originally there were some 100,000 Guanches; by 1530 only a handful was left, and in the seventeenth century they became extinct, spectacular victims of what has been called ecological imperialism.

The first epidemic, which struck Hispaniola in 1493, may have been swine influenza, carried by pigs aboard Columbus's ships. Other deadly diseases then struck in hammerblows, so that New World populations were reeling even before smallpox reached the Caribbean in 1518. That outbreak killed one third to one half of the Arawaks on Hispaniola and spread from there to Puerto Rico and Cuba. A few Spaniards fell sick but none died and, as ever, all was attributed to God's will, in support of the Christian conquest.

Smallpox accompanied Hernan Cortés (1485–1547) to Monte-zuma's Aztec Mexico, where the main town was Tenochtitlan (modern Mexico City); with some 300,000 people, it was three times the size of Seville. Contact spread the disease among the natives outside the city and then within. In 1521, Cortés attacked with 300 Spaniards. Three months later, when the city fell, the conqueror learned that half its people had died, including Montezuma and his successor: 'a man could not put his foot down unless on the corpse of an Indian.' The same happened when Pizarro (c. 1475–1541) took on the Incas: smallpox ran ahead of him to Peru. By 1533, when he entered Cuzco to plunder its treasure, the Incas were incapable of serious resistance.

Infections thus primed and sped conquest, rippling outwards to fell countless indigenes the Spanish troops did not have to butcher. The consequent epidemics did not merely exterminate vast numbers, they destroyed the will to resist – the psychological impact was as devastating as the physical. Between 1518 and 1531, perhaps one third of the total Indian population died of smallpox, while the Spanish hardly suffered. With allies like microbes, the Europeans did not require many soldiers or much military acumen.

These initial smallpox outbreaks were only the beginning of a long, mainly unintentional, but almost genocidal germ onslaught unleashed against the Amerindians. Waves of measles – 1519 (Santa Domingo), 1523 (Guatemala) and 1531 (Mexico) – influenza, and finally typhus followed, all bringing devastating mortalities. In 1529 measles killed two thirds of those who had just survived smallpox; two years later it had killed half the Hondurans, ravaged Mexico, raced through Central America and attacked the Incas. Repeated epidemics followed, one of the worst being that of typhus, which towards 1600 killed about two million people in the Mexican highlands. By then, 90 per cent of the local inhabitants had died in successive diseases, and the fabric of life had fallen to pieces.

Though the mainland populations of Mexico and the Andes gradu-ally recovered, in the Caribbean and in parts of Brazil decline verged upon extinction; from as early as 1520, the Spanish imported slaves from Africa to meet the labour shortages in their lucrative Peruvian silver mines. African slaves, in turn, brought malaria and yellow fever, creating further disasters. Guns and germs enabled small European bands to conquer half a continent in what might be called, to echo Gibbon, another victory of barbarism over civilization.

In later centuries the North American Indian population was similarly decimated by the English and French, sometimes by the fiendish distribution of smallpox-infected blankets and clothes. In 1645, smallpox killed half the Hurons; the same happened later with the Cherokees in the Charleston area, and with the Omahas and the Mandans. Not one European fell sick of smallpox in 1680, when the Revd Increase Mather (1639–1723) tersely recorded that 'the Indians began to be quarrelsome ... but God ended the controversy by sending the smallpox among the Indians'. The wholesale destruction of indigenous New World populations continued for over three hundred years; twenty million slaves had to be shipped to America to fill the vacuum, causing cruelty and suffering on a scale not matched until the regimes of Hitler and Stalin.

SYPHILIS

European expansion produced the 'Columbian exchange', a highly unequal disease trade-off in which Columbus may have brought one killer disease back from the Americas: syphilis. This broke out in 1493–4 during a war between Spain and France being waged in Italy. When Naples fell to the French, the conquerors indulged in the usual orgy of rape and pillage, and the troops and their camp-followers then scattered throughout Europe. Soon, a terrible venereal epidemic was raging. It began with genital sores, progressing to a general rash, to ulceration, and to revolting abscesses eating into bones and destroying the nose, lips and genitals, and often proving fatal.

Initially, it was called the 'disease of Naples', but rapidly became the 'French Pox' and other terms accusing this or that nation: the Spanish disease in Holland, the Polish disease in Russia, the Russian disease in Siberia, the Christian disease in Turkey and the Portuguese disease in India and Japan. For their part, the Portuguese called it the Castilian disease, and a couple of centuries later Captain Cook (1728–79), exploring the Pacific, rued that the Tahitians 'call the venereal disease *Apa no Britannia* – the British disease' (he thought they'd caught it from the French).

That some of the Spaniards at the siege of Naples had accompanied Columbus suggested an American origin for the pox (or 'great pox', to distinguish it from smallpox). It certainly behaved in Europe like a new disease, spreading like wildfire for a couple of decades. 'In recent times', reflected one sufferer, Joseph Gruenpeck (*c.* 1473–*c.* 1532):

> I have seen scourges, horrible sicknesses and many infirmities affect mankind from all corners of the earth. Amongst them has crept in, from the western shores of Gaul, a disease which is so cruel, so distressing, so appalling that until now nothing so horrifying, nothing more terrible or disgusting, has ever been known on this earth.

Syphilis, we now know, is one of several diseases caused by members of the *Treponema* group of spirochetes, a corkscrew-shaped bacterium.* There are four clinically distinct human treponematoses (the others are pinta, yaws and bejel) and their causative organisms are virtually identical, suggesting all are descendants of an ancestral spirochete which adapted to different climates and human behaviours.

What caused this terrible outbreak? Many epidemiological possibilities have been mooted. It is feasible that some American treponemal infection merged with a similar European one to become syphilis, with both initial infections subsequently disappearing. Others maintain that venereal infections had long been present in Europe but never properly distinguished from leprosy; treponemal infections (pinta, yaws, endemic and venereal syphilis) had, it is suggested, initially presented as mild childhood illnesses, spread by casual contact and producing a measure of immunity. With improved European living standards, treponemes dependent on skin contact had become disadvantaged, being replaced by hardier, sexually transmitted strains. Thus an initially mild disorder grew more serious. A related theory holds that the spirochete had long been present in both the Old World and the New; what would explain the sixteenth-century explosion were the social disruptions of the time, especially warfare.

Like the pox itself, the debate raged – and remains unresolved to this day. But whatever the precise epidemiology, syphilis, like typhus, should be regarded as typical of the new plagues of an age of conquest and turbulence, one spread by international warfare, rising population density, changed lifestyles and sexual behaviour, the migrations of soldiers and traders, and the ebb and flow of refugees and peasants. While

---

* Unlike syphilis, gonorrhoea is an ancient disease. An Assyrian tablet speaks of thick or cloudy urine, and the Hippocratic writers refer to 'strangury', that is, blockage of the urethra. There was no effective cure until sulfonamides became available in the 1930s.

Europeans were establishing their empires and exporting death to aboriginal peoples, they were caught in microbial civil wars at home. Bubonic plague bounced from the Balkans to Britain, malaria was on the increase, smallpox grew more virulent, while typhus and the 'bloody flux' (dysentery) became camp-followers of every army. Influenza epidemics raged, especially lethal being the 'English sweat' (*sudor Anglicus*) which struck in 1485 (delaying Henry VII's coronation), 1507, 1528, 1551 and 1578, and was described by Polydore Vergil, an Italian diplomat in London, as 'a pestilence horrible indeed, and before which no age could endure'. John Caius's (1510–73) *A Boke of Conseill against the Disease Commonly Called the Sweat or Sweating Sickness* (1552) noted the copious sweating, shivering, fever, nausea, headache, cramps, back pain, delirium and stupor. It came to crisis within twenty-four hours, with very high mortality. It was thought even worse than the plague, for plague:

> commonly giveth three or four, often seven, sometimes nine . . .
> sometimes eleven, and sometimes fourteen days' respect to whom
> it vexeth. But that [the sweating sickness] immediately killed some
> in opening their windows, some in playing with children in their
> street doors, some in one hour, many in two it destroyed, and at
> the longest, to they that merrily dined, it gave a sorrowful supper.

The 'English sweat' remains a riddle. Such calamities form a doleful backdrop to the Renaissance.

THE MEDICAL RENAISSANCE

From the fourteenth century Europe's cultural and intellectual life was undergoing a mighty rebirth. First in the bustling commercial cities of Italy and later in transalpine courts, the arts and humanities were being restored to a brilliance unknown for centuries. Glory would be achieved, enthusiasts proclaimed, by burying the immediate past and emulating the ancients. New inventions were changing material culture: gunpowder, the compass and Gutenberg's printing press. Books multiplied, and were cheered on by propagandists and educators.

Among these was the monk who quit his monastery, Desiderius Erasmus (1466–1536), who led European scholarship and culture for more than three decades. A supreme stylist, it was he who established Greek as the basis for literary and theological studies, not least through production of a restored Greek text for the New Testament. His example prompted others to produce the first Greek editions of the ancient medical authors, and he inspired young scholars and physicians to bring out the great Aldine edition of Galen (1525). He also took a keen personal interest in medicine, both as patient (he suffered from gout, kidney stone and hypochondria) and as author. His Latin versions of three of Galen's works, *The Protrepticus*, *The Best Method of Teaching*, and *The Best Doctor is also a Philosopher*, were the first to be based on the Greek of the Aldine edition, and enjoyed huge success. Yet, if Erasmus promoted medical learning, he was dubious about doctors, echoing that earlier humanist, Petrarch (1304–74), who had written, 'I have never believed in doctors nor ever will.'

Painters, philosophers and poets commended the beauty of the human form and the nobility of the human spirit, using the emblem of Vitruvian man, in which the idealized naked male human form was superimposed upon the cosmos at large. Above all perhaps, after centuries when the Church had taught mankind to renounce worldly goods for the sake of eternity, Renaissance man showed an insatiable curiosity for the materiality of the here and now, a Faustian itch to explore, know and possess every nook and cranny of creation. No wonder they became inquisitive about human bodies, which were judged to occupy a privileged status. According to the Venetian surgeon Alessandro Benedetti (*c.* 1450–1512),

> The human body was created for the sake of the soul and stands erect among other animals, as established by divine nature and reason so that it might look upward more comfortably. . . . The heart was first created since it contains the principle of life and sense. Next came the brain and liver. Then nature, performing like a painter, sketched out the other members with a life-giving fluid; they gradually receive their colours from the blood, which is very abundant in man and stirs up very much heat.

Art and nature thus both drew attention to the body, and in an intellectual climate that revered the classics, no wonder there was a revival of ancient medicine. For centuries, of course, Galen had been god: the Arabs had synthesized his works and the medieval West had translated these into Latin. So why was there a need for a Galen revival?

Admiration for all things Greek was in the air. Spurred by the fall of Constantinople in 1453, Greeks like Theodore Gaza (*fl.* 1430–80) and his student Demetrius Chalcondylas (d. 1511) went to Italy, taking manuscripts with them and passing their knowledge to Italian humanists eager to believe that truth was at its purest in Greek sources: Plato, Aristotle, the poets and orators. These ideas were obviously applicable to medicine too, for were not its first oracles Greek?

'Back to the sources' (*ad fontes*) acquired a further incentive. From 1517 Luther and his fellow Protestants were reforming the Church by returning to the Bible as the well-spring of true religion. Every doctrinal formulation of the Catholic Church was to be rejected unless sanctioned by the Bible, and the study of Greek manuscripts, it was argued, would purify the understanding of scripture. A return to the sources promised the key to progress, and philology (the study of language) was vital to rescue truth before it was engulfed in oblivion and error. This awakening prompted a medical parallel.

The first priority for medical humanists lay in sound new translations of original Greek texts, since the Arabic and medieval Latin editions were now judged incorrect and inelegant. Technical terms had been especially susceptible to adulteration. In 1492 Nicolaus Leoniceno (1428–1524), the doyen of Greek medical scholars at Ferrara, drew attention to this in his *De Plinii et aliorum in medicina erroribus* [On the Errors of Pliny and of Many Others in Medicine]. Criticizing Pliny's muddling of plant names, Leoniceno ordered a critical re-examination of medical knowledge through revitalized study of the classics. He urged the recovery and editing of ancient Greek medical texts, and promoted scholarly yet stylish new Latin versions. Scornful of the folios used in medical teaching, he criticized Arabic works such as Avicenna's *Canon* for corrupting the Greek treatises they purported to honour. It was he who provided the texts for the first Galenic works to be printed in Greek, and who published Latin versions of Galenic treatises, including the *Ars medica*.

Leoniceno delighted in exposing howlers resulting from inept scholarship, showing how mistranslations had clouded the terminology of diseases, plants and anatomy, with dangerous consequences – people would be prescribed the wrong drugs. One of the first treatises on syphilis, his *De epidemia quam vulgo morbum gallicum vocant* (1497) [On the Epidemic Vulgarly Called the French Disease] predictably denied it was new: he claimed classical texts should be scrutinized and provided a philological survey of Greek terminology for skin diseases.

In later years, much was done on texts and terms as part of a wider humanist attempt to dispel the medieval murk. Terminological exactitude was, for instance, crucial in a blood-letting controversy initiated by Pierre Brissot (d. 1522), who taught that the Greek texts of Hippocrates and Galen showed blood-letting was meant to be carried out on the *same* side as the source of illness rather than the *opposite* side, as in Avicenna's corrupt versions.

In 1525 the Aldine Press in Venice, Europe's leading printing house, published the complete works of Galen in Greek, a landmark in the retrieval of the pure word of the ancients. For workaday practitioners, it had little relevance, for few could read Greek; but they could use the new Latin translations, which after 1525 were mainly based upon the Aldine Greek. Galen's *On the Natural Faculties* was published in 1523 in a new translation by Thomas Linacre (c. 1460–1524), physician to Henry VII, and in 1531 Johann Guinther von Andernach (1487–1574) published the newly discovered text of Galen's *On Anatomical Procedures*, which sparked a reappraisal of dissection. During the sixteenth century an astonishing 590 editions of Galenic treatises appeared, the main publishing centres being Paris, Lyons, Venice and Basel. There was also a Hippocrates retrieval, the first humanist Latin edition appearing in 1525, and the first Greek edition, from the Aldine Press, a year later. In 1531 Guinther von Andernach, who was also one of Vesalius's teachers, praised the times as those when 'medicine has been raised from the dead', because Hippocrates and Galen – until recently 'almost utterly corrupt' – had 'at last been rescued from perpetual darkness'.

Greek texts were recovered: how did that affect medicine? It boosted the idea that ancient medicine was the true one and scholars its rightful guardians and interpreters. In Paris, the medical humanist Jacobus Sylvius (1478–1555) approached Hippocrates and Galen with religious awe, declaring 'they had never written anything in physiology or other parts of medicine that was not entirely true'. His pedantry and Galen worship culminated in an *Introduction to Anatomy* (1555), vindicating Galen against Vesalius. If what the eye saw at dissections did not correspond with what Galen had reported, the fault lay not with Galen but with the corpse! Puny moderns could not be expected to show so perfect a body structure as that displayed by the ancients.

Like many contemporary physicians, Sylvius was a bookworm. His *Order and Way of Reading Hippocrates and Galen* (1539) was one of the earliest attempts to evaluate the authenticity of the Hippocratic Corpus, as well as suggesting the best way for students to approach Galen. His enthusiasm for recovering the true Galen was widely shared. He marks the shift from Arabic to Greek Galenism, notably in his treatises on pharmacology, where he demanded a return to Galenic purity. Galen's remedies, he argued, were mainly composed of simples; the proliferation of compound medicines (ironically called Galenicals) was an Arab error. Not everyone, however, wanted to throw overboard the medical works of the Arabs and the medievals. Avicenna and Rhazes continued to be taught in most universities, and the tradition of medieval *practica* – handbooks listing disorders from head to toe with a description of symptoms and treatment – was too useful to be abandoned.

Scholarly study did not just give medical writings a classical authority and style; humanism spurred innovation as well. With the proliferation of medical discourse created by print culture, questions arose as to how medicine should be structured, taught and practised. Fifteenth-century medical teaching had become centred on the 'affections' (the ill happenings) of the body in terms of symptoms and cures, usually in a head-to-heels order; and the tried and tested *practica* supplied guides to diagnosis and remedies. But that hardly passed the crucial Galenic test: the conviction that therapy had to be rationally connected to aetiology. The *practica* contained little on disease causation, and failed to satisfy another Galenic requirement: the view that therapy should take into consideration the distinctive characteristics of each patient – constitution, temperament, strength, age and environment. Galen's *Methodus medendi* [Method of Healing], extremely influential once it was available in Thomas Linacre's translation (1519), declared that physicians had to assess not only the cause of the illness but all aspects of the patient.

Attempts were made to overcome this problem through that characteristic Renaissance solution, the application of method, an idea dear to the French philosopher Peter Ramus (1515–72). Scholars set about reducing Galenic medicine to 'method' and therefore certainty. The logical approach, they insisted, would help the physician to choose the correct 'indications' and so get the therapies right. The humanist faith in printed texts and academic methodologies encouraged encyclopaedic systematization, which could descend into the vain and verbose pedantry satirized by playwrights; Ben Jonson has one of his characters complain:

When he discourseth of *dissection*,
Or any point of *Anatomy*: that hee tells you,
Of *Vena cava*, and of *vena portam*,
The *Meseraicks*, and the *Mesenterium*,
What does hee else but cant? . . . Who here does understand him?

Giambatista da Monte (1498–1552), professor of the practice of medicine at Padua, was a pioneer of the new methodology. His 'universal method' involved proceeding, by systematic division and elimination, from the general to the particular, from broad disease classifications to specific disorder. His book helped the doctor to run through all possibilities until a full account of the indications for cure was reached.

The idea of a foolproof method for applying Galenic medicine to the individual (the parallel with computer diagnosis comes to mind) was taken further by Sanctorius Sanctorius (Santorio: 1561–1636), professor at Padua. In his *Methodi vitandorum errorum* (1603) [Methods for Avoiding Errors], he urged, echoing da Monte, that medicine should not begin with particulars; one had to work from general concepts, which were to be divided and divided again. What was being promoted was a teaching device exalting learning above empiricism.

Academic medicine was not totally conservative and in thrall to Galen, however; some new ideas were proposed about disease causation and remedies. Debates flared as to whether the traditional humours and temperaments could explain all sorts of illness. New diseases like the pox and the English sweat seemed to call for something beyond the old model of temperamental imbalance. And what of the influences of the heavens, or magic? Astrological powers, like the stars or moon, were 'occult', and thus by definition lay outside the Aristotelian–Galenic philosophy which addressed the natural, sensory world; they gained intellectual credit, however, from the neo-Platonic, Hermetic and magical currents popularized through such authors as Marsilio Ficino (1433–99) and Pico de la Mirandola (1463–94). Hidden qualities and sympathies which defied Aristotelian categories might be at work, such as magnetism and the electric discharge of the torpedo fish. These were explained by recourse to 'occult qualities' or to the action of what was known as the 'whole substance'.

Occult qualities were suspect in the eyes of many learned physicians, for they were the stock in trade of quacks, magicians and heretics. Nevertheless, thanks in part to the Platonic revival with its edifying vision of grand cosmic spiritual powers – and the undeniable fact that Plato preceded Aristotle and so was more 'pristine' and pure – they took hold.

Consider the career of Jean Fernel (1497–1558), one of the ornaments of the Paris medical faculty, who vowed there were some things 'beyond the power of the elements' (i.e., beyond Galen). Fernel devoted himself to philosophy, mathematics and classical writers such as Cicero, and wrote two major works of theoretical medicine. One was published in 1542 as *De naturali parte medicinae* [On the Natural Part of Medicine], reappearing in 1554 as the first book, *Physiologia*, of a general treatise, *Medicina*, which also included sections on pathology and therapeutics (Fernel introduced the terms 'physiology' and 'pathology'). The other was a speculative dialogue, *De abditis rerum causis* (1548) [On the Hidden Causes of Things], in which two friends, Brutus and Philiatros, question the physician Eudoxus on the 'hidden causes' of certain diseases. In particular they ask: Is there not something in disease which is divine? The discussion ranges widely over the philosophical basis of medicine.

Fernel was a reformer of Galenic medicine who interwove other philosophical and Christian strands. His physiology had recourse to the four elements; to the qualities; to the action of innate heat, found only in living things; and to a subtle substance, mediating soul and matter, which he called *spiritus* (spirit), present only where there was life; his emphasis upon the workings of spirit owed much to Platonists. Fernel's *Medicina* synthesized classical, medieval and Renaissance medical thought. By integrating Galenic medicine into wider Renaissance visions, his work achieved phenomenal popularity: ninety-seven complete editions or translations appeared between 1554 and 1680.

The problems posed by 'new diseases' forced Galenic theory to adapt. Debate raged about the nature and cause of syphilis. In his *Tractado contra el mal serpentino* (1539) [Treatise on the Serpentine Malady], the Spanish physician Ruy Diaz de Isla (1462–1542) judged that the great pox had been brought back from the New World, claiming he had treated Columbus's pilot in 1493. In 1530 the Veronese physician and humanist Girolamo Fracastoro (Hieronymus Fracastorus: 1478–1553) published his *Syphilis sive morbus gallicus* [Syphilis or the French Disease], describing in verse the disgusting symptoms and treatment of the disease to which he gave the modern name. The poem tells the story of a shepherd named Syphilis who, for insulting Apollo, was punished by a 'pestilence unknown', which brought out 'foul sores' upon his body that could be washed away only with quicksilver. Fracastoro offered a clear if poetical diagnostic portrait. While the disease 'arose in the generative organs', it would then 'eat away the groin' or race through the whole body. Severe pain arose in the bones; eruptions appeared, and 'unsightly scabs break forth, and foully defile the face and breast'.

In his more theoretical *De contagione et contagiosis morbis curatione*

(1546) [On Contagion and the Cure of Contagious Disease], Fracastoro developed the ideas of the Greek atomist Epicurus and the Roman philosopher-poet, Lucretius, to explain contagious diseases in general by the presence of 'seeds', which could infect by contact at a distance, or by 'fomites', substances such as textiles which harboured and transmitted 'disease seeds'. It is not likely that he thought of the *seminaria* (imperceptibly small particles) as micro-organisms – rather he imagined something more like a leaven or spores. A contagious disease like syphilis was, however, specific, retaining its character in person-to-person transmission.*

Whatever the cause, syphilis had to be treated – but how? Quacks offered nostrums, but the basic therapy, as recommended by Fracastoro, was the classically impeccable bleeding, together with the application to the sores of *unguentum Saracenicum*, a mercurial ointment long used for skin eruptions like scabies and leprosy ('a night with Venus, a lifetime with mercury', people quipped). Controversy raged as to how mercury cured – or rather seemed to bring improvement – but most agreed that by means of the copious salivation and sweating it raised, aided by fires and much 'rubbing and tubbing' in special heated barrels, the poison would be expelled. Humoralists argued that the pox produced an excess of phlegm; hence, mercury, which provoked evacuant drooling, seemed the right intervention. Therapeutic hyperthermia (induced fever) long remained popular.

Mercury treatment involved the isolation, tubbing and sweating of the patient for up to one month, though in that process the 'cure' might become almost indistinguishable from the disease, as mercury produced drastic side-effects, including gum ulcerations, tooth loss and bone deterioration. Given the lethality of syphilis, these side-effects could be viewed in a favourable light: had not Hippocrates taught that desperate diseases needed desperate cures? For those wary of mercury and seeking gentler specifics, sarsaparilla was recommended, as was guaiacum bark (see below). But nothing was truly effective against a frightening new disease associated with sex and partly responsible for the bleak, puritanical and often misogynistic mood pervading contemporary sermons and

---

* The ontological view of disease as produced by distinct entities had a few classical antecedents. In *Timaeus* Plato had compared diseases to creatures, and Varro (116–27 BC) had spoken of animals too small to be seen by the eye, 'which by mouth and nose through the air enter the body and cause severe diseases'.

plays. 'How long will a man lie i' the earth ere he rot?', asks Hamlet: 'Faith,' replies the grave-digger, 'if he be not rotten before he die, as we have many pocky corpses now-a-days.' The syphilis threat led authorities to close bath-houses and brothels and to victimize prostitutes; Henry VIII shut down the London 'stews'. Many believed that it was God's will that a disease due to vice should wreak great havoc – a view which has surfaced again today with AIDS.

ANATOMY

The theory and practice of Galenic medicine were under debate, but in essentials Galenism remained intact, queried by some, defied by quacks and mavericks, but challenged head-on only occasionally, notably by the Swiss iconoclast, Paracelsus (see Chapter 9). Substantial change did, however, occur in anatomy. For long but an antechamber in the palace of medicine, anatomy's rise owed much to Renaissance artists who grew fascinated with body form and developed the representational, naturalistic techniques so conspicuous in the magnificent illustrations of sixteenth-century anatomy texts.

In his *De statua* (c. 1435) [On the Statue], the humanist Leon Battista Alberti (1404–1472) argued that knowledge of the bodily parts was vital for the artist, providing him with insight into human proportion which echoed the harmonies of nature and art. Lorenzo Ghiberti (d. 1455) claimed that the artist had to be proficient in the 'liberal arts', including perspective, drawing-theory and anatomy. Knowledge of the skeleton conferred insight into proportion in both microcosm and macrocosm. Art theory and practice emphasized the value of anatomical knowledge and hence of dissecting experience. Underlying this was a naturalistic impulse, though one with its eye on the ideal beauty glimpsed in Graeco–Roman statues. Like the literary humanists, Renaissance artists believed the ancients had observed nature best.

Painters were soon pursuing anatomy as a matter of course. Leonardo da Vinci's teacher Andrea Verrocchio (1435–88), Andrea Mantegna (d. 1506) and Luca Signorelli (c. 1444–1524) all showed some knowledge of muscular and perhaps of deeper anatomy: Verrocchio had his pupils study flayed bodies. It was, however, da Vinci (1452–1519), Albrecht Dürer (1471–1528) and Michelangelo (1475–1564) who most clearly applied the knowledge gained from anatomy.

A brilliant anatomical illustrator, Leonardo was also a perceptive investigator of the mechanics of the human body. Ironically, given the humanist creed, he had no medical education, stumbled over Latin and knew no Greek. His anatomical notebooks show him comparing anatomy with architecture, and using it to probe the mysteries of the microcosm. Although it was never fully realized, from 1489 he planned an anatomical atlas of the stages of man from womb to tomb. His earliest investigations in the late 1480s centred upon a series of skull drawings, which outclassed all previous descriptions. He prized 'experience', but retained a traditional view of brain functions, attributing mental activity to three ventricles governing respectively sensation, intellect, and memory. The nervous system was rendered as a series of passages through which sensations and signals ebbed and flowed.

'Passing the night hours in the company of these corpses, quartered and flayed and horrible to behold', it was after 1506 that Leonardo made his main anatomical contributions, devoting his attention to embryonic development, the muscles, and the nervous, vascular, respiratory and urino-genital systems. The vessels and respiratory passages were compared to the branching of trees and river valleys, and the workings of the heart explained in terms of hydrodynamics and mechanics. Leonardo executed about 750 anatomical drawings, which in some respects are superior to those in Vesalius's *Fabrica* (1543), yet his thinking remained traditional. He continued to accept the Galenic doctrine that blood passed between the ventricles through invisible pores in the septum; and his drawings of the embryo were set within a 'traditional' womb. His career reflects the new involvement of artists with anatomy, though his work had no influence on contemporary medicine, since none of his anatomical manuscripts was published until the late eighteenth century.

As well as artists, medical men also anatomized. Among Renaissance anatomists the desire to see for oneself (the literal meaning of 'autopsy') arose from a variety of traditions. Berengario da Carpi (*c.* 1460–*c.* 1530) studied at Bologna, the cradle of dissection, and in 1502 became lecturer in surgery there. He made the basis for his lectures the *Anatomy* of his Bolognese predecessor, Mondino, and his *Introduction* follows earlier procedures for public dissection. Berengario was no slavish imitator. While often using Galen to disprove Mondino, he was prepared to criticize him on the basis of personal observations, denying the existence in humans of Galen's *rete mirabile*, that 'marvellous network' of blood vessels supposedly lying at the base of the brain (it is found in some animals but not in humans). Insisting on the need for frequent dissections, including humans, he gained a knowledge of female internal anatomy on the basis of postmortem examinations, including one of an executed pregnant woman.

The earliest truly Greek anatomical text was that of Alessandro Benedetti (d. 1512), who lived for sixteen years in Greece and Crete before returning to Padua in 1490 as professor of practical anatomy. In his *Historia corporis humani; sive anatomice* (1502) [The Account of the Human Body: Or Anatomy], the Greek *anatomice* in the title highlighted his hellenism. As a good humanist, Benedetti, like Leoniceno, weeded out Arabic terminology and self-consciously used Greek anatomical terms. Though his book was philological rather than substantive, it did provide an account of a well-ordered anatomy theatre.

Humanist anatomy was given a boost by the discovery of the first part of Galen's *On Anatomical Procedures* (his treatise on how to carry out a dissection) translated into Latin by Guinther von Andernach in 1531. Mondino had started with the internal organs, since these putrefied first. His procedures were rejected by humanists in favour of Galen, who had begun in a more logical fashion with the bones – they were like the walls of houses, he wrote, everything else took shape from the skeleton – next proceeding to the muscles, nerves, veins and arteries, before reaching the cavities of the belly, the chest and the brain, and the internal organs.

But if Galen's dissection strategy was more rational and the quality of his descriptions superior, its flaw was that it was animal not human. A challenge was thus thrown down to anatomists to outdo the master through hands-on investigation of the human corpse. The *Liber introductorius anatomiae* (1536) [Introductory Book of Anatomy] of the Venetian physician Niccolo Massa (c. 1485–1569) scolded those who pronounced on anatomy without having applied the knife to the things they wrote about.

By the 1520s increasing numbers of anatomical texts were being published, and Johannes Dryander (1500–60), professor of medicine at Marburg, carried out some of the first public dissections in Germany, writing these up in a treatise on the anatomy of the head. Andreas Vesalius (1514–64), however, restored Galenic anatomy in such a way as to transcend it. A true Galenic anatomist, in the sense of following the master's advice to see for oneself, Vesalius also presented himself in his *De humani corporis fabrica* (1543) [On the Fabric of the Human Body] as a critic who had no compunction about exposing Galen's errors: 'How much has been attributed to Galen, easily leader of the professors of dissection, by those physicians and anatomists who have followed him, and often against reason!'

Born Andreas van Wesele in Brussels, where his father was pharmacist to Emperor Charles V, Vesalius learned Latin and Greek and enrolled in the Paris Faculty of Medicine, studying under the conservative humanist Sylvius, then Galen's great champion. (In later years Sylvius became a scourge of Vesalius, wittily calling him *vesanus*: madman.) Vesalius learnt his dissecting skills from Guinther von Andernach, and when in 1536 war forced him to flee Paris, he returned to Louvain where he introduced dissection. He showed his anatomical zeal by robbing a wayside gibbet, smuggling the bones back home and reconstructing the skeleton.

In 1537 he moved to Padua, where he made his anatomical name. Dissection had previously been demonstrated there by surgeons, and had never been mandatory for physicians. The rediscovery of Galen's *On Anatomical Procedures* and the wider dissemination of his *On the Use of Parts* meant that humanists were beating the drum for the subject, and the appointment of the young physician was one consequence. Vesalius's *Tabulae anatomicae sex* (1538) [Six Anatomical Pictures] were among the first anatomical illustrations specifically designed for students. The first three sheets were drawn by Vesalius himself and represented the liver and its blood vessels, together with the male and female reproductive organs, the venous and the arterial system. He was still viewing the body through Galenic eyes: despite Berengario, he drew the *rete mirabile*; the liver was still five-lobed, and the heart an ape's.

Thereafter Vesalius grew more critical. Familiarity with human anatomy drove him to the unsettling conclusion that Galen had dissected only animals, and forced him to see that animal anatomy was no substitute for human. He now began to challenge the master on points of detail: for instance, the lower jaw comprised a single bone not two, as Galen, relying on animals, had stated. Evidently, human anatomy had to be learned from dead bodies not dead languages.

In 1539 he acquired a larger supply of cadavers of executed criminals and worked on his great masterpiece, the *De humani corporis fabrica*. Finishing it in 1542, he took it to Basel where the press of Joannes Oporinus published it in 1543 as one of the pearls of Renaissance printing. It presents exact descriptions of the skeleton and muscles, the nervous system, blood vessels and viscera. Though it contains no shattering discoveries, it marks a watershed in the medical understanding of bodily structures, for Vesalius interrogated Galen by reference to the human corpse. Others had criticized odds and ends of Galenic anatomy, but Vesalius was the first to do this systematically. The *Fabrica* gained immensely from the contribution of the artist, Jan Stephan van Calcar (1499–*c*. 1546), also from the Netherlands, who provided the text with technically accurate drawings displaying the dissected body in graceful lifelike poses. The work also enunciated clear methodological principles: the anatomist-lecturer must perform the dissection himself, the eye was preferable to authority, and anatomy was the skeleton key to medicine.

Book I of the *Fabrica* began in Galenic fashion with the bones rather than the internal organs. Various Galenic lapses were corrected: for example, the human sternum has three, not seven, segments. Book II dealt with the muscles and included the famous suite of illustrations showing 'muscle-men' at different stages of corporeal 'undress'. Book III, on the vascular system, was less accurate because Vesalius still based his descriptions partly on animal material. Book IV described the nervous system, following the Galenic classification of the cranial nerves into seven pairs.

Book V dealt with the abdominal and reproductive organs, where he corrected Galen's belief in the five-lobed human liver. He nevertheless still accepted the Galenic physiological tenet that the liver produced blood from chyle, while denying that the vena cava originated in the liver – an observation which, had Vesalius been more physiologically-minded, might have begun the erosion of the Galenic belief in two distinct vascular systems, the venous originating in the liver and the arterial stemming from the heart.

Book VI was devoted to the thorax. Examining the heart, Vesalius cast doubt on the permeability of the interventricular septum: 'We are driven to wonder at the handiwork of the Almighty by means of which the blood sweats from the right into the left ventricle through passages which escape the human vision.' In the second edition (1555), this implicit denial of the septum's permeability was made direct. Here lay a milestone of Renaissance anatomy, for it encouraged anatomists like Realdo Colombo (*c*. 1515–59) to conceive of the pulmonary transit, later used by William Harvey as evidence of the circulation of the blood. Another crucial correction of Galen came in Book VII, on the brain, where Vesalius denied the existence of the *rete mirabile* in humans.

In the end, Vesalius's importance lay in daring to think the unthinkable: that Galen might actually be wrong, and Galen worship with it:

> How much has been attributed to Galen, easily leader of the professors of dissection, by those physicians and anatomists who have followed him, and often against reason! . . . Indeed, I myself cannot wonder enough at my own stupidity and too great trust in the writings of Galen and other anatomists.

The *Fabrica* thus laid the groundwork for observation-based anatomy, announcing a new principle of fact-finding and truth-testing: all anatomical statements were to be subjected to the test of human cadavers.

Later anatomists corrected Vesalius as he had corrected Galen, and independent observation thus became sovereign. Anatomists also grew impatient to establish personal priority in discovering new structures. Amerigo Vespucci had his name immortalized in a continent; for an anatomist, naming a bodily part could be crucial for making his name.*

The frontispiece of the *Fabrica* presents the dreams, the programme, the agenda, of the new medicine. The cadaver is the central figure. Its abdomen has been opened so that everyone can peer in; it is as if death itself had been put on display. A faceless skeleton points towards the open abdomen. Then there is Vesalius, who looks out as if extending an invitation to anatomy. Medicine would thenceforth be about looking inside bodies for the truth of disease. The violation of the body would be the revelation of its truth.

By transference, the idea of anatomizing became a potent medical metaphor during the next couple of centuries, as in Robert Burton's *Anatomy of Melancholy* (1621) or John Donne's poem 'An Anatomy of the World' (1611), and modern medicine adopted the anatomy lesson as its signature: medicine was represented as a probe into nature's secrets, peeling away layer upon layer in the hunt for truth; nothing would resist its gaze. The knife also suggested other modes of mastery, not least sexual conquest, as when Donne likens the lover's caress to a surgeon's knife:

> And such in searching wounds the surgeon is
> As wee, when wee embrace, or touch, or kiss.

---

* The heyday of eponyms was the seventeenth century, with Aselli's pancreas, Graafian follicles, Haversian canals, the circle of Willis, Tulp's valve, Bartholin's duct and glands, and many lesser ones.

A new genre came into fashion: self-anatomy, introspection into one's own soul (*autopsy* means personal observation). 'I have cut up mine owne *Anatomy*,' declared Donne, 'dissected myselfe, and they are got to read upon me.'

Practical anatomy advanced on a broad front after the *Fabrica*. Accounts of the whole body continued to be published, for instance Charles Estienne's (1504–64) *De dissectione partium corporis humani* (1545) [On the Dissection of the Human Body]. Realdo Colombo, an apothecary's son who studied surgery at Padua, succeeding Vesalius there in 1544, corrected some of his errors in his *De re anatomica* [On Anatomy], published posthumously in 1559. He accused Vesalius of passing off descriptions of animal anatomy as human – precisely Vesalius's charge against Galen. Colombo's discovery of the pulmonary transit and elucidation of the heartbeat were momentous. Vivisection experiments showed that blood went from the right side of the heart through the lungs to the left side; that the pulmonary vein did not, as Galen had thought, contain air but blood; and that blood was mixed with air not in the left ventricle of the heart but in the lungs, where it took on the bright red hue of arterial blood. Describing the heartbeat, Colombo held, opposing former views, that the heart acted with greater force in systole (contraction) than in diastole (dilation); this too was crucial for Harvey.

Gabriele Falloppia (1523–63) was appointed in 1551 to perform the annual anatomies at Padua, and he produced more criticism of the *Fabrica* in his *Observationes anatomicae* (1561) [Anatomical Observations]. The tremendous kudos of the new anatomical teaching is illustrated by an incident in 1555, when the university authorities sought to revive the old style of anatomizing as ordained by the statutes. A junior lecturer was to read out Mondino's *Anatomia*, and the senior professor, Vettor Trincavella (1490–1563), was to deliver theoretical lectures. Falloppia's role as anatomist would thereby have been demeaned. In the event, Trincavella's orations were broken up by rowdy students chanting *vogliamo il Falloppio* ('we want Falloppia'), after which anatomy was entirely in his hands.

Falloppia's *Observationes* may be regarded as a coda to the *Fabrica*, adding new observations and correcting errors in both Galenic and Vesalian anatomy. Though not a systematic textbook, it covered a wide range of subjects, with emphasis on the skeleton, especially the skull, and the muscles. Particularly important were his descriptions of the structure of the inner ear, the carotid arteries, the head and neck muscles, and the orbital muscles of the eye. It also contains the famous description of the uterine tubes bearing his name. Falloppia meanwhile kept up a huge practice, claiming to have examined the genitals of 10,000 syphilitics.

Unlike Vesalius, later anatomists produced specialized studies of body parts, such as the treatises on the kidney, the ear and the venous system published by Bartolomeo Eustachio (*c.* 1500–74) in his *Opuscula anatomica* (1564) [Anatomical Studies]. He scolded Vesalius for depicting a dog's kidney instead of a human one, and produced figures of the ear ossicles and the *tensor tympani* in man and in dogs. The Eustachian tube from the throat to the middle ear was described, though priority really belonged to Giovanni Ingrassia (1510–80), who had discovered it in 1546.

Study of specific structures encouraged comparative anatomy, in which different animals were correlated in a self-consciously Aristotelian manner; Aristotle had been keen to compare animal anatomy for classification purposes and to discover essential structural/functional correlations. The greatest comparative anatomist was one of Falloppia's pupils, Hieronymus Fabricius ab Aquapendente (Fabrizio or Fabrici: *c.* 1533–1619), who succeeded to his Padua chair in 1565. Fabricius's aim was to produce a work to be called *Totius animalis fabricae theatrum* [The Theatre of the Entire Animal Structure], but only small sections emerged. As an anatomist he was less interested in Vesalian structural architecture than a comparative approach which stressed three aspects of anatomy: the description, action, and use of body parts. Although Vesalius had surpassed the ancients in *descriptive* accuracy, he had written little on the action and use of the parts; this was what Fabricius aimed to remedy.

Fabricius's most significant work was *De venarum ostiolis* (1603) [On the Valves of the Veins], for the venous valves were to be crucial for William Harvey's demonstration of the blood circulation. It was not Fabricius who discovered them, but he was the first to discuss them at any length. The valves, he maintained, were designed to prevent the extremities from being flooded with blood and to ensure that the other body parts would get their fair share. This theory tallied with the Galenic view that blood was attracted from the liver, the blood-making organ, by each part of the body when it needed nourishment. The valves thus helped the central and upper parts to get blood by preventing its tendency to gather at the extremities.

Fabricius's embryological treatises also influenced Harvey. *De formatione ovi et pulli* (1621) deals with the development of the egg and the generation of the chick, while *De formatu foetu* (1604) [On the Formation of the Foetus] describes how nature provides the means for foetal growth, nourishment and birth. His descriptions of foetal development lay within the Aristotelian theoretical framework of the female contributing the matter and the male the form.

A more idiosyncratic challenge to Galenic physiology had meanwhile come from the polymath Michael Servetus (1511–53). Sickened by the corruption of the Roman Church, Servetus went further than Luther along the road of heresy and developed anti-Trinitarian views, leading to condemnation by Catholics and Protestants alike. In Lyons he had met the medical humanist Symphorien Champier (c. 1471–1539), who advised him to study in Paris, where he worked with the cream of the faculty: Sylvius, Fernel and Guinther von Andernacht. But he soon fell under suspicion, and was condemned in 1538 by the Parlement of Paris for lecturing on astrology. In 1553 he anonymously published his major work, the 700-page *Christianismi restitutio* [The Restoration of Christianity], which was denounced by Calvin as heretical. Escaping the Inquisition, Servetus was nevertheless condemned for heresy on entering Calvin's Geneva, and burnt at the stake.

It was in *The Restoration of Christianity* that Servetus announced the pulmonary transit of the blood, within the framework of an heretical account of how the Holy Spirit entered man. The Bible taught that the blood was the seat of the soul and that the soul was breathed into man by God: there had therefore to be a contact point between air and blood. This led Servetus to denounce Galen's whole scheme. Blood did not go through the septum; he proposed instead a path from the right to the left heart through the lungs. Blood was mixed with air (that is, spirit) in the lungs, rather than in the left ventricle. Confirmation lay in the size of the pulmonary artery – its design was too large to transmit blood for the lungs alone. Servetus's views had no influence on the development of anatomy, not least because almost all copies of his book were burnt with their author.

Renaissance dissections increased knowledge of the structure of man and other animals. But while precipitating an anti-Galen reaction, Vesalian anatomy followed his precepts: without Galen no *Fabrica*. Humanist anatomy was conservative in *theory*. No anatomist opposed the traditional Galenic tripartite division of physiologic function (venous, centred on the liver; arterial, centred on the heart; and sensory/motor, centred on the brain), even when anatomical structures and vascular connections crucial to the scheme were being discredited (for instance, the *rete mirabile*). For all their radical rhetoric, Vesalius's generation shored up ancient medicine and philosophy even as they exposed its factual errors. All the same, Renaissance anatomists enormously elevated the standing of their subject. Its status had been low; it was not listed among the ancient major divisions of medicine, and was stigmatized by its surgical connexions; but the appointment of the physician Vesalius at Padua served notice that anatomy and surgery were to be incorporated into the wider humanist medical movement. The *Fabrica*'s preface argued for the unity of the different medical arts; physicians should not disdain to use their hands, an adage equally dear to contemporary experimental natural philosophers.

Anatomy became integrated into learned medicine – even in backward England, thanks to John Caius (1510–73). Caius was a Galenist physician and protégé of Thomas Linacre, who had been largely responsible for the founding of the College of Physicians in 1518, and for the medical lectureships at Oxford and Cambridge.

Educated at Gonville Hall in Cambridge, from 1539 Caius studied at Padua, teaching Greek and collecting manuscripts, particularly those of Galen, whom he idolized. On his return, he settled in the capital, being admitted Fellow of the College of Physicians in 1547. In his nine terms as president, Caius attempted to mould the college along continental lines, regulating medicine according to the best Galenic standards. He reorganized its statutes, and introduced formal anatomies into its lectures, also demonstrating anatomy before the Barber-Surgeons Company. In Cambridge he refounded his old hall in 1557 as Gonville and Caius College, serving as its master from 1559 and fostering a strong medical tradition, from which William Harvey (1578–1657) was to benefit. Through enthusiasts like Caius and his equivalent in Leiden, Pieter Pauw (1564–1617), anatomy became incorporated throughout Europe into the humanist revival.

Anatomists presented their subject as the cutting edge; the way to certain knowledge was through the senses, especially by 'autopsia', seeing for oneself. Though the Paduan Aristotelian philosopher Cesare Cremonini (1552–1631) was still insisting in 1627 that anatomy could never be the foundation of medicine (only *causes*, the domain of philosophy, and not *observation* could lead to certainty), the sheer success of anatomy swept this dogma aside. Dissections became public events: at Bologna they were staged during the annual carnival, the macabre fascination of the *memento mori*, juxtaposing life and death, contributing to the appeal. Rembrandt's 'The Anatomy Lesson of Dr Nicolaes Tulp' (1632), shows that anatomy had become one of the spectacles and symbols of the age. Not only the method of medicine, anatomy became accepted as a window onto the human condition.

SURGERY

Surgery saw fewer significant changes, and still played second fiddle to physic, being relatively unaffected by the new anatomy. Restricted largely to the body's surface, surgeons dealt with the many accidents of life. They set fractures, treated burns, contusions, knife wounds and the increasingly common gunshot wounds, tumours and swellings, ulcers and various skin diseases; syphilis was usually handled as a surgical condition. Surgery was seen as a skilled craft: 'A chirurgien should have three divers properties in his person,' judged John Halle (1529–68), 'that is to say, a heart as the heart of a lion, his eye like the eyes of an hawk, and his hands as the hands of a woman.'

Through most of Europe, surgery continued to be taught by apprenticeship and organized in guilds. In London a master surgeons' guild had been founded in 1368; the Mystery or Guild of the Barbers of London received its charter from Edward IV in 1462; and in 1540, by Act of Parliament, the Guild of Surgeons merged with the Barbers to form the Barber-Surgeons Company, its first master being Thomas Vicary (c. 1490–1561); Holbein painted Henry VIII chartering the company, which continued until 1745. An active member was William Clowes (1544–1603), who worked as a naval surgeon before setting up in practice in London and being appointed surgeon at St Bartholomew's Hospital in 1575. Military operations in the Low Countries (1586) gave him ample experience, and in 1588 he was appointed surgeon to the fleet. Clowes's treatises on wounds, venereal disease and scrofula were written in racy vernacular, with young surgeons in mind, presenting personal case histories.

Clowes was one of a line of able common-or-garden surgeons: John Woodall's (1556–1643) *The Surgeon's Mate* (1617) served as a manual of naval surgery, attacking the bad habits of 'blaspheming the name of the Almighty' and the 'dedication to the pot and Tobacco-pipe' which were all too common among apprentices; Richard Wiseman (1621–76) was honoured as the 'father of English surgery'. His *Several Chirurgical Treatises* (1676) dwelt on military and naval problems, while his *Treatise of Wounds* (1672), jocularly known as Wiseman's Book of Martyrs, advertised itself as specially for ships' doctors 'who seldom burden their cabin with many books'. He picked up much of his experience during the English Civil War, and his account of military surgery reveals its horrors: cannonballs and gunshot caused horrifying wounds, and amputation and trepanation were often the only remedies, conducted on the battlefield or on a storm-tossed vessel.

Fabricius left a graphic description of a sixteenth-century amputation:

> I was about to cut off the thigh of a man of forty yeares of age, and ready to use the saw, and Cauteries. For the sick man no sooner began to roare out, but all ranne away, except only my eldest Sonne, who was then but little, and to whom I had committed the holding of his thigh, for forme only; and but that my wife then great with child, came running out of the next chamber, and clapt hold of the Patient's Thorax, both he and myselfe had been in extreme danger.

This may not have been an uncommon scene before anaesthesia was available.

'He who wishes to be a surgeon should go to war,' Hippocrates had advised, and the battlefield became accepted as the school of surgery. Growing use of gunpowder had worsened the injuries confronting field-surgeons, because cannonballs and lead shot destroyed far more tissue than arrows or swords and left gaping wounds prone to infection. Many of the most popular vernacular handbooks, such as the *Buch der Wund-Artzney* (1497) [Book of Wound Dressing] of Hieronymus Brunschwig (1450–1533) and the *Feldbuch der Wundartzney* (1517) [Fieldbook of Wound Dressing] of Hans von Gersdorff (c. 1455–1529), were based on field experience. Brunschwig's work contains the earliest printed illustrations of surgical instruments, and endorsed the view that shot wounds were poisoned by gunpowder and so required cautery. Gersdorff explained how to extract bullets with special instruments and dress wounds with hot oil. Amputated stumps were to be enclosed in an animal bladder, after controlling haemorrhage by pressure and styptics.

Thomas Gale (1507–87) published *An Excellent Treatise of Wounds made with Gonneshot* (1563) – the first English work on the subject.

The most acclaimed Renaissance surgeon, Ambroise Paré (1510–90), also learned his craft through war. In 1533 he served as *aide-chirurgien* to the chief Paris hospital, the Hôtel Dieu; and from 1537, for almost thirty years, he divided his time between tending the Paris sick and following the army. Enrolled in 1554 into the confraternity of St Côme, the surgeons' college, five years later Paré attempted in vain to save the life of Henri II after he had been wounded in a jousting tournament.

Paré gave a conventional account of the 'five duties' of his art: 'to remove what is superfluous, to restore what has been dislocated, to separate what has grown together, to reunite what has been divided and to redress the defects of nature'. His prime innovation lay in rejection of the standard treatments for gunshot wounds: the use of cautery (the burning iron) or scalding oil ('potential cautery') to destroy poison and forestall putrefaction before beginning restorative therapy. In his *La methode de traicter leys playes faictes par hacquebutes et aultres bastons à feu* (1545) [Treatise on Gunshot Wounds], he described how, as a green-horn on campaign in Italy in 1537, he had been forced to innovate. Initially, as taught, he had used boiling oil on what were considered to be poisonous gunpowder wounds:

> But my oil ran out and I had to apply a healing salve made of egg-white, rose-oil and turpentine. The next night I slept badly, plagued by the thought that I would find the men dead whose wounds I had failed to burn, so I got up early to visit them. To my great surprise, those treated with salve felt little pain, showed no inflammation or swelling, and had passed the night rather calmly – while the ones on which seething oil had been used lay in high fever with aches, swelling and inflammation around the wound.
>
> At this, I resolved never again cruelly to burn poor people who had suffered shot wounds.

Thenceforth he relied on restorative methods, using a digestive (wound-dressing) made of egg, oil of roses and turpentine, justifying this on the supposition that the gunpowder and shot were not, after all, poisonous. Piously, he always said that he had dressed the wound but God had healed the patient: *Je le pansay; Dieu le guarit.*

Another innovation mentioned in his *Dix livres de la chirurgie* (1564) [Ten Books of Surgery] was the use of ligatures in conducting amputations. Other writers had recommended tying off the veins and arteries so as to stop the blood, but Paré worked out the practical details. This made successful thigh amputations possible – William Clowes reported performing one in 1588, as did Fabricius a little later. There was, however, one drawback. No fewer than fifty-three ligatures were necessary in a thigh amputation, and this required trained assistance. Consequently, ligatures could come into general use only after a method had been found to control blood flow until the surgeon could tie the blood vessels, something accomplished in eighteenth-century France when J. L. Petit invented the first effective tourniquet.

Paré's *Cinq livres de chirurgie* (1572) [Five Books of Surgery] dealt at length with fractures and dislocations, while in the *Deux livres de chirurgie* (1572) [Two Books of Surgery] he addressed the study of obstetrics, showing the art of podalic version (turning a baby in the womb, to facilitate feet-first delivery, as earlier described by Soranus) – and also seeking to explain monstrous births. His successes, however, did not go unchallenged. In 1575, the Paris faculty condemned him for publishing on 'medical' topics – an affront reflecting the tetchiness of physicians towards surgeons' encroachments on their turf.

The practice of early modern surgeons challenges the myth that before anaesthesia and antisepsis their craft was crude and often lethal. The case notes of the London surgeon Joseph Binns (d. 1664) present a different picture. In a career stretching from 1633 to 1663 he recorded 616 cases. Of these no fewer than 196 related to gonorrhoea or syphilis; 77 were of swellings and 61 were more properly medical – including ague, stomach-ache, headache, insomnia, diarrhoea and epilepsy. Fifteen individuals suffered battle wounds, 14 were hurt at work, 19 suffered from falls from horses and 41 were injured in fights. Of the 402 outcomes recorded, 265 were cured and 62 improved; 22 showed no improvement and 53 died.

As Binns's cases show, surgeons' work remained mainly routine, small-scale and fairly safe – if often agonizing. Next to dressing wounds, drawing teeth, dealing with venereal sores and chancres, treating skin abrasions and so forth, the most common surgical procedure (indeed the profession's badge) was blood-letting, often performed at the patient's request. Galenic medicine had warned about the dangers posed by a 'plethora', believing that fevers, apoplexy and headache followed from excessive build-up of blood. Venesection was the obvious corrective. The normal method for phlebotomy was to tie a bandage around the arm to make the forearm veins swell up, and then open the exposed

vein with a lancet: this was popularly called 'breathing a vein'. Cupping
with scarification was another procedure for drawing blood.

A few surgeons came up with ambitious new operations. In Italy
Gaspare Tagliacozzi (1545–99) described in his *De curtorum chirurgia
per insitionem* (1597) [On the Surgery of the Mutilated by Grafting] the
procedure of rhinoplasty or nose reconstruction, which was obviously
attractive in the era of syphilis. Rhinoplasty had been known in India
since ancient times; in southern Italy the operation was apparently practised by empirics. Tagliacozzi was thus far from the technique's inventor,
but he published and claimed to have perfected it. In his rhinoplastic
procedure, a skin flap was partially detached from the flesh of the upper
arm, and allowed to establish itself as a viable tissue. Then the flap, still
attached to the arm, was shaped and sewn to the remains of the nose.
The patient remained with his arm thus attached to his nose for fourteen
days, before the flap was severed from its original site. After a further
period, the process began of reshaping the flap to form the new nose.
The whole business took from three to five months.

Overall, however, with its deep-seated craft basis, surgery remained
rather traditional. Paré concluded:

> A Chirurgion must have a strong, stable and intrepide hand, and
> a minde resolute and mercilesse, so that to heale him he taketh in
> hand, he be not moved to make more haste than the thing requires;
> or to cut lesse than is needfull; but which doth all things as if
> he were nothing affected with their cries; not giving heed to the
> judgement of the common people, who speake ill of Chirurgions
> because of their ignorance.

Whether surgeons were ignorant or not, there remained severe limits
upon what they could achieve.

PHARMACY

Pharmacy underwent significant change as the range of remedies was
extended, thanks to the retrieval of classical drugs, the discovery of new
vegetable products from America and the Indies, and the increasing use
of chemical substances. Herbs – understood in the widest sense as the
leaves, seeds or fruits, bark and roots of plants, shrubs and trees –
had always been the prime ingredients of medical remedies. If used

individually, apothecaries called them 'simples'; combined into a compound drug, perhaps with animal and mineral ingredients, they would
be called 'Galenicals'. Herb gathering (simpling) and preparation of
remedies were domestic skills practised in the family, but there was also
a commercial side to herbal medicine.

With the Greek revival, physicians became concerned that the remedies then in use were inferior, and sought to recover the original *materia
medica* used by the ancients. This required the reform of botany, since
there was no uniform nomenclature, leaving plant identification chancy.
Botany enjoyed its own humanist renaissance: medieval authors were
denounced for their barbaric language and for corrupting ancient texts,
and there was a call for pure editions of classical botanical works. The
great scourge of the pharmacists was the Paris humanist Symphorien
Champier. About 1513 he issued his *Myroel des Apothecaires*, whose sub-
title reveals his position: *The Mirror of the Apothecaries and Druggists in
Which is Demonstrated How the Apothecaries Commonly Make Mistakes in
Several Medicines Contrary to the Intention of the Greeks . . . on the Basis of
the Wicked and Faulty Teachings of the Arabs.*

Around the mid fifteenth century manuscripts of Theophrastus'
Historia plantarum [The History of Plants] and *De causis plantarum* [On
the Causes of Plants] were brought from Constantinople and translated
into Latin by Theodore Gaza. Galen's *De simplicium medicamentorum
facultatibus* [On the Powers of Simple Remedies] had been used in the
medieval universities, but in 1530 a new Latin translation was published,
corrected by reference to 'old manuscripts'. More important, however,
as a vehicle for medical botany was the *De materia medica* of Dioscorides
(*fl.* AD 50–70), which galvanized the botanical revival. The work had
been known in Latin to the Middle Ages, but humanists collected Greek
manuscripts, and the Aldine Press published a Greek edition in 1499.

With the Dioscorides revival, herbals themselves changed. The
earliest printed ones were compiled from medieval sources, but later
works by William Turner (*c.* 1510–68), Leonhart Fuchs (1501–66) and
others became more naturalistic, both verbally and pictorially, mirroring
the Renaissance anatomy atlases. The first to abandon the old stylized
pictures was the *Herbarum vivae eicones* (1530) [Living Images of Plants]
of Otto Brunfels (d. 1534), town physician of Bern. The artist Hans
Weiditz (d. *c.* 1536) (school of Dürer) gave this herbal its innovative
look. When his plants did not tally with Dioscorides, Brunfels tried to
force identifications.

He described 258 different plants; ninety-seven years later, Caspar Bauhin's (1560–1624) *Pinax theatri botanici* (1627) [A Catalogue of Botanical Theatre] included around 6,000 specimens. This stupendous increase was achieved through individual and collaborative efforts. The first chair in botany was established in Padua in 1533; botanical gardens were created in Pisa and Padua in 1544–5, with other universities following: Bologna, Leiden, Leipzig, Basel and Montpellier. Plants, however, were not always available and altered with the seasons; this made the artificial or dry garden (*hortus siccus*) an invaluable invention, allowing rare plants to be preserved or exchanged, and providing teaching material and draughtsmen's models.

A great boost was provided by Pier Andrea Mattioli (1500–77), who in 1542 became physician to the province of Gorizia, where he worked on a commentary of Dioscorides. Published in 1544, his edition of *De materia medica* became the spur for botanical and pharmacological research, earning its author European celebrity. Like Linnaeus later, Mattioli had a gift for inspiring collaborators to travel, collect and send him specimens. Expanding with each edition, the work culminated in the version of 1565, a lavishly illustrated Latin folio running to nearly 1500 pages, bejewelled with full-page illustrations.

As the entrepôt of the Mediterranean, enjoying close links with the Middle East and the overland spice trade from the Indies, Venice was the natural centre for the humanist goal of recovering classical medicaments. Not least, the Venetian Republic controlled Crete and Cyprus, the herb gardens of the ancients. Drugs unknown to the latin West – balsam and myrrh for instance – were rediscovered. Famous for its purging powers, rhubarb had entered Europe through the overland trade routes from the East; by the early seventeenth century, seeds from Bulgaria allowed one medically valuable type of rhubarb (*Rhaponticum*, from the Pontus or Black Sea) to be grown in Europe, while search continued for the 'true' rhubarb which Marco Polo had reported in 1295 as deriving from China. Theriac, that panacea of the ancients, composed of up to a hundred herbal, animal and mineral ingredients, seemed in the 1540s quite impossible to compound; many of its ingredients were unknown and more than twenty substitutes were needed. But by 1566 the Veronese botanist-pharmacist Francesco Calzolari (1522–1609) was using only three proxies. Physicians grew confident that the remedies of the ancients had been recovered.

Thanks to Iberian voyages of discovery, new drugs filtered in,

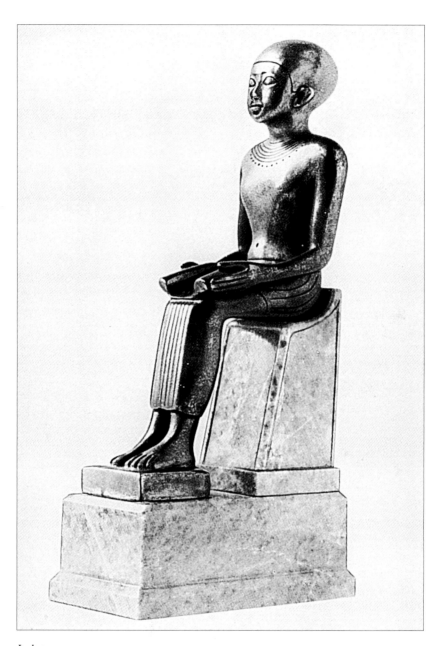

Imhotep.
Chief vizier to Pharaoh Zozer (*fl.* 27th century BC), Imhotep became hallowed as the physician-god of Egyptian medicine. He was associated with healing shrines and temple sleep (incubation cures). Statue, *c.* 650 BC.

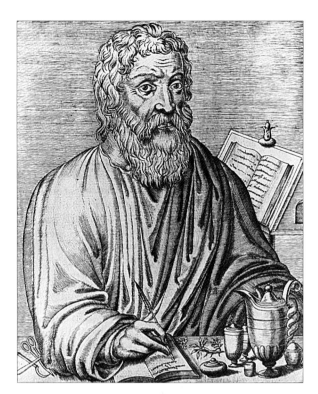

Hippocrates.

Though Hippocrates
(*c.* 460–377 BC) certainly existed,
all the biographical details about
him are legendary. Note how the
founder of bedside medicine was
turned by this Renaissance artist
into a scholar. Line drawing, 1584.

Galen.

Galen (AD 129–*c.* 216) was the
medical colossus of the Roman
era. Imaginative portraits of him
graced the numerous editions of
his works in the first age of print.
Georg Paul Busch, line drawing,
eighteenth century.

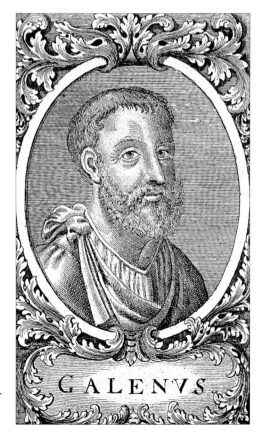

Hildegard of Bingen.
Hildegard of Bingen
(1098–1179), who began having
religious visions at an early age,
practised medicine in her role as
Abbess of Rupertsberg. Her
main work was on the curative
powers of herbs, stones and
animals. W. Marshall,
engraving, 1642.

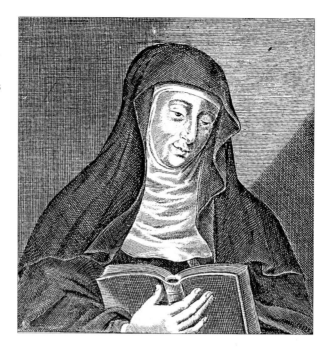

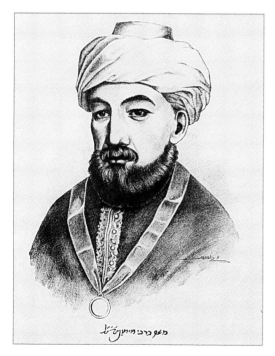

Moses Maimonides.
Moses Maimonides (1135–1204)
was the leading Jewish medical writer
of the medieval period. Born in
Cordova, he moved to Cairo,
becoming court physician to Saladin,
Sultan of Egypt. Photogravure by
M. Gur-Aryeh, Jerusalem (after
engraved portrait affixed to Ugolini,
Thesaurus antiquitatum sacrarum,
Venice, 1744).

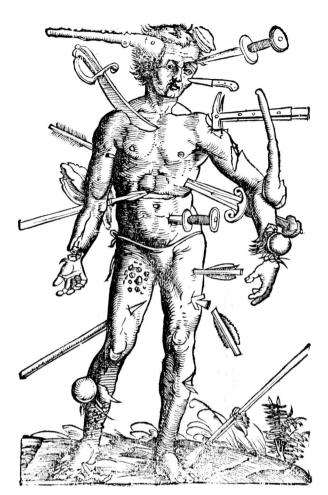

The Wound Man.
The Wound Man was a characteristic form of surgical illustration from medieval times onwards, demonstrating the wide range of injuries the surgeon claimed to be able to cure. Line drawing from H. von Gersdorf, *Feldtbuch der Wundartzney* (Strassburg: H Schott, 1530), fol. 22v.

The Common Willow.
Renaissance herbals were noted for their more naturalistic illustrations. According to Gerard, willow leaves 'do stay the spitting of bloud, and all other fluxes of bloud whatsoever in man or woman'. A later age would find in willow bark the essence of aspirin. Line drawing from J. Gerard, *The Herball, or General Historie of Plantes* (London: E. Bollifant for B. and J. Norton, 1597).

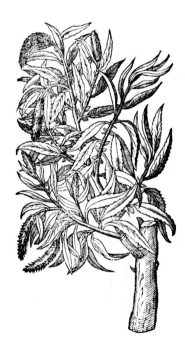

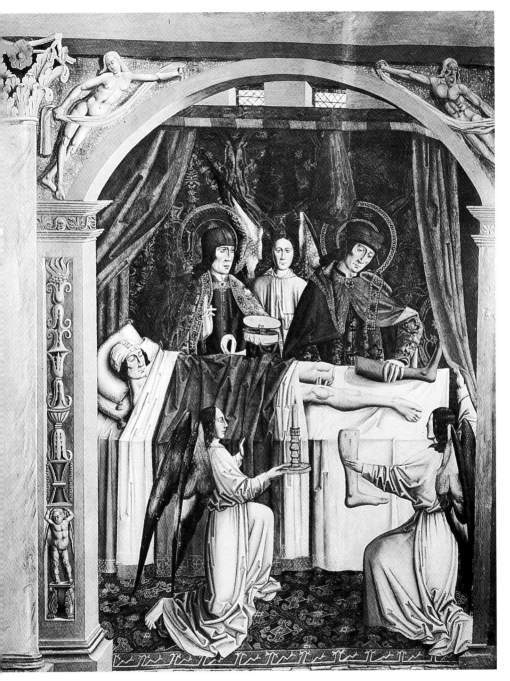

St Cosmas and St Damian performing the miracle of the black leg.

Damian and Cosmos became the patron saints of medicine. Brothers living in Asia Minor around the close of the third century, they were celebrated for their healing powers. Their chief medical miracle credits them with the first transplant: they amputated a (white) man's gangrenous leg and grafted in its place that of a dead Moor. Alonso de Sedano, oil painting, early sixteenth century.

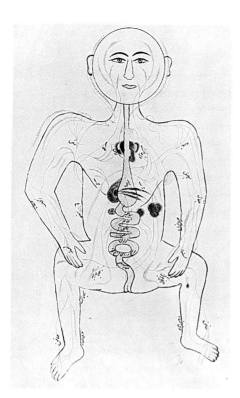

Medieval Persian anatomical drawing, showing the arterial system.

Both medieval European and Islamic anatomical illustrations favoured the squatting, arms-akimbo position. The aim was not naturalistic accuracy but the simplicity of a diagram. Line drawing, Persian MS no. 32427.

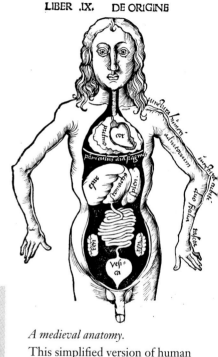

LIBER .IX. DE ORIGINE

A medieval anatomy.

This simplified version of human anatomy is less a mark of ignorance or lack of artistic skill than of the production of easy-to-memorize charts for student use. Gregorius Reisch, from *Margarita Philosophica* (Freiburg in Breisgau: J. Scott, 1503) IX, fol. F2v.

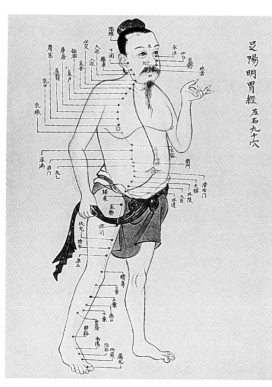

Chinese acupuncture chart.

This style of depicting acupuncture channels was well established by the seventeenth century. It principally represents the stomach meridian (*zu yang ming wei jing*). The stomach is viewed as a *yang* organ. Watercolour, eighteenth/nineteenth century.

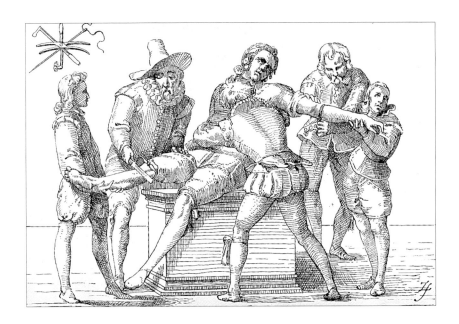

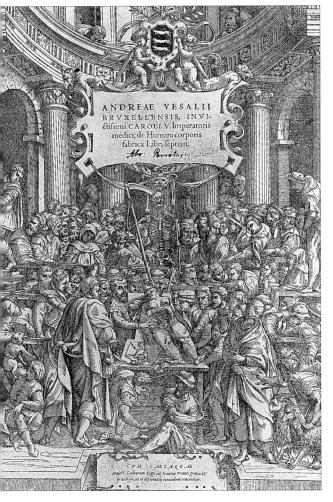

ABOVE *Two Surgeons Amputating the Leg and Arm of the Same Patient, who is being restrained by assistants.*

Early surgical illustrations of amputation are commonly stylized and comfortingly suggest a serenity in the patient and a gentleness in the surgeon which actual operating conditions must have belied. ZS, pen drawing, (after an engraving, 1597).

LEFT *The Frontispiece to Vesalius's* De humani corporis fabrica [On the Fabric of the Human Body: 1543].

This picture signals the new anatomy: the cadaver is the central figure. Its abdomen has been opened so that everyone can peer in. A skeleton points towards the opening. Notice how Vesalius looks out at us as if he were extending an invitation.

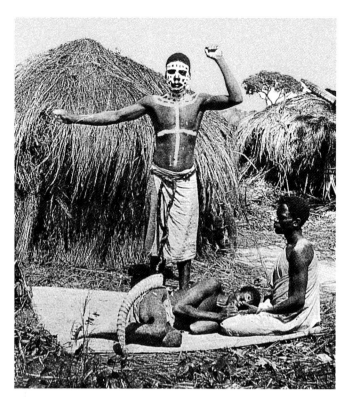

A medicine man or shaman, adorned with white paint, standing above a sick man trying to drive away the disease.

Early anthropologists witnessing and photographing scenes like this were dismissive. The original caption reads: 'Both doctor and patient believe in the farce.' Photograph, early twentieth century.

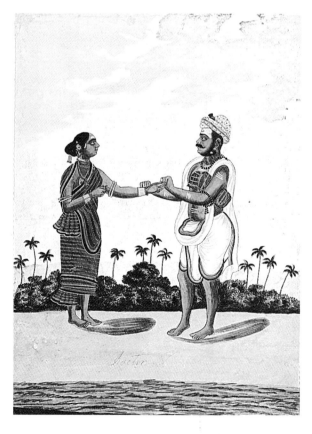

Indian doctor taking the pulse of a patient.

Pulse-taking was central to both the Indian and the Chinese clinical traditions. The hand was one of the few body parts (especially in a woman) that the physician might properly touch. Gouache drawing, nineteenth century.

together with foodstuffs like potatoes. Cocoa came back with Cortés in 1529, becoming a favourite drink, a specific for 'wasting diseases', a stimulant, and even the basis of cocoa-butter suppositories. Meanwhile the Portuguese had rounded the Cape of Good Hope in 1487–8 and reached India in 1499. By 1512–13 they landed in the legendary Spice Islands, the Moluccas, whose spices had traditionally arrived in Europe via the overland route.

Remedies from distant parts entered into scholarship, particularly through the writings of Nicolas Monardes (*c.* 1493–1588) and Garcia d'Orta (1501–68). Educated at Seville, Monardes commented that New World drugs were inferior to those of Spain (pharmaceutical chauvinism was strong), but he later changed his mind, enthusiastically praising their powers in his *Dos Libros* (1565–74). The book followed a standard format, giving for each plant its place of origin, appearance, colour, properties and uses. New World plants posed problems, for their virtues were uncertain. This led him to concentrate on the distinguishing marks of the new plants and to describe how they were processed by the American Indians. Together with coca, jalap, sarsaparilla and sassafras (these latter famed for blood-cleansing), one of his best-known descriptions was that of tobacco, which he praised for curing head pains, toothaches, bad breath, chilblains, worms, joint pains, swellings, poisoned wounds, kidney stones, carbuncles and fatigue. Its efficacy derived from its heating and drying qualities. Despite King James I's strictures against 'this filthy custom', tobacco enjoyed a high medicinal reputation in the seventeenth century.

In the face of the terrifying syphilis epidemic, imported plant remedies might appear godsends, for treatment with mercury was almost worse than the disease. In the Caribbean the Spaniards saw syphilis (more probably yaws) treated by decoctions made from guaiac wood (*Guaiacum officinalis*); by 1508 this was being imported into Spain and its use became widespread. Also known as 'holy wood', guaiac was obtained from evergreens indigenous to the West Indies and South America. The folk belief that God planted cures where diseases arose reinforced the conjectural New World origin for syphilis. Shiploads of guaiac were imported into Europe, organized by the Fuggers of Augsburg, the mercantile and banking family who monopolized the trade and profited mightily. The German humanist and soldier Ulrich von Hutten (1488–1523) experienced the horrors of the mercury treatment; he went through eleven mercury cures in nine years, then he heard of guaiac, and after repeated infusions believed he was cured. Von Hutten's *De guaiaci medicina et morbo gallico* (1519) [On the Guaiac Remedy and the French Disease] was translated into German and French, but by the time Monardes wrote in 1565 guaiac was losing support.

One key remedy from the East was opium, largely imported from Turkey. It had been in use in Egypt in the second millennium BC, and Avicenna called it 'the most powerful of stupefacients'. Ever the queen of drugs, it was profusely used in western medicine from the sixteenth century, and Thomas Sydenham (1624–89) later proclaimed that 'among the remedies which it has pleased the Almighty God to give to man to relieve his sufferings, none is so universal and so efficacious as opium.' It seemed the wonder drug; not just a pain-deadener, it also stopped dysentery and relieved respiratory disorders.

India supplied new remedies. In 1563 Garcia D'Orta published *Coloquios dos simples, e drogas he cousas mediçinais da India* [Dialogues on Simples and Drugs and Medical Matters from India] which described such eastern products as aloes, camphor, sandalwood, ginger, asafoetida and betel, and new fruits such as mangoes. Like the Italian humanist botanists, he had to confront identification problems. (Was modern cinnamon the 'canella', 'cinnamon' or 'cassia' of the ancients?) Other eastern drugs filtered to the West later, including Chinese rhubarb and ginseng, introduced in the eighteenth century by the Jesuits.

Thanks in part to the labours of the botanists and the importation of new drugs, the apothecary's trade boomed, though for many (witness Romeo's remarks) the apothecary remained a wretch vending poisons:

> I do remember an apothecary
> And hereabouts he dwells – whom late I noted
> In tatter'd weeds, with overwhelming brows,
> Culling of simples; meagre were his looks,
> Sharp misery had worn him to the bones;
> And in his needy shop a tortoise hung,
> An alligator stuff'd and other skins,
> Of ill-shap'd fishes . . .

Like other branches of medicine, apothecaries organized themselves. In England, James I recognized them as a special body in the Grocers' Company in 1607, and ten years later they gained their independence, organizing as the Masters, Wardens, and Society of the Art and Mystery of the Apothecaries of the City of London.

THE MIND

Renaissance humanism, mysticism, hermeticism and astrology fostered interest in the human soul, the spiritual fulcrum in a cosmos governed by supernatural forces – good and evil. It is not surprising, therefore, that one field in which Renaissance philosophy made a contribution to medicine was mental disorder. Theories remained complex, however. The neo-Platonist Ficino related melancholia to the sway of Saturn, but also to the action of black bile, the humour of genius and of depression.

Humanist moralists explored the mind, notably the French essayist, Michel de Montaigne (1533–92), twice mayor of Bordeaux. Suffering agony from a bladder stone* and sickened by religious and dynastic bloodshed, he retired from the world to compose his mind in tranquillity, only to find himself haunted by 'monsters' and 'chimeras'. Solitude sparked 'melancholy adust', a sick humour disposing his melancholic temperament towards madness. Composing his *Essais* (1580) was an antidote, a writing cure aimed at restoring balance through anatomizing his mind in quest of self-knowledge.

Montaigne kept his soul 'at home' in the body, studying both, hoping to grasp how man should live wisely and face death well. Yet in response to the old Socratic injunction of self-knowledge ('nosce te ipsum'), he was sceptical: *Que sçay-je?* (What do I know?), he asked. Such themes were relentlessly pursued, not least by Shakespeare, whose contemporary, Robert Burton (1557–1640), described himself as 'fatally driven' upon the rock of melancholy and mixed philosophy and medicine. His *Anatomy of Melancholy* (1621) was a satirical flagellation of folly but also a serious medical inquiry which included the following causes of depression: 'idleness, solitariness, overmuch study, passions, perturbations, discontents, cares, miseries, vehement desires, ambitions', and hundreds more.

---

* Montaigne wrote, 'I am in the grip of one of the worst diseases – painful, dreadful, and incurable. Yet even the pain itself, I find, is not so intolerable as to plunge a man of understanding into frenzy or despair. At least I have one advantage over the stone. It will gradually reconcile me to what I have always been loath to accept – the inevitable end. The more it presses and importunes me, the less I will fear to die.'

Self-possession in the face of sickness, he believed, was crucial. Physicians were of little use: 'no doctor takes pleasure in the health even of his friends,' he remarked; this was a long-standing humanist jibe.

Philosophical medicine explored sickness of the mind and its synergy with the body. Mingling suspicion with sympathy, paintings and plays made much of fools, melancholics and madmen. 'Bedlam' acquired its notoriety, and Tom o' Bedlam became a well-known figure, wandering the lanes, singing and begging. The period also brought the wave of mass hysteria and persecution known as the witch-craze. Despite the biblical injunction, 'thou shalt not suffer a witch to live' (Exodus 22:18), the medieval Church had long remained little concerned about witchcraft, but by the late fifteenth century this had changed, and a Papal Bull of 1484 condemned its spread and authorized a crackdown on its practitioners. Two years later, the *Malleus maleficarum* [Hammer of the Witches] of the Dominicans, Institoris and Sprenger, created a witchfinders' handbook that passed through more than twenty editions and translations. Accusations spread, especially where religious conflict and social tension were rife, and trials and executions mounted till around 1650. As late as 1692 the Salem, Massachusetts, trials resulted in thirty executions, and witches were still occasionally being executed in parts of Europe on the eve of the French Revolution.

Nineteenth-century psychiatrists retrospectively diagnosed witches as mentally disturbed, their confessions of compacts with the Devil being the progeny of delusions and hysterical personalities. More recently, such charges have been levelled primarily at the witch-hunters, for whipping up mass hysteria. Though most early-modern doctors supported the prosecution of witches, a few were sceptical, and doubts were particularly expressed in the *De praestigiis daemonum* (1563) [On the Conjuring Tricks of Demons] of Johannes Weyer (1515–88). Weyer was the town medical officer of Arnhem in the Netherlands, and he warned against mistaking sickness for Satan. The Devil had no power over the body; so-called witches imagined the enormities they confessed, perhaps in the throes of fever. He insisted that the deeds of which they were accused – causing sudden death, impotence or crop failure – were natural occurrences. Witches were to be pitied and healed rather than harried and punished.

Felix Platter (1536–1614), dean of the medical faculty at the University of Basel, left extensive accounts of psychiatric disorders in his *Praxis medica* (1602) [The Practice of Medicine] and *Observationum* (1614) [Observations]. From a medical viewpoint he downplayed diabolical agency, though advising the use of amulets in cases of madness. He discussed hysteria and sexual disorders, described cretinism (then common in Switzerland), and advocated a basket of psychological, pharmacological and physical therapies. Occasionally at witch trials, medical and theological interpretations of insanity clashed. Yet it was not until the triumph of the mechanical philosophy that a naturalistic theory of mind gained ground, ruling out the supernatural element in mental illness.

A window is offered onto the deranged by the case notes of the Revd Richard Napier (1559–1634), a contemporary of Shakespeare's who specialized in healing those afflicted in mind and spirit. A high proportion of the afflicted visiting him suffered family troubles, financial insecurities and religious torments, and many believed they were bewitched. Of the 134 cases of deep depression this Anglican clergyman handled, fifty-eight were attributed to deep grief following children's deaths ('Much grief for the death of two children', one parent related). Of Agnys Morton, who had murdered her illegitimate baby, evidently suffering from puerperal fever, Napier recorded,

> This woman is distracted of her wits ... went to make herself away, being tempted as she sayeth thereunto by the Tempter. Will not in any case say her prayers ... Very ravenous and greedy, and will say the foul Fiend lyeth at her heart, that she cannot feed him fast enough.

Napier cast horoscopes in forming his diagnoses, and healed with a mixture of herbal remedies, prayer and counsel, often giving patients sigils and talismans. He may be regarded as one of the last Renaissance magi.

MEDICINE IN SOCIETY

Renaissance humanism benefited the doctor more than the patient. The new learning hardly helped physicians to cure diseases. But it gave the medical profession an elevated sense of its proper dignity, and though playwrights loved poking fun at the pedantic pomposities of costly and useless physicians, medicine grew more status-conscious, and more dismissive of its rivals. 'All that falsely usurp this Title of Physitian', declared Richard Whitlock, 'take off their Visards, and underneath appeare Wicked Jewes, Murtherers of Christians, Monks, abdicant of their orders, &c. Unlearned Chymists, conceited Paedagogues, dull

Mechanicks, Pragmaticall Barbers, wandring Mountebancks, Cashiered Souldiers . . . Toothlesse-women, fudling Gossips, and Chare-women, talkative Midwives, &c. In summe . . . the scum of Mankind.'

This heightened sense of dignity was marked in public recognition. Earlier tendencies towards the public employment of physicians continued. The code of criminal procedure promulgated for the Habsburg empire by Charles V in 1532, known as the Carolina, required judges to consult surgeons in cases of suspected homicide, and midwives in infanticide. A landmark in forensic medicine, the Code was adopted in much of continental Europe. Medical authors were keen to display their expertise in the courtroom. Paré explained how to recognize the signs of virginity in women – important because under ecclesiastical law non-consummation was one of the very few grounds for annulment of marriage – and the indications of death by lightning, smothering, drowning, apoplexy, poison and infanticide; he also showed how to distinguish between wounds given to a body when dead and alive.

Medical institutions continued to develop under royal and municipal patronage. In 1518 Henry VIII chartered the College of Physicians, granting it examining, licensing and policing powers over medical practice in London. (It became 'Royal' from the time of Charles II.) Unlike some European counterparts, however, the college did not succeed in extending its jurisdiction to a wider region, nor did it have control over the licensing of surgeons and apothecaries.

In health care provision in England, the sixteenth century brought a major setback. The dissolution of the monasteries and chantries (rapacious asset-stripping carried out in the name of religious reform by Henry VIII and Edward VI) resulted in the closure of almost all the medieval hospitals, which, even if they had provided little treatment, at least had afforded shelter to the aged, sick and incapacitated. A few institutions survived the Reformation, being re-established on a new, secular basis. St Bartholomew's and St Thomas's passed to the City of London after the Dissolution, as did Bethlem for treating lunatics. Despite its burgeoning population, rising to 200,000 by 1600, London long possessed only these three hospitals, not in themselves very large (in 1569 St Thomas's housed 203 patients); beyond the capital, scarcely any medical institutions survived Henry VIII's destructive greed.

Shortcomings in institutional medical provision in England and elsewhere may have been counterbalanced by the growth, thanks to the development of printing, of writings popularizing health advice. These sprang largely from the regimen and hygiene traditions incorporated within the Salernitan Regime. Such works, stressing the non-naturals, instructed readers to monitor their constitutions. Andrewe Boorde (c. 1490–1549), an ex-monk turned physician, offered rules in his *Compendyous Regyment or a Dyetary of Healthe* (1547). He began by prescribing where to situate a house, how to organize a household, what to eat and drink and what to avoid, and what exercise to take, before moving on to more detailed physical methods of preserving and restoring health. The non-naturals were also stressed by André du Laurens (1558–1609), physician to Henri IV and professor at Montpellier. In 1597 he published a book translated as *Discourse of the Preservation of the Sight; of Melancholic Diseases; of Rheumes and of Old Age*, which contended that the causes of ageing were mental as well as physical: 'Nothing hastens old age more than idleness.' Early in the seventeenth century, Sir John Harington (1561–1612) brought out a popular English translation of the *Regimen sanitatis Salernitanum*. Addressed to King James, *The Englishman's Doctor* (1608) provided health advice to all:

> Salerne Schoole doth by these lines impart
> All health to England's King, and doth advise
> From care his head to keepe, from wrath his heart,
> Drinke not much wine, sup light, and soon arise,
> When meate is gone, long sitting breedeth smart:
> And after-noone still waking keepe your eyes.
> When mov'd you find your selfe to Natures Needs,
> Forbeare them not, for that much danger breeds,
> Use three Physicians still; first Doctor Quiet,
> Next Doctor Merry-man, and Doctor Dyet.

Temperance was the message of the highly successful *Discorsi della vita sobria* (1558–65) [Discourses on the Temperate Life] of Luigi Cornaro (c. 1464–1566), which he wrote in his eighties. Cornaro maintained that a temperate life would enable the body's finite supply of vital spirits to last until life ebbed peacefully away between the ages of five and six score. Practising what he preached, he attributed his longevity to moderation, exercise, keeping his mind occupied and heeding his diet. Old age aroused great interest. In 1635, William Harvey performed a post-mortem on Thomas Parr (c. 1483–1635), supposedly the oldest man in England. Brought to London, he was presented to Charles I and exhibited at taverns, but the smoky London atmosphere proved too much and he expired, allegedly at the ripe age of 152.

Printing made other sorts of health literature more widely available. Obstetrics and babycare books began to appear in many languages. The earliest published midwives' textbook written in the vernacular, Eucharius Rösslin's (d. 1526) *Der Swangern Frawen under Hebammen Rosengarten* (1513) [Garden of Roses for Pregnant Women and Mid-wives] appeared in English as the *Byrth of Mankynde* (1540) and was still in use in the eighteenth century. Its frontispiece pictures the mother in labour among relatives and midwives, groaning on a birth stool, while the attendant astrologer gazes through the window to cast the baby's horoscope.

Thanks to printing, stronger links were forged between medicine, learning and culture. Humanism's preoccupation with recovering the learned medicine of the ancients proved, however, a mixed blessing, and scepticism towards the profession remained deep-seated: 'Trust not the physician, his antidotes are poison,' warns Shakespeare's *Timon of Athens*. During the following century medicine was to build a new scientific basis.

CHAPTER IX

THE NEW SCIENCE

THE DREAM OF RENAISSANCE HUMANISTS was to restore medicine to its Greek purity, but a counter-view gained ground in the seventeenth century as the 'moderns' confronted the 'ancients': medicine could thrive only if the deadweight of the past were cast off. After centuries of stultifying homage to antiquity, a fresh start was needed. This was a subversive doctrine indeed, but support could be drawn from the Reformation: if Luther could break with Rome, how could it be impious to demand the reformation of medicine? Such revolutionary impulses first found expression in the work of the iconoclastic Paracelsus.

PARACELSUS

Meaning 'surpassing Celsus', Paracelsus was the cocksure name adopted in his early thirties by Theophrastus Philippus Aureolus Bombastus von Hohenheim (c. 1493–1542), a medical protestant if ever there was one – though, ironically, he never formally abandoned his native Catholicism. Paracelsus was born in Einsiedeln, Switzerland and educated by his physician father in botany, medicine and natural philosophy. Around the age of twenty he briefly studied medicine in Italy but subsequently led the life of a wandering student. All the while he picked up knowledge from artisans and miners ('I have not been ashamed to learn from tramps, butchers and barbers'), observed and thought for himself, and acquired a taste for the esoteric. The writings of Trithemius (1462–1516), an occultist who aspired to the wisdom of the mythic Hermes Trismegistus, convinced him of the workings of invisible powers as spiritual intercessors between God and man in an enchanted cosmos.

Paracelsus's off-beat education marked a drastic break with the orthodox university medical curriculum built on canonical texts; it helps explain how he repudiated Galenism and came up with new disease concepts in a twenty-year career that made him the scourge of the medical Establishment: 'When I saw that nothing resulted from [doctors'] practice but killing and laming, I determined to abandon such a miserable art and seek truth elsewhere.' But while there is no denying Paracelsus's break with the past, the common portrayal of him as the founder of scientific medicine is misleading, for his creed always involved mystical and esoteric doctrines quite alien to today's science. He thus appears a paradox. For while subscribing to popular beliefs and folk remedies, and lapping up the lore he heard from peasants about the nymphs and gnomes haunting mines and mountains, he also championed new chemical theories, dividing all substances into 'sulphur', 'mercury' and 'salt'. Yet these must be understood not as material elements but as hidden powers.

Paracelsus's fundamental conviction was that nature was sovereign, and the healer's prime duty was to know and obey her. Nature was illegible to proud professors, but clear to pious adepts. His teachings on remedies thus drew on the popular doctrine of signatures to identify curative powers: the orchid looked like a testicle to show it would heal venereal maladies, the plant eyebright (*Euphrasia officinalis*) had been made to resemble a blue eye to show it was good for eye diseases. Paracelsus was perhaps influenced by radical Protestantism and its faith in a priesthood of all believers: truth was to be found not in musty folios but in the fields, and in one's heart. Yet though he displayed a fiercely independent temper, kowtowing to none, unlike Servetus he cannily avoided getting ensnared in Reformation politics.

His fisticuffs mentality comes out clearly in his sublime contempt for academic pomposity: 'I tell you, one hair on my neck knows more than all you authors, and my shoe-buckles contain more wisdom than both Galen and Avicenna.' In 1526 he was appointed town physician and professor of medicine in Basel, a post requiring him to lecture to the medical faculty. This he did not in the customary Latin but in German, wearing not academic robes but the alchemist's leather apron, and his manifesto pronounced that he would not teach Hippocrates and Galen, since experience alone (which included his intuitive flights) would disclose the secrets of disease. Jeering at orthodox physicians, and taking his cue from Luther, he then publicly burned Avicenna's *Canon*, the

Bible of learned medicine, along with various Galenic texts on St John's day (24 June 1527). All this was quite unheard of.

Bloody-mindedness aside, Paracelsus's significance lay in pioneering a natural philosophy based on chemical principles. Salt, sulphur and mercury were for him the primary substances. These did not completely replace the Aristotelian–Galenic system of qualities, elements and humours, but he considered them superior because they were in alchemical terminology 'male' – that is active and spiritual – whereas the elements were 'female' and passive. His 'tria prima' are to be understood not as material substances but as principles: solidity or consistency were represented by salt; inflammability or combustibility by sulphur; and spirituousness or volatility by mercury. Drawing on the occult, he associated diseases with the spirits of particular minerals and metals: 'When you see erysipelas, say there is vitriol. When you see cancer, say there is colcothar' (peroxide of iron). But he also boldly deployed metals and minerals – mercury, antimony (stibium), iron, arsenic, lead, copper and sulphur – for therapeutic purposes, together with laudanum (tincture of opium).

Embodying spiritual and vital forces, Paracelsus's chemical principles explained living processes. These depended upon what he called *archei*, the internal living properties controlling processes like digestion; and also *semina* or seeds deriving from God, the great magus (magician) who orchestrated nature. The agents of disease, on the other hand, might be poisonous emanations from the stars or minerals from the earth, especially salts. His belief that there were as 'many diseases as pears, apples, nuts', and that each disease had a specific external cause sounds like an anticipation of ontological doctrines, but it must be remembered that he saw the essence of disease as spiritual.

Paracelsus ridiculed hidebound practices. Sickness was to be understood not by conventional urine inspection (uroscopy) but by chemical analysis using distillation and coagulation tests. He also enjoyed mocking innovations championed by others. Dissection, for instance, was worthless 'dead anatomy', for it could not reveal how the living body functioned. He died before Vesalius published his *Fabrica*, but he would probably have deemed it not worth a sausage. True physiology had to discover the nourishment each body part needed, while to fathom pathology stellar influences had to be probed and the presence of abnormal quantities of salt, sulphur and mercury tested. By disparaging humoral balance and stressing the prime role of particular organs in health and disease, he countered Galenist constitutionalism with a new notion of specificity and a pathology of disease as invasion from outside.*

He interpreted familiar diseases in new ways. Take gout, regarded by Hippocratic medicine as a classic humoral imbalance involving defluxion into the foot ('gutta' means 'flowing'). Paracelsus read gout not constitutionally but chemically, seeing it in terms of the wider category of 'tartaric disease' (diseases of incrustations). In *De morbis tartareis* (1531) [On Diseases of Tartar], he proposed that some local external factor, such as water supply, might produce the characteristic chemical depositions in the joints. He boasted patriotically that in Switzerland, 'the most healthy land, superior to Germany, Italy and France, nay all Western and Eastern Europe, there is no gout, no colic, no rheumatism and no stone'. Gouty nodules, he maintained, consisted of calcined synovia or an excremental salt (tartar) coagulated in a joint. Since the tartar coating wine casks was a product of fermentation, such material could be compared to bodily deposits like gallstones, kidney stones, and the dental incrustations still known as tartar. Bodily tartar was thus derived from food and released through digestion. In some individuals it failed to be excreted, tending instead to be transformed by 'spirit of salt' into stony substances like calculi or gouty tophi. This theory of 'tartarous disease' was one of the earliest attempts to advance a chemical aetiology for a malady.

Paracelsus sneered at bookworms ('not even a dog-killer can learn his trade from books'), and his copious writings taught that truth was to be found not in libraries but in the Book of Nature, and issued a health warning: 'the more learned, the more perverted'. Personal experience was what counted – 'he who would explore nature must tread her books with his feet.'

However ambivalent such views – Paracelsus was the classic dogmatic anti-dogmatist, the humble chap convinced everyone else was wrong, the inveterate scribbler who told readers to close their books –

---

* Paracelsus became and remains the patron saint of alternative medicine; in 1982 the Prince of Wales told the British Medical Association that 'we could do worse than to look ... at the principles he so desperately believed in, for they have a message for our time; a time in which science has tended to become estranged from nature – and that is the moment when we should remember Paracelsus.' But in his localism and advocacy of heavy-metal remedies, Paracelsus was a far cry from the kind of holism praised by today's alternative-medicine fans. Paracelsus has also attracted dubious supporters, not least among Nazis, who admired him for his commitment to folk wisdom.

his commitment to the discovery of truth through observation and experiment was a breath of fresh air. And it became the inspiration of the new medicine emerging in the 'scientific revolution' stirring at about the time of his death: 1543 brought not just Vesalius's *De fabrica* but also Copernicus's *De revolutionibus orbium coelestium* [On the Revolutions of the Heavenly Spheres] with its revolutionary heliocentric astronomy.

MEDICAL CHEMISTRY

Few of Paracelsus's medical writings were published before his death in 1542, but by the 1550s they were spreading in a blaze of controversy. His followers made an odd bunch. His writings appealed, as would be expected, to radical reformers, such as the Danish Lutheran Peter Severinus, whose *Idea medicinae philosophicae* (1571) [The Idea of Philosophical Medicine] mocked Galenism, and in true Paracelsan fashion told readers to burn their books (though presumably not the *Idea!*), sell their houses and go on their travels, studying plants and learning from peasants. But his teachings also found favour in more select circles.

Cold-shouldered by universities, followers sought friends in high places; princely patronage would give Paracelsanism its imprimatur, while royal largesse could equip the laboratories chemical medicine required. In any case, many Renaissance rulers had intellectual aspirations of their own. The elector of the palatinate, Otto Heinrich Duke of Neuburg, was probably the first German noble to favour Paracelsans, and they also found support alongside the astrologers and magicians at the Prague court of the mystically-minded Holy Roman emperor, Rudolf II.

Amongst the most courtly Paracelsan physicians was Theodore Turquet de Mayerne (1573–1655), educated at Geneva, Heidelberg and Montpellier. In a protracted controversy over chemical (or 'spagyric') medicines, Turquet de Mayerne ranged himself against the Paris Galenists on the side of the Calvinist Paracelsan Joseph Duchesne (known as Quercetanus: *c.* 1544–1609). A Protestant himself, he prudently moved to London following the assassination of the French king, Henri IV, and was appointed royal physician by successive Stuart monarchs. He proved active in the establishment of the Worshipful Society of Apothecaries, and was knighted by James I in 1624.

A moderate Paracelsan, Turquet de Mayerne maintained that

chemical cures were quite compatible with Hippocratic teachings. Late in life Guinther von Andernach, the humanist physician, anatomist and translator, had attempted a similar *via media* in his *De medicina veteri et nova* (1571) [Concerning the Ancient and the New Medicine]. While advocating chemical remedies, he squared the Paracelsan three principles of salt, sulphur and mercury with the Aristotelian elements, emphasizing that the Greeks no less than Paracelsus had believed in macro/microcosm correspondences and the heavenly harmonies.

As such compromises and syntheses suggest, it was not only hardline Paracelsans who embraced spagyric remedies. After all, distillation of plants for their 'essences' was ancient, bridging herbal and laboratory medicine by chemicalizing herbs; and chemical remedies received sanction in official pharmacopoeias. The Augsburg pharmacopoeia of 1564 listed distillations and some chemical remedies for external use. In England, assisted by Turquet de Mayerne, the College of Physicians published the first *Pharmacopoeia Londinensis* in 1618. This included sections on salts, metals, minerals; 122 chemical preparations were listed in the enlarged second edition appearing in the same year, and its 2140 remedies also included dried viper lozenges, foxes' lungs, live frogs, wolf oil and crabs' eyes. The *Pharmacopoeia* accepted the 'more recent' chemical remedies that 'might act as auxiliaries', amongst them *crocus metallorum* (crocus of antimony), *vitrum antimonii* (vitrified antimony), *mercurius vitae* (mercury of life, also known as butter of antimony), *turbith minerale* (mercuric sulfate), and *mercurius dolcis* (calomel).

Many advocates of chemical remedies, for instance the German Andreas Libavius (1540–1616), never regarded themselves as card-carrying Paracelsans. A man of wide interests, Libavius developed his own, rather idiosyncratic, creed: he defended Luther against Catholicism and late in life attacked Calvinism, while supporting Aristotelian logic against the radical logician Peter Ramus (1515–72). In the spagyric remedies controversy Libavius steered between the Paracelsan Scylla and the Galenic Charybdis. Chemical remedies should be used, he argued in his *Alchymia* (1606) [Alchemy], often regarded as the first chemistry textbook, but he deplored the 'obscurity' and 'mysticism' of the Paracelsans, calling for a 'true chemistry' purged of superstition. Nevertheless, like Turquet de Mayerne, he supported the Paracelsan Duchesne when his works were outlawed by the hardline Galenic Paris medical faculty, advocating 'a middle path between the rigid Paracelsan and the rigid Galenic'.

In this *via media*, the chemists' principles of salt, sulphur and mercury applied to chemistry but not to medicine as such; there the traditional four humours (blood, phlegm, yellow and black bile) still held sway. Chemistry was medicine's servant, and chemical treatments should plainly be promoted, but herbal remedies were valuable too. Research was needed to reveal the true nature of matter, and nature must not be rammed into any exclusive, preconceived system.

Another proponent of medical chemistry who learnt from Paracelsanism but moved beyond the Paracelsan magic circle was Daniel Sennert (1572–1637), appointed professor of medicine at Wittenberg in 1602. Sennert won recognition as one of the major thinkers of his day through his attempt to give chemistry an atomistic grounding. His influence was felt in Germany until the nineteenth century – there were at least 125 different editions of his books, including six of the complete works. His aim was to unite experience, reason and the best authorities, both ancient and modern. Although critical of certain precepts, he accepted many Paracelsan notions, blending them with humoralism. His disease theory, for example, adopted a position between the Galenic notion of dis-ease (humoral disequilibrium) and the Paracelsan ontological concept of disease as a real, local entity. Sickness was the result of an accident affecting the soul or vital powers of the body, impairing its normal organizing power and resulting in pathological disruption.

Paracelsus's most ardent disciple was Joan Baptista van Helmont (1579–1644), a key transitional figure who gave medical chemistry fresh impetus through his laboratory researches, while sustaining its Christian spiritual vision. Like Paracelsus, van Helmont appears Janus-faced: he rejected orthodox humoral pathology, preferring an ontological disease theory, yet should not be called a 'modern' chemist. For him chemical analysis was a means of achieving understanding of nature and union with God, the marriage of an enquiring mind with fervent mysticism.

Educated at Louvain in the Spanish Netherlands, at the tender age of seventeen van Helmont was already delivering medical lectures; in 1605 he bravely stayed to treat the sick during the plague in Antwerp and then, inspired by deep piety, undertook a programme of chemical analysis by the use of fire in a grail-like quest for the arcana of creation. From 1624 to 1642, however, he published nothing; these decades, amid the terrible Thirty Years War then tearing Christendom apart, were for him times of bitter controversy and religious persecution, in which he battled against traditionalists, particularly the Jesuits. He was denounced for heretical leanings in 1630, and proceedings against him continued until 1642, when he finally received an *imprimatur* for his treatise on fevers. The bulk of his works did not appear until four years after his death, as the *Ortus medicinae* (1648) [The Garden of Medicine]. In the eyes of some, he was as bad as Paracelsus, Gui Patin (1601/2 --72), the doyen of the Paris faculty, dubbing him 'a mad Flemish scoundrel'.

Van Helmont's 'Christian philosophy' rejected the Galenic elements, humours and qualities, seeing them as empty words. The quest for truth must be a search, in the Paracelsan manner, for invisible 'semina' (seeds), undertaken through the 'art of fire'. A vitalist, he believed all objects, minerals included, were alive, marriages of body and soul, matter and form. Matter (which he believed ultimately consisted of water, the unique element) was charged with a specific disposition (*archaeus*), which created life. In a celebrated experiment, he tried to prove this by showing a plant would grow if kept in water alone.*

Van Helmont has often been credited with the idea of 'gas'. But he did not anticipate the modern notion. Gas was for him a guiding spirit; distinct from mere atmospheric air, it could be seen as a ferment directing nutrition, digestion and other vital functions. He also postulated the existence of 'blas'. Rather like the Paracelsan *archaeus* – 'the heart of the elements', the natural reparative activity of the human body – this blas or life-force dominated all corporeal processes, all motion and change. It produced fever, sneezing and coughs in an effort to expel a disease entity, but as a health-defending property it might sometimes prove too energetic and require to be pacified by treatment.

In an elaborate pathological system van Helmont grappled with the complexities of general and local diseases, in both their physiological and spiritual dimensions. Each disease was an external thing (*ens*), possessing a specific morbid seed (*semen*) and capable of attacking the body, thereby causing irritation, like a thorn in the flesh. An ontological concept was thus crucial to his vision: every disease had a vital principle of its own (*archeus*) which could be treated by a specific medico-spiritual response. Medicines, especially minerals, targeted the disease and helped

---

* He placed 200 pounds of dried earth in an earthenware vessel, watered it, and planted in it a willow weighing 5 pounds. Water was added daily and at the end of 5 years the willow weighed 169 pounds and the earth had lost a negligible weight. He therefore assumed that the willow, and hence all vegetation, was composed only of water and that water was the primary element.

the host overcome its *archeus*. Such views led him to protest against excessive blood-letting – since plethora was not the cause of disease, phlebotomy only wasted the patient's vitality.

Overall van Helmont is an enigmatic figure; the more chemical aspects of his thinking were absorbed by later medical chemists (iatro-chemists), while his underlying spiritual quest was cast aside.

PARACELSAN PHYSIC AND POLITICS

Rebelling against the Galenic elite, Paracelsan iatrochemistry appealed to the rank and file: surgeons, apothecaries, empirics and irregulars. They might be cursed by their betters as brazen mountebanks peddling dangerous drugs, but such righteous indignation sounded like a pack of rationalizations coming from those desperate to preserve their monopoly.

The divisions in medicine resulting from the Paracelsan heresy were professionally scarring; in England, monarchs from Elizabeth to Charles II sometimes supported unlicensed practitioners against the College of Physicians, while in France the court afforded shelter to Paracelsan physicians, generally Montpellier-trained, against the hidebound Paris faculty. Thereafter medicine could rarely show a united professional front, and tended to factionalize.

Paracelsanism enjoyed a robust appeal; unlike Galenism, it was Christian through and through (a great asset in the Reformation era) and its teachings appealed to the people against the powerful, especially in its vision of medicine as a charitable vocation, a divine gift for the relief of suffering. Noteworthy were the philanthropic initiatives of the Montpellier-trained iatrochemist, royal physician and one-time Hugue-not, Théophraste Renaudot (1584–1653), who established a bureau d'adresse in Paris, which served as a labour exchange while offering free medical treatment to the sick poor. Extending its services, he came up with *La presence des absens* (1642) [The Presence of the Absent], a booklet designed to allow the sick from the provinces to have their illnesses diagnosed and treated by post, by providing lists of symptoms to be ticked and simple bodily diagrams for patients to mark where it hurt. The bureau was given royal sanction to establish laboratories for analysing therapeutic substances. The Paris faculty fumed, but could do nothing so long as Renaudot enjoyed Cardinal Richelieu's protection.

In England, too, political and medical radicalism joined forces in the Civil War and interregnum era (1642–60), leading to bold schemes for reform in health care, poverty relief and education. A leading figure, Nicholas Culpeper (1616–54) significantly had no university degree, being apprenticed to an apothecary before setting up as a doctor to the London poor. After supporting the Parliamentarians in the Civil War, he daringly produced *A Physicall Directory, or a Translation of the London Dispensatory* (1649), an unauthorized translation of the College of Physicians' Latin *Pharmacopoeia*. In his eyes the College's monopoly was unchristian because it drove up the costs of medical treatment beyond the pockets of the poor. Culpeper countered by recommending simple homegrown herbal remedies in a cheap, vernacular handbook. The College was outraged:

> By two yeeres drunken labour he hath Gallimawfred the apothecaries book into nonsense ... and to supply his drunkenness and leachery with a thirty shilling reward endeavoured to bring into obloquy the famous societies of apothecaries and chyrurgeons.

Riled by the College's reprisals, he issued a more controversial version, *The English Physician Enlarged* (1653), which went through scores of editions, becoming known simply as *Culpeper's Herbal* (revised editions are still in print). It prescribed over 500 plants, from agrimony to yucca, to deal with human ills from adder bites to wind. Elite physicians were berated as toadies of tyranny: princes, priests and physicians equally infringed the people's liberties, and Latin was the tongue of monopoly, greed and obscurantism. Indeed, from that time, English medical books were largely written in the vernacular rather than in Latin.

Paracelsan iatrochemistry sided with the reform of medicine, education and government. Puritans praised it as truly Christian, unmasking the heathen roots of Galenism. But though many radical reform schemes were broached (for example, to democratize or abolish the College of Physicians and fund state-provided health care), these came to little. Nor did the College or Galenic medicine at large regain their former standing after the Restoration in 1660, not least because Charles II patronized the new experimental natural philosophy, chartering the Royal Society in 1662. By the 1660s Galenism was in tatters, yet the Paracelsan movement was also on the wane, being overtaken by or absorbed into medical–chemical investigations pursued under the banner of the 'new philosophy' and associated in England with the

Royal Society, in France with the Académie Royale des Sciences, and in Italy with the Accademia del Cimento.

HARVEY

Renaissance anatomy further subverted the Greek medical legacy it admired through its finest achievement: William Harvey's demonstration of the circulation of the blood. Building on Vesalian anatomy and developing a new physiology, Harvey's revolutionary work convinced later investigators that medical science had to be put on a new footing.

To grasp the magnitude of his reconceptualization, it is worth recalling the ancient model of the blood system still authoritative around 1600. In traditional Galenic physiology there were two types of blood, the venous and the arterial, with distinct pathways and functions, relating to the three chief body centres: the liver (responsible for nutrition and growth), the heart (vitality), and the brain (sensation and reason). Nourishment and growth were secured by the venous blood originating in the liver, while vitality was conveyed to the body parts by the arterial blood originating in the heart. Arterial (life-giving) blood contained pneuma (spirituous air) and blood; and, like venous blood, was thought to spread to all parts of the body when needed, being there used up; it did not return to the heart. Given the quite distinct functions of venous and arterial blood, their different sources, and the belief that they were expended, there was no question of the blood circulating around the body. The heart did not even drive blood through the arteries – for Galen the active phase of the heart's motion was diastole (dilation), when, like a bladder filling, it sucked blood in. The heart did not pump blood out; the blood's movement through the arteries was explained by an innate 'pulsative faculty' in the arteries themselves.

One awkwardness in Galen's cardiovascular system lay in explaining how the ingredients of arterial blood (that is, venous blood and air) got into the left ventricle of the heart where they were changed into arterial blood. Evidently venous blood had to pass from the right side of the heart to the left. Galen had stated that this occurred by blood seeping through hidden pores in the interventricular septum, the fleshy wall separating the ventricles of the heart. He had no conception of the pulmonary transit of the blood: passing from the right to the left side of the heart by looping through the lungs (through the pulmonary artery into the lungs, then into the pulmonary vein, and finally into the heart). Hardly any blood (just enough to nourish the lungs) left the right side of the heart, he believed.

If air was necessary for making arterial blood, how did it get to the heart? Galenists believed the pulmonary vein's function was to convey air from the lungs to the left side of the heart. The end result of the mixture of pneuma and blood in the left ventricle was arterial blood – thinner and brighter than the dark-red venous blood. A by-product of this process were 'sooty vapours', which travelled back to the lungs along the same pulmonary vein and were then exhaled. The pulmonary vein was a two-way street: air went down into the heart, and sooty vapours returned up to the lungs. With hindsight, the lack of a sound observational basis for many of these particulars (the permeable septum, the paucity of blood in the pulmonary vein, and the sooty vapours there) appears problematic, but the Galenic cardiovascular system scored because it explained so much so coherently.

As noted earlier, Renaissance anatomists questioned aspects of Galen's model. In the *Fabrica*, Vesalius had observed that the vena cava did not, after all, originate in the liver, and in the second edition he denied the septum's permeability. Realdo Colombo brought to light the pulmonary transit, and vivisection experiments led him to conclude that the active phase of the heart was when it constricted (systole), not when it dilated (diastole). The heart discharged blood into the arteries when it constricted and the arteries then felt full – a discovery crucial for Harvey, as it led him to ponder the quantity of blood flowing out of the heart at every constriction.

Other anatomists also contributed observations that did not square with Galen: Servetus conceived of the pulmonary transit; Andrea Cesalpino (1519–1603) supported the pulmonary circulation, described the heart's valve action, and began to use the term *circulatio*; and in 1603, Fabricius published his description of venous valves. The culmination of such developments came in 1628, when Harvey published his *Exercitatio anatomica de motu cordis et sanguinis in animalibus* [An Anatomical Essay Concerning the Movement of the Heart and the Blood in Animals].

Born at Folkestone, William Harvey (1578–1657) attended Caius College, Cambridge. From 1600 he studied at Padua under Fabricius, from whom he absorbed Aristotelian approaches to the study of nature, especially in comparative anatomy and embryology. Like his teacher, he dissected animals to discover how particular organs worked, relating structure to function, concerned with the 'action, function and purpose' of the parts.

In 1602 he returned to England. A swarthy and testy man who habitually wore a dagger, he was elected a Fellow of the College of Physicians in 1607 and two years later physician to St Bartholomew's Hospital. He swiftly established himself; in 1615 he was appointed by the College its Lumleian lecturer, charged with lecturing on anatomy and conducting public dissections. By 1618 he was one of the royal physicians.

Harvey's Paduan experiences set him at the forefront of learned medicine, where neo-Aristotelian ideas were challenging Galenic ones. His 1616 Lumleian lectures significantly begin with the statement that anatomy deals with 'the uses and actions of the parts [of the body] by eyesight inspection and by dissection' – a clear sign that he had adopted Fabricius's Aristotelianism. He had also taken initial steps towards probing the blood system. Confirming Colombo's work on the pulmonary transit, he concluded that the heart worked as a muscle, with the ventricles contracting and expelling blood in systolic contractions rather than sucking it in during diastole (relaxation); the arteries pulsated because of the shockwave from the beating heart – they did not pulsate of their own intrinsic 'pulsative virtue'.

De motu cordis falls into two parts. Harvey first pointed out Galen's flaws. How could the air and sooty vapours be kept distinct in the pulmonary vein? When it was opened, neither the said air nor the vapours could be seen in that vein, but blood alone. Discussing the action of the auricles and the ventricles of the heart, he showed the reality of the pulmonary transit of the blood, pointing to vivisections he had performed on frogs whose hearts were simpler and beat more slowly than those of warm-blooded animals, thereby permitting slow-motion experiments.

He then turned to novel matters, announcing his discovery of the circulation. Experiments showed that so much blood left the heart in a minute that it could not conceivably be absorbed by the body and continually replaced by blood made in the liver from chyle. Like no one before him, Harvey noted that the amount of blood forced out of the heart in an hour far exceeded its volume in the whole animal. This

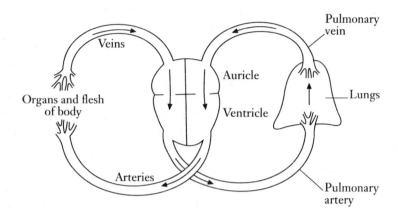

The heart and the circulation, as understood by Harvey.

quantitative evidence established that the blood must constantly move in a circuit, otherwise the arteries and body would explode under the pressure:

> Since all things, both argument and ocular demonstration, show that the blood passes through the lungs and heart by the force of the ventricles, and is sent for distribution to all parts of the body, where it makes its way into the veins and porosities of the flesh, and then flows by the veins from the circumference on every side to the centre, from the lesser to the greater veins, and is by them finally discharged into the vena cava and right auricle of the heart, and this in such a quantity or in such a flux and reflux thither by the arteries, hither by the veins, as cannot possibly be supplied by the ingesta, and is much greater than can be required for mere purposes of nutrition; it is absolutely necessary to conclude that the blood in the animal body is impelled in a circle, and is in a state of ceaseless motion.

What Harvey could not achieve was to display the complete pathways of the circular movement. He could not see with his eyes the minute connexions – the capillaries – between the arteries and the veins, and did not attempt to do so with the newly developed microscope. By means of a simple experiment, however, he showed that a connexion, albeit unknown, must exist. He ligated a forearm extremely tightly so that no arterial blood could flow below the ligature down the arm. He then loosened it so that arterial blood flowed down the arm, though it remained tight enough to stop venous blood moving back above the ligature. With the ligature very tight, the veins in the arm below it had appeared normal, but now they became swollen, showing that blood had poured down the arteries and then back up the arm within the veins; thus there had to be as yet undiscovered pathways at the extremities for the blood to pass from arteries to veins. Finally, he showed that the valves in the veins always directed blood back to the heart; *pace* Fabricius, they did not act to prevent the lower parts of the body from flooding with blood. Having displayed the circulation and its passages through the one-way valve system, Harvey was then able to explain, by means of the circulation theory, such previously puzzling phenomena as the rapid spread of poisons through the body.

Harvey's work appears very modern: he experimented and obeyed the injunction of the Paduan anatomists to see for oneself. 'I profess to learn and teach anatomy not from books but from dissections,' he declared, 'not from the tenets of Philosophers but from the fabric of Nature.' But that is only half true; certainly he looked for himself (and without the aid of the microscope), but he saw through Aristotelian spectacles.* Harvey did not, as sometimes supposed, conceive of the body in a 'modern' mechanical fashion: it was not a machine, but was moved by vital forces. In discussing the circulation, his terms and ideas were Aristotelian. The purpose of the circulation, he wrote, drawing on traditional macrocosm/microcosm correlations, was to transport life-giving blood to the periphery and then to return it to the heart where it could be re-enlivened:

> So in all likelihood it comes to pass in the body, that all the parts are nourished, cherished, and quickned with blood, which is warm, perfect, vaporous, full of spirit, and, that I may so say, alimentative: in the parts the blood is refrigerated, coagulated, and made as it were barren, from thence it returns to the heart, as to the fountain or dwelling-house of the body, to recover its perfection, and there again by naturall heat, powerfull, and vehement, it is melted, and is dispens'd again through the body from thence, being fraught

* In his final book, *De Generatione* (1651) [On Generation], Harvey revealed another aspect of his deep Aristotelianism. There he argued for a non-material process of generation, 'beyond the power of the elements', debating fertilization and the respective roles played by the male and female in it.

with spirits, as with balsam, and that all the things do depend upon the motional pulsation of the heart: So the heart is the beginning of life, the Sun of the Microcosm, as proportionably the Sun deserves to be call'd the heart of the world, by whose virtue, and pulsation, the blood is mov'd perfected, made vegetable, and is defended from corruption, and mattering; and this familiar household-god doth his duty to the whole body, by nourishing, cherishing, and vegetating, being the foundation of life, and author of all. [From the 1653 translation].

It was not, in other words, from the 'new philosophy' that Harvey drew his inspiration; indeed, according to John Aubrey's gossipy *Brief Lives*, Harvey slighted Francis Bacon ('he writes Philosophy like a Lord Chancellour'), while 'shitt-breeches' was his put-down for the 'neoteriques' (the Paracelsans). With Aristotle he shared a teleological view of the body and the belief that its workings depended upon the distinctive soul.

It is somewhat ironic, therefore, that the fiercest attack on Harvey came from an ultra-conservative, Jean Riolan the Younger (1580–1657), the leading Galenist in the Paris faculty. Riolan had studied medicine under his distinguished father, continuing his war against the Paracelsans and attaining formidable erudition in classical literature and philosophy. He grasped that Harvey's doctrine of the circulation had the potential to explode Galenic physiology. It would mean, for instance, that the liver was no longer the blood-making organ, and once the liver's function was questioned, what else would not be questioned? Even Galenic therapeutics would be challenged, because the rationale for bleeding had been undermined: what price all the old rules about the correct places to bleed if the same blood were streaming round the body?

In his *Opuscula anatomica* (1649) [Little Anatomical Work], Riolan fired salvoes while offering a few concessions: the blood still followed the old Galenic pathways and did not generally circulate, but he conceded a minor circulation in the aorta and vena cava. Harvey retaliated in his *Exercitatio anatomica de circulatione sanguinis* (1649) [Anatomical Exercise on the Circulation of the Blood], insisting that Riolan's position made observational nonsense, for the blood in *all* the arteries moved with considerable force and in great quantities, which pointed clearly to the circulation.

DESCARTES

Attacked by conservatives, Harvey's theories found favour, somewhat ironically, with 'new philosophers', notably Descartes, who were promoting the mechanical philosophy. The towering thinker of the Scientific Revolution, René Descartes (1596–1650) was born in Normandy and educated by the Jesuits, who introduced him to mathematics and physics, including Galileo's work. After enlisting as a gentleman-soldier and travelling, he settled in Amsterdam, living by the butchers' quarter and performing animal dissections.

Friendship with Isaac Beeckman (1588–1637) fired his love of mathematics and the physical sciences; by 1619 his fertile mind had glimpsed the possibility of combining algebra and geometry into analytical geometry; and on 10 November 1619, in a quasi-mystical experience recorded in his *Discours de la méthode* (1637) [Discourse on Method], he dedicated his life to the pursuit of truth, determining to doubt all and, on the basis of self-evident first principles, to reconstruct natural philosophy. Starting with the one thing he could not doubt – his own consciousness (*Cogito, ergo sum*: I am thinking, therefore I exist) – he aspired to establish principles so clear and distinct 'that the mind of man cannot doubt their truth'. Though his philosophical method was deductive, he recognized that in practice observation and experimentation were needed.

Descartes always regarded medicine as a key to the natural world. He often dissected animals, and produced three works devoted to the life sciences: *Tractatus de formatione foetus* (1664) [Treatise on the Formation of the Foetus], *La description du corps humain* (1648–9) [Description of the Human Body], and *Traité de l'homme* (1662) [Treatise of Man]. Other works, especially *Les passions de l'âme* (1649) [The Passions of the Soul], examined the psycho-physiological consequences of the radical dualism premised by his mechanical philosophy.

Mind and matter, he taught, were incommensurable: matter was extended, corpuscular and quantifiable, mind (or soul) was insubstantial and immortal, the source of consciousness. The two could (almost) never meet. In a thought experiment, the *Traité de l'homme* proposed a mechanical model of the human animal; drawing analogies with clocks and automata, he proposed that an 'artificial' man would have physiological processes identical to those of real humans, explicable only in terms of matter in motion. Animals did not possess souls and so were indeed to be viewed as automata pure and simple; mind distinguished humans from all other living beings, in a manner philosophically paralleling the Christian theology of the cosmic uniqueness of the human soul.

Descartes thus radically rethought the metaphysics of physiology and medicine – his mechanistic account of the nervous system included a model of the reflex concept. But he never worked out, at least to his critics' satisfaction, how mind and body could actually interact; for critics, his speculative localization of the link in the pineal gland, a unitary structure seated in the mid-brain just behind the main ventricle, merely compounded the problem. Mind had been made a mysterious ghost in the machine, while his notion of the passions as mediating mind and body was more holistic than his mind/body dualism seemed to sanction. Overall, however, Cartesianism's significance for bio-medicine was enormous: Descartes regarded the body exactly as he viewed the world, as a mechanism. Dismissing Aristotelian–Galenic elements and humours even more radically than Paracelsus, he postulated that matter in motion would explain both the human body and the system of nature at large. That was an audacious challenge.

In the *Discourse on Method* Descartes enlisted Harveian blood circulation in support of his new philosophy, but parted company with *De motu* on the operation of the heart. Harvey's vital forces were dismissed – all body actions had to have mechanical explanations. For Descartes, the heart was active in diastole (not, as for Harvey, in systole), when its innate heat rarefied drops of blood in its chambers and made them expand and force blood particles into the arteries. Minuscule blood particles became the animal spirits that flowed through the brain, nerves and muscles, conveying sensation and motion. The heart was thus an engine, imparting motion to the rest of the body.

Descartes and later mechanical philosophers were determined that their 'new philosophy' should replace the Aristotelian cosmos of qualities and elements with one composed of particles of matter in motion obeying mathematical laws. Descartes was himself no materialist, but materialists emerged who went further and denied the reality of anything but matter or body. To the orthodox, the most threatening was Thomas Hobbes (1588–1679), who drew inspiration from Galileo and Descartes and grappled with the formidable implications not simply of a mechanical physiology but of a materialistic psychology.

Between 1634 and 1636 Hobbes accompanied the Earl of Devonshire on the grand tour, meeting Galileo, and he was in France again between 1640 and 1651 as an exile during the English Civil War. It was then that he published much of his natural, moral and political philosophy, including *Leviathan* (1651) whose supposed atheism sparked an outcry. Hobbes regarded the universe as a material continuum, devoid of spirit. Knowledge was derived purely from sense impressions, and man's behaviour was determined by physical laws, grounded in self-preservation. While Hobbes was universally reviled, Descartes's philosophy was given a more respectable face in France by Pierre Gassendi (1592–1655), and in England by Walter Charleton (1619–1707), having an oblique influence upon the thinking of Robert Boyle (1627–91) and of John Locke (1632–1704) (discussed below).

Renaissance anatomy had revealed that the structures of the body were not strictly as Galen had stated, and Harvey showed that Galenic ideas of their functions were also flawed. The formation of the blood, the workings of the stomach, liver and lungs – these and other physiological matters were bound in their turn to come up for debate. And dissection was meanwhile revealing anatomical structures unknown to ancient authority.

RESEARCHING THE BODY

Opening up bodies – dead human cadavers, living animal ones – had become the prescription for true medical knowledge. One field undergoing change was understanding of digestion, in which thinking was transformed thanks first to Gaspare Aselli (1581–1625), a professor of anatomy at Pavia. Vivisecting a recently fed dog, he noticed white filaments throughout the mesentery and along the peritoneal surface of the intestine; when cut, a milky fluid emerged. He had hit upon the chyliferous vessels of the intestine, which he called lacteals ('white veins'). Observing their presence in various animal species, he went on to explore their function, proving experimentally that the chyliferous vessels became swollen after feeding.

Aselli related the vessels to the mesenteric glands, which were further traced through to the thoracic duct by Jean Pecquet (1622–74), helping to overthrow Galen's liver-centred physiology. About the same time Thomas Bartholin (1616–80) demonstrated the existence of the chyliferous vessels in man as well, and explored the lymphatic system in *Vasa lymphatica . . . et hepatis exsequiae* (1653) [The Lymphatic Vessels and the Secretion of the Liver] – this was the book which introduced colour plates into anatomical studies. The pancreatic duct was discovered in 1644, the submaxillary duct in 1656, and the parotid duct in 1659. In short, by the late seventeenth century, anatomists had laid bare the glandular structures of the digestive system, destroying the food-chyle-blood scheme so basic to Galenic physiology which centred on a blood-making liver.

In the light of such developments Franz de le Boë (Franciscus Sylvius: 1614–72) proposed an un-Galenic chemical theory of digestion. A French-born supporter of Harvey, teaching in Leiden, Sylvius grasped the significance of blood circulation for general physiology; he developed a more materialistic iatrochemistry critical of van Helmont's quasi-mystical ideas and strove to fuse chemical analysis with circulation theory. Drawing in part on van Helmont's teachings on digestion, Sylvius claimed that the essential element was acid, rather than (as for Galen) innate heat. Digestion was essentially a fermentational process taking place in the mouth, the stomach, the heart and in the blood.

It was, however, investigations into respiration conducted by a circle of English researchers that most spectacularly challenged Galenic physiology. Harvey had shown the flaws in the Galenic theory of respiration, maintaining that life was located in the blood rather than the heart, which was essentially just a pump, working by muscular force. But what precisely was life-giving in the blood? And how did it get there? These questions propelled post-Harveian research into respiration.

Air was already the subject of various investigations. In 1643 the Italian Galileans, Vincenzo Viviani (1621–1703) and Evangelista Torricelli (1608–47) demonstrated atmospheric pressure (the force or 'spring' of the air) through air-pump experiments. The Hon. Robert Boyle, aristocrat, puritan and experimenter, explored the behaviour of animals and birds in a bell-jar from which the air had been evacuated: in a vacuum they could not live, nor would a candle burn. From such experiments it became clear that there were different types and conditions of air. Experiments conducted by Robert Hooke (1635–1702) helped to challenge the old view that the lungs were basically bellows designed to cool the fiery heart. Against this background, Richard Lower (1631–91) overturned the Galenic belief that air united with blood in the left ventricle of the heart.

Of an old Cornish family, Lower studied medicine at Oxford, becoming an active member of the scientific circle there associated with Boyle and Hooke, attending Peter Stahl's (d. 1675) chemistry classes and working as an assistant to the pioneer neuro-anatomist Thomas Willis (1621–75). Fascinated by the life-sustaining properties of blood, Lower recognized the significance of its different types and sought to explain the clear difference in appearance between venous (dark) and arterial (bright) blood. He first surmised that blood received some form of stimulus while in the heart, imparting to arterial blood its scarlet look; he also suspected that the lungs supplied the blood with a nutrient (a 'nitrous pabulum') drawn from the air.

In October 1667, conducting experiments with Robert Hooke, Lower perceived the significance of the fact that the blood leaving the right ventricle of the heart to enter the lungs was venous, and had not been affected by its passage through the heart. The blood leaving the lungs to enter the left ventricle had, by contrast, already achieved its bright hue. Evidently, as he pointed out in his *Tractatus de corde* (1669) [Treatise on the Heart], it was the lungs that vivified the arterial blood; the heart was a pump rather than a chemical laboratory. Having thus refuted the old theories, he set about verifying experimentally that the air in the lungs caused the blood's colour change. There must be a 'nitrous spirit of the air', vital to life, which mixed with the blood during its transit through the lungs.

De corde was duly acclaimed, but the nature of that 'nitrous spirit' remained to be determined. That was taken up by John Mayow (1641–79). He too had studied medicine at Oxford, assisting Boyle in his air-pump investigations. The purpose of respiration, argued his *De respiratione* (1668) [On Respiration], was to communicate something from the air to the blood during the pulmonary circuit. Like Lower, he maintained that air abounded with 'nitrous particles' essential to life. Mixing with the sulphur believed to be present in the blood, 'aerial nitre' caused fermentation and heating. This continued as the blood coursed from the heart into the arterial system, maintaining body heat. Moreover aerial nitre was also essential for muscular contraction: contact between the nitrous particles and the animal spirits caused an 'explosion' which swelled the muscle, producing a corresponding shortening. Lack of air and its 'nitrous' constituent would, therefore, deprive the blood of its heat and result in the failure of the heart muscles, causing death. No breath, no life.

Mayow's final account of aerial nitre was given in his *Tractatus quinque* (1674) [Fifth Treatise], in which he elaborated upon the physico-chemical properties of this '*vital, igneous* and highly *fermentative spirit*'. The 'nitre-aerial particles' or 'nitre-aerial spirit' – his active principle – were also responsible for the combustible properties of gunpowder; fermentation was a motion of nitro-aerial particles occurring spontaneously whenever they encountered sulphur or salt particles; and all combustion was a kind of ferment. Mayow thus held there was something in the air necessary for the support both of life and of flame, but used up in respiration and combustion, thereby leaving 'vitiated' air. These links between respiration in the body and combustion in external nature set challenges to chemists which were resolved only a century later with the theory of oxygen.

Another contemporary grappling with ideas of vitality was Francis Glisson (1597–1677), Regius professor of physic at Cambridge and an early fellow of the Royal Society; his first publication, *De rachitide* (1650) [On Rickets], was a pioneering study of what was cast as a new disease. In his *Anatomia hepatis* (1654) [Anatomy of the Liver], Glisson explored its normal and morbid anatomy and developed a new concept of biological irritability. The sporadic excretion of bile into the intestines, he submitted, was brought about by the reaction to irritation of the gall-bladder and biliary ducts; such irritability implied the presence of nerves. He later became convinced that irritability was a property inherent in all tissue, independent of nerves, endowing all matter with an internal principle of motion, an elementary 'awareness' of change. The soul itself was dependent on sensation and could appear in a foetus only in conjunction with the development of the bodily organs, as a manifestation of the organization of 'animated' matter. These speculations provided the foundation for the mature doctrine of tissue irritability spelt out in *De ventriculo* (1677) [On the Ventricle].

The world remained unconvinced, however, and the doctrine of irritability was largely forgotten until Albrecht von Haller (1708–77) revived it, restricting it to muscle fibres. But Glisson's speculations attest the radical re-thinking of basic bodily functions prompted by Harvey's discoveries, by broader experimental impulses, and by the mechanical philosophy. A new physiology was taking shape.

THE MICROSCOPE

Other developments followed from the microscope, constructed around 1600 by three Dutch spectacle-makers, Hans Janssen, his son Zacharias, and Hans Lipperskey. Many naturalists used it to peer at gnats and grubs, but the work of Hooke, Marcello Malpighi (1628–94) and Antoni van Leeuwenhoek (1632–1723) stands out.

The hypochondriacal Hooke served as Robert Boyle's assistant and became curator of experiments for the new Royal Society. Echoing Francis Bacon, he held that the defects of human reason could be remedied only by 'the real, the mechanical, the experimental Philosophy' whose 'groundwork' was 'sense'. His microscopic studies, presented in his *Micrographia* (1665), a book containing thirty-eight plates, included investigations into lice, and featured the first biological use of the word 'cell' in describing the 'pores' in wood.

Malpighi, professor of medicine in Pisa, similarly used the microscope to advance an essentially mechanical model of the structure of living beings. Falling under the influence of the experimentalists Francesco Redi (1626–98) and Giovanni Borelli (1608–97), he was drawn away from Aristotelianism to a 'free and Democritean' (that is, atomistic) philosophy, applying the mechanical model to living things. Malpighi made many remarkable discoveries with the microscope. Dissecting frogs, he differentiated the fine structure of the lungs. Previously blood and air had been thought to mingle freely in the fleshy parenchyma of the lungs, but the microscope now revealed the membranous alveoli at the ends of the tracheo-bronchial ramifications. His *De pulmonibus* (1661) [On the Lungs] described this fine texture of blood vessels – the missing link in Harvey's theory – and thus provided decisive confirmation of the blood's circulation:

> I saw the blood, flowing in minute streams through the arteries, in the manner of a flood, and I might have believed that the blood itself escaped into an empty space and was collected up again by a gaping vessel, but an objection to the view was afforded by the movement of the blood being tortuous and scattered in different directions and by its being united again in a definite path. My doubt was changed to certainty by the dried lung of a frog which to a marked degree had preserved the redness of the blood in very

tiny tracts, which were afterwards found to be vessels, where by the help of a glass I saw not scattered points but vessels drawn together in a ring-like fashion . . . Thus it was clear that the blood flowed along sinuous vessels and did not empty into spaces, but was always contained within vessels, the paths of which produced its dispersion.

In *De lingua* (1665) [On the Tongue], Malpighi distinguished the horny outer layer of the tongue from the reticular mucous layer (now known as the Malpighian layer), and isolated the taste buds, the papillae of the tongue. *De externo tactus organo* (1665) [On the External Organ of Touch] described the papillae of the skin, the organs of touch. *De cerebro* (1665) [On the Brain] showed how the white matter of the nervous system consisted of bundles of fibres connecting the brain with the spinal cord. *De viscerum structura* (1666) [On the Structure of the Viscera] showed that the liver, not the gall bladder, secreted bile and that the kidneys worked like sieves. *De polypo cordis* (1666) [On the Polyp of the Heart] gave the first description of red blood corpuscles. Overall, Malpighi was convinced that the best model for interpreting such investigations was offered by machinery:

> the mechanisms of our bodies are composed of strings, thread, beams, levers, cloth, flowing fluids, cisterns, ducts, filters, sieves, and other similar mechanisms. Through studying these parts with the help of Anatomy, Philosophy and Mechanics, man has discovered their structure and function. . . . With this and the help of discourse, he apprehends the way nature acts and he lays the foundation of Physiology, Pathology, and eventually the art of Medicine.

The microscope's technical possibilities were most breathtakingly exploited by the Dutchman van Leeuwenhoek, a draper from Delft. The development of the instrument was to take two divergent forms: one, the forerunner of the modern microscope, was the compound version, relying on a combination of two or more lenses held in a tube; the other type, the simple version, consisted of a single tiny lens, and was essentially an extremely powerful magnifying-glass. Developed from about 1671, Leeuwenhoek's instruments (he made 247) were all of that simple type, using a tiny bead of glass as the lens. The fact that it required only one lens minimized the inescapable problems of spherical and chromatic aberration, while the tiny size of the lens (often less than

2mm across) permitted remarkably high magnification. The strongest of his extant microscopes, preserved in the Utrecht University Museum, has a linear magnifying power of 266 and a resolving power of 1.35×, which means that two features separated by only 0.00135mm can be distinguished by the user. Leeuwenhoek kept his lens-grinding techniques to himself, and his achievements remained unmatched until the nineteenth century.

He brought to his researches phenomenal eyesight, a remarkable dexterity in preparing samples and, as a tradesman without formal scientific education, a mind somewhat free from academic metaphysics – though his pious faith convinced him that the study of nature would demonstrate the existence of an 'All-wise Creator' and thus explode atheistic suppositions such as spontaneous generation. All things arose from living organisms and not from dew, mud or the products of putrefaction. Henry Oldenburg (c. 1615–1677), secretary of the Royal Society, initiated the correspondence with Leeuwenhoek which was to result in hundreds of his contributions being published in its *Philosophical Transactions*.

Leeuwenhoek studied the microscopic texture of wood, the cells of plants and the fine structure of animal bodies; he saw red blood corpuscles and blood capillaries and the crystals responsible for the agonies of gout; he noted the organization of nerves, muscles, bone, teeth and hair, and examined the fine structure of 67 species of insect, 11 species of spider and 10 of crustacea. His most remarkable discovery was the observation of 'animalcules' in various fluids, being the first person ever to see assorted spirogyra, hydra, protozoa, bacteria, infusoria and human spermatozoa. He estimated the population density of his animalcules at more than a million for each drop of water. These findings fuelled fierce disputes about the spontaneous generation of lower orders of animals – always denied by Leeuwenhoek – and about the respective roles of the sexes in reproduction.

Leeuwenhoek's early observations were known to Regnier de Graaf (1641–73), a fellow Dutch anatomist who explored the female mammalian reproductive organs. About the same time as the Dane Niels Stensen (1638–86), he described the 'Graafian follicle', the vesicle on the surface of the ovaries which cups the unfertilized egg. Applying the term 'ovary' to the female gonad, he contended that the ovum played the key role in reproduction, launching the 'ovist' school of thought, and giving rise to fierce embryological controversy.

Countering 'ovism', the rival 'animalculist' school regarded spermatozoa, discovered in semen by Leeuwenhoek, as the true source of conception. Enthusiasts like the Dutchman Jan Swammerdam (1637–80) claimed to see a miniature organism present within the unfertilized ovum (that is, the Graafian follicle); rivals professed to see an equivalent in the semen, giving rise to the 'preformation' or *emboîtement* theories which contended that the new individual was completely developed as a tiny *homunculus* from the moment of conception.

Both these ran counter to Harvey's Aristotelian concepts of generation. Through experiments on deer, graciously supplied to him from the royal park by Charles I, Harvey had attempted to show the successive appearance of the limbs and organs in the developing foetus, produced by a 'formative virtue', actualizing what was potential: the embryo thus developed by differentiation rather than being preformed in miniature. Preformationists rejoined that Harveian epigenesis was unscientific, for such a virtue could not be observed. The theological ramifications of preformationism – a biological analogue of Calvinist predestination – were long contested, and are continued by modern debates as to how far we are the puppets of our genes.

MEDICAL PRACTICE

By mid century, a new and often aggressive scientific spirit was rampant, debunking Aristotelian–Galenic learning as empty verbiage. Traditional medicine was ridiculed in the comedies of Molière (1622–73). In *Le médecin malgré lui* (1666–7) [The Doctor Despite Himself], Sganarelle, masquerading as a physician, is called in to treat a girl by her father, who has a credulous faith in medicine. The mock-doctor launches into a harangue to explain how the patient has lost her voice:

> These vapours of which I was speaking, passing from the left side, where the liver is situated, to the right side where the heart is, finds that the lung, which we call armyan in Latin, communicating with the brain, which we call nasmus in Greek, by means of the vena cava, which we call cubile in Hebrew, meets in its path the above-mentioned vapours, which fill the ventricles of the omoplate.

Molière had realized that fashionable audiences liked hearing old medical learning exposed as gibberish; he also sent up Galenism in *Le malade imaginaire* (1673) [The Hypochondriac], with its burlesque of a medical examination and the conferral of a medical degree. The doctoral candidate is subjected to stiff questioning: Why does opium cause sleep? The candidate replies,

> Mihi a docto doctore
> Demandatur causam et rationem quare
> Opium facit dormire.

> A quoi respondeo,
> Quia est in eo
> Virtus dormativa,
> Cujus est natura
> Sensus assoupire*

This dazzling answer won the plaudits of the elders:

> Dignus, dignus est intrare
> In nostro docto corpore.
> Bene, bene, respondere.†

Molière's joke suggests that new doctrines were timely. Simultaneously, in his popular *Cours de chémie* (1675) [Course of Chemistry], Nicholas Lémery (1645–1715) was giving the 'new' explanation of how opium worked: a 'gummy and earthy matter' in the drug produced sleep, acting like other mucilaginous substances which, when mixed with blood, emulsified and retarded the spirits flowing in the brain, producing somnolence. To us nowadays there might seem little to choose between this and the Galenic 'dormitive faculty' Molière mocked, yet Lemery's strong suit would have been the empirical evidence he could present, for the gum was the residue left by chemical analysis in the test-tube, so his findings seemed grounded on tangible experience.

Prizing things above words, the mechanical philosophy encouraged explorations of such material reality. A Galilean, Giovanni Borelli (1608–78), studied muscular action, gland secretions, respiration, heart rhythm, and neural response. His *De motu animalium* (1680) [On Animal Motion] recorded remarkable observations on birds in flight, fish swimming, muscular contraction, respiration, and a host of similar subjects, attempting to analyse body functions in terms of physics, while

---

* I have been asked by a learned doctor what is the cause and reason why opium induces sleep. To which I reply it is because there is in it a dormitive virtue, the nature of which is to sedate the senses.

† You are worthy, worthy, to enter into our learned body. You have responded well.

postulating a 'contractile element' in the muscles, their operation being triggered by processes similar to chemical fermentation. Respiration was a mechanical process driving air via the lungs into the bloodstream. Air possessed a life-sustaining function because it was a medium for 'elastic particles' entering the blood to impart internal motion to it. Iatrophysics (medical physics) and iatrochemistry together promised to reduce the mystery of life to questions of matter in motion. Whatever could not be weighed and measured was mysticism.

Experimentation brought to bear the precision of number. The pioneer of iatromathematics (medical mathematics) was Santorius, who studied at Padua and set up in practice in Venice where he associated with Galileo Galilei (1564–1642). His *Methodi vitandorum errorum omnium qui in arte medica contingunt* (1602) [Methods of Avoiding all Errors Pertaining to the Art of Medicine] asserted that credence should be given first to experience, second to reason, and only third to the ancients. He developed a thermometer to measure bodily temperature in physiological experiments and clinical practice, and his most influential book, *De statica medicina* (1614) [On Medical Statics], outlined experiments using other instruments as well – a pendulum for measuring pulse-rate, a hygrometer, a syringe to extract bladder stones, a trochar for tracheotomy, and the pulsilogium, a pulse watch.

His most ingenious device was the weighing machine or balance. Writing and even sleeping in this contraption, he monitored his body functions for some thirty years, documenting body weight after eating and drinking, evacuating and exercising, and correlating all these to his health. Discovering that the weight of his excreta was less than that of the food and drink he consumed, with no increase in his own weight to account for the difference, he explained it in terms of invisible perspiration, traditionally judged a salutary mode of bodily discharge.

The hope of wedding the new mathematical physics to medicine culminated in Giorgio Baglivi (1668–1707), who practised in Padua and Venice before settling in Bologna in 1691 as Malpighi's assistant. He pictured the body as a machine: the teeth were compared to scissors; the thorax, bellows; the heart and vessels, water-works; the stomach, a grinding-mill. A distinguished physiological researcher fascinated by the nerves, his microscopic studies enabled him to distinguish between smooth and striated muscles and distinct kinds of fibres, suggesting that health largely depended upon the condition of the muscle fibres (i.e., the active solids).

Yet there was another face to Baglivi; wearing his hat as a clinician, he pooh-poohed theoretical speculations and reiterated traditional Hippocratic ideals:

> Length of life does not depend so much on a good physical constitution as it does on the best use of the six non-natural things, which if we rule aright, we shall live long and healthy lives: to divide the day properly between sleep and waking; to adjust our air to the needs of the body; to take more or less food and drink according to our age, our temperament, and whether we live an active or inactive life; to take exercise or rest according to the quantity of our food and whether we are lean or fat; to know ourselves, and be able to rule our emotions, and subject them to our reason. Whoever handles these wisely will live long and seldom need a doctor.

Medicine was thus in flux, but one thing was clear: the new interpretive frameworks had discarded Galenism. When Thomas Willis reviewed the three philosophies available to medicine – the Aristotelian, the Epicurean (or mechanical) and the chemical – he was quite contemptuous of the first. Yet while experimental philosophers gloried in being 'moderns', in clinical medicine much of the ancient heritage remained intact, perhaps because the patients were conservative, preferring the therapeutic devil they knew. And if the arch-enemy was now Galen, now supposed to have sterilized medicine with his sophistry, Hippocrates maintained his olympian status as the champion of bedside experience. Thomas Sydenham (1624–89) was acclaimed as the 'English Hippocrates' since he prized observation, avoiding speculation but using his senses. Asked what were the best medical books, he replied 'Read *Don Quixote*'. He equally distrusted dissection and the speculations it provoked. 'This is all very fine,' he told a young student, 'but it won't do – Anatomy – Botany – Nonsense! Sir, I know an old woman in Covent Garden who understands botany better, and as for anatomy, my butcher can dissect a joint full and well; now, young man, all that is stuff; you must go to the bedside, it is there alone you can learn disease.' He summed up his philosophy:

> I became convinced that the physician who earnestly studies, with his own eyes – and not through the medium of books – the natural phenomena of the different diseases, must necessarily excel in the art of discovering what, in any given case, are the true indications as to the remedial measures that should be employed.

Oxford educated, Sydenham served in the Parliamentary Army. From 1655 he practised in London, investigating smallpox and other fevers. Revering Hippocrates, his programme was simple: medicine was a craft which would progress through observation of patients and monitoring of therapies. Drawing on experience, the goal was to discover (a modern touch here) specific remedies, the paradigm of which was cinchona (Peruvian or Jesuits' Bark), used against the ague (malaria). Conventional remedies were meant to purge the body of peccant humours, but the bark seemed to root out the disease at source. It was arguably the first effective specific drug. This action reinforced Sydenham's (modern) conviction that diseases were specific entities: 'all diseases should be reduced to definite and certain *Species*... with the same care which we see exhibited by Botanick Writers in their Phytologies.' In turn specificity boosted his hopes for a science of diseases:

> Nature, in the production of diseases, is uniform and consistent ... and the selfsame phenomena that you would observe in the sickness of a Socrates you would observe in the sickness of a simpleton. Just so the universal characters of a plant are extended to every individual of the species.

Diseases were thus distinct, possessing unique natural histories – citing mistletoe growing on trees, he emphasized how the disease was independent of the sufferer. Yet, at least for chronic diseases, he never abandoned his humoral framework.

Sydenham's thinking grew out of clinical experience, especially his careful observations of the epidemic diseases prevalent in London in the 1660s and 1670s, which he ascribed to changing environmental conditions or the 'epidemic constitution'. The prevalent fever, he noted, was the ague (benign tertian malaria), familiar as the annual epidemic of intermittent fever occurring from March to July. He judged it arose from the warmth of the sun acting on humours which had accumulated in the blood during the winter. For Sydenham, as for Hippocratic physicians in Greece two thousand years earlier, the regularity of intermittent fevers held the promise of setting clinical medicine on a sounder footing.

With fevers like smallpox, Sydenham pioneered 'cool therapy'. Physicians had standardly prescribed piles of blankets and heating cordials to sweat out the diseased matter. This orthodox heating regimen caused excessive 'ebullition' of blood, he judged, leading to confluent pustules, brain-fever and even death. Sydenham aimed by contrast to assist nature, prescribing a cooling regime, copious fluids and moderate bleeding. This advice proved influential and even beneficial.

Overall, however, it is a moot point whether bedside medicine was growing wiser or safer. The sixteenth and seventeenth centuries brought no revolution in medical services or treatments. There remained a mosaic of practitioners – learned physicians, herbalists, wise-women, astrologers, uroscopists, empirics, apothecaries, barber-surgeons and specialists like tooth-drawers and lithotomists. Moneyed patients shopped around, while the poor were restricted to the aid of family, neighbours and priests.

Women remained in charge of childbirth, except when a surgeon was called in to use his instruments to extract a dead foetus from the womb. Midwives, according to William Sermon's (*c.* 1629–1679) *Ladies Companion, or, The English Midwife* (1671) 'must be mild, gentle, courteous, sober, chaste and patient ... As concerning their minds, they must be wise and discreet.' Wise or not, most lacked formal training and learnt on the job; Perceval Willoughby (1596–1685), an English surgeon who specialized in difficult deliveries, was predictably critical of their lack of skill, bemoaning their tendency in a slow labour to tug upon a hand or a foot, sometimes yanking it off altogether.

But there was also an elite of the better-educated. Louise Bourgeois (1563–1636) married a surgeon and acquired a huge practice, serving Marie de Medici, wife to Henri IV, through six confinements and publishing books relating her experiences, one of which was translated as *The Compleat Midwife's Practice Enlarged* (1659). Partly thanks to her, from 1631 Paris midwives began to get some formal training at the Hôtel Dieu, and after 1679 Amsterdam midwives had to attend anatomy and obstetrics lectures. Alleging that many mothers and babies died through incompetent midwives, Elizabeth Cellier petitioned James II in 1687 to provide a lying-in hospital run by trained midwives, but, fearing rivals and belittling women, the College of Physicians scotched the scheme.

Gynaecological problems and obstetric skills were discussed in a stream of books. In 1661 Hendrik van Roonhuyze (1622–72), of Amsterdam, published a work describing caesarean section, and discussing cases of ectopic pregnancy and of vesico-vaginal fistula. François Mauriceau (1637–1709) produced his classic *Traité des maladies des femmes grosses* (1668) [Treatise on the Illnesses of Pregnant Women], which disposed, among other things, of the hoary myth that the pelvic bones separated during labour to enlarge the birth canal. Hendrik van Deventer (1651–1724), from the Hague, described how pelvic deformities obstructed labour in *Operationes chirurgicae novum lumen exhibentes obstetricantibus* (1716) [The Art of Midwifery Improved].

One development was the obstetrical forceps, introduced by a French Huguenot, William Chamberlen (*c.* 1540–96), who had fled to England. The two halves of the tongs could be separated at their crossover point, permitting each curved, hollowed, metal blade to be inserted separately into the pelvis to grasp the baby's head; a pin was then inserted, allowing the head to be gripped and drawn out. Chamberlen kept the instrument a family secret, passing it on to his son, Peter, who passed it on to his son, Peter (1601–83), who passed it on to his son, Hugh (1630–1720). When called to a confinement, they supposedly hid the forceps in a box to preserve their trade secret; and it was easy to conceal in the labour room, since modesty demanded that a sheet should cover the parturient woman.

CURING

Bedside practice changed little. Physicians would take a history in the Hippocratic manner, inquiring from the patient about his or her lifestyle and the onset of the complaint. They would feel the pulse and inspect urine samples – though uroscopy lost credit, becoming the trademark of the quackish 'pisse-prophet' and being attacked with 'cozening quacksalvers, women physitians and the like stuffe' by status-anxious physicians such as the Netherlander Pieter van Foreest (1522–97). New anatomical discoveries produced few therapeutic payoffs – perhaps they would have scared the patients. 'I have heard him say', John Aubrey reported of William Harvey, 'that, when his book on blood circulation came out, his practice suffered and people called him mad.'

Therapeutics remained grounded in tradition. Here is Shakespeare's son-in-law John Hall (1575–1635) recording a case.

> Esq. *Packinton*, as he was riding to *London*, in his Inne was suddenly and miserably afflicted with the Gout in hands and feet, so that he could neither stand nor handle any thing. Being called to him, I thus cured him: ℞ *Mallowes with the roots cut small, they were boyled*

in equal parts of Wine and Vinegar, to the wasting of the third part, to which was added Rye bran after a light boyling. They were laid to the pained Joints, with which he was well eased in one day, and delivered from the Inflammation by fomenting the parts with *Water of the spawn of Frogs.* After was applied *Emplast, Diachalcit.* The same day I gave ʒii *Pul. Sen. Montag. cum Hermodaci.* gr. xv. He was restored the third day, and rid towards *London.*

In other words, Hall applied a poultice of mallows, a fomentation of frog spawn and a plaster. The patient was purged with senna powder, a medicine attributed to the Paduan physician Bartolomeo Montagnana (d. 1460). To this powder Hall added the purgative hermodactylus, a species of colchicum, recommended by Paul of Aegina back in the seventh century for the treatment of pain in the joints.

If frog spawn seems odd, all sorts of other weird and wonderful ingredients continued in use. For instance, Henry Oldenburg, secretary of the Royal Society, wrote in 1664 to Robert Boyle, 'I owe you many thanks for a medicine against Fluxes, but give me leave to ask, whether the hot cinnamon and nutmeg may not claim as great a share in the effect as the cold deadman's skull.'

Sufferers from intermittent fevers (malaria) did benefit, however, from the use of cinchona (or Peruvian) bark. This (the source of quinine) was brought to Europe between about 1630 and 1640, perhaps by Jesuit missionaries, hence the name Jesuits' Bark and the refusal of staunch Protestants like Oliver Cromwell to take it. Galenists too objected, believing that a drug alleged to be hot was counterindicated in a fever. Cinchona was effective, however, and was introduced into the *London Pharmacopoeia* in 1677.

Ipecacuanha (*Cephaelis ipecacuanha*: 'the little plant which grows by the wayside and causes vomiting') reached Europe from Brazil. It remedied amoebic dysentery and proved a cough expectorant and an effective emetic in poisoning cases. Other new imported plants doubled as social amenities and as medicines: tea and coffee came from the East, while tobacco (*Nicotiana*) was brought to England from the Americas by Sir Walter Ralegh.

Critics denounced physicians as meddlesome, capriciously practising an often dangerous polypharmacy – a blunderbuss approach. Charles II's deathbed was a conspicuous instance of such medical overkill: after he suffered a stroke, the doctors moved in, and Sir Raymond Crawfurd (1865–1938) recreated the scene:

Sixteen ounces of blood were removed from a vein in his right arm with immediate good effect. As was the approved practice at this time, the King was allowed to remain in the chair in which the convulsions seized him; his teeth were held forcibly open to prevent him biting his tongue; the regimen was, as Roger North pithily describes it, 'first to get him to wake, and then to keep him from sleeping'. Urgent messages had been dispatched to the King's numerous personal physicians, who quickly came flocking to his assistance: they were summoned regardless of distinctions of creed and politics, and they came. They ordered cupping-glasses to be applied to his shoulders forthwith, and deep scarification to be carried out, by which they succeeded in removing another eight ounces of blood. A strong antimonial emetic was administered, but as the King could be got to swallow only a small portion of it, they determined to render assurance doubly sure by a full dose of Sulphate of Zinc. Strong purgatives were given, and supplemented by a succession of clysters. The hair was shorn close and pungent blistering agents were applied all over his head; and as though this were not enough, the red-hot cautery was requisitioned as well.

One of the dozen physicians attending, Dr Charles Scarburgh, ominously justified these practices by saying that 'nothing was left untried', and the Merrie Monarch graciously apologized for being 'an unconscionable time a-dying'.

Not all experiences were as grim, however, as the diary of Samuel Pepys (1633–1703) suggests. Cambridge educated, Pepys became one of England's most capable naval administrators. Keen on the 'new science', he was an early fellow of the Royal Society, where he witnessed some of the earliest blood transfusions. During the late 1650s, Christopher Wren (1632–1723) – primarily famous as an architect – had been attempting to introduce medicinal liquors directly into the bloodstream, and the French physician, Jean-Baptiste Denys (c. 1625–1704), transfused blood from dog to dog. And then, before the Royal Society, Richard Lower in November 1667 made a transfusion from a sheep to a divinity student, Arthur Coga, who was described as somewhat crack-brained; it was hoped a transfusion might cure him. The satirist Thomas Shadwell (1641–92) hinted in his play *The Virtuoso* that such patients would grow magnificent fleeces and prove good economic investments, while Pepys wondered what would happen if a Quaker's blood were given to an archbishop.

Pepys also experienced the great plague of 1665, giving an eye-witness account of the panic and terror and noting the flight from town of fashionable physicians, excusing themselves on the grounds that their duty was to follow their patients. On 7 June he saw red crosses springing up on houses in Drury Lane, bearing the words 'Lord, have mercy upon us.' Some days later, the hackney coachman driving him along Holborn suddenly grew delirious with plague. The outbreak spread like wildfire, and the wealthy couldn't get out fast enough. Pepys remained in London, exercising some caution but distrusting the remedies and prophylactics of both the regulars and the empirics, and using the opportunity to indulge his fondness for sexual escapades.

So what of Pepys's own health? Shortly before commencing his diary, he had been cut for a bladder stone by Thomas Hollyer, surgeon at St Thomas's Hospital; it came out intact, as big as a tennis ball. The proud (and lucky!) survivor had it set in a case, which cost him twenty-four shillings. 'This day,' he recorded on 26 March 1659, 'it is two years since it pleased God that I was cut for the stone at Mrs Turner's in Salisbury Court. And did resolve while I live to keep it a festival, as I did the last year at my house.' Pepys was also plagued by bad eyes, which caused him to leave off writing his diary in 1669, though his fears that he was going blind proved false.

Despite these and other troubles, Pepys did not often call upon professional medical advice, though he numbered doctors among his friends. Prevention was better than cure, and he attended (heeding the non-naturals) to such matters as diet, exercise, climate, avoiding draughts and damp. One of his great bugbears was cold: on no fewer than 102 occasions he recorded taking cold. He generally blamed it on the weather, but his own carelessness was often at fault: leaving off his wig, standing in draughts, wearing unaired clothes. Every move might be full of peril: '[2 November 1662] and so to home and to bed, with some pain in making water, having taken cold this morning in staying too long bare-legged to pare my cornes.' On occasion he wore a hare's foot around his neck in the hope of warding off sickness; but, unlike many of his contemporaries who pondered the mysteries of mortality and the divine or diabolical sources of affliction, his attitude was pragmatic and rather secular.

MEDICINE AND THE PEOPLE

From the sixteenth century the fog, which from time immemorial kept the lives of most of humanity hidden from history, parts a little because parish clergy in many kingdoms were ordered to keep registers of births, marriages and deaths (though such data obviously have drastic limitations). The development of what became demography and epidemiology became possible as part of the wider quest to apply science to society.

In England the pioneer of demography was the haberdasher John Graunt (1620–74), an enthusiast for the 'new science' and an early fellow of the Royal Society. His *Natural and Political Observations. . . upon the Bills of Mortality* (1662) was based on analysis of the weekly burial lists compiled by London's parish clerks, setting out the numbers and causes of death in each parish. His figures allowed him to recognize that more boys were born than girls, and that urban mortality exceeded rural, though it was virtually impossible to identify the true causes of death. In London the 'searchers of the dead', old crones employed by the parish, assigned causes using symptom-based categories, but their terms such as 'aged', 'fever', 'surfet' and 'suddenly' nowadays appear hopelessly vague.

Another pioneer of social statistics was William Petty (1623–87), who coined the term 'political arithmetic'. His early life was spent at sea, but in 1645 he moved to Paris where he joined Hobbes's circle of natural philosophers. On his return to England he pursued medical studies at Oxford and established himself as one of the leading lights of the Royal Society. In the preface to his *Political Anatomy of Ireland* (1691), he acknowledged he had been inspired by Bacon's observation that the preservation of the body politic and the body natural were of a piece. He collected data on population, trade, manufacture, education, diseases and revenue, as part of what he termed 'political anatomy'. An important tool of these new vital statistics was the life-table, devised in 1693 by the astronomer Edmond Halley (c.1656–1743). Projecting expectations about length of life in arithmetical form, it became invaluable to the new insurance and annuity industries.

Infant mortality – the number of babies dying in the first year of life – became accepted in the nineteenth century as a reliable index of the health of a population. In western Europe today an infant mortality rate of around 9 per 1000 live births is the norm. In early modern England it was some fifteen times higher, and elsewhere worse still: before 1750 France had over 200 deaths per 1000 live births, Geneva 296. Expectation of life at birth typically averaged under thirty years (though huge infant and childhood mortality rates skew that figure). In cities deaths exceeded births, and towns depended on an influx of incomers from the countryside to maintain the population. The young of all classes were at greatest risk – from the bloody flux, scarlet fever, whooping cough, influenza, smallpox, pneumonia; these and a multitude of now unidentifiable fevers killed perhaps 40 per cent of Europe's children before the age of fifteen.

Occasional but devastating mortality crises were caused by dearth and pestilence. Lethal famines remained common in continental Europe up to the mid eighteenth century, but England was more fortunate: subsistence crises still affected the northern region in the late sixteenth century, but disappeared within half a century because of better communications and food markets.

Bubonic plague continued to wreak havoc throughout the early-modern era, made worse by the continual movement of peoples through persecution and poverty. Once plague broke out, nothing was of avail, though both civic and religious measures were taken. In the desperately severe outbreaks of the 1570s the archbishop of Milan, Carlo Borromeo, staged penitential processions and decreed that health officials should not halt church services. In 1630 and 1631 plague raged through the Arno valley: Monte Lupo, a small, poverty-stricken village near Florence, was particularly hard hit. The Florence health authorities imposed strict quarantine and policing orders to contain the outbreak. Don Antonio Bontadi, the village priest, had other ideas. He brought the miraculous crucifix of Monte Lupo out of the church and paraded it through the town. People from nearby villages joined the locals in the processions, conducted in defiance of the health authorities. Compromise was possible, however, between pious acts and public health, and even the Papal States had their own health boards. In England a plague policy was implemented from 1578, when the Privy Council published its Plague Orders. As in Italy, administration fell not on physicians but on magistrates (Justices of the Peace).

With only occasional respite since the Black Death, plague brought grim mortality. Germany, Holland, Italy and Spain all had devastating visitations in the first half of the sixteenth century, while Muscovy experienced a particularly severe outbreak in 1572, in which 200,000 deaths were reported. In 1630–1 Venice lost over 30 per cent of its people; in Genoa plague and famine in 1656 led to the death of up to three quarters of the population; in the same year a staggering 300,000 people died in Naples in just five months. Around one fifth of London's population perished in each of the plague outbreaks of 1563, 1603, 1625 and 1665, the death toll in 1665 approaching 80,000. There were, however, no further outbreaks in London, and thereafter plague disappeared from English soil.

In the early eighteenth century plague remained active in Turkey, the Balkans, Poland, Galicia and the Ukraine. In 1713 it made its final assault on Germany, Scandinavia and Austria, with Vienna suffering badly, while the last severe western outbreak occurred in the south of France in 1720–2 killing between 50,000 and 100,000 in Marseilles and two thirds of the population of Toulon. Various reasons have been suggested for the retreat of the plague, including the ousting of the house or black rat (*rattus rattus*) by the brown rat (*rattus norvegicus*), the less-domesticated sewer rat. Perhaps local and national policies of exclusion through quarantine and the cordon sanitaire finally worked.

The devastating effects of plague, epidemics and social unrest heightened the problem of the management of the urban masses. The years after 1500 brought rocketing population growth and, especially when famine struck, cities were overwhelmed by starving peasants flocking from the countryside. Formerly viewed as God's holy ones, beggars became targeted as dangerous rogues requiring discipline and moral reformation, and destitution became equated with disease. In Juan Luis Vives's (1492–1540) *De subventione pauperum* (1526) [On the Relief of the Poor], vagabonds were blamed for introducing plague and syphilis – indeed, vagrants were seen almost as a disease in their own right. In response to these problems, north European towns began to organize poor relief, while banning non-residents, criminalizing begging, and trying to reform the able-bodied through sermons and houses of industry.

Poor-relief schemes often divided 'undeserving' rogues from the 'deserving' (who included the sick, orphans and widows). Measures designed for the undeserving poor were sometimes extended to the deserving, who might be swept into barrack-like hospitals and work-houses which kept the dregs off the streets while providing a modicum of care. Outdoor relief was also given, and charity organized by civic or parochial authorities.

In 1601 the English Poor Law was consolidated. The destitute, aged, infirm or sick were to be supported by a poor rate levied on householders in each parish. Parish midwives would be available, and babies might be sent to wet-nurses; funerals were provided. The Poor Law could be seen as the nationalization of religious charity in the post-Reformation Protestant state; it was also a form of social regulation and a prophylactic against disorder.

Needy people in Florence, Genoa, Rome, Venice and many other Italian cities continued to be served, as earlier, by private institutions run by religious confraternities. Shows of conspicuous philanthropy involved considerable powers of patronage and conferred status. Italy's hospitals remained the envy of Europe. In 1594 Fynes Moryson (1566–1629) wrote of Florence, 'The Hospitall of S. Maria Nova is said to passe all others in Italy, for all necessaries to cure and nourish the sicke, and for orderly attendance.' Hospitals commonly took in abandoned children, women, the indigent and incurables. In 1591 Rome had 3666 hospital residents out of a population of 116,695, Venice around 4000, and in the mid seventeenth century Florence housed 2500 orphans and beggars. In Turin the city government was becoming involved in hospital administration. Benefactors used their leverage to provide relief for clients and dependants.

From the 1620s a revitalized Catholicism set about reforming the charitable institutions of France. The Company of the Holy Sacrament proposed institutions for vagrants, down-and-outs and the deserving poor: the former would be reformed by punishment, the latter given shelter. In 1656 the company established its first institution, the Hôpital Général in Paris, under Cardinal Mazarin, intended to house all manner of problem people and furnished with detention powers. By 1700, more than one hundred *hôpitaux généraux* had been built throughout France, their inmates numbering over 100,000. Run on a mixture of religious discipline and forced labour, they were not primarily medical institutions but workhouses and old people's homes. This new drive for the contain-ment of nuisances, beggars, the insane, orphans, petty thieves, prosti-tutes, unmarried mothers and the chronic sick has been called by the

French historian Michel Foucault 'the great confinement'. It was a prototype for later medical institutions for the poor.

Another type of charitable institution, the Hôtel Dieu, a large city hospital which in medieval times had provided hospitality and medical assistance, grew more 'medicalized', employing surgeons and having an attendant physician. The sick poor could use the Hôtel Dieu for treatment, though syphilitics and other infectious patients were barred. Catholic reform also created nursing communities, usually female, notably the Daughters of Charity, founded in 1633 by Vincent de Paul and Louise de Marillac. Often drawn from the poorer sections of society, in contrast to the wealthier cloistered nuns, the sisters supplied practical nursing skills and labour in French and foreign hospitals. Vincent de Paul gave pious nursing advice:

> never forget to say a few good words such as 'Well, brother, how do you think you are going to make the journey to the other world?' or 'Well, my child, don't you wish to unite yourself with God? Don't you wish to make a good confession in order to dispose yourself to die well? Don't you wish to go and see Our Lord?' And so you should always say something to them which will raise their hearts to God.

The Daughters of Charity were not solely spiritual workers; they were taught a range of nursing skills, the uses of drugs and simple surgical procedures. Practice in the care of the sick was afforded, and teaching opportunities for literate sisters were provided by the parish school attached to the motherhouse.

All such municipal and philanthropic initiatives may be styled 'medicalization' and viewed as part of the wider development of social administration and control, especially under absolutist regimes. Yet medicalization had limits. No single group of practitioners anywhere achieved a monopoly of practice, and all agreed that healing could be a gift of God. An English statute of 1542–3 gave its blessing to pious charitable medicine performed by

> divers honest persons, as well men women, whom God hath embued with the knowledge of the nature, kind and operation of certain herbs, roots and waters, and the using and ministering of them to such as been pained with customable diseases . . . the said persons have not taken anything for their pains or cunning [skill]

but have ministered to poor people only for neighbourhood and God's sake, and of pity and charity.

Religious views on sickness were reinforced in Catholic nations by Counter-Reformation piety. Prayers to saints and the virgin, pilgrimages to miraculous shrines, votive offerings, use of the sacraments and the anointing of the sick with holy oil all remained extremely popular. For their part, soul-searching Protestants could regard illness as a divine punishment for sin or as a Job-like trial of faith.

Religion retained its hold at the death-bed. How a person died was crucial, for it determined whether they went to heaven or hell. From medieval times the *ars moriendi* (the art of dying) had taught believers how to die well. For Catholics it was essential to make a last confession and to receive the sacraments, and so die in a state of grace.

In a Christian society, dying was the passage from this vale of tears to life eternal, marked by traditional Christian icons charged with dramatic eloquence: the grim Reaper with scythe and hourglass, the skull or the skeleton. Death was not regarded as an abrupt, instantaneous, biological reversal; dying was a process, beginning at birth itself, with a sequence of stages marked by appropriate behaviour and reminders (*memento mori*: prepare to meet thy death). Aristocratic funerals were protracted and lavish, involving throngs of mourners, exchanges of gifts and tokens, embalming, erection of memorial tablets and heraldic effigies, and the intricate conventions of mourning. All these customs preserved memory, emphasized the continuity of past, present and future generations, and allowed the dead to lord it still among the living.

Beliefs and practices changed of course. By abolishing the doctrine of purgatory, Protestantism removed a great link between the living and the dead, and rendered obsolete the majestic Catholic prayers for the departed and the requiem masses. By the eighteenth century, tombs and headstones were making more of worldly virtues ('a good man and an excellent bowler' was how Alderman Nynn of Kent was described), and the hellfire terrors of the dance of death were yielding to the rococo refinement of urns and laurel sprays. Only from the eighteenth century did doctors encroach upon the rituals of death.

MADNESS

The seventeenth century saw controversies between religious and secular explanations for certain diseases, especially with the new rationalist stress on nature's clockwork and the replacement of the image of God as a loving or vengeful Father with the notion of a divine but distant Master Mind, presiding over celestial machinery that obeyed universal scientific laws. The new philosophy had crucial implications for understanding of the soul, of mind/body relations, and hence of mental illness.

On such questions, Descartes's mechanical philosophy threw down the gauntlet; his successors had to take up the Cartesian challenge. The implications of Cartesianism for insanity were momentous, for his dualistic philosophy ruled out primary mental disease: madness, he taught, could not lie in the immortal soul or mind but had to be in the body. Though Descartes was no materialist, his writings encouraged a search for the site of madness within the organism, indeed within the brain.

Distinguished investigations were pursued by Thomas Willis. Anglican by faith and royalist in politics, Willis became a prominent member of the Oxford Philosophical Club and an associate of Petty, Boyle, Wren and Hooke. He grasped that Harvey's discovery of the circulation of the blood called for a complete re-thinking of medical theory. Building on painstaking anatomical investigations, first-hand knowledge of the nervous system, vivisection experiments and clinical experience, his *Cerebri anatome* (1664) [Anatomy of the Brain] was highly influential. A companion study, the *Pathologiae cerebri et nervosi generis specimen* (1667) [Pathology of the Brain, and Specimen of the Nature of the Nerves], developed ideas about the nervous origins of convulsive disorders such as epilepsy, asthma and convulsive coughs, narcolepsy and apoplexy.

Willis coined the term 'neurologie', developed the Cartesian idea of reflex, and has been called the founder of neuroanatomy and neurophysiology in view of his attempts to map mental functions onto particular areas of the brain (he is remembered for his description of the Circle of Willis, the arterial circle at the base of the brain). His theories of neurological activity continued to rely on animal spirits viewed as intermediaries between body and mind distributed to all parts of the body through the nervous system.

Such views did not lead to any original therapies. Willis believed, rather traditionally, that maniacs should be restrained while other sufferers required drugs and bathing. Nevertheless, as a result of Descartes, Willis and others, a new paradigm of madness was emerging, discarding both humoralism and supernaturalism in favour of an organic hypothesis. Thomas Sydenham left a particularly full discussion of hysteria, a medical dignosis increasingly used by doctors to explain the so-called manifestations of bewitchment.

Sydenham's greatest admirer was John Locke (1632–1704), who advanced his own explanation of insanity – a psychological hypothesis about the association of ideas. Representative of the late seventeenth-century amalgam of medicine, science and philosophy, Locke's thinking proved fundamental to the later methods of science and medicine, his *Essay Concerning Humane Understanding* (1690) being among the most important influences on the Enlightenment.

Locke was initiated into the new medicine by his old school friend, Richard Lower; attending Willis's lectures, he became involved in the pioneering experiments of Boyle and Hooke, and soon after became a close friend of Sydenham. He treated Anthony Ashley Cooper, later first earl of Shaftesbury (1621–83); the patient turned patron and Locke eventually joined the Ashley household in London. When Ashley fell gravely ill in 1668 from a suppurating hydatid cyst of the liver, Locke, after consulting Sydenham, supervised the draining of the abscess through a silver tube.

If medicine drew his attention to the virtues of observation, Locke's thinking, in turn, had a considerable bearing on medicine and philosophical psychology. His *Essay* mounted a critique of innate ideas and examined the mental operations (sensory perception and reflection) attending the formation of concepts. The mind prior to the acquisition of knowledge was a blank sheet of paper (tabula rasa); it was then shaped by experience and developed by habit. As to the body, he was still Hippocratic when it came to practical advice, as he explained in *Some Thoughts Concerning Education* (1693):

> And thus I have done with what concerns the Body and Health, which reduces it self to these few and easily observable Rules. Plenty of open Air, Exercise and Sleep; Plain Diet, no Wine or Strong Drink, and very little or no Physick; not too Warm and strait Clothing, especially the Head and Feet kept cold, and the Feet often used to cold Water, and exposed to Wet.

In *Le Médecin malgré lui*, Molière presented the following exchange between a patient and a pretender:

> GÉRONTE: It was very clearly explained, but there was just one
> thing which surprised me – that was the positions of the
> liver and the heart. It seemed to me that you got them the
> wrong way about, that the heart should be on the left side,
> and the liver on the right.
> SGANARELLE: Yes, it used to be so but we have changed all
> that. Everything's quite different in medicine nowadays.

Molière got it right. There was still much that was laughable about seventeenth-century medicine; but it was changing fast. In *The Advancement of Learning*, Francis Bacon had proclaimed:

> Medicine is a science which hath been (as we have said) more
> professed than laboured, and yet more laboured than advanced;
> the labour having been, in my judgement, rather in circle than in
> progression. For I find much iteration, but small addition.

By the century's end, addition was more visible.

CHAPTER X

ENLIGHTENMENT

IN SEARCH OF MEDICAL SCIENCE

A MINOR EIGHTEENTH-CENTURY MEDICAL WRITER, Samuel Wood, looked back in his *Strictures on the Gout* (1775) over the previous 'two thousand years' and deplored the 'unenlightened state of the ancient Practitioners', with whom 'all was mere conjecture'. 'There could be no Physiology at all,' he insisted, 'before our immortal Harvey's Discovery of the Circulation of the Blood,' since when, he concluded, 'it is much more easy to account for life, for health, and for diseases.'

Early-modern times brought Harvey's and other brilliant breakthroughs in anatomy and physiology, but achievements proved more impressive on paper than in bedside practice; the war against death was stalled, and, to make matters worse, epidemics rained down on Europe in the decades around 1700 and mortality rates soared. Warfare, worldwide trading webs, giant cities and the thronging urban poor – the populations of cities like Naples, Paris and London were already topping half a million – all exacerbated health hazards.

Better times were on the way, however, according to the new philosophy of progress proclaimed by enlightened intellectuals in the Netherlands, Britain and France: original sin was a myth, and life's journey was not the preachers' vale of tears. Reason, proclaimed Enlightenment propagandists, would create a better future; science and technology, as Francis Bacon had taught, would enhance man's control over nature, and social progress, prosperity and the conquest of disease would follow. In the 1790s the Marquis de Condorcet (1743–94) declared that future medical advances, supported by the civilizing process, would extend longevity, even perhaps to the point of immortality. 'The improvement of medical practice,' he declared, which will become more efficacious with the progress of reason and of the social order, will mean the end of infectious and hereditary diseases and illnesses brought on by climate, food, or working conditions. It is reasonable to hope that all other diseases may likewise disappear as their distant causes are discovered.

The ogres of error and blind authority had already been challenged by heroes like Vesalius and William Harvey; further progress would make medicine yet more scientific.

What precisely this scientific medicine should be like was hotly disputed. Iatromathematicians like Giorgio Baglivi (1668–1707) set great store by quantification. His *De praxi medica* (1699) [On Medical Practice] held that 'the human body ... operates by number, weight, and measure'. God, he asserted, 'seems to have sketched the most ordered series of proportions in the human body by the pen of Mathematics alone'. And numbers counted. In 1707, Sir John Floyer (1649–1734) published *The Physician's Pulse Watch*, which acknowledged the Galenists' skill in interpreting the pulse, but sought to establish objective numerical standards for determining abnormality, recommending checking the pulse against a watch with a special second hand.

With the idolization of Isaac Newton (1642–1727), whose *Principia* had been published in 1687, experimental natural philosophy offered the most persuasive scientific model. Leading the application of physics to medicine was the Dutch professor, Herman Boerhaave (1668–1738), who construed health and sickness as expressions of such variables as forces, weights and hydrostatic pressures. Boerhaave was the preeminent early Enlightenment physician, holding a succession of chairs at Leiden University from 1702. His influence spread through print: his textbook, *Institutiones medicae* (1708) [The Institutes of Medicine], ran through ten editions and was translated into five languages; protégés like Gerhard van Swieten (1700–72) exported his teachings to Vienna, Edinburgh and Göttingen.

Boerhaave promoted mechanistic disease explanation within a corpuscularian matter theory, seeing health in terms of hydrostatic equilibrium, a balance of internal fluid pressures. He distinguished between disorders of the 'solids' and those of the 'blood and humours'. Tuberculosis was an example of weakness of the solid parts, blood clots an example of overly rigid fibres. Give milk and iron for weak fibres; let blood for rigid ones, he counselled.

Such views encouraged experimentation. The mathematically

inclined Anglican clergyman Stephen Hales (1677–1761) thus devised 'haemodynamic' experiments to measure blood circulation. Analysing the circulation in his *Haemastaticks* (1733), he measured the force of the blood by inserting into the jugular vein and carotid artery of a living horse a goose's trachea attached to a glass tube eleven feet long, to see how far up the tube the column of blood was carried. He recorded that the arterial pressure was far greater than the venous. A dauntless animal experimenter, Hales also explored Descartes's notions of nerve action. His method involved decapitating frogs and stimulating their reflexes by pricking the skin, noting that nervous responses continued. These experiments provoked anti-vivisection protests. The normally thick-skinned Samuel Johnson (1709–84) denounced doctors who 'extend the arts of torture'. 'I know not', he asserted, 'that by living dissection any discovery has been made by which a single malady is more easily cured.'

Boerhaave's hydraulic model of the body incurred criticism, however, and attention shifted from the vascular to the nervous system. Vital qualities like irritability and sensibility were highlighted in the work of Albrecht von Haller (1708–77) in Göttingen, William Cullen (1710–90) and his colleagues in Edinburgh, and Théophile de Bordeu (1722–76) and other Montpellier vitalists – all of whom developed a more dynamic life-force physiology than Boerhaave's, in which health was the co-ordination of the separate life of each organ in the body.

In other words, eighteenth-century scientific medicine was far from monolithic. Rival camps proliferated, and the traditional Italian and French centres of excellence were challenged by Halle, Leiden, London, Edinburgh, Vienna and Philadelphia, each with its own school. In Halle, Georg Ernst Stahl (1659–1734) denounced the materialism he detected in Boerhaavian mechanical philosophy, advocating instead an 'animism' which proposed a God-given, super-added soul (*anima*) as the prime mover of living beings. Highly influential in German-speaking lands, Stahl attacked reductionism: organisms were more than the sum of their parts, and purposive human actions could not be explained by mechanical chain-reactions alone; activity presupposed the guiding purposive power of a soul. This *anima* was the agent of consciousness and physiological regulation, and disease was the soul's attempt to expel morbid matter and re-establish bodily order. Stahlian animism made medical sense, but it was also the product of evangelical Lutheran Pietism.

Yet even in Halle Stahl did not reign unchallenged, for his colleague there, Friedrich Hoffmann (1660–1742), leant towards mechanism. 'Medicine', announced his *Fundamenta medicinae* (1695) [Fundamentals of Medicine], 'is the art of properly utilizing physico-mechanical principles, in order to conserve the health of man or to restore it if lost.' Occupying the middle ground was Boissier de Sauvages (1706–67), professor of medicine at Montpellier. He accepted that the body was a machine, mathematically understandable, but disease was the effort by nature or the soul to expel morbific matter, and physiology was the science of that struggle.

In their different ways, Boissier de Sauvages's successors – Théophile de Bordeu, Robert Whytt (1714–66) in Edinburgh, and John Hunter (1728–93) in London – also denied the sufficiency of mechanics for explaining the body, postulating some vital force or organization. Very few physicians (the anti-clerical *philosophe* Julien Offray de La Mettrie (1709–51) was one) went the whole hog and unashamedly reduced man to mechanism. Influenced by the spectacular working automata constructed by craftsmen like Jacques Vaucanson (1709–82), La Mettrie held in his *L'homme machine* (1748) [Man a Machine] that matter thinks; there was no need for a soul, for the body is 'a machine that winds its own springs'.

There were, in short, numerous ways in which medical authors sought to set their discipline on scientific rails; even so, that medicine failed to match the achievements of experimental physics or chemistry remained scandalous. Towards 1800, Thomas Beddoes (1760–1808), the Bristol practitioner who dreamed of curing lung disorders with respirable gases, rued that medicine was 'remote . . . from such perfection'.

Historians have sometimes explained this apparent paradox of Enlightenment medical science – great expectations, disappointing results – as the consequence of over-ambitious theorizing. Yet that judgment seems misguided; for one thing, highly practical investigation continued unabated in fields like anatomy. As Italy's star waned, the lights of science moved north, to France, the Netherlands, England, Scotland and certain German principalities. For long Leiden led the field, thanks to Boerhaave and his pupil, Bernhard Siegfried Albinus (1697–1770) – in a pious gesture, they re-published Vesalius's works. Albinus's own writings on the bones, muscles and the gravid uterus were exquisitely illustrated. Many other impressive anatomical atlases appeared, notably William Cheselden's (1688–1752) *Osteographia* (1733) [The Bones Illustrated], Haller's *Icones anatomicae* (1743–56)

[Anatomical Images], and William Hunter's (1718–83) *Anatomia uteri humani gravidi* (1774) [Anatomy of the Human Gravid Uterus], an astonishing depiction of the pregnant woman and her foetus in thirty-four copper-plates.

Knowledge of gross anatomy was by then well-established, but innovations were still possible respecting the softer and more concealed fibres: the lacteal, lymphatic and particularly the nervous systems. Building on Willis's 'neurologie', it was studies by Jacob Winslow (1669–1760) and the Prussian, Samuel Thomas von Sömmerring (1755–1830) that established the classification of the cranial nerves. A Göttingen contemporary of the great Johann Friedrich Blumenbach (see below), Sömmerring produced a major series of anatomical treatises on the sense organs, beginning with the eye (1801). Comparative anatomy received a boost from Petrus Camper (1722–89), who enrolled at Leiden at the tender age of twelve and went on to win fame for dissections of elephants, rhinoceroses and orang-utans. His attempt to measure 'facial angle' (the line of the brow and nose) was misused in later physical anthropology as an index of racial type.

Comparative studies led Caspar Friedrich Wolff (1734–94) to conclude that 'all parts of the plant except the stem are modified leaves,' a metaphysical tenet later endorsed by the poet and polymath Johann Wolfgang von Goethe (1749–1832), who interpreted insect jaws as modified limbs, believed the skull was composed of modified vertebrae, and rejected mechanistic views of life in favour of a philosophy of holism. Exponents of *Naturphilosophie*, like Blumenbach's student, Laurenz Oken (1779–1851), were soon suggesting that nature embodied a transcendental unity of plan, built upon elemental structural archetypes or anatomical building-blocks; this paved the way for philosophical morphology.

It was not only *Naturphilosophie* which insisted there was more to bodies than pipes and pulleys, for experimentation itself revealed the limits of the mechanical model, forcing recognition of the astounding powers of living things – quite transcending clockwork. René Réaumur (1683–1757) demonstrated the ability of lobster claws to regrow after being severed; Abraham Trembley (1710–84) chopped polyps into pieces and produced new individuals; in 1768 Lazzaro Spallanzani (1729–99) succeeded in regenerating the tails of salamanders, snails and tadpoles. There was more to life than the mechanical philosophy had dreamt of.

But how was it to be explained in an era no longer prepared to entertain miracles or Galenic innate virtues? Experimentation prompted new accounts of vitality and the relations between body and soul, a movement whose towering figure was Albrecht von Haller. Haller learned much from his mentor, Boerhaave – indeed, one of his first works was an edition of Boerhaave's *Institutes of Medicine* (1739–44) – but he went beyond, unifying anatomy and physiology into a single science of 'living anatomy' (*anatomia animata*).

An infant prodigy from Bern, Haller studied in Leiden and taught for seventeen years at the newly-founded University of Göttingen, before returning in 1753 to his native Switzerland. Linguist, poet, polymath and devout Christian, his forte was physiological experimentation. His early *Anatomical Images* depicted vascular anatomy, and continuing physiological researches led to a systematic physiology textbook, the *Primae lineae physiologiae* (1747) [First Lines of Physiology], which went through several editions and translations and long served as a standard text. There followed his vast synthesis, the *Elementa physiologiae corporis humani* (8 vols, 1757–66) [Elements of the Physiology of the Human Body]. Its organizing assumption was Boerhaave's principle that man possesses a physical body, analysable in terms of matter and forces, and an immaterial soul.

Ironically, it was the pious Haller who conducted experiments which challenged his religiously reassuring dualism. In his *De partibus corporis humani sensibilibus et irritabilibus* (1752) [On the Sensible and Irritable Parts of the Human Body], he made his key contribution to the study of animal economy by showing, rather in line with Glisson's hypothesis, that irritability (contractility) was a property inherent in *all* muscular fibres, whereas sensibility was the exclusive attribute of *nervous* fibres. He thus established the fundamental division of fibres according to their reactive properties: the irritable and the sensible. The sensibility of nervous fibres lay in their responsiveness to painful stimuli; the irritability of muscle fibres was their property of contracting in reaction to stimuli. Haller therefore had an explanation of why the heart pulsated: it was the most 'irritable' organ in the body; composed of layers of muscular fibres, it was stimulated by the influx of blood, responding with systolic contractions. On the basis of animal experiments, Haller graded organs according to their fibres, ascribing to them inherent sensitivities independent of any super-added soul. As to the causes of such living forces, these were beyond knowing, or at least unknown: as with Newton on gravity, it was sufficient to study the effects.

Haller's model of fibre sensibility and irritability was open to varied interpretations. Robert Whytt, for instance, was troubled by its implied reductionism, fearing it would lead to materialism and atheism. Indeed, Haller's findings were appropriated by radical philosophers like Denis Diderot (1713–84), eager for polemical reasons to develop a biological materialism which held that matter possessed vital properties.

In *On the Vital and Other Involuntary Motions of Animals* (1751), Whytt reiterated the role of the soul, understood naturalistically not religiously. Unlike the Cartesian unextended soul, Whytt's was energetic, sentient at a non-conscious level (and so, in a sense, automatic) and spatially extended in the body. The sentience of the soul was fundamental to his notion of bodily co-ordination by means of sympathy, the irreducible perceptive power of the body. These views brought him into conflict with Haller, who found the notion of non-conscious perception unintelligible.

The problem of vitality also informed Haller's work on embryological development, conducted in the context of the preformationist/epigenicist debate. Preformationists held that either the egg or the sperm contained a miniature representation (*homunculus*) of the adult organism, foetal formation being a growth of parts already present at the moment of fertilization; epigenesists believed that the various organs were not all present but appeared gradually during the formation of the foetus. Early in his career Haller espoused epigenesis, but in the 1750s, once the unsettling implications of the new biological materialism were surfacing, he turned to preformationism. His main antagonist was Caspar Friedrich Wolff, who elaborated a rather Harveian epigenetic doctrine in his influential *Theoria generationis* (1759) [Theory of Generation]: tissues and organs differentiated and developed, maintained Wolff, rather than being preformed and merely ballooning in size in the fertilized egg.

Experimental researches thus forced Haller to confront unpalatable alternatives: Boerhaavian dualistic mechanism (too crude for resolving the puzzles of life), Stahlian animism (concealed theology), or atheistic reductionism. His concepts of irritability and sensibility won support, however, and mainstream successors treated vitality as a property of the organized ensemble of living bodies. Modifying Haller, his Göttingen successor Johann Friedrich Blumenbach (1752–1840) delineated vital properties, including the *nisus formativus* or *Bildungstrieb*, an inherent life-force shaping growth and regeneration. Appointed professor in 1776, Blumenbach was to dominate bio-medical thinking in Germany for over sixty years. In *De generis humani varietate nativa* (1776) [On the Natural Variety of the Human Race], he accepted Linnaeus's belief that man (*Homo sapiens*) could not be exempted from the standard rules of primate taxonomy; nevertheless man should be housed in a separate zoological order (*Bimana*: two-handed). Committed to monogenesis (the single origin of the human race), he identified five racial varieties: the Caucasian, Mongolian, Ethiopian, Malay and American Indian.

Scottish-born but London-based, John Hunter proposed a 'life-principle' in the blood to account for the properties which distinguished living organisms from inanimate matter; in France, it was the Montpellier pupils of Jean Astruc (1684–1766), who took up the vitality question. While accepting Boissier de Sauvages's denial that mechanism could explain purposive action, they tended towards a more materialist stance, stressing the inherent vitality of living bodies. Bordeu in particular maintained that each organ was naturally endowed with an inherent responsivity to stimuli: vital function was intrinsic to the fibres. It is no accident that Bordeu pops up as a character in one of Diderot's philosophical *jeux d'esprit*, arguing that the new physiology had proved that matter itself was the secret of life.

In this speculative context the vogue for electrical experiments proved significant; Haller's doctrines of sensitivity and irritability suggested parallels between physiological and electrical events. What fired the nerves? The force might be mechanical, as with a bell-pull; or chemical, akin to a gunpowder trail; but many thought it electrical. Electrophysiology was pioneered by Luigi Galvani (1737–98). In his *De viribus electricitatis in motu musculari* (1792) [On Electrical Powers in the Movement of Muscles], the Italian described experiments in which he suspended the legs of skinned dead frogs by copper wire from an iron balcony. As the feet touched the iron uprights, the legs twitched and the muscles contracted: muscular activity and electricity went together and electricity could apparently simulate life.

These experiments were followed up by Alessandro Volta (1745–1827), professor at Pavia, whose *Memorie sull' elettricità animale* (1792) [Letters on Animal Electricity] showed that a muscle could be thrown into continuous contraction by successive electric stimulations. The electricity of life implied by such writings shaped later neurophysiology and inspired science-fiction fantasies like Mary Shelley's (1797–1851) *Frankenstein* (1818), which depicted life being artificially created with the aid of an electrical spark.

Post-Boerhaavian investigators thus probed the gap between the living and the inanimate, and many regarded the superior properties of living entities as deriving not from some super-added transcendental principle but from innate organization. Echoing the Great Chain of Being, a hierarchy of levels of organic complexity was suggested. All living things displayed powers of nutrition and reproduction; unlike mere vegetables, animals also had capacities for motility and sensitivity, associated with the sensory-motor system; 'higher' creatures (vertebrates, mammals), endowed with more sophisticated nervous organization, additionally had the potential for voluntary action. Blessed with consciousness, man was the apex of this pyramid of organized vital powers – albeit, Linnaeus insisted, only one primate among many.

This gradation of faculties was expressed in the idiom of 'development': higher forms were more developed. But for most that term carried no implication of species transmutation over historical time – that is, 'evolution' in the modern sense – being rather a plan of Creation pre-ordained in the Divine Mind, unfolding by divine law. However, Erasmus Darwin (1731–1802) in Britain and Jean Baptiste Lamarck (1744–1829) in France turned the 'stages' model of the hierarchy of organized powers into full-blown biological transformationism, showing lower forms transmuting into higher, thanks to inherent dynamic drives and a capacity to respond to environmental challenge.

Medicine's interactions with what was by 1800 acquiring the label 'biology' thus posed key questions about the scientific understanding of life itself. If these proved intractable, other more modest investigations bore fruit. How did digestion work? By some internal vital force? By the chemical action of gastric acids? Or by mechanical churning, mincing and pulverizing? Building on the work of Van Helmont and Sylvius, new inquiries were initiated by the French naturalist, René Réaumur. By training a pet kite to swallow and regurgitate small porous food-filled tubes, he demonstrated the powers of gastric juices: digestion was not a process of trituration and putrefaction of food, as then believed; gastric juice dissolved food. Testing whether digestion was essentially a chemical process, Spallanzani self-experimented by gulping down and regurgitating linen bags, establishing the solvent powers of saliva.

Drawing upon the iatrochemical tradition, chemists meanwhile explored fermentation and the links between respiration and combustion. Joseph Black (1728–99), who taught chemistry at Glasgow and later Edinburgh, framed the notion of latent heat and identified fixed air or what came to be known, with Lavoisier's chemical revolution, as carbon dioxide. Gas chemistry advanced rapidly, especially with the recognition that the atmosphere was not homogeneous but a cocktail of distinct gases. In 1766 Henry Cavendish (1731–1810) identified hydrogen, and Daniel Rutherford (1749–1819) nitrogen in 1772. Soon after, Joseph Priestley (1733–1804) and Karl Wilhelm Scheele (1742–86) independently isolated the gas Antoine-Laurent Lavoisier (1743–94) would name oxygen (1775).

All this led to a new understanding of respiration. Black noted that the fixed air given off by quicklime was also present in expired air; though non-toxic, it could not be breathed. Priestley grasped that vegetating plants renewed vitiated air, which, as an advocate of the phlogiston theory developed by Stahl, he called 'phlogisticated dephlogisticated air'. Lavoisier then elucidated the exchange of gases in the lungs: the air inhaled was converted into Black's fixed air, whereas the nitrogen ('azote') remained unchanged. Rather like John Mayow before him, Lavoisier believed respiration was the analogue within living bodies of combustion in the outside world; both needed oxygen, and both produced carbon dioxide and water. Oxygen was evidently indispensable for the human body; while engaged in physical activities like digestion, it consumed greater quantities than when at rest. A little later, Spallanzani revealed that oxidation occurred in the blood and throughout the entire physical system, and by 1800 it was accepted that oxygen combined with the carbon contained in food to generate animal heat.

These inquiries also led to attempts to measure the salubrity of the atmosphere, with a view to purifying the noxious air of towns and fetid buildings. Pneumatic chemistry, it was hoped, held the key not just to environmental medicine but to therapeutics. The aim of Thomas Beddoes's Pneumatic Institute, opened in 1799 in Clifton (Bristol), was to find by experimentation therapies for conditions such as tuberculosis. Beddoes developed a partnership with the engineer James Watt (1736–1819), jointly publishing *Considerations on the Medicinal Use of Factitious Airs* (1794), and with his apprentice, Humphry Davy (1778–1829), he discovered nitrous oxide (laughing gas), which he hoped would cure consumptives. In the event, aërotherapy or pneumotherapy achieved little, while the valuable anaesthetic properties of nitrous oxide lay oddly neglected.

MEDICINE IN PRACTICE

Anatomy and physiology thus engaged in dialogue with experimental science, but biomedical findings did not often deliver clinical success, and divisions were opening up between research and clinical practice. Certainly, science was not what secured top clinicians their fame. Some achieved their busy practices through personal considerations: Richard Mead (1673–1754) was known for suavity (according to Dr Johnson, he 'lived more in the broad sunshine of life than almost any other man'), whereas for John Radcliffe (1652–1714) what paid was bluntness (his infallible recipe for success was, 'use mankind ill'). Others, like Mark Akenside (1721–70) and Samuel Garth (1661–1719) combined physic with wit. An affable courtly coffee-house physician, Garth's literary star rose with *The Dispensary* (1699), a mock-*Iliad*, likening a petty squabble between the College of Physicians and the Society of Apothecaries to the Trojan War.

In a polite and enlightened age many physicians made their name as men of letters, philanthropists or improvers. Charles Darwin's grandfather, Erasmus, studied medicine at Cambridge and Edinburgh, and also in London with William Hunter. Settling in Lichfield, in 1766 he helped form the Lunar Society of Birmingham, which aimed to develop knowledge useful to an industrializing society and included among its luminaries the potter Josiah Wedgwood (1730–95), the physician William Withering (1741–99), the chemist Joseph Priestley, and James Watt. Darwin was an incurable inventor; claiming to travel 5000 miles a year on his medical rounds, it is small wonder he left plans for a steam-driven car. He expounded his medical ideas in *Zoonomia* (1794–96), advocating the use of electricity and corresponding with Beddoes about pneumatic medicine. His fame, however, derived mainly from his breezy and colourful verse, especially *The Botanic Garden*, part of which (*The Loves of the Plants*: 1789), was a droll popularization of the Linnaean classification.

Darwin's contemporary John Coakley Lettsom (1744–1815) built a massive London practice and a fortune to match; at times he was netting up to £12,000 a year – more than most noblemen. This he owed partly to sheer hard work; in 1783 he reflected that 'since 1769 when I first settled in London I have not taken one half day's relaxation'. But he also won public regard thanks to his philanthropic activities and his improving essays on lying-in, charities, prostitution, the deaf and mute, religious persecution, Sunday schools, dispensaries, hydrophobia, sea-bathing infirmaries, cheap porridge for the poor, the evils of tea-drinking and quackery, the virtues of smallpox inoculation and vaccination, and many more. Though a Quaker, he was a social climber, being caricatured in the press as 'Dr Wriggle'.

Every court and capital had its Dr Wriggle, in silver-buckled shoes, tricorn hat and sporting his gold-headed cane, skilled in 'the Art of Rising in Physic'. The doyen in France was the Geneva-born Théodore Tronchin (1709–81), an enlightened intellectual and Voltaire's favourite doctor – though this was not saying much, since Voltaire believed that doctors poured drugs of which they knew little to cure diseases of which they knew less into human beings of whom they knew nothing. An advocate of inoculation, Tronchin was one of many physicians to point out that the stomach disorder called Poitou colic (in England Devon colic) was the product of lead poisoning.

In polite circles public mien meant much, but physicians won their reputation primarily for their bedside care. William Heberden (1710–1801), who advanced knowledge of angina pectoris, arthritis and night-blindness, left in his *Medical Commentaries on the History and Cure of Diseases* (1802) clinical descriptions which were models of acumen and limpid prose. He believed the essence of a good physician lay in bedside sagacity; his devoted patients agreed.

Some new bedside skills were touted. In his *Inventum novum* (1761) [New Discovery], Leopold Auenbrugger (1722–1809) of Vienna announced the technique of percussion of the chest. An innkeeper's son, he had been familiar since childhood with the trick of thumping barrels to test their fullness. Moving from kegs to rib-cages, he noted that when struck with the finger, a healthy chest sounded like a cloth-covered drum; by contrast, a muffled sound or one of high pitch indicated pulmonary disease.

Auenbrugger's auscultation was ignored until the nineteenth century, however, and in conducting their diagnoses physicians generally rested content with the traditional uses of the 'five senses'; they would feel the pulse, sniff for gangrene, taste urine, listen for breathing irregularities and observe skin and eye colour. This time-honoured approach remained essentially qualitative. Despite Floyer's pulse watch, what counted in pulse lore was not the number of beats per minute but their 'feel'. Skilled practitioners could judge patients by close personal attention.

Diagnosis was an art of observation and inference. John Rutherford (1695–1779), professor at Edinburgh, impressed upon his students the value of inspecting the patient's facial appearance. Discussing a patient admitted to the Infirmary, he noted,

> If it had been daylight, I would have examined her gums and the internal canthus of her eyes ... for by looking into the internal canthus and the gums and finding them in a florid state then the blood is in a good state, but if they are pale or livid it is a sign that blood is dissolved and watery; if they have a yellowish cast it is frequently attended with a degree of acrimony, but when the cast is of a greenish colour, the acrimony is much greater as we see in scorbutick people.

His careful inspection of her face did not extend to other body parts. Though he concluded that her 'disease seems to be owing to the mismanagement she underwent in childbed. She says she was lacerated and probably it was her vagina', he made no attempt to check that for himself, thereby revealing the limits of physical examination – in Britain at least.

This hands-off approach owed something to social etiquette and sexual propriety, but traditional diagnostic thinking gave no reason to privilege physical examination. What counted most was interpretation of the patient's own 'history' – the common practice of postal diagnosis was perfectly reputable. Armed with a fine memory, the clinician was thus, rather like a Freudian psychoanalyst, to be a good listener, doing his detective work by astute questioning. 'Endeavor to get the history of the disease from the patient himself,' advised the American physician, Benjamin Rush (1745–1813):

> Begin to interrogate your patient. How long he has been sick? When attacked and in what manner? What are the probable causes, former habits and dress; likewise the diet, etc., for a week before especially in acute diseases ... In chronic diseases enquire their complaints far back and the habits of life.... Pay attention to the phraseology of your patients, for the same ideas are frequently conveyed in different words. A pain in the precordia is called by an Englishman a pain in his stomach, by a Scotchman in his breasts, an Irishman in his heart and by a Southern man mighty poorly. Patients often conceal the cause of their disease – therefore

interrogate them particularly when you suspect intemperance as the cause of disease.

If Galen had sat in, he might have viewed the American as his prize pupil.

THE STUDY OF DISEASE

The clinician had to know his diseases as well as his patients, and many trod in the Hippocratic footsteps of the revered Thomas Sydenham, charting epidemic disorders. John Fothergill (1712–80), a Yorkshire Quaker who attracted a lucrative London practice, gave a model clinical description of diphtheria, then growing more prevalent, in his *An Account of the Sore Throat* (1748). Understanding of scurvy was advanced by James Lind (1716–94), while in 1776 Matthew Dobson (d. 1784) reported experiments in which he evaporated urine and found a residue which smelled and tasted like sugar. Finding sugar in the blood suggested that diabetes (known since antiquity) was not principally a kidney problem.

Other conditions attracted fresh attention. An age of luxury not surprisingly led to a plethora of works on gout and other fashionable disorders, while George Cheyne's (1671–1743) *The English Malady* (1733) was only the most striking of many treatises addressing the 'nervous diseases' supposedly rife among the elite. Prosperous England was worst afflicted: 'Since our Wealth has increas'd, and our Navigation has been extended, we have ransack'd all the Parts of the *Globe* to bring together its whole Stock of Materials for *Riot*, *Luxury*, and to provoke *Excess*.' Sickness was the price of success. The remedy? A milk, seeds and greens diet, Cheyne advised, abstinence from alcohol in extreme cases, and plenty of exercise on horseback or on the eighteenth-century precursor of the exercise bike, the indoor wooden chamber horse.

In French-speaking Europe a similar message was conveyed by the Swiss physician, Samuel Tissot (1728–97), whose moralizing echoes his compatriot Jean-Jacques Rousseau's praise of healthy nature: 'Beneath the rustic garb of the plowman and not beneath the gildings of the courtier will strength and vigour of the body be found,' exclaimed the philosopher. Tissot's *Avis au peuple sur la santé* (1761) [Advice to People with Respect to their Health] broached the problem of 'depopulation' and luxury, which he attributed to the seductions of cities. Another complaint he and many other physicians believed rampant was masturbation. In a book translated into English as *Onanism or a Treatise Upon the Disorders Produced by Masturbation* (1766), Tissot depicted it as yet another disease of civilization, brought on by idleness and meretricious novels.

Piecemeal advances thus occurred, but the fundamentals remained contentious. What was disease? What was its true cause (*vera causa*)? In a clinical climate honouring Hippocrates, sickness was still largely attributed to personal factors such as diet and exercise. Such constitutional concepts made sense of the visibly uneven distribution of sickness (some people fell sick, others did not); they also underlined individual responsibility and strategies of containment through self-help.

Theories of contagion were also in circulation, backed by the evidence of diseases such as syphilis. But contagion hypotheses had their difficulties: why were some people stricken and others spared? This problem partly explained the lasting popularity of miasmatic models, holding that sickness typically originated in the environment. With intermittent fevers like 'ague' (malaria), it was common knowledge that those living by estuaries and in wetlands were especially susceptible to what was often called 'marsh fever'. Low, spotted and 'putrid' fevers, including our typhus, were recognized as infecting slum-dwellers and the occupants of barracks, ships and workhouses. Miasmatic disease was said to arise from poisonous exhalations exuded by putrefying animal remains, rotting vegetation and stagnant water: bad environments generated bad air which then turned pestilential. After 1750, reformers directed attention to 'septic' diseases like gangrene and erysipelas decimating the populations of gaols and hospitals.

Historians have tended to divide disease theorists into rival camps: miasmatists *versus* contagionists. But that is too crude; much theoretical finessing went on (for instance, emphasizing the distinction between predisposing and precipitating factors), and in any case investigators were less interested in theorizing a primary cause than in documenting the prevalence of sickness and controlling its spread. That is why the umbrella-term 'fevers' proved as useful to the eighteenth century as to the Hippocratics, forming the organizing principle of works like *On Fevers* (1750) by the Devon physician John Huxham (1692–1768). Fevers could be recognized as epidemic but also interpreted in classic humoral terms as a febrile 'crisis' in the individual, involving the patient's 'coction' of morbific matter, to be resolved by the expulsion of peccant humours. The time-honoured view that fever was a process requiring 'support' rather than suppression still found favour, for the risk with heroic intervention was that fevers would 'turn in' and prove far more menacing. In reality, as experience showed, there was little that could be done with epidemic fevers, apart from supporting the patient and trusting to the healing power of nature.

In the English-speaking world, the most influential attempt to set disease in a coherent framework lay in the teachings of William Cullen. After studying at Glasgow and Edinburgh, Cullen practised as a surgeon; in 1740 he took his MD at Glasgow and four years later began delivering lectures there on medicine, *materia medica*, botany and chemistry. He was formally admitted later as professor of medicine, and became friendly with Joseph Black, Adam Smith (1723–90) and David Hume (1711–76), leading lights of the Scottish Enlightenment. In 1755 he was appointed professor of chemistry in Edinburgh, whose medical school was rising thanks mainly to the anatomy teaching of the Monros. In 1766 he gained the chair of the Institutes of Medicine, which comprised physiology, general pathology and therapeutics; and from 1769 he alternated courses on the Practice of Physic with his colleague, John Gregory (1729–73), accepting that chair on Gregory's death.

Cullen broke with the Boerhaavians in viewing not the vascular but the nervous system as the key to the 'animal economy' (that is, physiological balance), and he attempted to describe the law-like behaviour of the organism while avoiding reduction of life to the mechanical. The fundamental physiological fact was that life consisted in a state of nervous excitement produced by environmental stimuli. These produced sensations (some conscious, some not) which provoked irritable tissues in the organism. According to Cullen, irritability was dependent upon the nervous system and not, as Haller maintained, on an autonomous muscular response. Though Cullen denied knowledge of the essence of the nervous power, he tended to identify it with an aetherial fluid which was also the basis of light, heat, magnetism and electricity. Rejecting humoralism, he held that all pathology originated in a disordered action ('spasm') of the nervous system – earning him the nickname 'Old Spasm'.

Partly for classroom reasons, Cullen tried to bring order to clinical medicine by drawing up his own nosology (disease classification) in which he treated diseases, like plants, as real entities, with characteristic pathognomonic signs or symptoms. Nosology was in vogue. Naturalists, such as the Swede Karl von Linné (Linnaeus: 1707–78) author of *Systema naturae* (1735) and inventor of the binomial system, had developed new taxonomies for natural history, and symptom-based medical classifications inevitably followed. In his *Nouvelles classes des maladies* (1731) [New Classes of Illnesses] and *Nosologia methodica* (1768) [Methodical Nosology], Boissier de Sauvages classified diseases into 10 classes, 295 genera and a daunting 2400 species. Cullen's nosology, set out in his influential *First Lines of the Practice of Physic* (1778–9), was far simpler. It reduced disease classes to 4, with the first 3 (pyrexias, neuroses, cachexias) based on disturbances of the traditional physiological functions: animal, vital, and natural. His fourth class (local disease) included local pathological changes.

Cullen placed most infectious diseases in the category of *Pyrexiae* or febrile diseases, differentiated by local inflammations. Among such fevers, conditions like smallpox with well-defined symptoms and spreading by contact were attributed to specific contagions. Intermediate between these and the diseases of locality at the other end of the spectrum (typified by ague or intermittent fever, associated with the rotting vegetation of marshes) lay the 'doubtful' diseases, which were 'sometimes contagious and sometimes not' – an *ad hoc* character quite alien to later bacteriological specificity, but compatible with ideas stressing filth and putrefaction as elements in disease.

The least defined pyrexiae were the continued fevers, divided mainly into typhus, enteric (typhoid) and relapsing. Possessing some of the same characteristics were diseases related to common putrefaction – the 'septic' diseases: gangrene, septicaemia, scarlet fever, diphtheria, erysipelas and puerperal fever. In his clinical teaching Cullen devoted particular attention to slow and nervous fevers, diseases then rife in gaols and hospitals, stressing the role of filth and poor ventilation rather than concentrating on traditional Galenic factors like diet. Since fevers of that kind were debilitating, blood-letting was contra-indicated.

A simple inflammatory fever (as in a cold or pneumonia) with a strong hard pulse but no delirium was labelled by Cullen *synocha*. If accompanied by delirium or stupor, he called it *typhus*. In Scotland the prevailing form of continued fever seemed to be a combination of synocha and typhus which he termed *synochus*. In short, fever was a general malady which might assume various forms, though its common underlying phenomenon was a spasm of the arteries. Fevers developed in three stages: debility with relaxation (*atony*) of the arteries; a stage of irritation; and third, the hot stage resulting from the arterial spasm.

A fever might be caused by atmospheric matter. If it arose from the bodies of the sick, it would be called contagion; if from marshes and standing water, miasma. Contagion or miasma exerted a sedative influence on the body, inducing debility. Cullen recommended supportive treatment to overcome weakness; blood-letting might be used to relieve spasm, and there was always the healing power of nature.

Though attempting a nosology, Cullen was not set upon the ontological view of disease. He believed most diseases to be caused by external influences – climate, foodstuffs, effluvia, humidity, and so on – and he taught that the same external factors could cause different diseases in different individuals, depending on the state of the nervous system. As the foremost teacher of his age, Cullen's disease framework shaped the beliefs and practice of thousands of doctors throughout the English-speaking world for the next fifty years; broadly comparable systems were meanwhile being taught to students in Montpellier, Halle and Vienna.

Some of the tendencies of Cullen's theory were taken to their logical conclusions by his one-time pupil and later foe, John Brown (1735–88), the Scottish Paracelsus, who insisted upon the unitary nature of sickness. There was only *one* disease, though it assumed myriad forms and forces. Brown reduced questions of health to variations of irritability (his word was 'excitability'). Life was thus to be understood not as a spontaneous state but as a 'forced condition', the product of the action of external stimuli. Sickness was disturbance of the proper functioning of excitement, and diseases were to be treated as 'sthenic' or 'asthenic' according as 'excitement' increased or diminished.

Attempting to distil disease into medicine-by-numbers, Brown envisaged a thermometer calibrated upon a single scale, rising from zero ('asthenic' disorders, lethal under-stimulation of the body) to 80 degrees (fatal over-excitement); the mid-point formed a healthy equilibrium. The device of a single axis objectified illness into something quantifiable, and pointed to a therapeutics dependent upon dosage size. For Brown, treatment was essentially a matter of larger or smaller measures of sedatives and stimulants, principally opiates and alcohol.

Though winning scant support in France and England, Brunonian medicine had the virtue of simplicity and was enthusiastically taken up in America by Benjamin Rush, and in Italy by Giovanni Rasori (1766–1837); Christoph Girtanner (1760–1800) and Johann Peter Frank (1745–1821) popularized it in German-speaking Europe.

PATHOLOGY

Cullen gathered, sifted and glossed available medical knowledge, his emphasis being on use rather than discovery. A new approach was, however, being developed which was to prove profoundly significant in transforming the very idea of disease aetiology. Since Vesalius, practitioners had pursued gross anatomy, and greater attention began to be paid to the connexions between the sick person and the disease signs afforded by the corpse. Anatomy thereby led to morbid anatomy in necropsy studies pursued by, among others, Johann Wepfer (1620–95) and Théophile Bonet (1620–89), both Swiss. The conviction that postmortem investigation was the key to the bodily changes brought about by disease (not least, cause of death) was largely due to Giovanni Battista Morgagni (1682–1771), professor of anatomy at Padua, who, aged almost eighty, published *De sedibus et causis morborum* (1761) [On the Sites and Causes of Disease]. Drawing on the findings of some 700 autopsies to show how bodily organs revealed the footprints of disease, this work achieved instant recognition; it was translated into English in 1769 and German in 1774.

Born at Forli, Morgagni had studied under Anton Maria Valsalva (1660–1723), a remarkable experimentalist from whom he acquired extensive dissection experience. In 1715, he moved to the chair of anatomy at Padua, becoming the leading Italian anatomist. *De sedibus* is divided into five sections, devoted respectively to diseases of the head, the chest, the abdomen and to surgical conditions, with addenda in the form of seventy letters to friends. Case histories, with their most striking symptoms and autopsy results, were followed by an elucidation of the relationships between the case history and morbid anatomy.

Morgagni's discoveries were numerous. He described the anatomical phenomena observable in angina pectoris and myocardial degeneration, the fibrinous clots found in the heart after death, and the heart-block syndrome now termed Stokes-Adams. He associated cyanosis (blueness of the skin) with pulmonary stenosis (narrowing of vessels) and made major observations on arteriosclerosis of the coronary and cerebral arteries and hypertrophy of the heart in mitral stenosis. He pointed out that apoplexy or stroke was not caused by a lesion of the brain but by alteration in the cerebral blood vessels. He accounted for aspects of gastric ulcers, the vermiform appendix, emphysema and numerous other conditions. *De sedibus* shifted emphasis from symptoms to site. Thinking anatomically, he demonstrated that diseases were located in specific organs, that symptoms tallied with anatomical lesions, and that such morbid organ changes were responsible for disease.

The great significance of his work was recognized and developed by others. In Britain, Matthew Baillie (1761–1823) was prominent. A nephew of the Hunters, Baillie trained at his uncle William's Great Windmill Street anatomy school and at St George's Hospital, where his other uncle, John, was surgeon. William's death in 1783 left the young Baillie the happy owner of the anatomy school, and by 1787 he was also physician at St George's, later becoming physician extra-ordinary to George III.

Arranged by organs, Baillie's *Morbid Anatomy of Some of the Most Important Parts of the Human Body* (1793) discussed the pathological changes caused by diseases. Working from autopsy evidence, Baillie confined himself to what he could see with his eyes without specu-lating on the ultimate causes of disease or bringing in symptom-based nosologies.

Building on Morgagni while incorporating the newer pathological methods emerging in France, *Morbid Anatomy* contains several classic descriptions, including emphysema and cirrhosis of the liver, which he linked to alcohol. He offered numerous new descriptions, including ovarian cysts, gastric ulcer and the hepatization of the lungs in pneu-monia. Illustrated by William Clift (1775–1849) with superb copper-plates, depicting, among other things, Samuel Johnson's emphysema, Baillie's was more of a textbook than Morgagni's, describing as it does the morbid appearances of each organ in succession. It went through eight English and three American editions and was translated into French, Italian, German and Russian. The second edition (1797) developed the idea of 'rheumatism of the heart' (rheumatic fever), con-tributing to the early study of heart disease. J. B. Sénac (1693–1770) had published important findings in 1749, and in 1799 Caleb Parry (1755–1822) brought out his *Inquiry into the Symptoms and Causes of the Syncope Anginosa, Commonly Called Angina Pectoris*, discussing cases with their postmortem results, including ossification and obstruction of the coronary arteries, together with gross pathology of the aorta.

Across the Channel, pathology's possibilities were being extended through the publication in 1799 of the *Traité des membranes* [Treatise on Membranes] by Marie François Xavier Bichat (1771–1802). A doctor's son from the Jura, Bichat studied at Lyon and Paris at the height of the Terror. Army service provided him with ample surgical practice, and from June 1794 he settled in Paris, becoming assistant to the leading surgeon, Pierre-Joseph Desault (1738–95). Bichat taught private courses and conducted some 600 anatomies, but never obtained a major hospital post and died tragically young.

Designed to set medicine on a sound anatomical basis, his *Traité* and his *Anatomie générale* (1801) focused attention on structures comparable in texture but found in different organs. Bichat's key innovation was the doctrine of tissues: he described twenty-one such membranes, including connective, muscle, and nerve tissue, distinguished by appearance and vital qualities. The most widespread were cellular tissue, nerves, arteries, veins, absorbent and exhalant vessels; these were found intermeshed in most other tissue systems. More restricted ones included skeletal muscle, involuntary muscle, gland, cartilage, bone, mucous and serous membranes. These, he proposed, should be the analytical building-blocks of anatomy, physiology and pathology, rather as elements were in Lavoisier's new chemistry, and he set about delineating their structure, vital properties, abnormalities and responsiveness. Bichat dismissed 'souls' or 'vital spirits' as metaphysical will-o'-the-wisps and avoided microscopes as machines of error. Tissues would provide a new map of the body, and henceforth diseases were to be lesions of specific tissues rather than simply of organs.

The vital properties of tissues formed the focus of Bichatian physiology. He distinguished between those of animal life (voluntary muscle, sense organs and their nervous connections) and those of organic life (comprising lungs, circulatory system, alimentary canal and excretory organs). The former were said to form paired structures and to show a higher degree of sensibility and contractility, whereas the latter showed only the contractility characterizing all living tissues.

Bichat saw pathology with fresh eyes. 'The more one will observe diseases and open cadavers,' he declared, 'the more one will be convinced of the necessity of considering local diseases not from the aspect of the complex organs [as with Morgagni] but from that of the individual tissues.' His work laid the foundations for nineteenth-century patho-anatomy, and helps to explain why, within a few decades, Cullen and his colleagues had gone the way of Galen.

THERAPEUTICS

Advances in pathology pinpointed a paradox: 'I know better perhaps than another man, from my knowledge of anatomy, how to discover disease,' Baillie remarked, 'but when I have done so, I don't know better how to cure it.' Indeed. Pathology did not open the door to cures – hardly any eighteenth-century scientific advance helped heal the sick directly. Therapeutics made herculean efforts, but the net contribution of physicians to the relief and cure of the sick remained marginal. 'Cur'd yesterday of my Disease, I died last night of my Physician,' quipped Matthew Prior in 1714.

Certain innovations were positively harmful. The new lying-in hospitals had horrendous mortality rates, for reasons little understood till the work of Ignaz Semmelweis in the following century (see Chapter 12). The fondness for heroic blood-letting, often coupled with heroic dosing, was deleterious. Phlebotomy won its most sanguine advocate in Rush, the 'founding father' of American medicine. Born in Philadelphia, Rush studied in Edinburgh and on his return to his native land was appointed professor first of chemistry and then of medicine at the College of Philadelphia. The American Revolution drew him into politics, and he was a signatory of the Declaration of Independence. Modifying Cullen, Rush concluded that a hyperactive state of the arteries (he called it 'hypertension') was the key to disease. This dictated an aggressively depletive therapeutics consisting of copious blood-letting.*

Calling mercury 'a safe and nearly a universal medicine', Rush also recommended calomel purges – dubious methods destined to remain favoured by American regulars, partly because of Rush's standing as the American Hippocrates. Calomel (mercurous chloride) appeared in every physician's bag throughout the nineteenth century, and was an active ingredient in the 'blue pills' prominent in nineteenth-century English therapeutics. Many physicians felt driven to caution against the worth-

---

* Le Sage had already turned the abuse of blood-letting into fine satire in his *Adventures of Gil Blas* (1715–35). He told of a cleric who consulted a Dr Sangrado for gout. The physician's favourite remedy was copious bleeding. 'It is a mere vulgar error, that the blood is of any use in the system', prated Sangrado, who instructed a surgeon to withdraw 'six porringers of blood' and 'as much more three hours hence' and then to repeat the process the next day.

lessness of the available drugs. 'I do not deny', wrote John Berkenhout in his *Symptomatology* (1784)

> that many lives might be saved by the skilful administration of proper medicine; but a thousand indisputable facts convince me, that the present established practice of physic in England is infinitely destructive of the lives of his Majesty's subjects. I prefer the practice of old women, because they do not sport with edged tools; being unacquainted with the powerful articles of the *Materia Medica*.

But, then, could old crones be trusted? Didn't they dabble in abortifacients and the like?

Genteel patients continued to be treated by top clinicians according to traditional learned medicine. Tailored to individual needs, therapeutic strategies centred upon temperance and hygiene, good air, diet, evacuations, sleep, exercise and equanimity. These factors (the ancient 'non-naturals') were essential for avoiding what pedants sometimes called the 'contra-naturals'; in common parlance, disease. The concept of health as natural balance pointed to various physical strategies, including dietetics, bathing and purging. Diet – still meaning a comprehensive ordering of life – was discussed down to the last lettuce leaf in works like the *Essay Concerning the Nature of Aliments* (1731) by John Arbuthnot (1667–1735).

The benefits of travel were also much touted, in accordance with the Hippocratic *Airs, Waters, Places* tradition. With the spread of tuberculosis, 'phthisical' or consumptive gentlefolk made winter pilgrimages to Lisbon or Livorno in search of balmy air, while travelling itself (colloquially 'Dr Horse') was said to recruit the constitution and strengthen the nerves. 'I must be on horseback for life, if I would be healthy,' claimed John Wesley (1703–91) – and indeed the founder of Methodism was still galloping round the country delivering hellfire sermons in his eighties.

For the fashionable, the benefits of travel were combined with taking the waters. Spas like Vichy, Bourbon and Baden Baden abounded across the Continent, but it was in England's burgeoning consumer society that they first became big business, promising elegant healing rituals, social contacts and rich pickings for hoteliers and doctors. Pre-eminently Bath, but also Tunbridge Wells, Buxton, Scarborough and Cheltenham, provided balls, gambling, diversions and assignations, to accompany dipping, pumping and drinking the waters. By 1801, Bath, mixing medicine and merriment, had astonishingly become England's seventh largest city.

After 1750, with England leading the way, the therapeutic virtues of the seaside were also being praised. Dr Richard Russell (1687–1759), the booster of Brighton, contended that sea water should preferably be *drunk* (the salts were beneficial), but most people settled less heroically for bathing, with the additional boon of sea air, for consumptives in particular. The Philadelphia polymath and inventor of bi-focals, Benjamin Franklin (1706–90), practised air-bathing, sitting naked each morning before an open window.

Yet, despite the medley of physical methods long popular, there are signs that, even then, healing was growing increasingly medication-centred. Prescription of medicines was the expected outcome of medical consultations, as was admitted in Bernard Mandeville's *A Treatise of Hypochondriack and Hysterick Passions* (1711), a witty exposé of unscrupulous practitioners. Routine prescribing of pills, rather than a comprehensive regimen, was still frowned upon in the best circles as the lazy practice of those who, so George Cheyne alleged, 'are continually cramming their Patients with nauseous and loathsome Potions, Pills and Bolus's, Electuaries, Powders and Juleps'. It was easier for practitioners to charge for their pills and boluses than for attendance or advice alone. In any case the new science was leading to pharmaceutical improvements, and large manufacturing druggists emerged, selling wholesale and retail. The London chemist Thomas Corbyn (1711–91), like many others in the trade a Quaker, stocked over 2500 different items of *materia medica*, employed a staff of ten, and by the 1780s was running a business with a capital of some £20,000. He traded extensively with North America, the West Indies and the Continent.

Whether used simply or in compound mixtures, distilled, dried, ground or decocted, herbs still constituted the bulk of the *materia medica* employed by apothecaries and in kitchen physic. Herbal remedies were designed largely to act as emetics and laxatives, although elite medicine also made a fancy parade of alteratives, diluents, deobstruents and similar hifalutin categories, each with its own action and rationale. Alteratives were supposed to strengthen the system, bitters were said to brace the solids – e.g., to clear the head and settle the stomach after a binge, and stimulate the appetite. Medications, learned physicians stressed, must be regarded not as panaceas but as auxiliaries in bespoke therapeutic regimes. Dosage had to be modified perhaps every day, explaining the habit of prescribing only a few measures at a time but prescribing extremely frequently – a recipe for profiteering, accused the cynics. The palaver of prescribing may have masked the fact that few drugs did much good.

Preparation of human cranium was still present in the *Pharmacia Antverpiensis* of 1661 and oil of earthworms in the Leiden *Pharmacopoeia Leodiensis* of 1741. Still prescribed was the bezoar, a concretion found in the alimentary organs of ruminants, recommended as an antidote against poison. In 1696 a noted German physician, Christian Paullini (1643–1712), published his *Dreckapotheke* [Filth Pharmacy]. Yet changes were coming about in the medical armamentarium. The fifth London *Pharmacopoeia* (1746) eliminated human fat, spider webs, moss from human skulls, unicorn's horn, virgin's milk (not the literal liquid but an alchemical remedy) and the like, but mithridate, woodlice, pearls, bezoar stones, vipers and coral remained. Most of the animal *materia medica* had disappeared from the sixth *Pharmacopoeia* (1788), while among the new drugs and compounds were aconite, castor oil, quassia, magnesia, ether, tartrate of iron, oxide of zinc, Dover's powder, sarsaparilla decoctions and paregoric (liquid opium). Chemistry popularized mineral and metallic drugs: antimony-based medicines circulated as febrifuges, in England being patented as Dr James's Powders; and calomel (the 'blue pill') became the purge of choice. The lumber-room of preparations inherited from antiquity was being sorted out at last.

Significant also was the publication in 1745 of William Heberden's *Antitheriaka: an Essay on Mithridatium and Theriac*, denying that these polypharmaceuticals had antidotal properties against poisons, venoms, or other harmful substances. The *Pharmacopoeia Edinburgensis* dropped theriac and mithridatium in 1756, but pharmacopoeias in France, Spain, and Germany found a place for them well into the nineteenth century.

Opium was freely available over the counter and widely used, often in liquid form as laudanum, as an analgesic, fever specific, sedative and diarrhoea corrective. 'Providence has been kind and gracious to us beyond all Expression', enthused Cheyne, 'in furnishing us with a certain *Relief,* if not a Remedy, even to our most *intense Pains* and *extreme Miseries*' – tortured patients surely agreed. Some doctors, however, suspected that opium created dependency: Samuel Crumpe (1766–96) recorded that users deprived even for a single day 'became languid, dejected, and uneasy', a view confirmed by the experience of the poet-philosopher Samuel Taylor Coleridge (1772–1834) and others who began by dosing themselves for medical reasons but ended up suffering the horrors of addiction.

A few significant innovations were achieved. In 1763 the Revd Edmund Stone (d. 1768) drew attention to willow bark (*Salix alba*). Its bitterness reminded him of Peruvian bark; moreover, the willow grew in the damp places where agues and fevers abounded, and pious folk belief had it that God planted cures where diseases originated. Hence he suspected it would serve as an ague remedy, giving it to some fifty persons who had rheumatic fever symptoms and reporting satisfactory results. (Salicin, the active ingredient in willow bark, has an effect similar to aspirin.) Stone communicated his discovery to the Royal Society, but it was ignored.

William Withering had better success. In 1785 he produced *An Account of the Foxglove and Some of its Medical Uses etc; With Practical Remarks on Dropsy and Other Diseases*, which demonstrated that digitalis had a powerful stimulant action on the heart, reducing the oedema commonly accompanying heart disease. A follower of Linnaeus and a medical botanist, Withering had heard from a Shropshire woman of a herbal tea (a secret 'family receipt') useful in treating swollen legs. Deducing that the effective element in her twenty-ingredient dropsy medicine must be foxglove, whose leaves yielded digitalis, he monitored its use to ascertain the best dosage for treating both dropsy and heart disease. On 8 December 1775, he gave foxglove tea to a fifty-year-old builder with asthma and fluid in the abdomen, who 'made a large quantity of water. His breath gradually drew easier, his belly subsided, and in about ten days he began to eat with a keen appetite.' Foxglove proved effective against cardiac dropsy though not renal dropsy – a distinction later grasped by Richard Bright. In 1783 digitalis entered the *Pharmacopoeia Edinburgensis*, and twenty-six years later the London *Pharmacopoeia*.

Overall, however, pharmacy left much to be desired. Proprietary nostrums were often unsafe, and polypharmacy – complex drug cocktails, some ingredients countering others – was a recipe for abuse. Violent purgatives and lead- or mercury-based medicines caused spasm and colic, often relieved by belladonna or other concoctions that induced further poisoning. The Scottish naval doctor Thomas Trotter (1760–1832) was not alone in warning that modern society was bingeing on harmful sedatives, tonics and narcotics, washed down with tea, brandy and other stimulants. Small wonder the German physician Samuel Hahnemann (1755–1843) reacted by developing his homoeopathic system, which valued purity of drugs and minimal dosage.

INSANITY

Particular forms of sickness also saw therapeutic developments. The theory and treatment of insanity had undergone a seachange; the notion of insanity as demonic possession was finally discredited among medical men and magistrates. Mania and melancholy, mad doctors argued, derived not from the heavens but from the body; insanity was organic. 'Every change of the mind', wrote the physician, Nicholas Robinson (1697–1775), '. . . indicates a Change in the Bodily Organs.'

They could build upon old humoral interpretations that emphasized the role of yellow bile (choler) in mania and black bile in melancholy. But humoral explanations also lost credit as the new science pictured the body as a machine and neuro-anatomy highlighted the role of the nerves. William Cullen thus defined insanity (vesania) as a type of dynamic neurological disorder (neurosis), but also regarded madness, following Locke, as a false association of ideas. The mad, according to Locke, 'do not appear to me to have lost the faculty of reasoning, but having joined together some ideas very wrongly, they mistake them for truths, and they err as men do that argue right from wrong principles'.

One of the most exemplary encounters with madness was that of George III. The king experienced his first attack in autumn 1788, and as his condition worsened and the physicians-in-ordinary proved unable to cope or cure, the Revd Dr Francis Willis (1717–1807), a clergyman doctor who ran a madhouse in Lincolnshire, was called in. Partly because he insisted upon exclusive medical control, Willis encountered bitter opposition from the regular physicians. They regarded him as little better than a quack – he was, after all, a clergyman, and running a lunatic asylum was rather a disreputable specialty.

From the first Willis expressed confidence that the king would recover if he were allowed to follow his favourite methods of moral management, involving complete physical and psychological domination over his patient. Madness, he believed, was essentially a product of over-excitation; hence the chief priorities were calm and control. A man of vast faith in his own powers, Willis proved fearless in asserting his authority over the king, when necessary using a straitjacket, a gag, and a restraining chair upon his royal patient, and a quasi-mesmerizing technique of fixing his patient with his eye. Apart from intimidation, Willis recognized the importance of winning the king's trust and cooperation; in due course, he permitted his patient to read Shakespeare and to shave himself and pare his nails with a penknife. The king resented Willis's bullying ways but was responsive to his optimism.

By February 1789 George had largely recovered (it has recently been argued that this was a spontaneous recovery from a bout of porphyria, and had little to do with Willis's therapies) and Willis was quick to claim the credit. The grateful prime minister, William Pitt, spared the prospect of a regency, had Parliament vote the mad doctor a pension of £1000 a year for twenty-one years. Willis himself had medallions struck with the inscription, 'Britons Rejoice, Your King's Restored'.

This confirmed the optimism of many who claimed that since insanity was a bodily disease, it should prove responsive to medical treatments. Certainly a great variety of medical 'cures' came into vogue, some designed to sedate maniacs, others to stimulate melancholics (opium might be prescribed for both). Physical treatments were used, such as blood-lettings, emetics, and violent purges to discharge toxins; shock treatments such as cold showers; new technologies such as rotatory chairs and swings, designed to disrupt *idées fixes*; and, when all else failed, shackles and straitjackets. Treating the body was meant to restore the mind.

Yet none of these had proved very effective; partly for this reason, new faith was vested in the madhouse. In particular, as the failure of drugging became clear and critics condemned manacles as cruel and counter-productive, the well-run asylum commended itself, and asylum design and management became part of the late Enlightenment utilitarian preoccupation with orderly institutions: schools, hospitals, gaols, warships. The total environmental control produced by the asylum, would, it was hoped, manage madness, while creating the family atmosphere that would rekindle civilized sentiments. Some of these establishments were hellholes, but others were quite civilized. At the superior and expensive end was the house kept in Lincolnshire by Willis himself. It was said that 'the unprepared traveller ... was astonished to find almost all the surrounding ploughmen, gardeners, threshers, thatchers, and other labourers, attired in black coats, white waistcoats, black silk breeches and stockings, and the head of each *bien poudrée, frisée et arrangée*. These were the doctor's patients.'

Such ideals of disciplined order and resocialization helped popularize psychological theories of insanity, which incorporated the new theories of Locke and Condillac (1714–80) in the influential *A Treatise on Madness* (1758) by William Battie (1704–76). He claimed that 'management' would achieve more than 'medicine', optimistically declared that 'madness is ... as manageable as many other distempers,' and insisted that 'such unhappy objects ought by no means to be abandoned, much less shut up in loathsome prisons as criminals or nuisances to society.' Battie called for the replacement of hidebound madhouses like Bethlem by purpose-built institutions such as St Luke's in London, which he helped to found.

Particularly in England, small private madhouses were set up, largely for bourgeois patients, in which a new interactive form of psychotherapy could be practised, called 'moral management'. This viewed madness as a psychological condition (a defect of the understanding, rather than of the soul or body) to be corrected by the superior will, personality and insights of the madhouse keeper.

CHILDBIRTH

Another area of change was childbirth. Birthing had essentially been a women-only event. Within polite circles first in England and then in North America, the traditional 'granny midwife' was now widely displaced by a male operator, called a 'man-midwife' or *accoucheur*, who claimed superior expertise. As a qualified medical practitioner, his anatomical skill made him confident that he could let nature take her course in case of normal deliveries: man-midwives like William Hunter prided themselves upon being *less* interventionist than fiddling old midwives. Yet unlike the midwife, *accoucheurs* possessed surgical instruments, above all, the new forceps (*tire-tête*), for difficult and emergency labours. Once the secret of the Chamberlen family, these had become common property by 1730.

Developing their new specialty, *accoucheurs* set up obstetric schools or taught in the newly founded lying-in charities. In London the leaders were Scots: the down-to-earth William Smellie (1697–1763) – 'a great horse godmother of a he-midwife', according to the midwife, Elizabeth

Nihell (*fl.* 1760) – and his suave pupil, William Hunter. Paris-trained, Smellie settled in London in 1739, taught his craft, streamlined forceps design, and published his practical *Midwifery* (1752), which included the first systematic discussion of forceps. Hunter had five years' training at Glasgow, three as Cullen's pupil, before giving private lecture courses on dissecting, surgery, and obstetrics. He trained many of the surgeon-obstetricians who were to introduce man-midwifery into town and country practices, while he delivered the babies of the *bon ton*. *Accoucheurs* won trade but not status, as is suggested by the gross caricature of Dr Slop in Laurence Sterne's *Tristram Shandy* (1760), who bungles the hero's birth with his forceps.

In America, medical midwifery developed under the influence of William Shippen (1736–1808), who studied anatomy in London with the Hunters and on his return to Philadelphia began anatomical instruction on the Hunterian model. Three years later he opened a small lying-in hospital. The aggressive entrepreneurialism of American surgeon-obstetricians led to male operators dominating the field.

Where such *accoucheurs* flourished, the procedures of childbirth were transformed. Under male influence, fashionable ladies were encouraged to give birth in rooms into which daylight and fresh air were admitted. Their newborns were no longer swaddled: new theories claimed that leaving infant limbs free would strengthen bones and promote development. Books like *An Essay upon Nursing, and the Management of Children* (1748) by William Cadogan (1711–97), encouraged modern women to dismiss their wet-nurses and to breast feed: mother's milk was natural and would encourage mother-baby bonding.

Thus Enlightenment values could promote changes in childbirth and baby-care. But these were by no means universal. In France, for instance, wet-nursing remained common; in the German principalities, midwives secured improved training, attending lectures and gaining licences; and male obstetricians made no headway at all in Catholic Italy and Spain where the Church upheld female modesty.

THE PREVENTION OF SMALLPOX

The one eighteenth-century improvement in practical medicine which decisively saved lives was the introduction first of inoculation and then of vaccination against smallpox. 'The speckled monster' had become virulent throughout Europe, responsible in bad years for perhaps a tenth of all deaths; Queen Mary of England (1662–94) died of it, as did Louis XV (1710–74) of France.

There had long been awareness of the immunizing properties of an attack, but elites were slow to take notice. Widespread publicity was achieved thanks to the observations of Lady Mary Wortley Montagu (1689–1762), wife of the British consul in Constantinople, who reported how Turkish peasant women held smallpox parties at which they routinely performed inoculations, describing this procedure to a friend in 1717:

> *Apropos* of distempers, I am going to tell you a thing that will make you wish yourself here. The *smallpox*, so fatal and so general among us, is here entirely harmless by the invention of *engrafting*, which is the term they give it. There is a set of old women who make it their business to perform the operation every autumn in the month of September when the great heat is abated. . . . They make parties for the purpose . . . the old woman comes with a nutshell full of the matter of the best sort of smallpox, and asks what veins you please to have open'd. She immediately rips open . . . and puts into the vein as much [smallpox] matter as can lie upon the head of her needle.

The aim was to induce a mild dose so as to confer lifelong protection without pock-marking. Back in Britain, Lady Mary had her five-year-old daughter inoculated in 1721 by the surgeon Charles Maitland (1677–1748). Experiments followed with condemned felons, and the Prince of Wales, later George II (1683–1760), had his two daughters inoculated.

The innovation won influential allies. The physician James Jurin (1684–1750), secretary of the Royal Society of London, tried to promote it with the aid of statistics. He found that smallpox had killed one fourteenth of the inhabitants of London during the forty-two-year period before 1723; during bad epidemics up to 40 per cent of those stricken died. Prompted by Jurin, in 1722 the Yorkshire physician Thomas Nettleton (1683–1742) reported to the Society his calculations of mortality ratios in natural and in inoculated smallpox in a number of communities. Jurin extended Nettleton's studies, using numbers 'to give plain Proof from Experience and Matters of Fact that the Small Pox procured by inoculation . . . is far less Dangerous than the same Distemper has been for many Years in the Natural Way'.

Elite physicians predictably developed complex and costly techniques, beginning with purging and bleeding. The real breakthrough came after 1750 with the activities of the Sutton family, Robert (1707–88) and his sons, especially Daniel (1735–1819). Humble surgeons, the Suttons devised an easy, safe and cheap way, leading to mass inoculation. Between them, they claimed to have inoculated in about thirty years around 400,000 people, with a minuscule death-rate. Dispensaries were founded in Chester and other towns, where the public health activist, John Haygarth (1740–1827) hoped for blanket inoculation.

Variolation spread to other countries; in France it found the support of the *philosophes*. In Prussia, Austria and Russia, inoculation of members of the royal household publicized the measure; Catherine the Great (1729–96) had her family done by Thomas Dimsdale (1712–1800), an English surgeon who was awarded £10,000 and a Russian barony for his services. But it was slow to spread to much of the Continent, due to a mixture of medical, moral and religious misgivings (there was some resistance from Calvinists in Scotland, who feared that inoculation interfered with Divine Providence). In North America, however, the preacher Cotton Mather (1663–1728) was a champion; he knew about suffering, having had to watch as two wives and thirteen of his fifteen children succumbed to disease.

Edward Jenner (1749–1823) was an English country doctor who performed inoculations. A clergyman's son, he had studied in London under John Hunter, who gave him a taste for experiment. 'I think your solution is just', Hunter once told him, 'but why think? Why not try the experiment?'. Jenner learned that among the countryfolk in his native Gloucestershire it was known that cowpox, a cattle disease occasionally contracted by humans, particularly dairy-maids, conferred immunity against smallpox. Suspecting that it might be possible to produce this immunity by arm-to-arm inoculation from the cowpox pustule, and surmising it would be safer than inoculation, since in humans cowpox was benign, Jenner tried the experiment. On 14 May 1796 he inoculated eight-year-old James Phipps with some matter taken from the cowpox pustule of a dairy-maid, Sarah Nelmes. The boy developed a slight fever from which he soon recovered. Six weeks later Jenner inoculated him with smallpox 'virus': the inoculation did not take. Clearly, Jenner's surmise was correct.

In 1798 he published his discovery in *An Inquiry into the Causes and Effects of the Variolae Vaccinae*. This attracted immediate attention, running to a third edition by 1801, an American in 1802, and Latin, German, French, Italian, Dutch, Spanish and Portuguese translations by 1803. By 1799, over 5000 individuals had been vaccinated in England and abroad the practice was taken up remarkably swiftly, being made compulsory in Sweden and supported by Napoleon, who had his army vaccinated. 'Anything Jenner wants shall be granted. He has been my most faithful servant in the European campaigns,' declared the emperor when Jenner wrote to ask for the release of an imprisoned British officer. In 1802 Parliament granted Jenner £10,000, and one year later the Royal Jennerian Society was founded to promote vaccination – signs that rulers were awakening to the view that health promotion was integral to a well-run state.

SURGERY

Meanwhile surgery was undergoing changes in techniques, scope and status. Judged a manual skill rather than a liberal science, the cutter's art had traditionally carried scant prestige. After all, the surgeon was habitually handling nasty tumours, wens, gangrene and syphilitic chancres, and his means were invasive: the knife, cauterizing instruments and the amputating saw. Surgeons normally passed through a practical, not a liberal education; often yoked in guilds with barbers, they were scathingly compared to butchers. The caricature, however, tells but a partial truth.

The traditional surgeon's day-to-day business did not revolve around high-risk operations like amputations; it was a round of minor running-repairs: blood-letting, lancing boils, dressing skin abrasions, pulling teeth, managing whitlows, trussing ruptures, treating skin ulcers and so forth. Their fatality rates were low, for surgeons understood their limits, and the repertoire of operative surgery they took on was small, because of the well-known risks of trauma, blood-loss and sepsis. Internal malfunctions were treated not by the knife but by medicines and management, for major internal surgery was unthinkable before anaesthetics and antiseptic procedures. A surgeon would occasionally slit open a woman dying in labour to deliver a baby, but caesarians were desperate measures and there is no record of a mother surviving one in Britain until the close of the eighteenth century.

Improvements occurred, however, in certain operations, for instance lithotomy. For centuries, surgical treatment of bladder stones had followed the method described by Celsus (*methodus Celsiana*) in the first century AD – the surgeon cut down onto the base of the bladder through the perineum, a finger in the rectum making the stone bulge into the perineum – a technique known as the 'apparatus minor', implying that it needed no special instruments. Early in the sixteenth century the method of Mariano Santo of Barletta (1488–*c.* 1550) became widely adopted. This involved dilating and incising the urethra just anterior to the bladder neck to allow the introduction of instruments to extract the stone. Known as the 'apparatus major', this avoided the prostate gland damage which frequently led to haemorrhage and incontinence after the Celsan operation.

Lateral cystotomy was introduced by the itinerant practitioner, Jacques de Beaulieu (1651–1719), styled Frère Jacques because he travelled for safety in the habit and broad-brimmed hat of a Franciscan friar. A man sometimes called a quack yet clearly gifted, his lithotomy from the side involved cutting into the perineum and opening up both bladder and bladder neck. In Paris he became an overnight sensation thanks to the virtuosity and speed with which he worked; he is reputed to have performed some 4500 lithotomies and 2000 hernia operations in his nineteen-year career.

Johannes Rau (1688–1719) in Amsterdam and William Cheselden in London took up the Frenchman's method. An outstanding practical operator, Cheselden lectured on anatomy and served as surgeon at St Thomas's Hospital, making the stone his specialty. After publishing his *Treatise on the High Operation for the Stone* in 1723, he shifted his lithotomy technique to the 'lateral operation', rendering the operation safer and speedy – he could remove a stone in less than a minute. 'If I have any reputation in this way I have earned it dearly,' he wrote, reflecting upon his career,

> for no one ever endured more anxiety and sickness before an operation, yet from the time I began to operate all uneasiness ceased and if I have had better success than some others I do not impute it to more knowledge but to the happiness of mind that was never ruffled or disconcerted and a hand that never trembled during any operation.

Other techniques appeared, for instance for eye diseases. It was recognized that cataracts involved a hardening of the lens. The French oculist Jacques Daviel (1696–1762) found a way to extract the lens, performing the operation several hundred times with good results. Also skilled in that operation was the British oculist, John ('Chevalier') Taylor (1703–72), but he was a different kettle of fish, being an itinerant who practised with great razzmatazz at many of the courts of Europe (enemies alleged he contributed to the blindness of both Bach and Handel).

War brought developments in surgery, in particular in the management of gunshot wounds. Warfare and colonial expansion created insatiable demands for junior surgeons. By 1713, the British fleet had 247 vessels, each carrying a surgeon and his mate. For those with strong stomachs, like the surgeon-hero of Tobias Smollett's (1721–71) novel, *Roderick Random* (1748), naval or military service provided boundless experience and a leg-up into the profession.

At last surgery began to enjoy a rise in professional standing, notably in France. In 1687 French surgeons had a lucky break when Louis XIV developed an anal fistula. The success of the operation performed on the Sun King by C. F. Félix (1650–1703) – he had first practised on the poor – contributed to surgery's growing prestige. 'When Lewis XIV happened to have a fistula', William Heberden later commented,

> the French surgeons of that time complain of their being incessantly teased by people, who pretended, whatever their complaints were, that they proceeded from a fistula: and if there had been in France a mineral water reputed capable of giving it them, they would perhaps have flocked thither as eagerly as Englishmen resort to Bath in order to get the gout.

Félix's success earned him an estate and 300,000 livres.

By the early eighteenth century, surgery was widely taught in Paris through lectures and demonstrations, leading to the ending in 1768 of conventional apprenticeship training. Meanwhile in 1724 Louis XV granted the College of Saint-Côme in Paris (since medieval times, the elite organization of 'academic' surgeons) permission for public surgical courses. Senior Parisian surgeons used this royal favour to establish a school, lecturing on anatomy, surgery and *materia medica*, and undermining the guild mentality: instead of 'secret' knowledge passing from master to apprentice, lectures opened surgical theories and techniques to professional scrutiny. The most eminent teacher was Jean Louis Petit (1674–1750), inventor of the screw tourniquet – invaluable for thigh amputations and for controlling blood flow while the surgeon carried out Paré's ligatures – and the first to perform a successful operation for mastoiditis.

Thereafter surgeons jockeyed with physicians for status, maintaining that surgery possessed its own body of theory and so was no mere handicraft but a science. Such claims squared with the Enlightenment bent for the useful, and with the new pathology's view of disease as localized.

The radical reform of French medical education imposed in 1794 crowned surgery's rise; thenceforth it was taught to all students together with medicine. The prominence of the hospital in the post-1789 medical system and the prestige of pathological anatomy further elevated its status.

France was not alone in these developments. Alexander Monro (primus) (1697–1767), first incumbent of the Edinburgh chair of anatomy and surgery, was himself a surgeon who gave instruction in operations to medical students and surgical apprentices as well as pioneering anatomy teaching. Edinburgh education thus eroded the old divisions between physic and surgery, and its students equipped themselves in both skills, since most were likely to become surgeon-apothecaries or, as they would soon be called, general practitioners.

Other institutional developments in Britain gave surgery a fillip. The hospital movement led to the infirmary becoming a major site for accident and emergency cases, which were treated by surgeons, who could thereby control admissions. Hospitals also provided supplies of unclaimed bodies, which they could dissect. And, most significantly, the lustre of anatomy benefited surgery, both being arts of the knife. The celebrated anatomy school established in Piccadilly by William Hunter offered instruction in surgery, physiology, pathology and midwifery. And William's younger brother, John, the leading surgeon-physiologist of his age, became a prolific dissector, devoting his wealth and energies to research. The junior Hunter symbolized, for later practitioners, the arrival of surgery as physic's peer.

John Hunter was an indefatigable experimentalist. Addressing topics such as inflammation, shock and disorders of the vascular system, his main treatises – *Natural History of the Human Teeth* (1771), *Observations on Certain Parts of the Animal Oeconomy* (1786), and *Treatise on the Blood, Inflammation and Gunshot Wounds* (1794) – contributed to surgery's emergence from a manual craft into a scientific discipline involving physiological investigation. He was also energetic in investigating venereal disease, a field racked by controversy between 'dualists', arguing for specificity, and 'unicists', claiming a single affliction. He tried an experiment to settle the question. When a subject (perhaps himself), injected with pus from a gonorrhoeic patient, developed a typical syphilitic chancre, he logically concluded, in *On Venereal Disease* (1786), that the two diseases were really one, as had often been presumed. (As it turned out, the patient must have been infected with both gonorrhoea and syphilis, and Hunter's research muddied the waters for another seventy years.)

He amassed a huge collection of anatomical and biological specimens, including the skeleton of the Irish giant, John Byrne; about 13,000 of these became the basis of the Hunterian Museum of the Royal College of Surgeons. He also trained many eminent pupils, including Jenner, Astley Cooper (1768–1841), John Abernethy (1764–1831), Henry Cline (1750–1827), William Clift (1775–1849), and Philip Syng Physick (1768–1837), the latter importing Hunterian surgery into the New World. As in France where surgeons vied with physicians for professional distinction, in Britain Hunter was seen to embody surgery's claim to be the true basis of experimental physiology and, through the cultivation of anatomy, the model of medical instruction and research.

MEDICINE AND THE PEOPLE

Discussion so far has focused upon professional medical men – and a tiny number of women. But they comprised only the tip of the healing iceberg. From peasants to princes, people had views and practices of their own in health, sickness and remedies. Across vast tracts of Europe and its overseas empires, professional help might be far distant, but disease was always lurking. In this biological *ancien régime*, life expectations might be barely more than one third of today's – in 1750 the average Frenchman lived around twenty-seven years, his English equivalent around thirty-six. Ordinary people mainly treated themselves, at least in the first instance. There was nothing new about this in the eighteenth century, but better survival of records allows us more of a glimpse of the 'medicine without doctors' which was a necessity for many and a preference for some.

Religious healing continued to be practised, and not only by so-called ignorant peasants. Healing and holiness still criss-crossed. In Europe and Latin America, the Catholic Church upheld familiar healing rituals: holy water and wells, shrines, saints' relics, *ex voto* offerings, processions and pilgrimages. Even in Protestant nations where such 'superstitions' were censured, seventh sons of seventh sons and 'strokers' might claim 'miracle' cures, while Bourbon and Stuart monarchs flaunted their 'divine right' powers by touching for the 'king's evil' (scrofula). In England such thaumaturgical healing lapsed in 1714 with the Hanoverian succession (the infant Samuel Johnson was one of the last to be touched by the last Stuart, Queen Anne), but the ritual went on in France. At his coronation in 1722, Louis XV touched more than 2000 scrofula victims, and as late as the Bourbon restoration in 1815 touching was revived in hopes of strengthening the monarchy if not of healing the sick. Charles X gave the last performance on 31 May 1825.

Magic still underlay much vernacular healing. The touch of an executed man's hand, for instance, or the rope that hanged him at the scaffold were popularly credited with curative powers. The antiquarian fellow of the Royal Society, John Aubrey (1626–97), recorded numerous magic formulae such as: 'write these characters + Zada + Zadash + Zadathan + Abira + in virgin paper, I beleeve parchment, carry it always with you, and no gun-shott can hurt you.' And where does one draw the divide between magic and natural healing practices? In case of a painful stye, it was customary to stroke the eye with a black cat's tail: was that an empirical remedy or a relic of black magic? A common cure for inflammation of the brain was to 'cut open a live Chicken or Pigeon, and apply it to the Head': was this a medical therapy drawing upon the virtue of heat, or did its efficacy lie in the blood sacrifice?

Similarly with the evergreen doctrine of signatures in herbal healing. Paracelsus had been recommending the plant eyebright for bad eyes in the sixteenth century; it was still in widespread use in the eighteenth. Family recipe books show heaps of healing salves, prophylactics and remedial practices, some of which – the use of dead toads or vipers' blood, for example – had their origins in the occult. Everyone had a cure for everything, and some may have worked, if only as placebos.

Diaries and letters show that when people fell sick, they often framed their own diagnoses, helping them to make their next decision: whether to summon professional help. Many had recourse to folk healers. 'I would rather have the advice or take physick from an experienced old woman that had been at many sick people's bedsides,' Thomas Hobbes avowed, 'than from the learnedst but unexperienced physician'; and Robert Southey (1774–1843) could note over a century later that 'a cunning man, or a cunning woman, as they are termed, is to be found near every town.'

But, like witchcraft and astrology, magic was waning, at least among the growing ranks of the literate. This decline marks what Max Weber called the 'demystification of the world'; it also shows the withdrawal of the elite from popular ways. Education, books and travel were spreading a literate metropolitan culture prizing science and rationality, and dismissive of the old values.

Print brought simplified versions of elite medicine to the people, cheap texts with titles like *The Poor Man's Medicine Chest* (1791). In his immensely popular *Primitive Physick* (1747), John Wesley taught common folks how to treat their ills with the aid of simple kitchen ingredients like onions and honey; liquorice was good for pacifying a consumptive cough, and a deep cut could be stopped by binding on toasted cheese. William Buchan's *Domestic Medicine* (1769) and Samuel Tissot's *Avis au peuple sur la santé* (1761) [Advice to the People Regarding their Health] ran to scores of editions, and were translated into many languages.

Like many such works, Buchan's carried a radical message. Though himself a trained physician, he denounced the medical profession as oligarchic. Aiming to 'lay open' medicine to all, he espoused medical democracy as a fulfilment of the rights of man declared by the French Revolution: for far too long healing had been monopolized by a clique. Like Wesley, Buchan set great store by simple treatments, regarding diet, hygiene and temperance as preferable to exorbitant polypharmacy. Yet Buchan also deplored old wives' tales and folk-myth.

Throughout Europe authors ploughed similar furrows. In *Gesundheits-Katechismus* (1794) [Catechism of Health], the German physician Bernhard Faust (1755–1842) used a question-and-answer format to impart his advice and, like Wesley, portrayed health as next to godliness. A preventative regime was recommended by Christian Wilhelm Hufeland (1762–1836), professor in Berlin and friend of Goethe. In *Makrobiotik, oder die Kunst das menschliche Leben zu Verlängern* (1796), translated as *The Art of Prolonging Life* (1797), he gave advice for conserving the vital energies to attain longevity. The impact of all such writings (indeed, print culture in general) might be highly ambiguous: they could reinforce the authority of the medical elite or they might encourage independence of judgment, breeding that 'health protestantism' which fired nineteenth-century alternative medicine.

In the commercial economies of north-west Europe, kitchen physic was supplemented by shop-bought items: purges, emetics, cordials and febrifuges. In late eighteenth-century England, readymade medicine chests became popular, and it was common for middle-class families to stock up with patent medicines. Some were respectable, like Dr James's Powders, the Georgian equivalent of aspirin, or the Scotch Pills, a mixture of aloes, jalap, gamboge and anise; many were frauds, such as Solomon's Balm of Gilead, Brodum's Cordial and similar much-hyped 'restoratives' which purported to rectify the damage done by masturbation and other youthful indiscretions.

The eighteenth century has been dubbed the golden age of quackery.* Through most of continental Europe laws kept the most brazen in check, and from the 1780s the French state attempted to control quack medicines through the Société Royale de Médecine, whose prerogatives included the right to assay and validate proprietary preparations. English common law, by contrast, followed the free-market maxim of *caveat emptor* (let the buyer beware), and irregulars, quacks and nostrum-mongers cashed in.

To speak of quackery is not automatically to impugn the motives of unqualified practitioners, nor to deny their powers. Many quacks – such as the Scot, James Graham (1745–94), who claimed that long life and sexual rejuvenation could be achieved by mud-bathing and the use of his special electrified Celestial Bed, available at his Temple of Health off London's Strand – were not so much swindlers as entrepreneurs or fanatics. From the 1780s the one medicine which would truly relieve an attack of gout – it contained colchicum – was a secret remedy: the *Eau médicinale*, marketed by a French army officer, Nicolas Husson, and opposed by the profession.

Quacks excelled in the arts of publicity. Rose's Balsamic Elixir, its vendors claimed, would cure 'the English Frenchify'd' (i.e., venereal patients) beyond all other medicines: 'It removes all pains in 3 or 4 doses.' In short, that elixir, like all the rest, worked like magic. Itinerants had to put on a show; gaudily dressed and flanked by a zany and a monkey, they would erect their stage in the market-place, drawing first

---

* The origins of that term are obscure; it may come from the Dutch 'quacksalver', meaning a quicksilver doctor, since mercury was widely used to treat syphilis.

a crowd and then perhaps some teeth, both to the accompaniment of drums and trumpets, giving out gratis a few bottles of julep or cordial, selling a few dozen more, and then riding out of town. Many claimed to come from faraway places: from Turkey or, in the nineteenth century, the North American prairies.

Most charlatans were small-timers, but some irregulars made big killings. Joanna Stephens (d. 1774) hawked a remedy that promised to dissolve painful bladder stones without the need for lithotomy. Parliament raised a £5000 subscription to buy the recipe from her. Joshua Ward (1685–1761) made a fortune out of his 'pill and drop'. The pill was an antimony compound which acted as an expectorant, an antipyretic and an emetic; the drop was a violent purgative. In many cases, the knack was to address needs that regulars (perhaps understandably) failed to supply. Thus patent medicines promised to cure cancer, to restore lost youth and potency, or to alleviate conditions like venereal disease, for which patients might be embarrassed to consult the family physician.

With the rise of a literate public eager to exercise its judgment and consumer power, demand welled up for all sorts of healing, and the more the state and the medical authorities tried to clamp down on them, the greater their popularity. This is illustrated by the chequered career of Franz Anton Mesmer (1734–1815). After studying in Vienna, Mesmer received his doctorate for a thesis on the medical effects of the influence of the planets. Going into practice, he developed unorthodox healing methods almost by accident. His inspiration was Franzisca Oesterlin, who suffered crippling periodic seizures which produced vomiting, convulsions, fainting fits, temporary blindness and occasional paralysis. He placed three magnets over critical positions on her body, producing convulsive responses and a remission of symptoms. When she repeatedly reacted in the same way, Mesmer was sure he had hit upon one of nature's fundamental secrets, a Newtonian aetherial fluid which he called animal magnetism and which he saw as 'permeating the entire universe and infusing both matter and spirit with its vital force'. Health continued while that fluid flowed freely through the body, disease resulted from obstructions, which his healing processes claimed to remove.

Though a qualified physician, friendly with the Mozarts, Mesmer was drummed out of Vienna by faculty opposition for what was deemed quackish practice. He migrated to Paris, winning celebrity for his fashionable *séances*, at which he cured nervously-afflicted women through animal magnetism. At group sessions in ornately furnished treatment rooms, patients gathered round a central tub filled with 'magnetized water'. They grasped iron rods protuding from the tub, placing them near their diseased bodily part. During the treatment, many patients were 'cured' through a convulsive fit while others were 'mesmerized' into a hypnotic trance.

Commissions established by Louis XVI found Mesmer guilty of charlatanry (his cures might work, but they were scientifically groundless and therefore unacceptable), and he was obliged to leave Paris as well. By contrast, Mesmerists were able to perform in London with no obstructions whatsoever.

In many respects eighteenth-century medicine operated more like a trade than the lofty profession with which it has since sought to be identified. Patient-doctor relations were fluid; in a social regime dominated by patronage and clientage, physicians inevitably deferred to social superiors, and powerful patients expected doctors to fall in with their self-diagnoses and pet treatments. Scorning 'popgun' remedies, Samuel Johnson bullied his medical attendants, on one occasion insisting against advice that his surgeon bleed him. The sick felt no compunction about shopping around for second and third opinions, and made free use of quack, family and unorthodox remedies as well, adopting a try-anything mentality.

Yet doctors also agonized over professional status and respect, and here lies the significance of the emergence in late eighteenth-century Britain of a new body of writings on medical ethics. The way was paved in 1772 by the *Lectures on the Duties and Qualifications of a Physician* of John Gregory (1725–73). A doctor had a duty to be humane, stressed Gregory: 'It is as much the business of a physician to alleviate pain, and to smooth the avenues of death, when unavoidable, as to cure diseases.' The main text, however, was the work of Thomas Percival (1740–1804). Belonging to a network of reforming physicians centred on early industrial Manchester, Percival offers an interesting example of the new physician. He undertook demographic studies, wrote on hospitals and prisons, promoted medical charities and public health, and became an early member of the Manchester Literary and Philosophical Society, the focus of middle-class provincial science. When professional conflicts flared, he turned to medical ethics, publishing in 1794 his *Medical Jurisprudence*, expanded in 1803 as *Medical Ethics*. This code aimed to avoid damaging intra-professional conflict between the various sectors of the profession, deploring price-cutting competition and resolving pecking orders. It also presented practical advice on how doctors could reinforce paternalism, frankly admitting that charity patients in hospitals could be treated with a degree of authority impractical with wealthy private patients whose foibles had to be humoured. Percival emphasized the personal qualities of the good physician: 'Every case, committed to the charge of a physician or surgeon, should be treated with attention, steadiness and humanity.'

MEDICINE, STATE AND SOCIETY: THE PROFESSION AND ITS INSTITUTIONS

Medicine today is organized through structures that grant the profession considerable autonomy under state protection, while claiming to protect the public from malpractice and quackery.

These crystallized in the nineteenth century. Before then, medicine was organized differently. From late medieval times, professionals had achieved a measure of self-regulation and corporate identity. For the lesser ranks – (small-town practitioners, apothecaries and surgeons) this involved apprenticeship to a master for five to seven years, followed by admission to a guild conferring a licence to practice. Elite physicians enjoyed a university training culminating in an academic degree, followed by admission to a faculty or a college, and often a court or official appointment. Such arrangements, ratified by princes or municipalities, conferred prestige and quasi-monopolistic rights to practise within a defined region and to prosecute interlopers.

In *ancien régime* France, medical regulation lay in the hands of faculties attached to the main universities: Paris, Montpellier, Rheims, Toulouse, Tours and so forth. Candidates who fulfilled prescribed criteria, passed examinations and paid dues, were licensed to practice within the local jurisdiction. To reduce competition and raise rewards, entry was restricted. The corporate rights and privileges of the French profession laid it open to attack in the Revolution and, condemning professions as selfish monopolies, the Jacobins abolished all the traditional medical faculties.

Medicine was regulated in the German-speaking principalities and the Austrian (Habsburg) empire through a system requiring academic qualifications. In states like Prussia where princes promoted a service ideal, physicians tended to pride themselves on operating as civil servants. Top physicians and medical professors typically belonged to a medical college (*collegium medicum*) attached to the royal court. Formal qualifications counted. In Prussia, for example, candidates for the MD were required to present a clinical case (*casus medicopracticus*) before the Collegium Medicum and the Medicochirurgicum (state board of health). Similar requirements applied in the Habsburg empire, where licences were conferred by the universities of Vienna and Prague.

In the German principalities, chains of command and responsibility descended from the Collegium Medicum through city councils to town and village physicians, whose local status was dignified by bureaucratic titles and sheaves of parchment diplomas. Official title conferred upon the licensed practitioner the exclusive right to local practice. It also meant a welter of trivial and irksome paperwork and administrative obligations: attending law courts, sanctioning military exemptions, regulating poisons, conducting examinations of lunacy, pregnancy and paternity, inspecting the poor and military recruits for venereal disease, documenting epidemic outbreaks and serving as public witness – all for paltry pecuniary reward.

In England, the formal regulation of the medical profession instigated in the sixteenth century was weakened by socio-economic change. The Royal College of Physicians of London subsided into a gentlemen's club, reserved for the fashionable. Its statutes restricted the fellowship to graduates of Oxford and Cambridge and members of the Church of England, and resisted reformist pressures, despite the fact that by 1750 the finest physicians were Dissenters by religion and trained either at Leiden or at Edinburgh. Eminences like William Hunter, John Fothergill and John Coakley Lettsom resented being relegated to the status of mere non-voting 'licentiates', or second-class citizens.

Yet if the college did little to promote medicine, it also had little power to restrict it. Its jurisdiction did not extend beyond the capital, and it rarely acted against interlopers. Following the House of Lords' judgment in the Rose Case (1704), the college lost its monopoly in prescribing medicines; henceforth apothecaries might also prescribe and, in effect, act as doctors.

London's Company (later College) of Surgeons failed to evolve into a modern teaching and examining body, though it formally separated in 1745 from the Barbers, signalling that surgery was a craft in its own right. The Society of Apothecaries officially regulated pharmacy in the capital, but unregulated chemists and druggists blossomed, together with quacks and unorthodox practitioners. Beyond London, there was *de facto* liberty to practise, and a free-for-all ensued.

In Britain, no uniform system of medical education prevailed. A few had degrees or diplomas from English universities, but medical graduates from Oxford and Cambridge dwindled to a trickle. Many possessed degrees from Leiden or a French or Italian university, and more and more gained their education in Scotland, mainly Edinburgh. Many practised without any formal qualifications at all. There was no regional system of medical licensing, partly because, unlike France, there were no provincial medical faculties. Prosecution for unauthorized healing was unusual, and the market regulated practice. Success depended upon a capacity to satisfy the public – by being inexpensive, by flattery, or by cutting a dash.

Developments in America resembled those in England. Medicine emerged without a supporting or restrictive framework of guild or university requirements, though a few medical bodies spluttered into being from the 1730s. Fresh developments in the 1760s are associated with John Morgan (1735–89), a Philadelphian who learnt his medicine from the Monros, Cullen and Whytt. Returning from Edinburgh, he published a *Discourse upon the Institution of Medical Schools in America* (1765), calling for qualifying examinations to ensure minimum standards. In the same year, he founded the medical department of the University of Pennsylvania, where he held the chair of practice of medicine. Another Philadelphia-born Edinburgh graduate, William Shippen Jr (1736–1808), worked with him, becoming professor of anatomy and surgery. In 1769 Benjamin Rush was elected professor of chemistry there, also becoming physician to the Pennsylvania Hospital (1783–1813) and founder of the Philadelphia Dispensary.

Despite attempts to erect institutions similar to those in Europe, American regulars faced an uphill struggle for recognition, especially as Congress and the state legislatures were unwilling to reinstate old-world monopolies after 1783; medical sects proliferated, individualism prevailed, and only slowly did some semblance of licensing emerge. The Harvard medical school was established in 1783, and twenty years later it was agreed that either a Harvard diploma or a qualifying examination would serve as a Massachusetts licence; in 1810 similar rules were formulated in Connecticut, and South Carolina followed in 1817.

After the Revolutionary War, settlers began to push through the mountains and to establish outposts in Kentucky, Tennessee, Ohio,

Illinois and Missouri. There were never enough doctors in the western settlements, and many settlers relied on books like *Every Man His Own Doctor* written in the 1730s by a Virginian, John Tennent (*c.* 1700–60).

With its pragmatic acceptance of a medical market-place within liberal political values, Anglo-American medicine diverged from the Continent. But everywhere education had to be demand-responsive in a medical sphere in which students still commonly went abroad for their medical training, aided by the *lingua franca* of Latin, and would-be doctors were seeking a training that would combine scientific prestige with practical bedside skills.

Early in the century Leiden assumed prominence, thanks to Boerhaave, a man who (if no great discoverer) became known as 'communis Europae praeceptor', the medical instructor of Europe. His *Institutiones medicae* (1708) [Medical Institutes] and *Elementa chemiae* (1731) [Elements of Chemistry] became evergreen teaching texts, and his personality inspired students who valued his clarity and orderliness. Like Cullen later, Boerhaave aimed to breed good clinicians: his inaugural lecture was significantly a call for a return to the study of Hippocrates.

Leiden owed its popularity in part to the promotion of clinical teaching. Two small wards were earmarked in a local charity hospital, where six men and six women were placed as demonstration material for clinical lectures. Though these cases served primarily to display book knowledge, such exercises underscored the importance of seeing real patients. This 'proto-clinic' was a major innovation, because traditional hospitals had rarely, because of their religious ethos, become teaching sites. Leiden's example was soon followed; in Vienna, for example, the hospital reforms carried through in the 1770s by Anton Stoerck (1731–1803) led to instruction on the wards.

Edinburgh became the British Leiden. Its medical school dates from the appointment in 1726 of the Leiden-trained Alexander Monro, primus, as professor of anatomy. By any standards, Edinburgh medicine was a stunning success in the following century. It boasted a galaxy of talent: the Monro family in anatomy (three, all Alexander, were professors in succession, Monro II (1733–1817) succeeding his father in 1758, and Monro III (1773–1859) following *his* father in 1798; he stayed till 1846, the three thus holding one chair for some 120 years.). There was also Black in chemistry, Cullen and Gregory in theoretical and practical medicine, and other lesser lights besides – and the attractions of Edinburgh's teachings in philosophy and the human sciences.

What did the average student get out of Edinburgh? Not primarily an intensive bedside training. Though it pioneered infirmary-based teaching, only around one third of the students signed up for clinical lectures. Nor did they get prolonged personal dissecting practice. There was always a shortage of corpses, and illegal acquisition of cadavers led to scandals which implicated anatomists and surgeons in body-snatching and finally murder. (For Burke and Hare, see Chapter Eleven.) The strength of an Edinburgh education lay in imparting the elements of anatomy, surgery, chemistry, medical theory and practice. After three years, an Edinburgh man trained in medicine and surgery was ready to go out into the world to practise the new trade of 'general practitioner' or family doctor. Those falling sick in 1810 in Newcastle, Newfoundland or New South Wales would most probably have been seen by Edinburgh doctors.

By the 1780s, when medicine was moribund at Oxford and Cambridge, Edinburgh University was attracting around two hundred medical students a year, and twice as many again by the 1820s. A staggering 17,000 medical students studied in the first century of the school, and there were additionally apprentices taking surgery at what was known from 1778 as the Edinburgh Royal College of Surgeons. The university had many attractions: it was cheap, there were no religious restrictions, and the lectures were in English. There was no obligation to graduate, students attended only the courses they desired, and paid for those alone. This demand-led regime kept the professors on their toes, and Edinburgh flourished because it offered the practical training students needed. The same applied to Montpellier where student demand led to the provision of new teaching in practical medicine, replacing the old bookish courses associated with Paris Galenism.

In England, innovations in medical education took place entirely outside the universities. Two sorts of medical instruction emerged to meet students' needs. One was the private anatomy school. From the 1720s medical lecture courses mushroomed in London, delivered by front-rank instructors and open to all. At least twenty-six medical lecturers had performed in the metropolis before William Hunter started up in the mid 1740s; by the 1780s, over twenty classes were running in a single year. The core course was anatomy, but practical physic, *materia medica*, chemistry, and specialisms like obstetrics were also taught.

In 1768, as we have noted, William Hunter set up the capital's top anatomy and obstetrics school, training leading anatomists and surgeons, including his brother, John, William Hewson (1739–74), William Cruikshank (1745–1800), and Matthew Baillie. His series ran to 112 meetings, held six days a week for three and a half months, ensuring comprehensive coverage of anatomy, practical surgery and midwifery. He prized his position as a 'breeder of anatomists'.

Such courses had special attractions, imparting discoveries unavailable elsewhere. William Hunter's auditors heard of his researches on aneurysm, the placental circulation, the lymphatic system and the gravid uterus – nowhere available in print. They also benefited from the specimens of Hewson, who had made over two hundred preparations, dry and wet (still surviving, these yield good-quality images with modern instruments). Private lecture schools could be centres of research excellence and proved popular with students because of the superb opportunities they offered for practical anatomy. 'The young Surgeon', noted Robert Campbell,

> must be an accurate Anatomist, not only as a speculative but practical Anatomist; without which he must turn out a mere Bungler. It is not sufficient for him to attend Anatomical Lectures, and see two or three Subjects cursorily dissected; but he must put his Hand to it himself, and be able to dissect every part, with the same Accuracy that the Professor performs.

Yet this was easier said than done. For the law and popular sentiment restricted the supply of cadavers. From 1752, the Company of Surgeons was granted the corpses of all executed felons, but Surgeons' Hall dissections were formal exercises, students being mere spectators. By contrast, private anatomy instructors ensured personal access to bodies. By turning a blind eye to legal niceties, private lecturers offered matchless hands-on anatomical experience.

The other new site for medical teaching was the hospital. In eighteenth-century Britain hospitals opened to students for the first time as places to learn, and teachers used clinical cases as training material. The Edinburgh medical school benefited from its links with the town infirmary. Professor John Rutherford (1695–1779) inaugurated clinical lecturing in the 1740s, and from 1750 a special clinical ward was set up. Students were also expected to visit patients' bedsides for themselves, studying the professors' reports. John Aikin (1747–1822), studying there in the 1770s, noted,

A number of such cases as are likely to prove instructive are selected and disposed in separate rooms in the Infirmary, and attended by one of the college professors. The students go round with him every day, and mark down the state of each patient and the medicines prescribed. At certain times lectures are read upon these cases . . .

Similar developments occurred south of the border, where hospitals developed on-site lecturing. In London, William Cheselden commenced private surgical lectures in 1711. From 1718, he moved them to St Thomas's, delivering four courses a year. The practice spread. Student training was essential to specialist institutions like maternity hospitals. By 1800 London was, according to Thomas Beddoes, 'the best spot in Great Britain, and probably in the whole world where medicine may be taught as well as cultivated to most advantage'.

Primary health care remained a matter for sick people to decide; but governments increasingly looked to works like the *Medicus politicus* (1738) [The State Doctor] of the Halle professor Friedrich Hoffmann to define the role of medicine within legal procedures.

The goal of promoting the people's health stemmed in part from the desire of Catholic rulers to supplant the Church as the primary regulatory agency. In Austria, Joseph II (1741–90) dissolved the monasteries to re-channel charity, and reformed Vienna's hospitals. Enlightened rulers such as Frederick the Great of Prussia prized 'cameralism', that is, rational administration. Medicine and law were seen as sister professions, serving the ruler and benefiting the nation. Influential thinkers publicized welfare questions, developing the science of 'statistics' (*Statistik*, derived from *Staat*, state), in which data would be tabulated on population, topography, climate, natural resources, trade, manufactures, military strength, education and religion. The Prussian army chaplain Johann Peter Süssmilch (1707–77) was a pioneer of vital statistics, assembling data relating to public hygiene, life-insurance and epidemics. His *Göttliche Ordnung* (1732) [Divine Ordering] was the first thorough demographic study using population statistics.

Of prime significance was the concept of medical police, expounded by Johann Peter Frank (1745–1821). After serving as district medical officer of Baden, Frank brought out the first volume of his comprehensive *System einer vollständigen medicinischen Polizey* (1779–1826) [System of a Complete Medical Police]. He adopted a cradle-to-grave approach; his first volume dealt with marriage, fertility, pregnancy, midwifery services and state action to ensure a healthy, populous citizenry, predicated on the mercantilist assumption that populous nations were economically and militarily strong, and that subjects were national assets. Subsequent volumes dealt with issues such as prostitution, venereal disease, abortion, foundling hospitals, nutrition, food control, clothing and housing.

Frank's great work was rooted in Enlightenment ideals. A faith in nature inspired his comments on the value of breast-feeding, fresh air, loose clothing and affectionate marriages. He made detailed comments on health and its promotion; on the importance of education, housing, food and wages; on hospitals, dispensaries and lying-in services; on medical education and medical licensing, and favoured central administrative measures to enhance welfare.

His full vision was never implemented, but aspects of it were becoming routine, including censuses. The 'westernizing' czar, Peter the Great (1672–1725), initiated a nationwide Russian census, characteristically for taxation purposes. From 1748, Sweden established a centralized system for compiling statistics, enabling Pehr Wargentin (1717–83) to publish in 1766 the first mortality table for an entire country. The United Kingdom established its national census only from 1801; earlier proposals had been frustrated by anti-centralizing scare rhetoric of 'liberty in danger'.

Statecraft required attention to health in many fields, not least military hygiene. For centuries, as James Lind observed, armies had lost 'more of their men by sickness, than by the sword', especially through insanitary camp conditions. Influential in efforts to change this was Sir John Pringle (1707–82), a Leiden-trained Scotsman who was physician-general of the British army from 1742 to 1758. He undertook a series of observations, communicated to the Royal Society, on the nature of antisepsis, and the relationship between putrefaction, infection, contagion and fever. Fevers were attributed to material generated by putrefaction, a process exacerbated by dirt and overcrowding. His 'Account of Several Persons Seized with the Gaol Fever, Working at Newgate' drew out the practical implications of his work on typhus. Personal hygiene and clean clothes were the best preventatives; prisoners should have their old clothes burnt and be supplied at public expense with clean ones; clothes and bodies should be 'washed from time to time'.

This 'gospel of cleanliness' permeated Pringle's *Observations on the Diseases of the Army* (1752), a work based on personal military experience and filled with advice on ways to prevent the most common disorders:

typhus, dysentery, 'bilious' fever, scabies, etc. While not strikingly original, it captured the Enlightenment concern for hygiene, public health and the value of life. Pringle is also remembered for developing the idea of the neutrality of the military hospital. At the battle of Dettingen (1743), he proposed to the French commanding officer that the hospital tents on each side should be immune from attack. The idea stuck.

The health of sailors also received great attention, especially once scurvy ravaged the crew of Lord Anson's (1697–1762) round-the-world expedition of 1740–44. Out of the 1955 men who set out, 320 had died from fevers and dysentery and 997 from scurvy by the time Anson returned to England in 1744. Involving swollen, spongy, bleeding gums, huge bruises, swollen joints, lassitude, heart failure and death, scurvy was investigated notably by James Lind (1716–91), a Scottish naval surgeon who bravely protested against the poor accommodation, rancid food, and foul water characterizing navy life. In his *Treatise on the Scurvy* (1753) he drew upon personal experience to reason that citrus fruits were effective antiscorbutics, supporting his hypothesis by the world's first controlled clinical trial on board HMS *Salisbury* in 1754.

Twelve scurvy patients were chosen. Lind gave two of them a quart of cider a day; two had oil of vitriol; two vinegar; two sea-water; two had oranges and lemons; and two an electuary of garlic, radish, Peru balsam and myrrh. The pair on oranges and lemons were fit for duty in six days, and put to nurse the others, who remained sick. Lind did *not* regard the condition, in the modern manner, as a deficiency disease – rather antiscorbutic fruits were thought to cure scurvy in a way analogous to the action of Jesuit's bark in malaria. Lind believed scurvy was associated with moist air, and that it operated by blocking normal perspiration. Lemon juice acted as a detergent which divided the toxic particles so that they could slip through the constricted sweating pores in the skin.

No immediate action followed from Lind's findings, and the voyages of James Cook (1728–79) show that scurvy remained part of the larger question of the health and management of sailors. Cook and other enlightened commanders recommended an integrated regime, emphasizing proper diet, cleanliness, ventilation and good morale. On his first circumnavigation in 1770, good management ensured there was only one death among his seamen. With fresh lemons, limes and oranges, Cook extolled the antiscorbutic virtues of onions, cabbage, sauerkraut and malt, and his preference was for a comprehensive 'managerial' strategy of cleanliness: scrubbing, fumigation, whitewashing, sprinkling with 'antiseptics' like vinegar, free ventilation and discipline. Within two years of the general issue of lemon juice to the navy in 1795, thanks to the publicizing efforts of Sir Gilbert Blane (1749–1834) scurvy had virtually disappeared from the British fleet. Lemons perhaps did as much as Nelson to defeat Napoleon. (Later the less effective limes were used, giving rise to the identification of the English abroad as 'limeys'.)

Army and navy experience suggested analogues for civilian sickness. Paralleling the work of Pringle, Lind and Blane, John Howard (1726–90) pioneered investigations into prisons, bridewells and lazarettos. On the basis of extensive gaol and hospital visiting in Britain and the Continent in the 1770s and 1780s, Howard concluded that filth and a close atmosphere were responsible for endemic conditions like gaol fever (typhus). Practical hygiene measures proved moderately effective. Contemplating improvements in street sanitation and personal hygiene in London, John Coakley Lettsom (1744–1815) declared in the 1790s,

> In the space of a very few years I have observed a total revolution in the conduct of the common people respecting their diseased friends. They have learned that most diseases are mitigated by a free admission of air, by cleanliness and by promoting instead of restraining the indulgence and care of the sick.

That Quaker physician and philanthropist had a reputation for looking on the bright side.

Attention was also paid to occupational disorders, thanks to the inquiries of Bernardino Ramazzini (1633–1714), from 1682 professor of medical theory at Modena. His *De constitutione anni 1690* [On the Constitution of the Year 1690] discussed the epidemiological consequences, notably malaria, of heavy rainfall and flooding in the Italian countryside. Over many years he collected material for his major work, *De morbis artificium* (1700) [On the Diseases of Workers], the first sustained study of occupational diseases. It dealt with the working conditions and ailments associated with more than fifty different trades, discussing miners, soap-makers, farmers, fishermen, laundresses, wet-nurses, writers and cesspit cleaners, noting diseases resulting from mercury poisoning as well as others caused by bad working postures. The English surgeon Percival Pott (1714–88) linked scrotal cancer to the soot to which young chimneysweeps were exposed. But little was done to counter occupational diseases – governments rarely hinder trade.

In Britain the improvement of urban hygiene remained largely a voluntary and local matter. John Bellers (1654–1725), a Quaker cloth merchant living in London, wrote perceptively on the health of towns. He urged street cleaning, refuse collection, regulation of dairies, abattoirs and noxious trades, and other measures which, initially considered visionary, found their way onto the statute book during the next two centuries. Bellers suggested that Parliament make provision for the improvement of medicine so that 'the Number of People in the Kingdom . . . may be doubled'. Sickness was a gross national waste: 'Every Able Industrious Labourer, that is capable to have Children, who so Untimely Dies, may be accounted Two Hundred Pound Loss to the *Kingdom.*'

Pivotal to the public provision of health-care facilities was the hospital, but it was also perhaps the nub of the problem. Nominally a site of recuperation, it became a spreader of disease. Hospitals took many forms and served many functions. In France, the *hôpital général*, an institution similar to the English poorhouse, sheltered beggars, orphans, vagabonds and prostitutes, together with the sick and mad. The Paris Hôtel Dieu was a healing institution, but had an atrocious reputation as a hotbed of infection. Howard called the Hôpital St Louis and Hôtel Dieu 'the two worst hospitals' he had ever visited. He often saw five or six patients to a bed, some of them dying. By contrast he commended the Leeds Infirmary, which, he said, had 'no bugs in the beds'.

The most notable new continental hospital was the Vienna Allgemeines Krankenhaus, rebuilt by Joseph II in 1784, an expression of the absolutist drive towards centralization. Planned for 1600 patients, this general hospital was divided into 6 medical, 4 surgical and 4 clinical sections; 86 clinical beds met teaching needs. Its administration was carried out by a director, an assistant director and a physician in charge of teaching. There were 6 physicians, 3 surgeons, 13 assistant physicians, and 7 assistant surgeons. Though sheltering the poor, it marked the growing conviction that hospitals were primarily institutions for the sick. Serving Joseph II's grand Enlightenment design, provincial hospitals were also built in Prague (1789), Olmütz (now Alamouc: 1787) and Linz (1788). Comparable institutions were set up in other states: Berlin's Charité Hospital was built in 1768, and in St Petersburg Catherine the Great (1762–96) erected the huge Obuchov Hospital.

Georgian England saw energetic hospital foundation. In London, only St Thomas's, St Bartholomew's and Bethlem Hospital (popularly called Bedlam, for long England's only madhouse) had survived the Reformation and, by European standards, England in 1700 was exceptionally ill-endowed with hospitals and sister institutions like orphanages. Enlightened philanthropy, secular and religious, raised new foundations, typically meant for the poor (but not paupers), who would receive care without charge, so as to reinforce ties of deference and gratitude to benefactors. London profited first. To the metropolis's ancient hospitals, five more general hospitals were added: the Westminster (1720), Guy's (1724), St George's (1733), the London (1740) and the Middlesex (1745). These spurred similar institutions in the provinces, where no genuinely medical hospitals had previously existed. The Edinburgh Royal Infirmary was set up in 1729, followed by Winchester and Bristol (1737), York (1740), Exeter (1741), Bath (1742), Northampton (1743) and some twenty others, until by 1800 twenty-eight English provincial towns had a general hospital.

Augmenting these general foundations, Georgian philanthropy supported specialist institutions. St Luke's Hospital was opened in London in 1751 amid optimistic fanfares. Its physician, William Battie (1703–76), asserted that, if treated with humanity, lunacy was no less curable than any other disease. By 1800, Manchester, Liverpool and York had philanthropically supported lunatic asylums. London's Lock Hospital for venereal cases opened in 1746, and in 1791 the brewer Samuel Whitbread endowed a cancer ward at Middlesex Hospital.

Another new institution was the lying-in hospital, four being set up in London between 1749 and 1765. Such maternity hospitals guaranteed a few days' bed-rest to poor women, while enabling unmarried mothers, usually servant girls, to deliver their babies with few questions asked. By 1800, London's hospitals were handling over 20,000 patients a year.

Similar developments occurred in North America. The first general hospital catering for the sick poor was founded in Philadelphia in 1751. Soliciting private subscriptions, Benjamin Franklin found people reluctant to give, and the Pennsylvania General Hospital became possible only when the Assembly agreed to match £2000 from private subscriptions; Franklin was thus the inventor of the matching grant. The New York Hospital was established some twenty years later, and the Massachusetts General Hospital in 1811.

Hospitals provided treatment, food, rest and convalescence, but they restricted themselves to complaints that would respond to treatment, excluded infectious cases and, in any case, could treat only a fraction of the sick. Their effects were consequently somewhat slight.

Alongside hospitals, supplementary medical institutions opened. The first London dispensary was set up in 1773; by 1800, sixteen existed, treating up to 50,000 outpatient cases a year, and many in the provinces besides. In the 1760s, George Armstrong founded his Dispensary for the Infant Poor, where in the course of twelve years he distributed advice and medicines to over 35,000 children. Dispensaries provided outpatient services, supplying advice and free medicine to the sick poor who did not require hospitalization. They also provided visits by physicians into the homes of the poor. Such first-hand experience of how the other half lived fired the reforming zeal of progressive doctors for improved housing, better sanitation and popular health education.

Also in England, where the philanthropic, voluntarist ethic was strong, the Humane Society (1773) aimed to heighten awareness of industrial hazards through teaching life-saving techniques to resuscitate the drowned (the proverbially suicidal English were said to make a habit of drowning themselves). Others were set up to provide free surgical appliances to labourers with hernias. All such initiatives changed the British medical landscape, since the voluntary hospital movement and its spin-offs signalled a new recognition of the people's health. Subscriptions generally came from nobles, gentry and civic worthies, and management remained mainly in the hands of lay governors, with physicians taking a back seat.

DISEASE AND THE LARGER PICTURE

Public action to promote health prompts the wider question: what was the balance sheet of health? What impact was civilization making on global epidemiology? The most momentous eighteenth-century development was the consolidation of the slave plantation economy in the New World, involving a massive triangular exchange of peoples between Africa, Europe and America. The transatlantic slave trade had got under way in the early sixteenth century. The arriving Africans possessed much the same immunities as the Europeans but were additionally resistant to the tropical illnesses of their own part of the world, notably falciparum malaria, thanks to the sickle-cell trait. Black slaves proved more fever

resistant in mosquito-infested America than whites, though their working conditions inevitably meant appalling disease rates overall. White
settlers were often crippled by malaria, a disease of the moving frontier,
spread through forest clearing and turning the soil. 'The washed coun-
tenances of the people standing at their doors,' observed a visitor to
Maryland in the 1690s, 'like so many standing ghosts . . . every house was
an infirmary.' Malaria was the price of 'development' – high-investment,
capital-intensive monocultures.

Perhaps the most spectacular disease spread by new trade patterns
was yellow fever. Its principal vector, the *Aedes aegypti* mosquito, was
taken to America by slave ships from Africa. From 1647, when an
epidemic in Barbados spread throughout the Caribbean, yellow fever
scourged the eastern coasts of the Americas. It struck Pernambuco in
Brazil in 1685, killing thousands in Recife and Olinda; it entered New
York in 1668, Philadelphia and Charleston in 1690, and in 1691 got as
far north as Boston. In the eighteenth century it became a regular visitor
to Colombia, Peru and Ecuador – and to a lesser degree Iberia. It
played a key part in Caribbean military campaigns and political fortunes,
thwarting Admiral Vernon's 1741 assault on Cartagena in Colombia
(half his force of 19,000 was lost), and accounting for many of the
40,000 French dead in their abortive attempt to re-occupy Haiti after
its slave-led revolt in 1790.

Yellow fever proved a lasting threat to the eastern seaboard of North
America. Charleston had six severe epidemics between 1790 and 1799,
and in 1793 Philadelphia suffered a terrible epidemic, with over 4000
deaths. 'Many never walked on the foot path', reported Matthew Carey
(1760–1839):

> but went into the middle of the streets, to avoid being infected in
> passing by houses wherein people had died. Acquaintances and
> friends avoided each other in the streets, and only signified their
> regard by a cold nod. The old custom of shaking hands fell into
> such general disuse, that many were affronted at even the offer of
> the hand.

Though originally believing yellow fever was contagious, Benjamin
Rush later abandoned that view, implicating a cargo of coffee dumped
on the Philadelphia quayside as the source of an infectious miasma,
and he firmly opposed quarantine measures. His free-trade views not
surprisingly won approval among the merchant community.

Europeans also exported their diseases to the South Seas once the Pacific was opened up following the voyages of Samuel Wallis (1766–68), Louis-Antoine de Bougainville (1766–69), and James Cook (1768–70, 1772–75, 1776–80). These had the same lethal outcome as in the Americas. The mortality of the Hawaiian natives was perhaps 90 per cent; in Australia, New Zealand and the remainder of Oceania the die-off precipitated by reunion with the rest of the world was also high. Epidemics, especially measles, decimated the Pacific islanders and the Maoris in New Zealand, who were also killed by tuberculosis. The peoples of islands like Tahiti, admired by eighteenth-century Europeans as paradises populated by noble savages, went into rapid decline, thanks to newly imported diseases such as syphilis, and the impact of Western civilization upon societies whose resistance to alcohol, guns and missionaries was as low as their resistance to European diseases. Tahiti's population declined from approximately 40,000 in 1769 to 9000 by 1830; the Maoris decreased from 150,000 in 1814 to 56,000 by 1857.

By 1800 Europe was on the brink of industrialization and population was climbing inexorably. First in Britain, but soon in France, the Low Countries and the USA, urban and commercial expansion, technological innovation and manufactures transformed material civilization. The population rise indispensable to industrialization was nowhere due to any significant decline in the death rate: rising birth rates were the cause. Chiefly due to social changes like earlier marriage, relaxed sexual mores and the economic incentive of the greater earning power of children, these owed little to medical factors.

The health profile around 1800 defies easy generalization. After four centuries of terror, bubonic plague had receded from Western Europe, but on the Continent, at least until 1760, crisis mortality remained severe, associated with periodic winter famines. Unregulated urban growth was spreading filth diseases such as typhoid and urban maladies like tuberculosis.

The Enlightenment brought transformations in perceptions of healthiness. It opened with mercantilist fears of depopulation. It was the duty of the monarch, all agreed, to take measures to boost the population. At least in Britain, however, the century ended with this reversed. In his *Essay on Population* (1798), the Revd Thomas Malthus (1766–1834) prophesied runaway population growth leading inexorably to wars, plague, famine, vice and social catastrophe. He was right, at least in part. By 1800, Europe was indeed beginning a population explosion. He also correctly attributed this demographic new regime to a rising birth rate.

Faith in medical science probably made its contribution to a new confidence in man's capacity to master his environment, natural and social. Science and medicine were challenging religion as meanings of existence. More people were being born in the presence of a medical attendant, more were dying with the ministrations of a physician rather than a priest, gliding perhaps into a peaceful death, thanks to opiate cocktails. The Enlightenment, as we have seen, sped the medicalization of life and death. If widely satirized, medicine was gaining cultural authority.

Seeking to understand and change society, Enlightenment thinkers looked to science for their model. It was seen as an incomparable engine of analysis: objective, critical, progressive. Natural order promised models of social order for many *philosophes*: a vision of free individual activity informed by natural law. Medical men, for their part, were gazing at society. The scientific spirit encouraged medicine to search out the wider laws of health and sickness, examining climate, environment and epidemics. Certain physicians acquired an enlarged social awareness, confronting the interplay of sickness, medicine and society. What governed the pathways of community illness? Why did sickness vary from society to society, from region to region, from group to group? Pondering such variables, physicians felt driven to be more than bedside healers; they had to become anatomists and doctors of society itself. The eighteenth century witnessed advances in medicine, but more importantly it began to transform perceptions of medicine's place in society.

In that context even Parson Malthus's melancholy is telling. The Bible had envisaged global disaster in terms of the Four Horsemen of the Apocalypse. The first horseman was the emblem of God, life and hope; the second was War; the third was Famine; the last was Pestilence and Death. By 1798, birth and death, so long the mysteries of Providence, could be reduced by a clergyman to a matter of arithmetic and geometry. Quantification pointed to a dilemma whose key lay not in Divine Providence but in equations. Enlightenment medicine made few positive advances but it became the basis of a new, materially based science of man, an anthropology in the widest sense, and a far from optimistic one.

Here are two voices from the end of the *ancien régime*. In 1794 William Heberden could write to his friend, Thomas Percival,

> I please myself with thinking that the method of teaching the art of healing is becoming every day more conformable to what reason and nature require; that the errors introduced by superstition and false philosophy are gradually retreating; and that medical knowledge, as well as all other dependent upon observation and experience, is continually increasing in the world. The present race of physicians is possessed of several most important rules of practice, utterly unknown to the ablest in former ages, not excepting Hippocrates himself, or even Aesculapius.

By contrast, the third president of the United States, Thomas Jefferson, a lover of enlightened learning yet no friend of the professions, pointed out in 1806:

> Harvey's discovery of the circulation of the blood was a beautiful addition to our knowledge of the animal economy, but on a review of the practice of medicine before and since that epoch, I do not see any great amelioration which has been derived from that discovery.

There was truth in both views.

CHAPTER XI

SCIENTIFIC MEDICINE IN THE NINETEENTH CENTURY

MODERN TIMES DAWNED with the nineteenth century. In the New World a nation had just been born. Declaring independence in 1776, the United States of America was the first to break with kings, nobles and prelates; the first bearing in its own constitution the seeds of democracy, though far from complete, since women did not have the vote and its economy ran on the blood of slaves. Founding fathers such as Thomas Jefferson trusted the new republic would be immune to Old World vices.

Europe was not to be outdone. From the storming of the Bastille on 14 July 1789, the French Revolution fought to realize the Enlightenment vision of the rights of man: liberty, equality and fraternity. To mark its clean break with the past, the Revolution set up a republic of virtue and a cult of the Supreme Being, and marked it all with a new calendar, opening with *An* 1 – and beheaded Louis XVI on 21 January 1793. The Revolution's clarion call of freedom from despotism and injustice resounded round the world, making tyrants tremble.

'Bliss was it in that dawn to be alive / But to be young was very heaven,' recalled the Romantic poet William Wordsworth of the time when he crossed the Channel in 1791 to rejoice in the birth of a nation; amid the spires of Oxford, the radical physician Thomas Beddoes addressed his friends as *citoyen*. The euphoria was shortlived, however, being depleted by the judicial blood-letting of the Committee of Public Safety and the atrocious carnage of the Revolutionary and Napoleonic Wars. The guillotine, that high-tech tool of the Jacobin Terror, was ironically the invention of a progressive Paris physician, Dr Joseph Guillotin (1738–1814), whose praise of its humanity (it was fast and foolproof) illustrates the Revolution's chilling blend of idealism and inhumanity. Like others, Wordsworth soon disowned the Revolution, but friend and foe alike agreed the world would never be the same again.

The nineteenth-century 'age of revolutions' which culminated in the First World War (1914–18) and the Russian Revolution (1917) brought unremitting, irresistible change. Erupting first in Britain, industrialization transformed the environment, natural and human, promising man's conquest over nature – or, in the eyes of critics, creating a Moloch of mechanization to gratify futile greed. Everyday life was transformed by technological innovations: steam engines and printing-presses, steam ships and the iron horse, and later electricity, the motor car and finally powered flight, with the Wright brothers becoming airborne in 1903. Throughout Europe and North America, population took off too, especially in industrial boom-towns blazing with opportunities for work and wealth but riddled with poverty, misery, disease and death – all products of a cut-throat competitive system in which masters and men alike were enslaved to the market.

Were they on the bloodied battlefields of liberty or in the squalid slums of Liverpool, all such changes made pressing demands upon medicine, nor could medicine itself escape transformation, thanks largely to the march of science. Bacon, Harvey, Galileo, Descartes and Newton had launched the New Science; the Enlightenment popularized it; but it was the age post-1800 that bankrolled public science, bringing new manpower, institutions, teaching, training and expectations. The state turned patron; new scientific bodies were founded; and reformers declared science the dynamo of progress. Directly and indirectly, medicine benefited from such transformations. It gained standing for being scientific, and ambitious medical men pressed to learn its procedures and speak its slogans. 'The physician without physiology and chemistry', remarked the eminent Canadian physician William Osler in 1894, 'flounders along in an aimless fashion, never able to gain any accurate conception of disease, practising a sort of popgun pharmacy.' Scientific medicine, by contrast, meant to get its magic bullets on target, though there was little agreement as to what it was or how it was to be practised.

PARIS MEDICINE

The mother of revolution, Paris also gave birth to the new medicine as reforms in medical policies and institutions afforded golden opportunities to ambitious physicians. New programmes of medical inquiry, new disease concepts and research practices were introduced. The outcome was a distinctive Parisian hospital medicine characterized by scientific observation and raised on pathological anatomy, the paradigm of the lesion, quantification and, not least, sublime faith in its own superiority.

The Revolution and its aftermath removed hospitals from the hands of the Church into those of the nation. The medical revolution was the work of a cadre of physicians seizing the opportunities afforded by salaried appointments in Paris's vast public hospitals – their 20,000 beds outnumbered England's entire in-patient population. French hospitals had traditionally been pious foundations devoted to tending the sick; elite physicians were to turn them into scientific machines for investigating diseases and for teaching the vast numbers of students (up to five thousand at a time) flocking to the capital for medical training. Perhaps taking their cue from Napoleon himself, they promoted themselves as captains of destiny, one of them, Jean Nicolas Corvisart (1755–1821), serving as the emperor's personal physician. 'I do not believe in medicine,' declared the emperor, 'but I do believe in Corvisart.'

This hospital milieu bred new priorities. Clinical practice had always leant heavily on traditional bookish teachings and the physician's personal sagacity; but yesterday's authorities went the way of the *ancien régime* as the revolutionary doctors put bodies before books, prizing the hands-on experience gained through indefatigable examination of the diseased, and later of their cadavers. Endorsing the Enlightenment empiricism of the philosopher-doctor Pierre Cabanis (1757–1808), Paris medicine's golden rule was 'read little, see much, do much'.

Objective and analytic in spirit, and completing the programme of Vesalian anatomy, it used autopsies to corroborate bedside diagnoses. The nuances of this or that patient were brushed aside, for such symptoms were now viewed as mere foam on the surface of what Jean Louis Alibert (1768–1837) called the 'uncharted ocean of disease'. What killed were underlying lesions – tumours, inflammation, gangrene – so attention had to focus on diseases understood as conditions with laws of their own, afflicting all alike; medicine's job was to establish the patterns of pathology. The new doctor was a detective, using the investigative tool of clinical-pathological correlation to be tirelessly on disease's trail.

Though these shifts in medical outlook were momentous, their abruptness should not be exaggerated. Earlier doctors had walked the woeful wards, displaying charity patients to their students and, as we have seen, clinical lecturing had grown up in eighteenth-century Leiden, Vienna and Edinburgh. The convergence of surgical with medical training encouraged anatomical knifework and fostered solidist and localist thinking. Thomas Sydenham and others had insisted that diseases were not simply patchworks of symptoms but clear and distinct entities ripe for taxonomy; from the 1760s Morgagni had made morbid anatomy the clue to sickness in the living. Thus the localized disease concepts promoted in Paris were not spontaneously generated, nor for that matter did the procedures pioneered in its showcase hospitals transform medicine at a stroke. Elite private practice drifted on much as before, and the new hospital medicine brought no quick therapeutic gains. Even so, Paris fashions, as always, made the world stare, and the new model of a science of disease enjoyed remarkable sway.

Dubbed anatomico-pathological to distinguish it from the age-old holistic stress on humoral balance, Paris medicine built upon the tissue pathology developed by Bichat. His *Traité de membranes* (1799) [Treatise on Membranes] viewed the human body in health, and particularly disease, through new eyes. In place of symptoms or organs, tissues assumed primacy, regarded as basic building-blocks and as pathological sites. Even as the guillotine was dispensing its political medicine, this outlook made death the essence of medical inquiry. In Bichat's view, life ('the sum of all the functions by which death is resisted') became somehow contingent, evanescent and, in the end, a loser. No longer was dying, as the Hippocratics taught, a natural terminus; like the Terror, indeed like the Grim Reaper, death ruled the world.

Bichat told doctors what to do: 'You may take notes for twenty years from morning to night at the bedside of the sick,' his *Anatomie générale* (1801) [General Anatomy] drily observed, 'and all will be to you only a confusion of symptoms . . . a train of incoherent phenomena.' But start cutting bodies open and, hey presto, 'this obscurity will soon disappear'. Here was the medicine of the all-powerful gaze.

Of those who took up Bichat's challenge to 'look and see', the physician who especially stamped his mark on the future was René Théophile Hyacinthe Laennec (1781–1826). He became physician to the Salpêtrière Hospital in 1814 and two years later chief at the Hôpital Necker – both vast infirmaries affording boundless access to the sick poor, or what tellingly became commodified as 'clinical material'. In 1816 Laennec devised the stethoscope, the chief tool of this new medicine of objective signs until the discovery of X-rays. By giving access to body noises – the sounds of breathing, the blood gurgling around the heart – the stethoscope changed approaches to internal disease and hence doctor-patient relations. At last, the living body was no longer a closed book: pathology could now be done on the living.

Clinical observation had previously been restricted to externals and diagnosis reliant on what the patient's history yielded. Auenbrugger's percussion technique – rapping the chest and listening to the different tones given off, to gauge the state of the internal organs – might have altered that. But it lay neglected until Corvisart translated his treatise, proceeding, on the basis of personal clinical experience, to publish the *Essai sur les maladies et les lésions organiques du coeur et des gros vaisseaux* (1806) [An Essay on the Organic Diseases and Lesions of the Heart and Great Vessels], a toehold in the arduous terrain of heart disease.

Why had physicians neglected internal diseases? The problem, judged the testy Corvisart, lay in ignorance of anatomy. The result? Myopic physicians had gone on misdiagnosing disease. The old rituals for determining symptoms would not do. Symptoms had to be correlated with the lesions found in the body postmortem – the smoking gun. Knowing how the tissues and organs functioned during life was equally vital. Aware that certain heart conditions produced sounds audible some distance from the patient, Corvisart would place his ear directly to the chest (*immediate* auscultation). However, it was Laennec who really capitalized on the opportunities provided by auscultation; he recorded a particular *Eureka!* moment:

> In 1816 I was consulted by a young woman presenting general symptoms of disease of the heart. Owing to her stoutness little information could be gathered by application of the hand and percussion. The patient's age and sex did not permit me to resort to [direct application of ear to chest]. I recalled a well-known acoustic phenomenon: namely, if you place your ear against one end of a wooden beam the scratch of a pin at the other extremity

is distinctly audible. It occurred to me that this physical property might serve a useful purpose in the case with which I was then dealing. Taking a sheet of paper I rolled it into a very tight roll, one end of which I placed on the precordial region, whilst I put my ear to the other. I was both surprised and gratified at being able to hear the beating of the heart with much greater clearness and distinctness than I had ever before by direct application of my ear.

Instantly, Laennec tells us, he grasped the significance of his discovery: it would be the key for 'studying, not only the beating of the heart, but likewise all movements capable of producing sound in the thoracic cavity'.

The first stethoscope was described in his 900-page *Traité de l'auscultation médiate* (1819) [Treatise on Mediate Auscultation]. It was a one-ear wooden instrument, 9 inches long and 1½ inches in diameter, made in two pieces which screwed together, with detachable ear- and chest-pieces. Minor modifications followed; by mid century, rubber tubing had been introduced to create a flexible monaural stethoscope, and in 1852 an American physician, George P. Cammann, devised our familiar two-ear instrument.

Attuning himself to normal and abnormal breath sounds audible through the instrument, Laennec developed exquisite skills for diagnosing pulmonary ailments such as bronchitis, pneumonia and above all tuberculosis (phthisis or consumption), the 'white plague' that was the age's greatest scourge. (Laennec was himself to succumb, with many other contemporaries, including the surgical student and poet, John Keats (1795–1821), and two of opera's tragic heroines, *La Traviata*'s Violetta and Mimi in *La Bohème*.) By bypassing the patient's unreliable account, diagnosis could be rendered objective. Thus of the sensations reported by patients Laennec noted that 'none suffices to characterize disease of the heart', and so 'for a certain diagnosis we must recur to mediate auscultation.' To underscore the difference this made, it is worth contrasting old and new. The fine eighteenth-century clinician William Heberden left this account of consumption based upon a lifetime of taking histories and close observation:

> The phthisis pulmonum usually begins with a dry cough, so light and inconsiderable, that little or no notice is taken of it, till its continuance, and gradual increase, begin to make it regarded. Such a cough has lasted for a few years without bringing on other complaints. It has sometimes wholly ceased, and after a truce of a very

uncertain length it has returned, and after frequent recoveries and relapses the patient begins at last to find an accession of other symptoms, which in bad cases will very soon follow the appearance of the first cough. These are shortness of breath, hoarseness, loss of appetite, wasting of the flesh and strength, pains in the breast, profuse sweats during sleep, spitting of blood and matter, shiverings succeeded by hot fits, with flushings of the face, and burning of the hands and feet, and a pulse constantly above ninety, a swelling of the legs, and an obstruction of the menstrua in women; a very small stone has sometimes been coughed up, and in the last stages of this illness a diarrhoea helps to waste the little remainder of flesh and strength.

Laennec's approach could not have been more different, homing in on physical change beneath the skin and manifesting the disease-centredness of the new medicine:

A woman, aged 40, came in the Hospital 29th January, having been affected with cough for five months, and which had increased since her confinement, three months ago. At this time the respiration was short and quick, and difficult; the chest resounded pretty well in the back and left side before, – but better on the right side; there was distinct pectoriloquism near the junction of the sternum and left clavicle, and the same phenomenon, but less distinct, on the same side where the arm joined the chest; the sound of the ventricles was dull, and the heart gave hardly any impulse. Two days after, by means of the cylinder, we distinguished a sound resembling fluctuation, in the left side, when the patient coughed, and the metallick tinkling when she spoke. Succussion of the trunk did not produce the sound of fluctuation. From these results the following diagnostic was given: very large tuberculous excavation in the middle of the left lung, containing a small quantity of very liquid tuberculous matter. The patient died five days after this.

Dissection twenty-four hours after death. In the right lung, through its whole extent, there were innumerable tubercles of a yellowish white colour, and varying in size from that of a hemp-seed to a cherry-stone, and even a large filbert. These last were evidently formed by the reunion of several small ones, and, for the most part, were more or less softened ... The left lung adhered closely to the pleura of the ribs and pericardium. On its anterior and lateral part it contained, near its surface, three cavities, one above the other, and communicating by two large openings ...

Heberden's sick person, gradually wasting away, has effectively disappeared, having been replaced by the patient's pleural cavity. The disease is revealed through auscultation; the diagnosis is encoded in anatomical technicalities; and the speedy autopsy proves the diagnosis was spot on. The long-term implications of this new way of seeing were pointed out later by the German physician Robert Volz (1806–82): 'The sick person has become a thing.'

Laennec provided the inspiration, instrument, techniques and programme for a generation of outstanding students of respiratory conditions. Stethoscopy won acclaim, and translations of his book spread the procedure no less than the foreigners flocking into Paris to share his rounds. The device became scientific medicine's hallmark. In George Eliot's novel *Middlemarch*, set in the early 1830s, the hero Tertius Lydgate, just back from his medical training in Paris, irks his stick-in-the-mud colleagues by singing the praises of this new-fangled foreign 'toy', and divides the community.

The high point of Laennec's treatise was the 200-page section on pulmonary tuberculosis. Clear descriptions were provided of the clinical course of 'phthisis', as well as guidance for diagnosing its early stages. Holding that the tubercle (the tuberculous nodule) was the mark of a single condition, be it found in the lungs, gut, liver or brain, he created the idea of a unified disease, tuberculosis, though this view remained contestable until bacteriologists discovered the bacillus. Laennec thought it had hereditary aspects and denied it was contagious, believing that in many cases a psychosomatic element ('sad passions') played a part. His own temper and losing battle with the disease perhaps prompted such beliefs.

Laennec's work complemented that of his colleague, Gaspard Laurent Bayle (1774–1816), who also died of the disease he studied. Enjoying the luxury of financial independence, Bayle had dabbled in theology, law and politics before making medicine his vocation. Joining the prestigious Charité hospital in 1807, he was later appointed physician to Napoleon's household. In his *Recherches sur la phthisie pulmonaire* (1810) [Researches on Pulmonary Phthisis], he preceded Laennec in proposing tuberculosis as a specific disease – not, as accepted, a generalized morbid wasting process (consumption) following a previous malady – establishing that tubercles would develop prior to the appearance of any symptoms. But though it was a single disease, the apostle of localism distinguished different forms, dependent on place, including tuberculosis of the ovaries, tubercular laryngitis, lymphadenitis (inflammation of the lymph nodes) and acute miliary tuberculosis (involving lesions resembling millet seeds). His *Traité des maladies cancereuses* (1833) [Treatise on Cancer] used similar methods to pioneer the study of cancer pathology.

Determined by physical diagnosis and appallingly swiftly confirmed by autopsy – for what was to be done about such lethal diseases? – lesions were prized by Paris medicine as the key to pathogenesis. Hospitals had 'clinical material' galore, and the signs and lesions there repeated, ward after ward, week after week, proved surer guides to pathogenesis than subjective symptoms. Corvisart, Laennec, Bayle and their *protégés* achieved diagnostic eminence through scrutiny of more bodies than any physicians had ever seen. Clinical medicine aimed to be a science; it hinged on the 'gaze' (clinical detachment), and was to be imbibed through the vigil of countless hours in the ward and the morgue.

Medical training, it followed, had therefore to be a matter of drilling students to interpret the sights, sounds and smells of disease – in short, a morbid education of the senses. Clinical judgment was the elucidation of what trained senses perceived, its end being to designate disease. Other departments of medicine came a distant second – even physiology, to say nothing of poor relations like pharmacy. With the cases filling the Paris hospitals, therapeutics was often beside the point, though Laennec, perhaps prompted by his own coughing, expressed a faith in the Hippocratic healing power of nature.

The youngest member of the cohort, Pierre Louis (1787–1872), drove this outlook one stage further, championing the use of numerical methods. Inheriting the quantifying spirit of the Enlightenment, as mediated through Condorcet's and Laplace's work on probability, Louis used simple arithmetic to put therapies to the test, for 'it is precisely because of the impossibility of judging each individual case with any sort of mathematical accuracy that it is necessary to count.' A single case taught nothing, but if two large batches of blindly selected patients underwent distinct treatments, differential mortality figures would assume genuine significance. In invoking arithmetic to evaluate therapeutics, Louis paved the way for the clinical trial, while providing models for the social statistics employed by Adolphe Quetelet (1796–1874) and more sophisticated biometricians like Karl Pearson (1857–1936).

Using *la méthode numérique* to test phlebotomy, Louis revealed that it made no difference to the outcome of pneumonia whether venesection was performed early or late, or whether large or small draughts of blood were let; in fact, nothing had much effect. Likewise, no therapies did much good with various fevers. Louis has sometimes been dubbed a therapeutic nihilist; his early medical experience in Russia had indeed taught him the sobering fact that medicine rarely cured. A pessimistic pall seemed to hang over Paris: medicine, mused Corvisart, 'is not the art of curing diseases', leading his editor to call his *oeuvre* 'a meditation on death'. Louis, however, was less a dogmatic nihilist than one distrustful of extravagant success claims; in this his particular *bête noire* was F. J. V. Broussais (1772–1838) who, like Galen, cried up blood-letting for virtually everything.

Paris medicine's meticulousness in documenting pathologies underscored the ontological model of diseases as discrete entities – real things. The shift from reliance upon the symptoms sufferers reported (now depreciated as subjective) to signs (praised as objective signifiers of lesions) bolstered the idea that disease was quite a different state from health. Not all agreed. Broussais accused his Paris peers of perverting medicine by localizing pathological anatomy, their obsessive creed of specificity and their therapeutic gloom. How could one understand disease without first grasping normal functioning?

Chief physician at the Paris Val de Grace military hospital, Broussais fired off polemical salvos. Bichat's true legacy, he argued, lay not in localism but in recognition of the primacy of physiology, and hence in furthering the notion that the difference between the normal and the pathological lay on a continuum. Disease was not distinct from health as black from white; rather illnesses occurred when normal functions went awry: they were shades of grey. Broussais set the dynamics of pathophysiology above pathological anatomy – a palpable hit at localism's Achilles' heel.

Broussais' *Examen des doctrines médicales et des systèmes de nosologie* (1821) [Examination of the Medical Doctrines and the Systems of Nosology] held that disease was not an ontological 'other' but the result of altered functions – too much or too little of regular processes. The prime source of such changes was excessive gastro-intestinal irritation, local manifestations elsewhere being sympathetic inflammatory reactions to the primary trouble. And if all diseases were ultimately the outcome of one fundamental cause, gastroenteritis, all, he reasoned, were to be treated by one therapy: blood-letting, preferably by leeches. Perhaps the most sanguinary physician in history – though Benjamin

Rush must have run him close – Broussais recommended applying leeches* fifty at a time, all over the skin. His disciple, Jean Baptiste Bouillard (1796–1881), followed suit, recommending copious phlebotomy, bleeding his patients time and again, removing up to three litres from those stricken with pneumonia. In some ways Broussais' views echoed John Brown's seductive doctrine of the unitary nature of disease; and, like Brunonianism, his *idée fixe*, inflammation, seemed cranky to many.

But though Broussais' star soon waned, he proved of lasting importance, not for his obsession with gastric inflammation but for his critique of hospital medicine in the light of Bichatian physiology. His idea of a slope from health to sickness was later persuasive for the towering figures of Claude Bernard and Rudolf Virchow, feeding the insight that physiological phenomena – the concentration of chemicals in the blood or urine, the ratio of red and white blood cells, body temperature or blood pressure – varied around a mean to be correlated by age, sex or physique. If the patho-anatomists were consumed with disease and death, Broussais' physiology opened windows onto the laws of life – and incidentally influenced the positivist philosophy of Auguste Comte (1798–1857), who analysed society in physiological terms as an organism.

THE INFLUENCE OF PARIS

Though not exactly a coterie, the Paris professors assumed some collective identity, and from the end of the Napoleonic Wars students converged from Europe and North America to learn from them first-hand, Laennec alone teaching some 300 foreign pupils. Apart from the wine, women and song, one great inducement for students to study in Paris

---

* *Hirudo medicinalis*, the slug-like leech used to suck blood, is 1½ inches long, expanding to 6 inches on feeding. It has 10 stomachs down each side. Wordsworth celebrated a leech-gatherer in 1807:

> He told, that to these waters he had come
> To gather leeches, being old and poor:
> Employment hazardous and wearisome!

In 1825 France was a leech-exporting country; by 1837 it was importing 33 million leeches: what had Broussais done to the balance of payments?

was that they had free run of the public hospitals; it was easier to get ample bedside and dissection experience there than anywhere else. Instructed and inspired, students then returned to London or Lisbon, Vienna or Philadelphia to beat the drum for French medicine. Pioneering English stethoscopists like Thomas Hodgkin (1798–1866) were proud to have learned the art directly from the master.

Hodgkin had a career pattern typical of the time. A Quaker like many other English medical students of his generation (Friends were excluded from politics and the military), he went to Edinburgh, but broke his studies with a year in Paris; and so inspired was he by Laennec that he went back for more. In 1825 he settled in London as lecturer in morbid anatomy at Guy's Hospital, introducing the stethoscope and giving the first systematic lectures in English on the new French pathology. Deploying the techniques of morbid anatomy, his paper 'On Some Morbid Appearances of the Absorbent Glands and Spleen' (1832) described what was later called Hodgkin's Disease, a malignant disease of the lymph glands, involving enlargement of the lymph nodes and lymphatic tissue.

Following the French, medical education everywhere grew more systematic and scientific, drilling students in the stern discipline of diagnosis. Through such means, Vienna recouped its fading fortunes. Though its university had been one of the early pioneers of bedside teaching in the Boerhaavian era, thanks to Van Swieten and de Haen, decay had set in before revival by the Paris-inspired Carl von Rokitansky (1804–78), who made pathological anatomy compulsory. Rokitansky was the age's champion dissector – his institute did over 1,500 necropsies a year and he supposedly performed 60,000 autopsies in the course of his career. He was a master of patho-anatomy, making notable studies of congenital malformations and conditions like peptic ulcer, pneumonia and valvular heart disease, written up in his *Handbuch der pathologische Anatomie* (1842–6) [Handbook of Pathological Anatomy]. 'Pathological anatomy must constitute the groundwork, not only of all medical knowledge, but also of all medical treatment,' he taught, 'it embraces all that medicine has to offer of positive knowledge.' On that basis he would reason from end-stage disease backwards, to reconstruct the sequence of changes which must have led to the necropsy findings.

Alongside Rokitansky worked the more clinically oriented Joseph Skoda (1805–81), a blacksmith's son who had walked all the way from Pilsen in Bohemia to study in Vienna. In the French manner, he devoted his attention to chest diseases, writing a major work on percussion and auscultation which assigned to each of the sounds its musical pitch and medical meaning. As well as doing much to further physical diagnosis, Skoda was the first Viennese professor to follow the example of Paracelsus three centuries earlier and abandon Latin, to lecture in German.

At a time when its population was racing past the million mark, London medicine was also developing, stimulated by the founding of London University and its associated teaching hospitals and by rivalry with Paris. Since around 1750 the capital's hospitals had been taking physicians' and surgeons' pupils in growing numbers, though their governors regarded this with some qualms, anxious lest patient care might be jeopardized and donors deterred. Hence, while the Paris hospitals frankly became machines for teaching and research, in Britain patients were less likely to be turned into 'clinical material' to satisfy students, and autopsies, as Americans in London complained, were not so frequent. In retrospect, as James Paget was to recall, a medical training in London seemed pretty disorganized:

> I entered at St Bartholomew's Hospital on the 3rd or 4th of October, 1834. . . . There was very little, or no, personal guidance; the demonstrators had some private pupils, whom they 'ground' for the College examinations, but these were only a small portion of the school; the surgeons had apprentices, to whom they seldom taught more than to other students; for the most part, the students guided themselves or one another to evil or to good, to various degrees of work or of idleness. No one was, in any sense, responsible for them. I am not sure that, being well disposed for work, I was the worse for this.
>
> The dead-house (it was never called by any better name) was a miserable kind of shed, stonefloored, damp and dirty, where all stood around a table on which the examinations were made. And these were usually made in the roughest and least instructive way; and, unless one of the physicians were present, nothing was carefully looked at, nothing was taught. Pathology, in any fair sense of the word, was hardly considered.

London, however, was in the process of modernizing and restructuring its medical teaching. The 1815 Apothecaries Act specified that all apothecaries (in effect, general practitioners) must henceforth possess the Licence of the Society of Apothecaries (LSA); candidates were required to attend lectures on anatomy, botany, chemistry, *materia medica*, and the theory and practice of physic, and also to undertake six months' hospital bedside work. By the 1830s more than 400 students per year were taking the LSA, and demand for clinical training soared, forcing hospitals to expand teaching facilities. By 1841 St Bartholomew's had 300 pupils; there were scores of students in other London hospital schools too; and the new London University possessed two colleges, University and King's, each with a new hospital, opened in 1837 and 1840 respectively.

As with Bichat in Paris, London bathed in the reflected glory of John Hunter. His devoted disciples ran the private anatomy schools that upheld the Hunterian gospel of anatomy, an orientation rather different from the Paris accent on pathology. The crown prince of that tradition was the surgeon Charles Bell; migrating from Edinburgh to London, in 1812 he acquired William Hunter's old Windmill Street anatomy school. Like other British anatomists, he was distrustful of animal vivisection on both moral and medical grounds, so his scope as an experimenter had limits. His *Essays on the Anatomy of Expression in Painting* (1806) reaffirmed the old alliance between art and anatomy.

The career of Robert Knox (1791–1862) exemplifies the strengths and weaknesses of British anatomy. Appealing to medical students and gentlemen alike, his inspiring extra-mural lectures attracted classes of five hundred in Edinburgh. But at the peak of his fame, he fell foul of a snare threatening British anatomy. Brisk demand for bodies to dissect but lack of an adequate legal supply had ensured good business for the 'resurrectionists', who robbed new graves to sell their spoils to anatomists like Knox.

In 1827 an old man died in William Hare's (1792–1870) boarding-house. Assisted by his lodger, William Burke (1792–1829), Hare hit upon the idea of direct selling to anatomists, bypassing the grave altogether. Spurred by success, they turned next to murder, luring victims in and suffocating them, so that the corpse betrayed no trace of violence. Sixteen were done to death and their bodies sold, fetching around £7 each, before Burke and Hare were brought to justice in 1829. Hare turned King's evidence and Burke was hanged, his body being publicly anatomized and flayed, and his skin tanned and sold by the strip. The final cadaver had been discovered in Knox's dissecting rooms; despite his howls of innocence, the incensed crowd burned down his house, and he fled to London with his career in tatters, eventually dying in obscurity.

One outcome of such body-snatching outrages was the passing of the 1832 Anatomy Act, which, over the protests of a public distrustful of anatomists, awarded the medical profession rights to 'unclaimed bodies' – in effect, paupers without family dying in workhouses and hospitals. Despite the Burke and Hare débâcle, the anatomical tradition retained its vitality in Britain, explaining among other things an immortal work produced by Henry Gray (1827–61), an anatomy lecturer at St George's Hospital who suffered an early death from smallpox. *Gray's Anatomy, Descriptive and Applied* first appeared in 1858, and in time became the anatomist's bible. An updated version is still in print at the end of the twentieth century.

Alongside Hunterian anatomy Britain was absorbing the new French medicine. One pioneer, already mentioned, was Thomas Hodgkin; another was Thomas Addison (1793–1860). An Edinburgh graduate, Addison practised in London, becoming assistant physician at Guy's Hospital in 1824. While characteristically averse to specialization ('it savoured of quackery'), he followed Laennec and applied the stethoscope to chest disorders. Later he gave the first description of 'a remarkable form of anaemia' which often resulted in death, postmortems revealing disease in the suprarenals, organs just above the kidneys. His *On the Constitutional and Local Effects of Disease of the Suprarenal Capsules* (1855) distinguished two kinds of anaemia: one, that known later as 'pernicious anaemia' in which no organic lesion could be found; the other, the version involving darkened skin and diseased suprarenal capsules, since known as Addison's disease, from which Jane Austen died.

Another of the 'great men of Guy's' was Addison's colleague Richard Bright (1789–1858). The son of a Bristol banker, he too received his medical education at Edinburgh before settling in London to become assistant physician at Guy's in 1820. Investigating the pathology of dropsy, a common disease marked by accumulation of fluid in the tissues, his *Reports of Medical Cases Selected with a View of Illustrating the Symptoms and Cure of Disease by Reference to Morbid Anatomy* (1827) described twenty-three cases which postmortem showed to be due to renal disease. Since heating a sufferer's urine precipitated albumen as an opaque white material, and dropsy was accompanied by shrinking of the kidneys, a connexion was established between a patient's symptoms and lesions visible at autopsy. French methods once again proved effective in linking symptoms, signs and pathogenesis. At Guy's, Bright set aside two wards for kidney patients, with a laboratory and a consulting room attached, a precursor of the clinical research unit.

Irish medicine too fell under continental influence. Before becoming physician to the Meath Hospital in Dublin, Robert Graves (1796–1853) spent several years studying on the Continent, as his chief work, *Clinical Lectures on the Practice of Medicine* (1843), makes clear. He is famous for describing the bulging eyes (exophthalmus) and other symptoms linked to toxic goitre (Graves' disease or hyperthyroidism). His colleague William Stokes (1804–78), while only twenty-one, published a treatise on the stethoscope, inspired by Laennec. He collaborated with Graves in developing the new system of clinical instruction, and his *The Diagnosis and Treatment of Diseases of the Chest* (1837) made his name as a clinician. Stokes described the type of breathing since known as 'Cheyne-Stokes respiration', and noted its ominousness. With Robert Adams (1791–1875), he also recorded cases of slow pulse, accompanied by syncope (loss of consciousness): the 'Stokes-Adams syndrome'.

While the new French hospital medicine was being naturalized into Britain, American medical students, largely from Boston, Philadelphia and New York, were sailing (or later steaming) across the Atlantic. Three mid-century luminaries of the Philadelphia Hospital and Medical College – Alfred Stillé (1813–1900), William Gerhard (1809–72) and Samuel Morton (1799–1851) had studied in Paris, going on to produce French-style researches on consumption, typhus and typhoid. The *laissez-faire* climate of the US was not, however, congenial for high-quality medical schools and investigations; most of the sixty or so proprietary colleges which sprang up before 1875 were poorly staffed and blatantly commercial, offering quick degrees on the cheap. Owen Tully Stratton (1868–1950), who in 1895 attended the Barnes Medical College in St Louis, recalled that, on graduation, 'I'd never had the advantage of practicing under a preceptor, never dressed a serious wound, had never given a hypodermic, had never been present when a baby was born. I had no bedside manner, since I had never attended a bedside in a professional capacity.'

In the United States well-educated regulars were in a bind. Not only were they at risk of losing out to rivals from teaching factories but they faced hot competition from medical sects which ran their own colleges. Not least, the therapeutic nihilism of Paris medicine, which was well-adapted to French charity hospitals, was hopeless for a nation of intrepid pioneers. Following Rush's lead, regulars went to the opposite extreme, making heroic therapeutics their trademark, partly to demarcate themselves from the irregulars' pious trust in nature, herbs and water. The formation of the American Medical Association in 1847, with Stillé as one of its secretaries, gave the regulars an institutional anchor, but overall they remained on the defensive.

GERMANY AND THE LABORATORY

Paris teachings turned the morgue into a shrine. Another site of medical worship emerged, challenging and to some degree supplanting the hospital as the hub of discovery: the laboratory. By 1850, laboratories were creating a new physiology and pathology and beginning to reshape medical education. Laboratory medicine was of course not new – it went back at least to the seventeenth century – but nineteenth-century laboratory lions prided themselves on creating a distinct scientific medicine based on microscopy, vivisection, chemical investigations and everything else measurable, weighable and testable in its uniquely controlled environment. The hospital, they admitted, was fine for observing, but the laboratory was tailormade for experiment. The stethoscope was thus challenged by the microscope, whose improvements ushered in a new discipline, histology, which bridged anatomy and physiology. 'Learn to see microscopically,' Rudolf Virchow told his pupils, insisting that 'experiment is the final and highest court of pathological physiology, for experiment alone shows the specific phenomenon in its dependency on specific conditions, for these conditions are arranged by choice.'

As late as 1819, when the word histology was coined, the value of the microscope was still disputed – had not brilliant investigators like Bichat preferred the naked eye? Microscopists might purport to show how all tissues were composed of tiny globules, but were not these phenomena rank optical distortions? Major technical improvements were on the way, however, being introduced by Joseph Jackson Lister (1786–1869), father of the illustrious surgeon. In 1826 he produced an instrument with a far superior high-magnification performance, and thanks to this was able to publish with Thomas Hodgkin in 1827 the paper often credited with founding modern histology, revealing the structure of tissues to be fibres not globules. Further design improvements followed until, by 1890, resolution had reached a high point.

Overawed perhaps by Bichat's scepticism, French researchers were slow to respond, and it was in Germany that microscopy was most warmly welcomed, spurring the new cell biology and pathology which were quite unthinkable without it. Though German lens-making initially lagged, in 1846 Carl Zeiss (1816–88) established his workshop in Jena, and within half a century the firms of Zeiss and Leitz had achieved industrial supremacy. Before long, Germany was envied for its instruments, which became cheaper and simpler to handle, and thus were suitable for student use. Expert fixing of tissues, to render specimens permanent and highlight their parts, was established by about 1870, while colour-staining was standard by 1880; sectioning of specimens was achieved soon after, and formaldehyde was introduced in 1893. Together, these provided the necessary preparative techniques. Even so, the practical challenges facing microscopists demanded great skill and patience.

Among the trailblazers was Jacob Henle (1809–85), one of Johannes Müller's many protégés, who was to hold anatomy chairs successively at Zürich, Heidelberg and Göttingen. His three-volume *Handbuch der systematischen Anatomie des Menschen* (1866–71) [Handbook of Systematic Human Anatomy] addressed the body from an architectural standpoint, describing its macro- and microscopic structure. As the discoverer of the tubules of the kidney, and the first to describe the muscular coat of the arteries, the minute anatomy of the eye and various skin structures, Henle gained a name as the Vesalius of histology, but his real importance was as an educator. He was among the first to make the microscope a tool used by students themselves, thus pointing to experimental physiology as central to medical training.

Another Müller man, Albert von Kölliker (1817–1905), produced the first histological textbook in his *Handbuch der Gewebelehre des Menschen* (1852) [Handbook of the Tissues of Man], applying cell theory to descriptive embryology. 'Medicine has reached a point', he proclaimed, 'at which microscopical anatomy appears to constitute its foundation, quite as much as the anatomy of the organs and systems.' In Britain, the first work devoted to microscopic preparations was brought out in 1848 by John Quekett (1815–61), who initiated histology courses at the Royal College of Surgeons as well as making thousands of preparations, many of which survive. By mid century, the microscope was giving medicine new eyes.

Technological improvements mean little, however, without matching advances in ideas and opportunities – recall how Leeuwenhoek's stunning observations founded no tradition. Such openings were provided by German universities, which were then developing a research ethos with momentous implications for medical investigation, training and (finally) practice. Impressed by the educational reforms brought about in Prussia by Wilhelm von Humboldt (1769–1859), rulers looked to investment in academic science (*Wissenschaft*) as the highroad to national prestige and industrial progress. German universities and their attached specialist scientific institutes blossomed into research centres, whose budgets and staffing levels were the envy of the world. Professors were granted freedom to teach their specialities (*Lehrfreiheit*), while students could tramp from one campus to another (*Lernfreiheit*). All this amounted to a recipe for research unparalleled in France or Britain, where universities were less engines of inquiry than extensions of high-school or finishing schools for gentlemen.

A model for laboratory science was provided by Liebig's Institute of Chemistry at Giessen University. After studying at Bonn and Erlangen, Justus von Liebig (1803–73) passed two years in Paris before being appointed in 1824 (when barely twenty-one) chemistry professor at Giessen, where his institute was a magnet for students seeking practical training in chemical analysis. Success bred success, until the University of Munich lured him away in 1852.

Liebig's life work lay in experimental study of the energy-producing function of food through techniques of controlled measurement; 'God has ordered all His Creation by Weight and Measure,' announced the motto over his laboratory door. It was not a completely unploughed field. Between 1809 and 1825 an Animal Chemistry Society in London investigated animal heat, and William Prout (1785–1850) delivered lectures on animal chemistry, predicting that, though physiology had hitherto gained little from chemistry, it could prove 'one of the most powerful instruments'.

Addressing nutrition, Prout showed that the contents of the stomach contained hydrochloric acid, and hypothesized that, since mother's milk was the basic nutrient, its constituents should provide a classification of foodstuffs: oleaginous materials (fats), saccharinous substances (carbohydrates) and albuminous or nitrogenous matter (proteins). From this he formulated a speculative physiological chemistry in which fats, sugars and nitrogenous substances were chemically transformed by adding or removing water, electrolytes and tiny quantities of minerals, the underlying idea being to establish the chemical basis of an adequate diet.

Like most contemporaries, Prout was a vitalist who believed the chemistry of living beings was altogether different from that of un-organized materials, such differences being explained by a 'principle of organization'. 'Imbued by the Creator with a faculty little short of Intelligence', this vital principle synthesized organic substances from inorganic elements into combinations unlike those in the mineral kingdom. Living systems could be sustained only by 'the constant and unremitting agency of the vital principle'; otherwise death resulted, releasing the atoms into their original inorganic state.

Another who made nutrition his study, albeit only thanks to a bizarre stroke of luck, was William Beaumont (1785–1853). This US army surgeon, stationed at Fort Mackinac on Lake Erie, was summoned in 1822 to a trading post on the Canadian border to treat Alexis St Martin, a nineteen-year-old trapper who had received a gaping shotgun wound in the abdomen. He recovered, except for a permanent stomach fistula, open to the outside (it had to be plugged during meals to stop the food oozing out).

Though without academic training, Beaumont took advantage of his patient's unique window to conduct experiments on digestive processes, investigating the appearance and properties of digestive fluid. He introduced into St Martin raw and cooked meat and other foods, rather as with Réaumur's earlier experiments with his pet kite, tying pieces of thread to them so that they could be recovered. The digestibility of different types of edibles was put to the test:

> August 1 1825. At 12 o'clock I introduced through the perforation, into the stomach, the following articles of diet, suspended with a silk string, so as to pass in without pain: viz. a piece of high seasoned *à la mode beef*; a piece of *raw, salted fat pork*; a piece of *raw, salted, lean beef*; a piece of *boiled, salted beef*; a piece of *stale bread*; and a bunch of *raw, sliced cabbage*.

The cabbage and bread were digested first, then the pork and boiled beef; the *boeuf à la mode* took longest. From numerous experiments Beaumont showed how the digestive processes worked not through maceration or putrefaction of foodstuffs but through the stomach dissolving – that is, beginning to digest – them through its gastric juice. His *Observations on the Gastric Juice and the Physiology of Digestion* (1833), a work used by Claude Bernard and other later investigators of metabolism, confirmed Prout's notion of the presence in the stomach of hydrochloric acid and located the ferment later identified as the protein-breaking enzyme, pepsin. The constraint on Beaumont's work was that he had only St Martin's stomach as his laboratory.

Physiological chemistry was thus not barren. But while advances were being made here and there, it was Liebig who launched the first programme for systematically subjecting experimental animals to rigorous laboratory analysis. Early in his career he introduced a method for determining the amount of urea (which is produced by the breakdown of nitrogenous substances or proteins) in a solution. With Friedrich Wöhler (1800–82), he showed that a small organic group of atoms (or 'radical') was capable of forming an unchanging constituent through a long series of compounds, behaving like an element. This discovery of the benzoyl radical (many more were later distinguished) proved a key to biochemical change.

Liebig read the organism in terms of physico-chemical systems: thus animal heat was not innate, as Galenism had held, but the outcome of Lavoisierian combustion (oxidation). Respiration introduced oxygen, which combined with starches to liberate energy, carbon dioxide and water; nitrogenous material turned into muscle and similar tissues; and the end results included urine, together with phosphates and assorted chemical by-products. Study of input (food, gases, water) and output (acids, salts, water, urea and carbon dioxide) would decipher the 'black box' of the innards. To this end, Liebig drilled his students to perform exhaustive chemical analyses of animal tissues such as liver and muscle, and of fluids such as sweat and urine, measuring the ratios between food intake, oxygen consumption and energy production. Methodical investigation of nutrition and metabolism laid the foundations for what would be called biochemistry.

His friend Wöhler's demonstration that salts or organic acids were transformed into carbonates when passed through an animal's system, and Wöhler's discovery in 1828 that urea could be produced from ammonium nitrate, led Liebig, unlike Prout, to view the distinction between the inorganic and the organic as one of degree not kind, and hence as open to further exploration. His forte lay in the painstaking pursuit of an essentially simple programme designed to lay bare the chemical relationships between the inorganic world and plant and animal life.

Liebig did not just grind out data; he had an entrepreneurial side as well. In 1847 he described an 'extract of meat' prepared by low-pressure evaporation of soup from lean meat, claiming it would be a valuable restorative for the sick. Where cattle were chiefly slaughtered for their hides, as on the pampas, such a food could be cheaply prepared. This suggestion was taken up in the 1860s by an enterprising Brazilian, George Giebert (d. 1874) who worked for Fray Bentos in Uruguay and, with Liebig's assistance, marketed 'Liebig's Extract of Beef' as an invalid food.

Liebig was also speculative, envisaging a grand system governing the economy of nature. Plants, he maintained, derived their food (nitrogen and carbon), from atmospheric carbon dioxide and ammonia, and these compounds were restored to the atmosphere by putrefaction. This pointed to a natural cycle of composition, decomposition and recomposition. Somewhat like Prout, he distinguished 'plastic' foods (nitrogenous substances) from 'respiratory' ones. Carbon-containing fats could be likened to coal, while sugars and starches, derived from fibrous plants, were like wood; fats and sugars were fuels.

He formulated conjectures about disease causation too, maintaining in his *Die organische Chemie in ihrer Anwendung auf Physiologie und Pathologie* (1842) [Animal Chemistry] that when a decomposing substance came into contact with another body, vibratory motion could destabilize the latter. Pathology was thus a question of ferments, consisting of self-reproducing chemical particles spontaneously generated during the decomposition of organic matter. Like the fermentation of sugar to alcohol by yeast, disease was putrefaction; this 'zymotic' theory was popular in mid-century public health circles, until undermined by Pasteur's bacteriology.

The age's great chemist-breeder, Liebig drilled platoons of students in research methods, systematized laboratory research, and revealed how physico-chemical analysis could illuminate biological processes. His reductionist agenda of applying physical science to living organisms encouraged promoters of scientific materialism, who repudiated the idealistic *Naturphilosophie* favoured by Romantics. Liebigians dismissed theories about the meaning of life as speculative rhapsodies. Thanks to Liebig and Wöhler, chemical methods became widely employed in medical research, especially as study of *materia medica* was transformed into pharmacology. But it was physiology which became the high-prestige laboratory discipline that promised to unveil the laws of life.

One branch, relating somewhat tangentially to medicine, was embryology, set on a sound footing as a science of development by Karl Ernst von Baer (1792–1876). Born in Estonia, then part of Prussia, von Baer studied at Dorpat (Tartu) under the influential physiologist Karl

Friedrich Burdach (1776–1847), an exponent of Romantic *Naturphilosophie*, imbibing from him a sense of the importance of *Entwicklungsgeschichte* (development). In 1815 he moved to Würzburg, where he forged his techniques of embryological investigation, while using the Frenchman Georges Cuvier's comparative anatomy as a corrective to the visionary flights of *Naturphilosophie*.

Von Baer's main achievement was establishing the function of the mammalian ovary, resolving one of the great mysteries of the female reproductive system. Sheep experiments had led the great Haller to reaffirm preformationism, but von Baer overturned this by experimenting on his chief's pet bitch, demonstrating the essential role of ovulation in mammalian reproduction. Von Baer also sketched the emergence of life forms from the egg. There was an initial blastoderm that originally comprised four layers: the upper two comprised the 'animal' (serous) layers; the lower the 'vegetative' (plastic). From these 'germ-layers' (*Keimblätter*) arose the different organ systems. The top generated the external coverings of the embryo and the central nervous system; the next gave rise to the muscular and skeletal systems; the third produced the blood-vessels; and the fourth the mucous membrane of the alimentary canal and its processes. These layers became bent over to form tubes, which constituted the body's fundamental organs. Such speculations provided starting-points for later theories respecting the building-blocks of life.

Von Baer stressed that the embryos of various species initially share highly analogous and even indistinguishable forms, gradually differentiating, so that in embryonic development general characters appear before special ones. Nevertheless his *Entwicklungsgeschichte der Thiere* (1828–37) [Developmental History of Animals] rejected the suggestion that the developing human embryo faithfully recapitulated the structures of the lower animals – there was no single path to perfection which the human embryo had to ascend.

Despite such strictures upon the theory of parallelism (the idea that ontogeny recapitulates phylogeny), von Baer retained much of the cast of mind of the *Naturphilosophen*. Convinced of the fundamental unity of the living world, he believed the diversity of animal forms arose from the branching of originally simple models. Since homogeneity led to heterogeneity, embryology offered the best window onto morphology, because it was only by developmental thinking that the true homologies of parts could be grasped.

Whereas Liebig privileged chemistry, von Baer made the embryo-logical or developmental viewpoint basic, linking it to morphology and pointing the way to later versions of 'evolution'. Which was the more fundamental science for explaining life was passionately debated. Never-theless, general physiology could assert pride of place, and its claims were never better staked than by Johannes Müller (1801–58), professor of physiology and anatomy first at Bonn and then from 1833 at Berlin. A gifted neurophysiological researcher, his *Handbuch der Physiologie des Menschen* (2 vols, 1833–40) [Handbook of Human Physiology] became the physiologists' bible, despite what were later seen as certain aberra-tions, such as his vitalistic view of the soul.

Addressing the laws and relationships governing motion in animals, Müller's early studies gave particular attention to glands and their secretions, genital structures, blood and blood vessels, voice and colour vision. In neuro-physiology, he confirmed Bell's and Magendie's experi-ments by tracing electrical paths along the nerve roots: the dorsal roots carried information about sensations, and the front ones controlled movements. Such researches led him to his law of specific nerve energies: that each sensory nerve, however stimulated, gave rise to a single specific sensation. Thus, when applied to the optic nerve, electrical, mechanical and thermal heat would produce only the sensation of light. The human mind, in other words, did not perceive the processes of the external world but only the alterations produced by the sensory systems.

Müller's prime importance was not his discoveries; he achieved for experimental physiology what Liebig did for chemistry: systematizing laboratory inquiry. His methods set great store by microscopy and ani-mal experimentation, even though he grew doubtful about the latter, on practical and moral grounds alike. An early advocate of the micro-scope in pathology, his great work on tumours was built on study of the cell as the basic functional unit.

He was an inspiring teacher and his many brilliant students went on to dominate laboratory research, though significantly abandoning his vitalism; the disciplines of the laboratory encouraged reductionist approaches. Four of his protégés – Helmholtz, du Bois-Reymond, Brücke and Ludwig – published a manifesto in 1847 proclaiming physi-ology's goal to be the explanation of all vital phenomena through physico-chemical laws, thereby distancing themselves somewhat from their teacher.

Hermann von Helmholtz (1821–94) was descended on his mother's side from William Penn, the Quaker founder of Pennsylvania. His first love was physics, but poor career prospects led him to become an army surgeon. Grounded upon physiological studies of the heat generated in muscle, his seminal paper on the conservation of energy, published in Müller's *Archiv*, made his name and led to his appointment in 1849 as professor of physiology at Königsberg. One of his achievements, utterly characteristic of the new breed of laboratory physiology, lay in establishing the transmission rate of nervous impulses. Müller had stated in his *Handbuch* that he could not detect electric currents in nerves, doubting whether the speed of the nerve impulse was capable of measurement. Within twenty years his student had predictably risen to the challenge and done the impossible, developing new instruments and finding that in frogs the speed was about twenty metres per second. Instrumentation held the key to progress: in 1851 his new ophthalmoscope gave him 'the great joy of being the first to see a living human retina' (that is, to see to the back of the eye, to the end of the optic nerve).

Emil du Bois-Reymond (1818–96) came from Neuchâtel in Switzerland, then under Prussian control, and studied with Müller in Berlin, where he remained all his life. His great passion was the investigation of animal electricity. Building on earlier work on the electric organs of torpedo fish, he showed the individual nerve impulse to be electrical in nature. As with Helmholtz, his innovations in neuromuscular physiology owed much to dexterity in designing new laboratory equipment. He was a staunch anti-vitalist, though he conceded, in a rather Newtonian manner, that fundamental questions concerning the origin of life and consciousness lay beyond science's reach. Ernst Brücke (1819–92) taught in Vienna, where his concerns spanned physiological chemistry, histology and neuromuscular physiology. Committed to scientific naturalism, he is today remembered largely for being one of Freud's mentors and heroes.

It was Karl Ludwig (1816–95), however, who was the supreme physiological teacher after Müller. Abandoning his mentor's vitalism, he became a champion of the positivistic, materialistic science which toppled Romantic views: his early monograph (1842) on urine secretion signalled his reductionist approach to physiology. After spells at Marburg, Zürich and Vienna, he was appointed in 1865 director of the Physiological Institute in Leipzig, an institution on the grand scale. It was built in the form of an E, one wing being devoted to histology and anatomy, another to physiological chemistry and the third to the physical study of physiological problems. Research and teaching went hand in hand, and his students spread the gospel of experimental physiology far and wide: Pavlov and Sechenov in Russia; Gaskell, Lauder Brunton and Gotch in Britain; and Bowditch and Welch in America.

Ludwig's message – physiological science must ditch vitalism and become quantitative, analytical and physico-chemical – was expressly stated in his *Lehrbuch der Physiologie des Menschen* (1852–6) [Textbook of Human Physiology], the first sentence defining its task as that of 'determining the functions of the animal body and of deriving them consequentially from its elementary conditions'. In his view (quite unlike Paris hospital medicine) there could be no medicine without physiology, since 'every case of illness is a physiological experiment, . . . and each physiological experiment is an artificially produced illness.'

Ludwigian physiology exploited the laboratory's potential to the full. His prime invention was the kymograph (1846), the pen-and-drum instrument designed to measure and record continuous variations in fluid pressure. Initially used to show respiration patterns and variations in arterial pressure, it was subsequently adapted to trace all manner of physiological responses. His *Stromuhr* measured blood-flow rate, while his mercury pump metered blood gas concentrations, leading to a new understanding of respiration chemistry. A dedicated vivisector, he also pioneered the use of isolated, perfused hearts, kidneys and other organs in research, devising ingenious ways to keep them functioning.

As conducted by Ludwig's school and its satellites, experimental physiology aimed to understand life 'from the elementary conditions inherent in the organism itself'. The materialism implicit in such strategies was left to others to trumpet: 'The brain secretes thought', announced Karl Vogt (1817–95), 'as the stomach secretes gastric juice, the liver bile, and the kidneys urine.' Medical materialism, as least as a *modus operandi* and sometimes as a metaphysic, was the child of the physiological laboratory.

One of those 'elementary conditions' being explored by laboratory life was the cell. Made possible by the new microscopy, study of cells became associated with yet another of Müller's pupils, Theodor Schwann (1810–82), famous also for discovering the enzyme pepsin and investigating the role of micro-organisms in putrefaction. The idea of cells was nothing new, since Robert Hooke had used the term in a biological context as far back as 1664, referring to the 'pores' in wood. But it had been applied in Hooke's sense to denote not an entity in its own right but an enclosed space: 'cellular tissue' was thus connective tissue which could be inflated with air or fluid to fill the spaces (cells) between membranes.

Modern cell theories began in botany. The Jena botanist Matthias Schleiden (1804–81) declared that plants were aggregates of cells, existing as self-reproducing living units. Exploring analogies between animals and plants in structure and growth, Schwann took up this idea, maintaining that all these phenomena could also 'be demonstrated in animal structures': living cells were basic to living things.

Cells, Schleiden and Schwann judged, were the fundamental units of zoological and botanical action, incorporating a nucleus (its reproductive unit) and an outer membrane. But what was their origin? How did they grow? Were they derived from an elemental 'life stuff'? Somewhat reflecting von Baer's concerns with germs, they connected cell reproduction with the concept of a nurturing fluid or matrix, out of which cells initially arose through a kind of spontaneous generation, comparing them to crystals growing in solutions. This fluid or blastema (in some ways a descendant of humoralism and of John Hunter's coagulable lymph) was pictured by Schwann in a reductionist way as a 'structureless substance, which lies either within or between already present cells'.

The medical implications of cell theory were taken up by Rudolf Virchow (1821–1902), who dominated German biomedical research for half a century. Studying under Müller, Virchow acquired a taste for laboratory life; J. L. Schoenlein (1793–1864) introduced him to clinical problems and to French hospital pathology. Based at the Charité hospital in Berlin, he broadened his practical experience, brought lab techniques to bear on clinical problems, and in 1847 founded the journal later known as *Virchows Archiv*. Forced from Berlin following his courageous support for the 1848 liberal revolution, he moved to Würzburg where, making the best of internal exile, he devoted himself for seven years to the study of cells.

Schwann had argued that, in embryological development and in certain pathological situations such as inflammation or tubercle formation, new cells formed out of blastema. Similar possibilities were proposed by Rokitansky, who speculated that conditions affecting the blood sometimes caused the blastema to spawn abnormal cells, leading to disease. He developed a neo-humoralism which held that diseases originated in an imbalance of protein substances such as fibrin and albumin in the blood. This was partly to explain the awkward fact that autopsy often revealed no evident gross pathological changes sufficient to account for death. Such ideas, appearing in his *Handbuch der pathologische Anatomie* (1846) [Handbook of Pathological Anatomy], made blastema theory the cornerstone for a comprehensive haemato-humoral pathogenesis.

Together with Robert Remak (1815–65),* Virchow distrusted all such notions, maintaining that cells always arose from pre-existing cells through cellular division. In cases of inflammation, for instance, he contended that the 'pus cells' were identical to white blood cells (leucocytes) circulating in the blood. The proliferation of these cells Virchow called 'leucocytosis', and in 1847, at about the same time as the Edinburgh professor John Hughes Bennett (1812–75), he described the pathological condition which he named leukaemia.

Virchow soon abandoned blastema theory altogether, asserting that 'there is no life but through direct succession,' and producing the ringing aphorism: *omnis cellula a cellula* (each cell from a cell). All cells were multiples of one original; back through an ancestral line, life was a hereditary succession of cells. Drawing a pointed political analogy, cells lived in what Virchow called a 'cellular democracy' or 'republic of the cells'.

Cells explained pathology. Diseases, stated his *Die Cellularpathologie* (1858) [Cell Pathology], came from abnormal changes within cells, and abnormal cells in turn multiplied through division – diseases were thus the result of disturbances in the body's cellular structures. Cell analysis was basic to the understanding of tumour formation and metastasis in cancer. Morgagni had highlighted the organ, Bichat the tissue; Virchow had now given pride of place to the cell.

Virchow's views were attacked, not least by Rokitansky who clung to his neo-humoral pathology, warning that all diseases should not be attributed to the 'solid pathology' of such body parts as cells. Nor were converts to the new bacteriology happy with Virchovian cellular pathology. Edwin Klebs (1834–1913) condemned it as 'an extreme doctrine which regards all morbid processes as purely internal events and

---

* A practising Jew, Remak's career shows how a talented medical scientist could be denied due rewards in Germany at this time because of anti-semitism. Though making distinguished contributions in many fields, notably histology and neurology, he never gained a chair, supporting himself by private practice.

completely neglects the importance of external factors which provoke diseases.' Deeming germ theory superficial, Virchow feared that such views would rekindle the Romantic concept of disease as a 'living entity'; correlating disease symptoms with cellular effects, he reaffirmed his morphological approach to pathology.

Alongside his contributions to thinking about cancers, Virchow clarified cardiovascular conditions in his work on thrombosis and embolism. Through animal experiments, autopsies and clinical observations, he elucidated the nature of phlebitis. In most cases of vascular inflammation associated with blood clots, what formed first was the clot (or thrombus), the surrounding vascular inflammation being the secondary and local result of mechanical, obstructive factors in the clot. The 'emboli' commonly found in the lungs at autopsy did not result from general vascular disorder or a vague 'dyscrasia', but were thrown off by venous thrombi elsewhere in the body and transported via the right ventricle into the lungs, where they set off local vascular reactions which were often fatal. Producing such emboli in experimental animals, he studied them chemically and microscopically. Virchow's chemical interests also led to work on body pigments such as bilirubin and haematin, and on proteins and amino-acids. His emphasis on the importance of chemical pathology and of the chemical components of cells was continued in work conducted by his pupil Felix Hoppe-Seyler (1825–95) and others.

Virchow's astonishingly productive and wide-ranging academic career attests the strength of the German university system. In 1856 he returned to Berlin to become director of the Pathological Institute, where he trained the new generation of pathologists. Like many other German academics, he was also a man of broad culture; though doubtful about Darwin, he was deeply fascinated by anthropology in its widest sense. In 1879 he accompanied Heinrich Schliemann (1822–90) to excavate what was believed to be Troy.

In politics a staunch liberal, Virchow co-founded the Progressive Party and was for many years its leader, being elected in 1860 to the Prussian House of Representatives, where his disputes with the conservative Bismarck almost provoked a duel. A champion of public hygiene and social reform, he conducted an investigation into the physiques of six million German children, concluding that fitness was a product of living conditions not race. Criticizing the emergent Teutonic racial theories, he denied there was any such thing as a pure Aryan race; blond hair, blue eyes and other supposed virtues were distributed through people from a variety of geographical or ethnic origins, Jews included.

In 1902, this erstwhile rebel was honoured with a state funeral in Berlin. Virchow's career shows how research had become far more than a matter of laboratory experiments; for better or worse, in Virchow's Berlin as in Pasteur's Paris, medicine had grown inseparable from politics, prestige and nationalism.

PHARMACOLOGY

One of the branches of medicine profoundly altered by the laboratory was *materia medica*. Drug-therapy had long been a jumble of items and uses lacking unity, relegated to the apothecary's backroom. Their study had seen uneven advances in the eighteenth century: chemical, animal and human experiments had led, for instance, to better understanding of opiates, lithontriptics (stone-dissolving medicines) and cinchona bark. But it was only in the nineteenth century that new laboratory skills brought the systematic advances dignified by the name of pharmacology.

Various developments played a part. Forensic medicine's profile was heightened by the Minorca-born physician Joseph Orfila (1787–1853), who went to Paris and successively held the chairs of legal medicine and medical chemistry. His encyclopaedic *Traité des poisons* (1814) [Treatise of Poisons] systematized toxicology, and he gave his subject visibility through testifying in poisoning cases in the courts, helping to raise the profile of medical expertise in medico-legal matters. One who studied with Orfila was Robert Christison (1797–1882), who then passed a long career as professor in Edinburgh. Christison investigated poisonous seeds, partly by self-experimentation, and published a *Treatise on Poisons* in 1829, while his successor Thomas Fraser (1841–1920) isolated the alkaloid eserine and made the important discovery that another alkaloid, atropine, blocked some of eserine's actions.

Organized experimentation into the action of drugs was most successfully undertaken in France, however, inspired by François Magendie (1783–1855), professor of anatomy at the Collège de France, who conducted major studies of nerve physiology. In 1809 he carried out the first experiments with the Javanese arrow poison whose active constituent was later shown to be strychnine. In 1817, with Pierre Joseph Pelletier (1788–1842), Magendie performed experiments on emetics and the nature of vomiting, and showed that the emetic properties of ipecacuanha were due to a substance he named emetine.

Together with Joseph Caventou (1795–1877), Pelletier enjoyed a series of spectacular successes in refining the active therapeutic agents in natural drugs: between 1818 and 1821 they obtained strychnine, brucine, veratrine, cinchonine, quinine and caffeine. Nicotine followed in 1828, atropine in 1833. Above all, opium was subjected to analysis. In 1803–4 the French pharmacists C. L. Derosne (1780–1846) and Armand Seguin (1767–1835) isolated from raw opium a crystalline substance whose chemical nature they could not elucidate. The German pharmacist Friedrich Wilhelm Sertürner (1783–1841) showed it was alkaline, and called it *Morphium* (morphine).

Through such experiments in alkaloid chemistry, the active principle was being extracted from many vegetable substances long used in pharmacy; and once this was concentrated in chemical form, purity, strength and dosage could at last be regulated. Many new alkaloids were brought to light. Pierre Jean Robiquet (1780–1840) introduced codeine in 1832, Philip Lorenz Geiger (1785–1836) explored aconitine, atropine, colchicine, daturine and hyoscyamine, and in 1860 Albert Niemann (1834–61) isolated cocaine.

These alkaloids set the stage for a pharmacological transformation. The pharmacist and the physician now had potent medicaments which included morphine, codeine, quinine, cocaine, colchicine, ephedrine, atropine, reserpine and digitoxin. The therapeutic potential of the alkaloids was stressed in works such as Magendie's *Formulaire pour la préparation et l'emploi de plusieurs nouveaux médicamens* (1821) [Formulary for the Preparation and Use of Several New Drugs]; this pocket book for practising physicians dealt almost entirely with the clinical use of the new alkaloid remedies.

The first chair of pharmacology was established in 1847 at the University of Dorpat (now Tartu, Estonia) and held by Rudolf Buchheim (1820–79), a Leipzig graduate who translated the drugs manual written by the London chemist, Jonathan Pereira (1804–53). Training students in his new pharmacological institute, Buchheim helped launch the science as a laboratory discipline. One of his pupils, Oswald Schmiedeberg (1838–1921), succeeded him at Dorpat and later moved to Strasbourg in 1872, which was then being turned into a

German showcase after its seizure in the Franco-Prussian War. Schmiedeberg set up a major centre for experimental pharmacology, studying chloroform and other anaesthetics and narcotics, digitalis, and drugs such as nicotine and muscarine with actions related to the autonomic nervous system. Pharmacology had been put on the academic map, and the pharmacologists he trained went elsewhere in Germany and further afield, creating new pharmacology departments.

EXPERIMENTAL SCIENCE IN BRITAIN AND AMERICA

These laboratory-based research traditions in physiology, histology, cytology, pharmacology and cognate fields found their perfect habitat on the German campus. Anglo-American pastures were arid by contrast. Around 1830 British savants launched a 'Science in Decline' scare campaign, blaming backwardness on lack of public funding, but politicians raised the counter-scare of jobbery, aware that there were no votes in funding science and medicine, and relying on the ritual incantation of Newton, Harvey and other heroes.

The situation for medical researchers was not helped by the rise of anti-vivisection agitation, encouraged by Queen Victoria. This came to a head at the 1874 meeting of the British Medical Association after an experiment by the French psychiatrist Valentin Magnan (1835–1916) on two unanaesthetized dogs led to a cruelty prosecution. Though this failed, a Royal Commission followed. The resulting 1876 Cruelty to Animals Act, a classic British compromise, permitted licensed doctors to undertake vivisection, but only under strict conditions; continuing protests help to explain why the public was not minded to give for medical research.

Gradually English-speaking medical students deserted the hospitals of Paris for the laboratories of Germany. In the 1830s a few would-be chemists were seeking out Liebig in Giessen and some microscopists were enrolling with Müller in Berlin. Within fifty years, however, droves were pursuing biology and medicine in Heidelberg, Vienna, Leipzig, Munich and half a dozen other centres. There were about 15,000 Americans alone by 1914, mostly going for clinical instruction, though some made a bee-line for the laboratories, like the pathologist William Henry Welch (1850–1934), who studied physiology under Ludwig.

Welch's later career was associated with the university that planted the German ideal in the USA: Johns Hopkins in Baltimore. On his return in 1878, after establishing a pathology laboratory at Bellevue Hospital Medical School, New York, he accepted the pathology chair at Johns Hopkins, which he occupied for thirty-four years, building up a research tradition and making a major discovery: the anaerobic bacillus of gas gangrene, *Bacillus aerogenes capsulatus*. Though the number of American medical schools investing in science remained small, by 1900 there was a ferment of scientific activity at Harvard, Pennsylvania, Ann Arbor (Michigan) as well as at Johns Hopkins, where the medical staff were full-time and so were spared the distractions of private practice. In 1896 Welch helped to start the *Journal of Experimental Medicine*.

English medical students flocked to Germany too, but in Britain medicine remained heavily clinical, dictated by the demands of bread-and-butter private practice; pure research independent of healing was somewhat suspect and attracted scant state support. *Laissez-faire* and utilitarian politics combined with Oxbridge's genteel traditions were not conducive to careers in medical research. William Prout had conducted his animal chemical researches privately; and the talented neuro-physiologist Marshall Hall (1790–1857) never obtained an academic post, doing all his experiments at home and funding them with patients' guineas. From the 1830s, however, the founding of University College and King's College London began to change things. William Sharpey (1802–80), an Edinburgh graduate who had studied in Paris, was appointed in 1836 to the University College chair in anatomy and physiology, a post he held for thirty-eight years. The father of British academic physiology, he trained fine students, including Joseph Lister (1827–1912) and Michael Foster (1836–1907).

By the 1870s English physiology was beginning to thrive – indeed, as Ludwig's generation died off in the 1890s, leadership passed to Britain, thanks largely to Foster, who set physiology on its feet as an autonomous discipline. Moving in 1870 to Trinity College, Cambridge, he bred a research school that included Sherrington, Dale and Adrian, and these in turn promoted the discipline in the universities and medical schools. Foster's studies of the heartbeat (was it muscular or neurological in nature?) were expanded by these *protégés* into wider explorations of the physiology of the autonomic nervous system and the chemical transmission of nerve impulses. He also helped to set up the British

Physiological Society (1876), founded the *Journal of Physiology* (1878) and organized the physiologists' first international congress (1889). Meanwhile at University College London, John Burdon Sanderson (1828–1905) taught physiology, and when he moved to Oxford as the first Waynflete professor of physiology, his place was taken by Edward Schäfer (later Sharpey-Schäfer) (1850–1935), who played a pioneering role in the investigation of hormones.

FRANCE: CLAUDE BERNARD

And what of France? French medicine was so closely identified with the hospital that it was slow to assimilate the new German initiatives; the newly nationalized universities remained engines for instruction, examining and accreditation rather than research. In the German-speaking world, the jigsaw of diverse small principalities (political unification did not occur until 1871) nurtured local pride, the upshot being a score of prestigious university departments and institutes, pursuing distinctive research programmes, stimulating competition and creating a lively job market. In France, by contrast, Paris stood alone; extreme centralization, the product of the Revolution, produced uniformity, and the ensconced hospital tradition discouraged new initiatives.

Nevertheless, Laennec, Louis and Broussais had worthy successors. Pierre-François Rayer (1793–1867), who became dean of the Paris Medical School and physician successively to King Louis Philippe and Napoleon III, researched the gouty kidney; and Jean Cruveilhier (1791–1874) presented the first description of multiple sclerosis in his *Anatomie pathologique du corps humain* (1829–42) [Pathological Anatomy of the Human Body]. Pick of the bunch was Gabriel Andral (1797–1876), who succeeded Broussais at the Charité. An eclectic ('by necessity', he wrily commented), he aimed to reconcile the pathology of Laennec, the statistics of Louis and Broussais' physiology, while rejecting the *idée fixe* of inflammation as the root of all disease. The attempts he made in his *Traité d'anatomie pathologique* (1829) [Treatise of Pathological Anatomy] to integrate physiology and pathology proved fruitful (see below).

Beyond the hospital system, France created few niches for researchers, as is revealed by the chequered career of François Magendie who, though a brilliant experimentalist, long languished in clinical posts. But the fact that lavish facilities are not everything is shown by the career of his great *protégé*, Claude Bernard (1813–78). Though he never enjoyed the establishment of a Liebig or a Virchow and, lacking such an institutional base, did not create a research school in the Ludwigian manner, Bernard proved second to none as an experimentalist and thinker.

The youthful Burgundian's ambition was to shine as a dramatist, and one of his plays, *Rose du Rhône*, was performed in Lyon when he was just twenty. But a shrewd critic persuaded him that his *métier* lay elsewhere, and so he turned to medicine, moving to Paris to become in 1841 Magendie's assistant at the Collège de France. There was no looking back: in a dazzling career he gained chairs at the Sorbonne and the Museum of Natural History, the presidency of the French Academy and a seat in the Senate. Bernard's brilliance lay in his superb experimental techniques, based, as with Magendie, on bold animal experimentation. (His wife turned anti-vivisectionist; they separated in 1870, but not before he had spent her dowry to finance his research.)

Bernard's experiments covered many aspects of physiology: the oxygenation of blood; blood temperature and its changes; the opium alkaloids and the sympathetic nerves; the vasodilator nerves and their role in regulating blood-flow; and the action of poisons like carbon monoxide (which he found killed by displacing oxygen from haemoglobin) and curare, the South American alkaloid which killed by muscular paralysis.

Curare studies led Bernard to conclude that certain drugs acted at strictly localized and well-defined sites, discounting old convictions that drugs had some general bodily influence. Curare worked only where a nerve met the muscle on which it acted, causing paralysis by preventing the nerve impulse from making the muscle contract. Similar specific action points became recognized for other drugs; such drug 'receptors' later assumed huge importance in pharmacological research.

His key investigations overturned an old tenet: that whereas plants could synthesize complex substances, in animals fats, sugars and proteins could be broken down (as Liebig's animal chemistry attempted to show) but not built up. Experiments Bernard conducted in 1855 showed that if an animal were fed on a sugar diet, glucose could be recovered from the portal vein leading from the gut to the liver, and from the hepatic veins carrying blood from the liver to the circulation. Sugar had evidently passed through the liver. Feeding it on a sugarless diet, he found, as expected, no sugar in the portal vein; but the blood in the hepatic veins surprisingly contained high glucose concentrations, and sugar could be extracted from liver tissue itself. Evidently the liver was producing sugar independently. In other words, the body could make its own chemicals in normal functioning – for the sugar here produced was not pathological, as in diabetes. The process was called by Bernard 'internal secretion', the first use of a term later fundamental to endocrinology.

Further experiments confirmed that the sugar was not formed in the blood, but was a result of some sugar-forming substance in the liver; in 1857 he discovered this and called it glycogen (a kind of 'animal starch'), showing it was stored for later use by the organism as glucose and broken down when needed. Extending these carbohydrate metabolism researches, he found sugar in amniotic and cerebro-spinal fluid, and explored the breakdown of sugar by the tissues. In similar studies he examined the function of pancreatic juice. Juice from a living animal had first been collected in the seventeenth century by Regnier de Graaf who, finding it acid, had held that its function was to separate out the nutritious parts of the food. Bernard's teacher Magendie had also obtained pancreatic juice from a living animal but, while suspecting that the pancreas was a salivary gland, was baffled as to its physiological function.

Once again, Bernard performed a series of ingenious experiments. He found there was no secretion in a fasting dog but that, once it had eaten, the descent of the acid chyle into the duodenum stimulated the flow of pancreatic juice which transformed starch into sugar (maltose). In other words, digestion in the stomach was only a preliminary to the further digestive action of the juices released from the pancreas.

The *Introduction à l'étude de la médecine expérimentale* (1865) [Introduction to the Study of Experimental Medicine] spelt out Bernard's philosophy in a grand vindication of the experimental method for biomedicine. Hospital medicine, he insisted, had two limitations. Being an observational science it was essentially passive, akin to natural history; and the sickbed involved too many imponderables to permit precise scientific understanding. Scientific progress demanded active experimentation in strictly controlled environments. Moreover, the pathological lesion which the clinicians had fetishized was not the ideal *entrée* to disease, since it was its end-point. In short, pathology was blind without physiology; pathological processes could best be studied in experimental animals in regulated laboratory surroundings.

Taken together, physiology, pathology and pharmacology formed the triumvirate of experimental medicine, allowing exploration of the relations between normal and pathological functions, in particular at the biochemical level. Rather as with charity among the Christian virtues, of the three sciences physiology was the foremost, because diseases, Bernard taught, were not ontological but the result of excessive or defective physiological functions; conversely, as his curare experiments had shown, drugs or poisons acted only by altering such normal or abnormal functions.

Science should proceed by testing hypotheses through experimentation. Although (he conceded) the life sciences were not strictly reducible to physics and chemistry in the manner suggested by the German materialists, science would stand or fall by one golden rule: determinism. If physiological events were in some ways less certain than physical ones, that was a consequence of the multiplicity of variables encountered in complex living organisms.

Bernard was no reductionist or materialist; animals and humans were not puppets or Cartesian automata, and this was because higher organisms created their own internal environment (*milieu intérieur*), their living cell communities. Complex physiological mechanisms adjusted the sugar, oxygen and salt concentrations of the blood and tissue fluids. Body temperature was equilibriated in response to external fluctuations through temperature regulation (e.g., sweating), alterations in blood pressure and oxygen supply (e.g., panting), and changes in the water and chemicals (electrolytes) in the bloodstream. It was thanks to these sustaining mechanisms – later termed 'homeostasis' by the Harvard physiologist Walter Cannon (1871–1945) – that higher organisms achieved a measure of autonomy within the determinism imposed by natural law. 'The stability of the internal environment', Bernard declared, 'is the prime requirement for free, independent existence.' Physiology's key role for future medical investigation was thus established, and hospital medicine somewhat sidelined. 'An author has defined sickness as "a function that leads to death", as opposed to a normal function that sustains life,' he observed.

> I do not need to say that this definition of sickness seems to me pure fantasy. All functions have as their object the sustaining of life and tend constantly to restore the physiological condition when it is disturbed. The tendency persists in all morbid conditions, and it is this that already constituted for Hippocrates the healing power of nature.

Like Virchow, Bernard thus elevated the physiological model of disease above the anato-pathological. 'Medicine is the science of sickness; physiology is the science of life; thus physiology must be the scientific basis of medicine.'

CLINICAL PRACTICE AND CLINICAL SCIENCE

The pathological gaze penetrating the diseased body and the eye of microscopy formed part of wider attempts to apply the methods of science to the whole medical enterprise, including the regular business of clinical medicine. Alongside failures in the body's structure or architecture, defects in its functioning would also be studied.

For a long time practical medicine got by almost without technology. 'We had few instruments of precision,' recalled Robert Morris (1857–1945), looking back on the beginning of his medical career in New York in the 1880s:

> There was the stethoscope which, then as now, gave inside information in accordance with the sort of ear that was behind it. The clinical thermometer required three minutes for registering temperature, and people in general were more or less unfamiliar with its meaning. An old Irish lady in one of our Bellevue Hospital wards would not allow a thermometer to be put in her mouth on the ground that the doctor had put it in that of a patient in the next bed who had died less than an hour afterward. . . .
>
> Before the year 1870, in this country there were no laboratories excepting those of anatomy, because the expense of laboratories seemed too great for the teachers who divided fees that were received from students.

But the desire was expressed for more precise recording of physiological processes and pathological events, and this was to materialize in new visualizing and measuring devices like Ludwig's kymograph. The piecemeal observations typical of earlier investigations were transformed into systematic bodies of knowledge; take for instance what became the specialty of haematology.

In the seventeenth century the microscope had first afforded glimpses into the composition of blood. Swammerdam and Malpighi noted 'small globules' which were red blood cells, and Leeuwenhoek found that most mammals had circular red globules, while those of frogs, fish and birds were oval. The French physician Jean Sénac (1693–1770) mentioned 'white globules of pus' in the lymph (i.e., white blood cells), while in his *Experimental Enquiry into the Properties of the Blood* (1771), Hewson described such globules forming in the lymph glands and thymus and reaching the bloodstream by way of the thoracic duct – though he mistakenly thought red globules changed to white in the spleen.

Such studies were at an impasse, however, until Lister improved the microscopes. Working with Hodgkin, Lister verified the variety of cell shapes. Soon afterwards William Addison described the escape (diapedesis) of the white cells from the blood vessels into the tissues when attracted by inflammation, oozing into the infected area and form-ing pus. Magendie drew attention to the 'large white globules' which became known as leucocytes, while Alfred Donné (1801–78) identified platelets, another physical component in the blood.

Understanding of blood composition was taken further by Gabriel Andral. Aware of the relative proportions of its four constituents – globules, fibrin, solids and water – he observed how they varied between sickness and health. Establishing normal ratios, he linked fluctuations from the norm to different diseases. An excess of red globules (plethora) was accompanied by fever, dizziness and rapid heartbeat; anaemia (then being investigated by Addison) was quite different: the red globules were in meagre supply, producing low vitality. In Edinburgh John Hughes Bennett found that in leukaemia the normal ratio of red to white blood cells was reversed.

Measuring and counting the components of the blood became re-cognized as possessing diagnostic value. Hermann Welcker (1822–97) developed a method for counting white corpuscles. William Gowers (1845–1915), who maintained in his *On the Numeration of the Red Cor-puscles* (1877) that an accurate red blood cell count provided the best index for diagnosing anaemia, devised a counter, the haemocytometer, attachable to a microscope, to give a more precise count of the red blood cells. However, it proved difficult to use and unreliable.

Blood composition was just one field among many in which it became recognized that understanding of diseases must hinge not just on the discovery of tangible lesions (tubercles, tumours, etc.) but upon a knowledge of deviations from normal functioning. After all, post-mortems often revealed no obvious cause; dysfunction did not always correlate with structural defects – and pain without lesion could not in every case be blamed on hypochondria! Since pathological anatomy's dogmas were simplistic, physiology must come first for, in Virchow's dictum, 'disease is nothing but life under altered conditions.'

Physiology gave a new breadth to clinical thinking by presupposing that medical science had to understand the normal no less than the pathological; indeed the latter depended on the former. Hence vital actions had to be analysed through studies of the varying composition of blood and other indices of illness, such as blood pressure, temperature and breathing rates. To this end, experimental physiology developed techniques for monitoring organ functions, building on devices like Ludwig's kymograph, that unsleeping stethoscope which constantly surveyed and provided readings on the body. Whereas the stethoscope needed a trained auditor, the kymograph and its kin would objectively trace lines onto graph-paper – though skills were needed to interpret the inked marks.

Instruments recording normal functions and vital actions were physiology's assault on the dilemmas left unsolved by pathological anatomy. Another device was the spirometer, described by John Hutchinson (1811–61) in 1846, designed to measure the quantity of air breathed by registering motions in the chest wall. Among other readings it metered the air expelled in the greatest possible expiration following the deepest possible intake of air. Recording the vital capacity of more than 2000 healthy subjects, Hutchinson claimed his instrument could detect lung disease earlier than either percussion or auscultation. Moreover, unlike the stethoscope, the spirometer was purely mechanical and needed no expert to read the results.

Another vital sign increasingly tested for diagnostic purposes was the pulse. Traditional Galenic and Chinese pulse lore demanded qualitative judgments that could be made only by experts. Sanctorius devised a pulsilogium for counting the pulse, and Sir John Floyer's *The Physician's Pulse Watch* (1707) recommended timing the pulse against a clock, but these proved bright ideas that fell on sand. Deeming the pulse an unreliable pathological indicator, Laennec warned against its use.

The opposite view bore some fruit after 1835 when Julius Hèrisson devised a sphygmomanometer which displayed the pulse beat in a mercury column. This was clumsy and undependable; Ludwig modified it by adding a pen-and-drum arrangement to record the pulse beat automatically, though his 'kymographion' was used only for animal experiments. In 1854, Karl Vierordt (1818–84) linked Ludwig's recording apparatus with Hèrisson's machine to create the sphygmograph, a pulse recorder usable for routine monitoring on humans. Étienne-Jules Marey (1830–1904), a man preoccupied with monitoring all human activities to gauge the efficiency of the human machine, refined this in 1860, thanks to which evidence of real clinical significance could be accumulated, with the potential for giving early warning against some heart conditions.

Diagnostic monitoring of the pulse became linked to study of blood pressure, for which the sphygmomanometer was devised. Its basic design was established in 1896 by Scipione Riva-Rocci (1863–1937): an inflatable band was wrapped around the upper arm; air was pumped in until the pulse disappeared; it was then released from the band until the pulse reappeared, and the reading was taken. Blood pressure measurement was becoming an accepted clinical technique around the turn of the century and, as data increased, physicians were able to establish the normal blood pressure range and identify abnormalities pointing toward specific pathological conditions in the cardiovascular system. The American brain surgeon Harvey Cushing (1869–1939) would take readings in the course of surgery to check heart strength, while from 1912 the Massachusetts General Hospital started measuring the blood pressure of all admissions.

Another key vital sign to be recognized was temperature. Though the pathological significance of heat in fever was proverbial, measurement of temperatures was slow in coming. Galileo and Sanctorius attempted to calibrate body heat, but in 1683 Robert Boyle could still scorn it as 'a work of needless curiosity'. The eighteenth century brought a few pioneering advances. Gabriel Daniel Fahrenheit (1686–1736) developed first an alcohol and then a mercury thermometer with a temperature scale calibrated to three points: 0°, determined by a mixture of ice, water, and sal ammoniac or sea salt; 32°, the freezing point of water; and 96°, external human body temperature. Boerhaave used it with fever cases, and his student Anton de Haen regarded movement toward a normal temperature as a sign of recovery.

Few, however, showed much interest before the mid nineteenth century. As in other fields, Andral proved an innovator. In 1841 he published recordings of temperature variations in certain diseases; others followed, and around 1850 F. W. F. von Bärensprung (1822–64) and Ludwig Traube (1818–76) compiled all available readings to argue that body temperature was a key indicator in diagnosis and therapy. The classic work, however, was Carl Wunderlich's (1815–77) *Das Verhalten der Eigenwärme in Krankheiten* (1868) [The Temperature in Diseases], which presented data on nearly 25,000 patients and analysed temperature variations in thirty-two diseases, showing that temperature readings could differentiate fevers. What was important for understanding the course of disease, he insisted, was frequency of reading – at least twice a day. Absolute accuracy was unnecessary, so nurses and even relatives could take temperatures. Normal temperature signified health, fluctuations indicated disease, and certain temperature oscillations were signs of particular maladies. Initially somewhat controversial, thermometry established itself, reinforcing the notion that specific, objective and preferably graphic data were fundamental to clinical practice. In certain respects, pathology was being translated into recordings made by instruments.

Promoted by Liebig, chemistry also played an increasing part in checking normal function and pathological deviation. In the eighteenth century, Matthew Dobson developed tests for diabetes; in 1827, Richard Bright showed how the kidney complaint subsequently called Bright's disease could be diagnosed by a single, simple chemical test. Chemical analysis was crucial to Alfred Becquerel's (1814–62) 1841 urinalysis studies, establishing the average amounts of water, urea, uric acid, lactic acid, albumin and inorganic salts secreted over twenty-four hours, and correlating these with various disease conditions. In 1859, Alfred Garrod (1819–1907) devised a simple chemical test pathognomic for gout.

Bedside monitoring raised questions as to the best method of recording and representing data. Wunderlich believed thermometric observations – discontinuous, dotted recordings of biological events, taken at time intervals – should appear sequentially on a chart as a continuous oscillating line, accompanied by similar depictions of the frequency of the pulse and respiration. The whole course of the disease could be read at a glance.

Marey, by contrast, was in favour of representing on paper continuous, real-time, biological motions, such as the beating of a heart. The line based on such real-time recording was the best expression of medical changes:

To render accessible . . . all the phenomena of life – movements which are so light and fleeting, changes of form so slow or rapid, that they escape the senses – an objective form must be given to them. . . . The graphic curve of a movement . . . characterizes completely the act which it represents.

Whichever, objectifying such findings made bedside medicine more scientific: Wunderlich spoke of discovering 'laws that regulate the cause of disease'. By 1900 it was becoming possible to understand a patient not by his story, nor even simply through pathological signs ascertained by the 'medical gaze', but by ceaseless physiological monitoring. The apparatus for numerical and chemical readings was generally simple and easily accommodated to the bedside and the general practitioner's surgery.

Just as with the stethoscope over half a century earlier, the uptake of readings of temperature, blood pressure and so forth was uneven. Some physicians were keen, or believed patients craved the latest gadgets science could offer. Others regarded it as higher quackery or a form of de-skilling, believing there was no substitute for the trained senses and finger of the experienced clinician. One enthusiast in England was Clifford Allbutt (1836–1925), a general physician who developed a particular interest in nervous, cardiac and arterial disorders and after practising in Leeds finally became Regius professor of physic in Cambridge. Taking up Helmholtz's invention, his *Use of the Ophthalmoscope in Diseases of the Nervous System and of the Kidneys* (1871) contained original observations. He also modified the thermometer. When he commenced in practice, these were one foot long and took twenty minutes to get a reading. In 1867 he had a 'short' clinical thermometer made, six inches long, which registered its maximum in five minutes; a three-inch version followed.

If uptake among private doctors was patchy, such measuring devices *were* incorporated into the more enterprising hospitals which lent themselves to routines, had trained nurses and paramedics to take the readings, and were often keen to accumulate data for research. Later and more complex forms of monitoring machinery were suitable only for hospital and institutional use.

The latter part of the nineteenth century thus put 'low-tech' scientific testing on the agenda. The laboratory ceased to be only for basic research – diagnostic laboratories were being created to conduct routine clinical examinations. Clinical laboratories were the vehicles that transformed the new physiology into practical methods for diagnosing and treating illness. In hospitals the ward laboratory was developed, becoming more complex and employing technicians; these were now, opined Sir William Osler (1849–1919) – writing in the era of Henry Ford and of scientific management – 'as essential to the proper equipment of the hospital as the interns. They are to the physician just as the knife and scalpel are to the surgeon.'

Through such developments the gap between the hospital and the laboratory was bridged, though new chasms might open between the hospital and general practice. The stethoscope began the opening up of the living body to science and the medical gaze, biomedical research was being put to good effect, and the hospital was beginning to resemble a factory.

CHAPTER XII

NINETEENTH-CENTURY MEDICAL CARE

'I hope that Lord Grey and you are well – no easy thing seeing that there are above 1500 diseases to which Man is subjected.'

Sydney Smith to Lady Grey, February, 1836

THE MEDICAL PROFESSION

INDUSTRIALIZATION, THE RISE OF MARKET SOCIETY and the middle classes, the inexorable pressure of numbers and the reform of the state – all these and other modes of modernization made their mark upon the medical profession during the 'age of improvement', posing problems yet offering opportunities.

More doctors were needed; there was more money to buy their services; and, with aristocratic nepotism and patronage being challenged by bourgeois ideals of merit and achievement, the profession could collectively aspire to higher status and individual practitioners could hope for success in a career open to talent.

Private practice operated within an economic nexus in which doctors were self-employed petty capitalists; it was a market which could be lucrative but which was also competitive and insecure. The small-time practitioner might not be very different from the shopkeepers he looked down upon – indeed he might actually call the practice his 'shop', earning his daily bread by dispensing brightly coloured medicines. Medical practice was, nevertheless, a going concern. Its overheads were modest: training was admittedly expensive, but the surgeon needed only his tool-bag and the family doctor a horse and a drugs cabinet; before the twentieth century there was no call for costly premises, expensive equipment and insurance policies. Medicine wasn't a hazardous boom-

or-bust venture like running a factory or a theatre. Product demand never failed, reasonable patients would not hold out excessive expectations of miracles, and *caveat emptor* was the watchword.

Like tailors and landscape gardeners, prudent doctors deferred to their betters. 'Fine folks use their physicians', groused Dr George Cheyne in the 1730s, 'as they do their laundresses and send their linen to be cleaned in order only to be dirtied again,' and the nineteenth-century doctor might still be put in his place. The 'quality' might admit doctors only by the tradesmen's entrance and pay their bills appallingly late. George Eliot had Lady Chettam remark in *Middlemarch* (1872), 'For my own part, I like a medical man more on a footing with the servants.' But the social slights fashionable doctors bore might still be preferable to the plight of those practising in the sticks or in the slum quarters of the festering ports and industrial towns, the much put-upon '6d doctors', and those serving more or less gratis at dispensaries and charities in hopes of getting their name around. Life was also hard for many a 'horse and buggy' doctor in the American midwest; in rural Russia, the Australian outback and wherever else conditions were raw, patients formed a floating, feckless, hardbitten population, and passing irregulars and medicine-show hucksters spelt rivalry.

Some struck it lucky, like Sir Henry Halford (1766–1844), the courtly attendant to four successive British monarchs, who enjoyed entrée into the highest circles and the income of a peer. So suave was his bedside manner that aristocratic women were said to prefer dying with Sir Henry than living with lesser physicians. Another success story – not quite rags-to-riches but 'bright lad made good' – was that of Sir William Jenner (1815–98). Of modest background, he gained his medical education at the new London University, soon to challenge Edinburgh as the favourite medical school for the petty bourgeoisie. In 1837, the year Victoria came to the throne, he started up in private practice, combining it with a junior post as surgeon-accoucheur to a maternity charity. He became professor of pathology at University College Hospital, where he had clinical duties; at the London Fever Hospital and at the Hospital for Sick Children in Great Ormond Street.

Jenner was a good diagnostician and teacher, and spoke up for preventive medicine. He left a modest mark on medical science, differentiating typhus from typhoid fever on the basis of postmortem examinations (1849) and publishing on diphtheria, rickets, tuberculosis and other diseases. But his income came from private practice and, becoming overloaded, he began shedding the public appointments which had given him his leg-up. His reputation could bear this because in 1861 he became physician-extraordinary to the queen. The superior rank of physician-in-ordinary followed the next year; and for thirty years he managed the medical affairs of the royal household, tending Prince Albert during his fatal illness from typhoid, and the Prince of Wales for the same disease in 1871. In due course he got his baronetcy, numerous decorations and (the ultimate professional accolade) the presidency of the Royal College of Physicians.

Everywhere the cream did very well. Thirty-six British doctors were knighted between 1850 and 1883, and fifteen others given baronetcies; Joseph Lister (1827–1912) was the first to be made a peer. A few, like Virchow and Koch, Bernard and Charcot, achieved hero status and had *Strassen* and *rues* named after them – though none so many as Pasteur who was not actually a physician. The emergence of Harley Street as the consultants' quarter in London's West End – the 36 doctors it housed in 1873 leapt to almost 150 by 1900 – marked the consolidation of an inner circle of well-heeled consultants, well-respected in the profession and well-connected in society, dining at the best clubs and marrying off their daughters advantageously. Harley Street's reputation was chequered; some of its consultants shone for fashionability rather than ability, and Archibald Cronin (1896–1981), himself a physician, used his novel *The Citadel* (1937) to expose its mercenary and seedy side. More modestly, many a general practitioner achieved respectability as a pillar of provincial society: earnest, upright and public-spirited, sitting on church and charity committees, invited to the mayor's ball, or captain of the village cricket team.

In the social stakes doctors on the whole fared less well than their professional cousins, the lawyers, who had more opportunities for money-making and whose skills gave better opportunities for lucrative public office. In Somerset Maugham's *Of Human Bondage* (1915) a snobbish old lady remarks that in her youth, around 1850, medicine was regarded as not fit for a gentleman's son; other commentators allude to its insecure social status. Gustave Flaubert, himself a Rouen surgeon's son, mercilessly mocked the pompous *officier de santé*, Charles Bovary, and was happy to show him getting his come-uppance. Bovary and his ilk were unable to compete with an upstart drugs vendor – who was then awarded the *Légion d'honneur*. Likewise, George Eliot's Tertius Lydgate in *Middlemarch* had a spanking new Paris medical education and spoke passionately of progress, being fired with 'the conviction that the medical profession as it might be was the finest in the world; presenting the most perfect interchange between science and art; offering the most direct alliance between intellectual conquest and the social good'. Yet he was not quite accepted in society and made a hash of his life. If jokes and cartoons ceased to present doctors as lethal and lecherous, their later image in *Punch* was of a tribe steeped in snobbery and devoted to self-advancement.

Amid the rank-and-file, the anxiety was that medicine was growing 'overstocked'. With a plethora of doctors jostling for affluent invalids and faced by brisk competition from druggists, chemists and hucksters, medicine risked becoming a cut-throat, cut-price trade. 'Overcrowding', however, was less an objective fact than the gripe of vulnerable practitioners trying to convince legislators to restrict professional entry or ban rivals; many strata of the population rarely saw a doctor in a system in which purse-strings rather than need determined access. Yet professional insecurity was real enough on both sides of the Atlantic until well into the twentieth century. With the choice of eligible professions so limited, medicine was a magnet for the middle classes. Purchasing a desirable practice might involve an awesome outlay; junior partners often had to chafe under a senior colleague who hogged all the better-paying patients; and a young doctor without connexions might take years to get established. We owe Sherlock Holmes and Dr Watson to the fact that Dr Arthur Conan Doyle (1859–1930) had a slack surgery in his early years, giving him both the time and the need to write.

And it was for these reasons – career insecurities – that reformers like Thomas Wakley (1795–1862), founder of the *Lancet* (1823), battled to raise medicine into a respected profession, with structured, regulated entry and lofty ethical ideals – called restrictive practices by their foes. These might prove double-edged. While limiting damaging competition, professional regulations also tended to curtail lucrative sidelines like marketing nostrums, running rest-cure establishments or performing abortions; professionalization might thus raise status more than income. In the UK at least, it was only when the state began to underwrite general practice following the 1911 National Insurance Act and the National Health Service (1948), that medicine paid well for all. From the inter-war years, third party insurance helped do the same in the USA.

Although historians speak of the rise of professional society, the nineteenth-century state was not particularly accommodating to the medical profession. Statesmen sought to avoid being bogged down in medical regulation and reform. Politicians preaching economy and radicals denouncing jobbery were not likely to lend sympathetic ears to ancient chartered corporations wanting their privileges shored up by statute, or even to reformers seeking to promote the public health at taxpayers' cost.

FRANCE

In France the Revolution's medical legacy was the abolition of the university licensing faculties which had been the bastions of *ancien régime* medicine. By ending these and all the other old guilds and royal academies, the Revolution briefly embraced an exceptionally anti-elitist ideal of *liberté* and *égalité*, with practice thrown open to all, formally trained or irregulars. For a modest fee, anyone could acquire a legal permit to practise – a degree of openness unmatched in Europe.

This did not last and, while abolition of the old corporate regulation was ratified, medicine was rapidly brought under central control. In 1794, the National Convention decreed the establishment of an *école de santé* (school of health) in Paris, with twelve professors; others (with six professors) were formed at Montpellier and Strasbourg. Lower grade *officiers de santé* (health officers) were also to be trained, to meet wartime crises and provide basic medical cover. Teaching at the schools united physic and surgery and valued learning by doing, the accent being on practical dissection and bedside teaching. Thereafter, French medical education lay in state hands.

Napoleon went further to restore professional order to French medicine. In 1803 direct state examination and licensing of both tiers of practitioners were introduced: doctors of medicine or surgery holding degrees certifying four years of medical education were thenceforth qualified to practise anywhere, while *officiers de santé* were restricted to elementary practice in the region where they had been certified. This nationalization of training and licensing gave medicine a boost. Schooled in the new patho-anatomy, Paris-trained doctors could pride themselves upon being the scientific and professional top dogs. French medicine thus passed from *ancien régime* provincial corporate control, through

anarchy, to a rigidly centralized licensing system, with similar developments occurring in the Netherlands, the Rhineland, Italy and other
regions subjected to Napoleonic conquest, medical reforms being
exported with empire.

Throughout the nineteenth century the French medical profession
remained essentially as ordained by Napoleon, with distinctions
enforced between authorized professionals and irregular healers. The
profession thereby gained effective monopoly over urban practice and,
despite the persistence of peasant and religious healers (*maiges*), it infiltrated the countryside. Benefiting from state sanction and from the
superb clinical experience afforded by the teaching hospitals, it emerged
strengthened. The health officers dwindled until they were wound up
in 1893.

GERMANY

Developments took a different direction in the German-speaking lands.
There medicine had long been bureaucratically regulated, with the
princes' medical councils licensing practice. Physicians were function-
aries, holding quasi-official status, and medical policing authorized
health supervision of everyday life. This was to change, first in Prussia
and then, after German unification (1871), throughout the Reich.

By an act of 21 June 1869 Prussia established freedom of healing
(*Kurierfreiheit*), with liberals like Virchow and conservatives like Bismarck joining in unwonted alliance to end the old monopoly and throw
practice open. Progressives were convinced that, with the spread of
enlightened opinion, the public would turn only to qualified doctors,
while abolition of privileges offered the regime an easy way to curry
popular favour. Deregulation brought more openings but competition
all round and, right up to the Nazi era, alternative healers flourished
in Germany, rather as in the USA, with the state's blessing. In Prussia
alone (excluding Berlin) the total of recognized irregulars rose from
269 in 1876 to 4104 in 1902: one for every five qualified doctors.
Irregulars were nevertheless barred from official medical duties and
offices; they could not issue certificates, perform vaccinations, prescribe
dangerous drugs, become district physicians or (from 1883) treat panel
patients; apothecaries who kept shop and midwives were also denied
the right to practise medicine.

Two developments palliated the effects of this free-trade ordinance. In 1883 Bismarck established a sweeping system of medical insurance, which in effect offered state employment to regular doctors who so wished. And a law of 1899 extended the powers of the *Kreisarzt* or district physician, a post open only to regulars. It became his job to supervise apothecaries and hospitals; to assume public health and social hygiene duties in fields like school medical inspection, infant welfare, provision for physical defectives, mental patients and the infirm; and to act for the state in a medico-legal capacity.

BRITAIN

In Britain no reforms matched the toppling of the old medical corporations in revolutionary France, and indignation seethed among rank-and-file practitioners who felt denied a control over their own professional lives. They resented being undercut by untrained chemists, druggists and quacks, against whom the state afforded them (or, as they phrased it, the *public*) no protection. They resented the lordly Royal Colleges of Physicians and of Surgeons, who pretended to represent their interests while defending only the perks and privileges of the metropolitan elite.

Unlike Germany or post-revolutionary France, British practitioners continued to be licensed not by the state but by their respective royal colleges. Resisting reform, these oligarchic bodies were subjected to ferocious censure, notably from Thomas Wakley's *Lancet*, which stabbed away at medical grandees and quacks alike. To gain some voice, doctors set up local medical societies, calling for the abolition or democratization of the colleges, bans on unqualified practice, and a single national register for all qualified medical men (the admission of women never crossed their minds). The Provincial Medical and Surgical Association, founded in 1832 by Charles Hastings (1794–1866), gave expression to provincial and then also to metropolitan opinion, becoming in 1855 the British Medical Association, the general practitioners' platform. From 1857 its organ was known as the *British Medical Journal*.

Comparable bids for professional solidarity were made elsewhere, as national medical societies became established: the American Medical Association (1847), the Association Générale des Médecins de France (1858) and the Canadian Medical Association (1867). Such national societies built up professional strength, crusaded against irregulars and lobbied governments. By 1900, they had grown in numbers and standing. Success varied, however, as medics strove for state protection in a climate often antagonistic to monopoly and unconvinced that regular medicine was best.

It was in the United States that regulars faced the most daunting challenge. Congress accepted no responsibility for medical licensing or policing, and state legislatures had small reason to privilege allopaths when medical sects enjoyed popularity in the new nation's anti-elitist atmosphere. With medical schools unregulated and practice unlicensed, well might the American physician look enviously to Europe, where his colleagues faced less aggressive competition from sectaries, could count on some deference towards learning and were less likely to have to cope with the blunt frontier mentality. The autobiography of Edward Jarvis (1803–84), who practised in Louisville, Kentucky and various New England towns in the 1830s and 1840s, reveals how vulnerable a doctor was to small-town political and sectarian religious prejudices.

In Britain, reform stalled because Parliament regarded medical regulation as a minefield. But gradually *laissez-faire* yielded to the neo-paternalism of a Victorian administrative state prepared to shoulder greater responsibilities, in part to placate a more democratic electorate. Parliament's growing promotion of public health led to official appointments for medical men, forging links between the profession and the state, though public employment itself bred new intra-professional tensions.

Meanwhile the licensing system had been overhauled. Agitation led to the Apothecaries Act in 1815, the first attempt to set standards of professional education in England and Wales. All apothecaries (in effect, general practitioners) were to be licensed, after attendance at approved lectures and six months' hospital clinical work. Though critics disowned it as a reform which essentially confirmed the *status quo*, general practitioners would at least have undergone some academic and clinical training, thereby raising their standing.

A further forty years' pressure, prevarication and politicking were required to produce the Medical Act of 1858, another compromise which pleased no one but which worked. This established a unified medical register of all approved practitioners, who alone would be eligible for public employment, specified entry qualifications, and created the General Medical Council (GMC) as an ethico-legal watchdog, with jurisdiction over malpractice and 'infamous conduct' including advertising and collaboration with irregulars. The first Medical Register (1859) contained the names of about 15,000 doctors – a century later there were six times as many.

As the GMC was dominated by the (as yet unreformed and oligarchic) colleges, and unlicensed practice continued to be lawful, bodies like the BMA still felt aggrieved, especially as elite physicians and surgeons were further strengthening their position in hospitals. Nevertheless medical licensing, and the threat of removal from the register, at least marginalized quacks and irregulars. And the boisterous, jovial sporting atmosphere of the all-male medical school with its student high-jinks and horseplay was consolidating an *esprit de corps* that helped doctors to present some kind of united front:

> 'Nothing like dissecting, to give one an appetite,' said Mr Bob Sawyer, looking round the table.
> Mr Pickwick slightly shuddered.
> 'Bye the bye, Bob,' said Mr Allen, 'have you finished that leg yet?'
> 'Nearly,' replied Sawyer, helping himself to half a fowl as he spoke. 'It's a very muscular one for a child's.'
> 'Is it?' inquired Mr Allen, carelessly.
> 'Very,' said Bob Sawyer, with his mouth full.
> 'I've put my name down for an arm, at our place,' said Mr Allen. 'We're clubbing for a subject, and the list is nearly full, only we can't get hold of any fellow that wants a head. I wish you'd take it.'
> 'No,' replied Bob Sawyer, 'can't afford expensive luxuries.'

For Dickens, medical students were 'young gentlemen who smoke in the streets by day, shout and scream in the same by night, call waiters by their christian names, and do various other acts and deeds of a facetious description'.

THE ADMISSION OF WOMEN

A modest breach was made in this clubby, chummy male monopoly when women stormed the medical citadel. Women had always been engaged in practical healing, but in 1800 they were everywhere professionally excluded, not least because they were also barred from university. Reactionaries warned that young ladies were gynaecologically and psychologically unfit for higher education: dominated by her ovaries, a woman's place was in the home as wife and mother. Over-exercise of the brain would divert energy from the womb and lead to sterility and hysteria – and anyway, with its blood and guts, medicine was no profession for ladies!

It is no accident that the first woman doctor graduated in America, since that was where licensing was least stringent.* A Bristol sugar-refiner's daughter, Elizabeth Blackwell (1821–1910) graduated in 1849 top of the class from the Geneva Medical School in New York. Blackwell, who believed nature made women better healers than men, went on to found the New York Infirmary for Indigent Women (1857) and to organize nurses in the American Civil War. 1850 brought the foundation in Philadelphia of the Women's Medical College of Pennsylvania. Also early in admitting female medical students were Berne and Zürich, where many Russian and German women studied.

The first woman to qualify in Britain was Elizabeth Garrett (1836–1917), who exploited various legal loopholes to obtain the diploma of the Society of Apothecaries in 1865, thereby securing enrolment on the Medical Register. Indefatigable in pressing for women's acceptance in the profession, by 1870 she had developed an extensive private practice, established St Mary's Dispensary for Women, received a medical degree from the University of Paris and married the wealthy James Anderson. She was instrumental in the establishment in 1874 of the London School of Medicine for Women, and through a further bureaucratic oversight was admitted to the British Medical Association, which did not officially enrol women until 1892.

The main battleground in the educational war was Edinburgh University, thanks to campaigns waged by Sophia Jex-Blake (1840–1913) whose desire to become a doctor had been fired by meeting Blackwell. Refused by London University, she was admitted as a student to Edinburgh, matriculating in 1869 with four other women students. But complaints to the university court led to their being disqualified from graduation and offered mere 'certificates of proficiency'. Amid student riots, an appeal against this ruling was first upheld then overturned.

---

* A unique exception was Dr James Barry (1797–1865), who practised as a medical officer in the British army and enjoyed a reputation as a crack marksman as well as a skilled surgeon. The autopsy performed after his death revealed that Dr Barry was female.

The battling Jex-Blake, who had meanwhile taken her MD in Berne, eventually became licensed through the College of Physicians in Ireland. She opened the London School of Medicine for Women in 1874, and three years later female medical students gained access to clinical experience through the London (later the Royal) Free Hospital. An Act of Parliament in 1876 finally empowered examining bodies to allow women to qualify.

In due course entry rights for women were won everywhere (in Germany only at the beginning of the twentieth century), but resistance remained strong. St Mary's Hospital Medical School in London, which let female students in during the crisis of the First World War, barred them again later (the school prided itself on its rugby team). The reforms in American medical education following the Flexner Report (1910) also resulted in the closure of some women's medical schools; it was only after the Second World War that the Harvard and Yale medical schools opened their doors to women. By 1976, 20 per cent of British doctors were women, and in 1996 for the first time more than half the intake to British medical schools was female.

PRIVATE PRACTICE

The Bismarckian reforms, as we have seen, established a national insurance scheme in Germany which foreshadowed the assimilation of the medical profession within a state-run health care system. But medical practice everywhere remained grounded on the ideal and reality of the private system, fee-for-service and market-driven. The personal relationship between physician and patient, perhaps sanctified by a framed copy of the Hippocratic Oath hanging above the physician's desk, confirmed cherished ideals of individual freedom, confidentiality and male honour. At its best, it was a system in which the doctor became a trusted family friend and, like the priest or pastor, a pillar of the community. Care, courtesy and compassion were valued even though the doctor's medications could do little against the dysentery, scarlet fever, puerperal fever and pneumonia which still, in 1900 as in 1800, wreaked countless family tragedies among rich and poor alike.*

Private practice had its merits, and many have looked back nostal-

---

* Changes in bedside practice since 1800 are surveyed in Chapter 21.

gically upon the old-time family doctor who rode out in all weathers to help babies into this world and the dying into the next. 'I had enormous admiration for him,' a modern British general practitioner has written about his senior partner around 1950, because 'like so many of his generation, he was *there*. . . . He was just in his practice every morning and every evening, day in and day out, week in and week out, year after year.' That tribute might equally have been paid in 1850 or 1900.

But provision was patchy. Aspiring physicians clustered in capital and cathedral cities, spa and health resorts like Bath, Biarritz and Marienbad, awash with affluent valetudinarians and convalescents; but they could be few and far between in the slumlands where they were really needed. Endemic poor health and high levels of peri-natal deaths showed that health care needs were not being met by market mechanisms. But, Germany excepted, the new century dawned without solutions on the statute book for the daunting problem of the distribution of medicine through society. Prizing their independence, the profession was suspicious of public employment. 'State medicine' was a concept which, though touted by some, was widely feared: Darwin's bulldog Thomas Huxley (1825–95) declared that, when it came to the choice of a doctor, government should 'let everybody do as he likes'; indeed, in 1909 Parliament bowed to protests and ended compulsory smallpox vaccination (the threat was admittedly declining).

Medicine was deeply divided about its future. For every Virchow advocating state medicine there were thousands of doctors wanting to be left alone; for every Virchow granted a state funeral there were thousands of anonymous, unsung, overworked practitioners haunted by bad debts and dying patients. George Bernard Shaw's *The Doctor's Dilemma* (1906) poked fun at a profession which was a queer mix of science and sham, idealism and cupidity. 'Have we lost faith?', he quizzed. 'Certainly not; but we have transferred it from God to the General Medical Council.' Yet the very fact that Shaw – a health crank who embraced vegetarianism and dreamed of man and superman – was driven to write this play suggests that the doctor's dilemma was becoming society's problem.

SURGERY

If bedside practice remained largely business as usual, one branch of medicine broke free of its ancient chains. Thanks to bold individuals and some epochal innovations, surgery changed more in the nineteenth century than in the previous two thousand years, paving the way for today's high-profile, high-tech, sky's-the-limit specialty.

In 1800, as in Paré's time, operative surgery rarely went beyond breakages, fractures and amputations, and even these were highly chancy, on account of infection. For all that, the old image of the brutal sawbones was disappearing. Well-trained general practitioners were pouring off the assembly lines in Paris, London and Edinburgh, Vienna and Leiden; the merger of surgical and medical education worked to surgery's benefit; and a generation of European warfare gave beginners boundless practice on battlefields and the quarterdeck.

The hospitals of London and Paris provided theatres for virtuoso surgeons rated and fêted rather like stars ('actors and surgeons . . . are all heroes of the moment,' commented Balzac). Operating day was a weekly show with celebrities performing before colleagues, students and the public at large; scores of spectators might flock in, applauding the surgeon as he approached the wooden operating table with its leather straps and sawdust to soak up the blood. Top operators commanded top fees for their private operations, performed of course in patients' homes: Astley Cooper (1768–1841) of Guy's, for example, earned the stupendous sum of £15,000 each year, thanks to his legendary brilliance.

The range of operations attempted was narrow and their total small – even a large teaching hospital might have just a handful each week. The most common was amputation, necessitated by accidents and by tubercular infections producing bone necrosis. Post-operative infection meant that mortality might be as high as 40 per cent. The surgeon's only answers to the excruciating pain attending all knife-and-saw work were skill and speed. In 1824, Astley Cooper took twenty minutes to amputate a leg through the hip joint; ten years later, James Syme (1799–1870) was doing it in ninety seconds. Brilliance was timed by the stopwatch. 'Look out sharp,' it was said of Sir William Fergusson (1808–77) at work, 'because if you only wink, you'll miss the operation altogether.'

The most influential English surgeons were John Hunter's apostles. John Abernethy (1764–1831), like his mentor, placed great emphasis on anatomy, seeking to turn surgery from craft into science. In 1814 he was made professor at the College of Surgeons, newly moved to magnificent new premises in Lincoln's Inn Fields. Another was Henry Cline (1750–1827), a man so dedicated that he even lectured on his wedding-day. But the leader was Cooper: for him, as for Hunter his hero, a day without dissecting was a day lost. Unlike the blunt Hunter, however, Cooper was a debonair man of the world who hobnobbed in the highest circles (removal of a cyst from George IV's head made him Sir Astley Cooper, Bart). His most famous operation involved an attempt to overcome the problem of aneurysm, a ballooning in one of the large arteries – a field explored by Hunter. Finding a pulsating tumour in a man suffering from abdominal pain, he diagnosed an aneurysm, knowing it would soon burst and bleed him to death. After testing on a cadaver in the dead-room, he operated and technically succeeded, although the patient later died. His *Anatomy and Surgical Treatise of Inguinal and Congenital Hernia* (1804–7) was based upon years of dissections and operations.

Among the rising generation, Robert Liston (1794–1847) was a lion of a man with a sharp knife and a sharper temper. Speed was his forte, biting his blade between his teeth like a butcher so as to free his hands and save time. Lithotomy, he declared, 'should not occupy more than two or three minutes at most'. From 1818 he taught anatomy in Edinburgh, assisted by Syme (who 'never wasted . . . a drop of ink or a drop of blood') until they quarrelled. The operations Liston performed in the homes of his private patients included the removal of a scrotum tumour, weighing forty-four pounds, which boosted his fame. In 1835 he moved to University College London, where he became celebrated as a teacher.

Many surgeons won honours at war. In England, George James Guthrie (1765–1856) sought to humanize the treatment of the wounded. The surgeon-anatomist Charles Bell was present at the Battle of Waterloo (1815), which gave him unique opportunities for treating gunshot wounds:

> It is impossible to convey to you the picture of human misery continually before my eye. . . . While I amputated one man's thigh, there lay at one time thirteen, all beseeching to be taken next. . . .

It was a strange thing to feel my clothes stiff with blood, and my arms powerless with the exertion of using the knife!

In France, Dominique Jean Larrey (1766–1842), became chief surgeon to the army, went on all Napoleon's campaigns, gained the emperor's friendship (and a barony), and recorded his adventures in his memoirs. Serving with the army of the Rhine he introduced his *ambulances volantes* (flying ambulances) – light, two-horse, two-wheeled, well-sprung vehicles – which enabled the wounded to be whisked from the thick of the fighting rather than bleeding in agony until it was over. A champion of early amputation, Larrey claimed that at the Battle of Borodino 'I performed in the first 24 hours, about 200': one every seven minutes! Their fate is not recorded.

Others made their mark in France: Joseph François Malgaigne (1806–65), surgeon to the Hôpital Saint-Louis of Paris, became a knee-cap specialist, while his colleague at the Hôpital, Auguste Nélaton (1807–73), invented a porcelain-tipped probe to locate bullets. He treated both Garibaldi and Napoleon III. Most illustrious was Guillaume Dupuytren (1777–1835); Of humble stock, he joined the Paris Hôtel Dieu in 1802, rising to chief surgeon. The first to classify burns systematically, he developed new plastic surgery for repairing skin defects and scars. A dazzling technician and eloquent lecturer, Dupuytren was eccentric (he operated in a cloth cap and carpet slippers) and notorious for his arrogance and cynicism. Eminent surgeons and anatomists had a reputation for aggression, William Hunter suggesting it was because 'the passive submission of dead bodies, their common objects, may render them less able to bear contradiction.' On his death-bed, Dupuytren spurned surgery, declaring he would rather die by God's hand.

Innovation was in the air. Johann Friedrich Dieffenbach (1794–1847), professor at the Berlin Charité, developed surgery for cleft palate and for squinting, and then turned to stammering. 'The idea lately suggested itself to me,' he observed in 1841, 'that an incision carried completely through the root of the tongue might be useful in stuttering which had resisted other means of cure.' His operation consisted of making a horizontal section, and excising a triangular wedge – rather a drastic procedure. He tried it out on a thirteen-year-old boy who 'stuttered in Latin and French as well as in his own language'. The first thing the boy said after the operation (we may admire his *sang froid*) was, 'There is some blood running down my shirt'.

Surgeons of all nationalities took up the stammering operation. Two Frenchmen, Alfred Velpeau (1795–1867) and Jean Amussat (1796–1856), were soon incising tongues; the fad spread to England, and later surgeons extracted the adenoids, and even occasionally tried trephining the skull to stop speech defects. The craze started by Dieffenbach was denounced by the *Lancet* as 'a perfect mania for operating', condemning 'the frightful attendant haemorrhage, the great risk of losing the tongue, or life itself'. Never short of critics, such surgical fashions were caricatured in Flaubert's portrait of Charles Bovary's disastrous attempt to correct clubfoot with the knife.

Breaches were being made in surgical conservatism, and it was predictably in America that the boldest operations were ventured, notably in gynaecological surgery, with Ephraim McDowell (1771–1830) and James Marion Sims (1813–83) leading the field. Having studied under John Bell (1763–1820) in Edinburgh, McDowell practised near the frontier in Danville, Kentucky. In 1809, he was called to a forty-seven-year-old woman, Jane Todd. She seemed pregnant, but he realized that her abdomen was swollen by a huge ovarian cyst. Though discussed by Bell, ovariotomy had never actually been done, but 'she appeared willing to undergo an experiment'. Working at home, McDowell took twenty-five minutes to remove the fifteen-pound water-filled tumour from the fully conscious Mrs Todd, who sang hymns to drown the pain, and lived for a further thirty-one years.

McDowell performed ovariotomy on thirteen patients, eight of whom recovered. The Attlee brothers in Pennsylvania then made it routine. John (1799–1885) did 78 between 1843 and 1883, with 64 recoveries, while Washington (1808–1878) reported 387. Like all risky innovations, it met with a mixed reception. Liston lashed the ovariotomists as 'belly rippers', and critics suggested it was done only to allow surgeons to practise pelvic surgery. All the same it was performed in England at least 200 times between 1838 and 1855, being regularly done by Spencer Wells (1818–97) in London (he notched up his 1000th in 1880). Although keen on cleanliness, Wells had a mortality rate of 25 per cent until he adopted Listerian antiseptic techniques in 1878.

James Marion Sims was responsible for a second dramatic achievement, the treatment of vesico-vaginal fistula, a condition common after mismanaged labour, in which a tear develops in the vagina, the bladder or rectum, resulting in permanent incontinence. An innkeeper's son, Sims studied at the new Jefferson College in Philadelphia, settled in

Alabama and built a reputation. Slave-women came to him with fistulas, but operations to correct these had never succeeded, and Sims did nothing. Soon afterwards, attending a woman who had suffered a uterine displacement in a riding accident, he put her into a lateral position ('Sims' position'), thus facilitating vaginal examination. With the aid of a special curved speculum, he now found he could see the fistula 'as no man had ever seen it before'; thus encouraged, he began trying out an operation on slaves to mend such tears in the vagina and bladder. He operated on his first patient no fewer than thirty-three times before the leak was stopped, in what he modestly called 'one of the most important discoveries of the age for suffering humanity'. In 1853 he moved to New York; there he established the Women's Hospital, which became a major gynaecological centre. Sims displayed his operation in Europe in the 1860s.

Hysterectomies also grew more common, and from 1872 another American, Robert Battey, popularized a further operation called 'normal ovariotomy', in which *healthy* ovaries were removed to relieve symptoms in women diagnosed hysterical or neurotic. Elizabeth Blackwell claimed Battey's operation betrayed an 'itch to cut', as surgical 'cures' for women's 'complaints' grew widespread. Abuse of gynaecological surgery to control women culminated in the work of Isaac Baker Brown (1812–73), a London surgeon who specialized in clitoridectomies on women whom he or their husbands judged oversexed, as evinced by masturbation or 'nymphomania'. Controversy blew up, and in 1867 Brown was expelled from the Obstetrical Society of London – not for performing the operation but because he had done so without informed consent and, no less importantly to his peers, because he had indulged in unseeemly self-promotion. Brown migrated to the United States, where professional regulation was laxer.

Despite such innovations, severe constraints limited what surgery could attempt, at least before two epochal breakthroughs. 'That beautiful dream has become a reality: operations can now be performed painlessly,' declared Dieffenbach on first witnessing the use of ether. Anaesthesia was vital for all future developments.

Pain had not prevented surgery in the past, but it had made it almost unbearable, and the accompanying trauma often proved dangerous. In 1810 Larrey performed a mastectomy without anaesthetic on the novelist Fanny Burney. She later wrote a long account of the operation, recording the excruciating agony she had suffered, and also evoking the ghastly, gothic and macabre ritual (a woman in the hands of a male executioner?) of an experience which she believed had nevertheless saved her life:

> M. Dubois placed me upon the Mattress, & spread a cambric handkerchief upon my face. It was transparent, however, & I saw through it that the Bed stead was instantly surrounded by the 7 men and my nurse, I refused to be held; but when, bright through the cambric, I saw the glitter of polished steel – I closed my eyes . . .
>
> Yet – when the dreadful steel was plunged into the breast – cutting through veins – arteries – flesh – nerves – I needed no injunctions not to restrain my cries. I began a scream that lasted unintermittingly during the whole time of the incision – & I almost marvel that it rings not in my Ears still! so excruciating was the agony. When the wound was made, & the instrument was withdrawn, the pain seemed undiminished, for the air that suddenly rushed into those delicate parts felt like a mass of minute but sharp & forked poniards, that were tearing the edges of the wound, – but when again I felt the instrument – describing a curve – cutting against the grain, if I may so say, while the flesh resisted in a manner so forcible as to oppose & tire the hand of the operator, who was forced to change from the right to the left – then, indeed, I thought I must have expired, I attempted no more to open my eyes. . . . The instrument this second time withdrawn, I concluded the operation over – Oh no! presently the terrible cutting was renewed – & worse than ever, to separate the bottom, the foundation of this dreadful gland from the parts to which it adhered . . . yet again all was not over.

The chilling account continued for several more pages.

Since antiquity doctors had attempted to deaden surgical pain. Opium and alcohol had long been used as analgesics, and Dioscorides urged that mandragora root (mandrake) steeped in wine be given to patients before facing the knife. (In *Romeo and Juliet* Shakespeare's heroine was sent into deathlike coma by a mandrake decoction). Medieval patients might be given a 'soporific sponge', soaked in opium, mandragora and hyoscyamine (popularly known as henbane, the poor man's opium). Experience, however, taught the dangers of dulling pains by plying patients with alcohol or opium, and few further developments followed until the chemical revolution produced the first anaesthetic gas.

In 1795 the young Humphry Davy (1778–1829), then Thomas

Beddoes's assistant, tried inhaling nitrous oxide; producing giggling and a 'tendency to dizziness', it became dubbed 'laughing gas'. Davy's *Researches, Chemical and Philosophical, Chiefly Concerning Nitrous Oxide and its Respiration* (1800) reported that the neat gas killed animals, but mixed with oxygen it induced reversible unconsciousness. Finding that when inhaled it relieved an inflamed gum, he noted that nitrous oxide 'seemed capable of destroying pain' and 'may probably be used with advantage during surgical operations'. But there it rested.

Henry Hill Hickman (1800–30), an enthusiastic young Shropshire doctor, experimented on animals with carbon dioxide, inducing what he called 'suspended animation'. He hoped to progress to humans, but his suggestion was slighted and never tried out – perhaps fortunately, since carbon dioxide can cause fatal suffocation. He died early, probably from consumption.

Unlike carbon dioxide, laughing gas had a vogue, especially in the USA, becoming part of the fun of the fair; out for amusement, people would sniff it, get giddy and fall down, apparently drunk. Laughing gas parties caught on, and such frolics probably inspired William E. Clarke (b. 1818), a chemist and doctor from Rochester, New York, to promote a tooth extraction under ether. (The 'sweet oil of vitriol' discovered in 1540 by the German botanist Valerius Cordus (1515–44), which had properties like nitrous oxide, was renamed 'ether' in 1730, its pungent vapour being used to bring up phlegm.) The operation in January 1842 was a success. Two months later this was taken further by Crawford Long (1815–78), a country doctor from Danielsville, Georgia, who had taken part in 'ether frolics', enjoying 'sweet kisses' from the girls. Noticing that under ether people felt no pain, in 1842 he successfully gave it to a boy named James Venable before cutting a cyst from his neck.

In December 1844, the dentist Horace Wells (1815–48) went to a fair in Hartford, Connecticut, where 'Professor' Gardner Colton (1814–98) was giving an exhibition of 'Exhilarating or Laughing Gas'. Curious whether it could be used for painless tooth extraction, Wells offered himself: Colton administered the gas while Dr John Riggs yanked out a molar. 'A new era of tooth-pulling!', Wells exclaimed, on coming round. Eager to exploit his breakthrough, he built a laughing gas apparatus: a bellows with a tube stuck into the patient's mouth. Demonstrating it in the dentistry class of John C. Warren (1778–1856) at the Massachusetts General Hospital, he botched the procedure, however, and his patient suffered agony. Wells lost medical support, grew depressed, became addicted to chloroform and, after arrest in New York for hurling sulphuric acid at two prostitutes, committed suicide in jail.

The key American ether pioneer was a Boston dentist, William Thomas Green Morton (1819–68). Following experiments on his pet dog, on himself and on a patient, on 16 October 1846 he persuaded Warren to allow him to anaesthetize a patient before removal of a neck tumour. Morton's new inhaler succeeded perfectly: 'Gentlemen, this is no humbug', Warren declared. Aiming to get rich, however, Morton descended to humbug, adding ingredients to colour the ether and mask its smell, and then announcing he had discovered a new gas: Letheon. But doctors rumbled him, and he never regained their confidence. The dismal fate of Wells and Morton says much about the commercial opportunism bedevilling medicine at that time, especially in America.

More powerful than nitrous oxide, ether spread to Europe. It was tried in Paris on 15 December 1846, in London four days later, and on 21 December Liston amputated a diseased thigh from a patient under ether, watched by a crowd of students, including Joseph Lister. 'This Yankee dodge, gentlemen, beats mesmerism hollow,' Liston pronounced. 'HAIL HAPPY HOUR! WE HAVE CONQUERED PAIN!' sang the newspaper headlines. Within a couple of months, Napoleon's old surgeon Malgaigne had notched up five ether anaesthetics in Paris; Dieffenbach used it in Berlin; in Edinburgh Syme followed, as did Nikolai Pirogoff (1810–81) in St Petersburg, using it extensively during the Crimean War.

Anaesthesia became accepted, but ether, which irritated the lungs and caused vomiting, was soon displaced by chloroform which, discovered in 1831, was powerful and easy to administer. Tradition has it that James Young Simpson (1811–70), professor of surgery in Edinburgh, had been testing chemicals with his assistants when somebody upset a bottle of chloroform. On bringing in dinner, his wife found them all asleep. Simpson tried it out on a woman in labour (half a teaspoon on a rag, applied to the nose), and was so pleased that he had given it to some thirty patients within a week.

The key event happened on 7 April 1853: Queen Victoria took chloroform for the birth of Prince Leopold; John Snow (1813–58) administered the anaesthetic. 'The effect was soothing, quieting & delightful beyond measure,' Her Majesty recorded in her journal. Protests followed; some were religious (the Bible taught women were to bring forth in pain) but most were medical, on safety grounds. 'In no case', boomed the *Lancet*, 'could it be justifiable to administer chloroform in perfectly ordinary labour.'

General anaesthesia could indeed prove dangerous, and deep unconsciousness was not needed for less invasive operations; so a search developed for substances that would numb a particular area for local surgery. Coca leaves had traditionally been used in South America for their analgesic and stimulating properties. The active chemical, cocaine, was isolated in 1859 – it was soon used as an ingredient in Coca-Cola and other soft drinks. In his pre-psychoanalysis days, Sigmund Freud (1856–1939) experimented with it. 'In my last severe depression,' he wrote in 1884 to his future wife, 'I took coca again and a small dose lifted me to the heights in a wonderful fashion. I am now busy collecting the literature for a song of praise to this magical substance.' Freud believed he could cure morphine addicts with cocaine, and mentioned its tongue-numbing capacity to the ophthalmologist Dr Carl Koller (1857–1944), who needed something to dull pain and keep the eye still during operations. Cocaine succeeded and became the first local anaesthetic, being synthesized in 1885 by the Merck drug company.

Anaesthesia proved invaluable for deadening pain, but it did not get to the root of the problem hindering surgery: infection.* The patient lay on a wooden table, with sawdust beneath. Operating in an old blood-caked frock-coat, the surgeon certainly washed his pus-coated hands *after* operating but not necessarily before. Sepsis was a common consequence; indeed hospital gangrene sometimes assumed such epi-

---

* Contemporaries had no doubt that 'dirt' of some kind was implicated in infection, but cleanliness is a culturally relative concept, and there was no agreement about proper standards of hygiene. Practising in America in the 1830s, Edward Jarvis (here writing in the third person in his autobiography) asked a medical student to make a plaster. The student answered, 'I do not know that we have any exactly like that in the drawer.'

'Do you have plasters on hand already spread?'
'Yes! There is a drawer full.'

He opened a drawer about 2 ft. long, 18 in. wide and 6 in. deep, filled with plasters of every sort ever used in medical practice -- blisters, pitch, resin, mercurial, olivine, etc. – that had been applied to patient after patient, for any and every cause; and, when taken off, put back into the drawer to be used again when occasion might require. Dr J. was struck with surprise and even indignation, and said, 'In no hospital or sick chamber should the exuviae of sickness be kept. Nothing from one diseased person should ever be offered or applied to another, but everything that has been so used should at once be destroyed.'

demic proportions that, as Simpson candidly admitted, those entering hospital for surgery were 'exposed to more chances of death than was the English soldier on the field of Waterloo'. The problem was all too familiar and seemed insoluble: fatalism resulted.

Sepsis was singularly tragic in the puerperal fever that struck mothers after childbirth. Everyone knew that the infection was much more likely with hospital than with home deliveries. Studying such cases, Alexander Gordon (1752–99) had argued in his *A Treatise on the Epidemic Puerperal Fever of Aberdeen* (1795) that the fever was caused by 'putrid matter' introduced into the uterus by the midwife or doctor. To prevent this he recommended the washing of the operator's person. In 1843 Oliver Wendell Holmes (1809–94) in Boston similarly regarded childbed fever as an infection, whose 'germs' were transmitted by birth attendants. A doctor should wait at least a day between an autopsy and a birth, he advised, and should change his suit and wash with chlorinated water – but two influential Philadelphia obstetricians, Charles D. Meigs (1792–1869) and Hugh L. Hodge (1796–1873), rebutted him with the orthodox wisdom that puerperal fever was neither contagious nor – perish the thought! – caused by doctors.

The sepsis problem came to a head in the 1840s at the Vienna General Hospital, where the maternity clinic, the world's biggest, was divided into two. In Ward One childbed fever raged, and the mortality rate hit a catastrophic 29 per cent. In Ward Two, the rate was only around 3 per cent. Why? Pondering the contrast, the assistant physician Ignaz Semmelweis (1818–65) judged the only difference between the two was that births in Ward One were handled by medical students and those in Ward Two by midwifery pupils. As an experiment, they were made to exchange places: the high mortality rate followed the medical students. Semmelweis's suspicion that infection was communicated during delivery was confirmed when Jakob Kolletschka (1803–47), professor of forensic medicine, cut his finger during an autopsy and died from septicaemia.

'Day and night, the image of Kolletschka's illness pursued me,' Semmelweis recalled. 'As we found identical changes in his body and those of the childbed women, it can be concluded that Kolletschka died of the same disease.' Since medical students came directly from autopsies with soiled hands and instruments, was it not obvious that 'puerperal fever is caused by conveyance to the pregnant woman of putrid particles derived from living organisms, through the agency of the examining fingers'? In May 1847 Semmelweis ordered hand-washing with chlorinated water before deliveries; in both wards mortality plummeted.

Meeting resistance from disbelieving colleagues, Semmelweis grew frustrated, finally resigning and leaving Vienna for Budapest, where in 1851 he became head of the obstetrical division of St Rochus Hospital. On introducing chlorine disinfection, puerperal fever mortality rates fell below 1 per cent, and in 1861 he published his *Die Aetiologie, der Begriff und die Prophylaxis des Kindbettfiebers* [The Cause, Concept and Prophylaxis of Childbed Fever]. He seems to have grown mentally unstable, however; in 1865 he was admitted to a Viennese mental hospital, where he died, perhaps the victim of the same type of streptococcal infection he had identified with puerperal fever.

Childbed tragedies highlighted the sepsis problem, but what was to be done? 'Antiseptics' of the general kind used by Semmelweis had long been discussed, the word being widely used by sanitarians to describe any substance impeding corruption. Greek medicine had employed wine and vinegar in wound care; alcohol gained favour; iodine became popular in France for bathing wounds; other antiseptics included bromine, creosote, zinc chloride and nitric acid, while sanitarians such as Florence Nightingale set store by scrupulous spotlessness. Whitewashing walls became common, and surgical cleanliness through dressing changes and soap was urged. Such disinfective moves carried no bacteriological implications: they were simply an attempt to counter contagious diseases. In short, Lister did not invent antisepsis; his achievement lay in making routine an effective form of it, and thus making surgery safe.

Joseph Lister (1827–1912) came from a well-off Yorkshire Quaker background; his father, Joseph Jackson Lister, had developed improved microscopes with achromatic lenses (see Chapter Eleven). After studying at University College, he became assistant surgeon in Edinburgh under Syme in 1854. (On marrying Syme's daughter, he was compelled to leave the Society of Friends, who did not accept marrying out.) After six years, he gained the Regius chair of surgery in Glasgow.

Lister found surgery there bedevilled by sepsis. In wound infection exposed tissues (for instance in the case of a compound fracture) were said to be affected by some stinking atmospheric 'miasma'. A new operation he had developed on tuberculous changes in the wrist had good results, Lister found, so long as the wound remained infection-free; but six out of sixteen patients developed fatal gangrene. Frog experiments showed Lister that gangrene was associated with the process of rotting: both involved the 'decomposition' of organic material. Pondering blood poisoning, erysipelas, pyaemia, septicaemia and hospital gangrene, he learned from reading Pasteur that such putrefaction was a fermentation caused by air-borne bacteria; it was not the air that caused post-operative sepsis but the microbes in it. Pasteur had also shown that rotting and fermentation could occur even without oxygen if anaerobic micro-organisms were present. The Frenchman's 'beautiful researches' won Lister over.

But what could be done? After considering its effectiveness in reducing infection among cattle on sewage farms and its use against typhoid, Lister concluded that bacteria were affected by carbolic acid (phenol). This had been isolated in the 1830s by a German industrial chemist, Friedlieb Runge (1797–1867), through coal tar distillation. Found to have antiseptic properties, it became extensively used in sewage treatment. Lister became convinced that it was necessary to cleanse the wound and keep out further infection, and tried various ways to do so. In the absence of the skin barrier, there had to be a chemical barrier. His first trial was on 12 August 1865, when he dressed a compound tibia fracture in James Greenlees, a boy who had been run over by a cart; Lister used lint soaked in carbolic acid and linseed oil. The dressing remained in place four days and the wound stayed infection-free; the boy walked out of the infirmary after six weeks. Nine months later Lister took up another case. Carbolic treatment was again applied and the wound again healed without infection: a serious condition had 'been entirely deprived of its most dangerous element'.

Lister developed an antiseptic ritual: the clotted blood was removed; the wound bathed with carbolic; carbolic-soaked lint applied; tinfoil added to prevent evaporation; absorbent wool packed around the wound; and when a new dressing was needed, the foil was lifted and fresh carbolic applied. Meanwhile, during the operation, the atmosphere was constantly sprayed with carbolic, saturating all present. The technique involved both antisepsis (killing infective agents in the wound) and asepsis – preventing infective bacteria getting into the wound.

He published his procedure and his first results in the *Lancet* on 16 March 1867, showing that in eleven compound fracture cases, none of the patients had died of sepsis. Nevertheless, criticism followed from those sceptical of the carbolic acid palaver. The Birmingham gynaecologist Robert Lawson Tait (1845–99) denied the existence of bacteria, was a stickler for operating theatre cleanliness and claimed equally good results: 'Let us hear no more of the nonsense about the bad results in surgery of pre-Listerian times as having been cured by Lister,' he growled in 1898, 'it is not the truth.'

Lister's post-amputation death rate dived, as the following table suggests:

Years	Total Cases	Lived	Died	Mortality %
1864–66	35	19	16	45.7 without antiseptics
1867–70	40	34	6	15.0 with antiseptics

He went on refining his techniques: surgeons were to wash with carbolic solutions before and during operations, and assistants were to spray it around the theatre. Starting with a scent spray, he graduated to a 'donkey engine', a jar of carbolic acid vaporized by a pump and driven by steam.

Some surgeons guffawed: 'Where are these little beasts?' rasped John Hughes Bennett, professor in Edinburgh. 'Show them to us, and we shall believe in them. Has anyone seen them yet?' But Lister firmly believed bacteria were the source of surgical trouble. By the 1880s his explanations of wound infection had been overtaken by Koch's researches on the role of specific micro-organisms. Lister clung to his earlier convictions that abscesses were generally germ-free and that the nervous system was involved in inflammation; he also thought (wrongly) that the two main bacteria found in wound infections – staphylococci and streptococci – were ubiquitous and often nonpathogenic.

Lister's 1867 report was supported by Carl Thiersch (1822–95) in Germany, and his technique spread, though too slowly for the Franco-Prussian War (1870). In that war the French amputated some 13,200 limbs, with 10,000 gangrene and fever deaths – a mortality rate of 76 per cent. Every single one of the seventy amputations the aged Nélaton performed during the Commune (1871) resulted in death. Such grim figures concentrated surgeons' minds. Among them was Johann Ritter von Nussbaum (1829–90). In the early 1870s, post-operative mortality at his Munich clinic rose to 80 per cent, but plummeted after his assistant Lindpainter returned from Glasgow with the new method. 'Behold now my wards,' he exclaimed, 'which so recently were ravaged by death. I can only say that I and my assistants and nurses are overwhelmed with joy and gladly submit to all the trouble this treatment involves.'

Another convert was the Prussian Ernst von Bergmann (1836–1907) who, disturbed at how carbolic acid irritated the skin, developed new aseptic techniques of cleaning the operation room, surgeon and patient, as well as the steam sterilization of instruments. Just Lucas-Championnière (1843–1913), who watched Lister perform, introduced the technique into France. 'Listerism' had further champions, Billroth in Vienna and Bassini (1844–1924) in Italy, for example. But although Marion Sims and William Halsted (1852–1922) grasped its value, uptake was slow in North America. Halsted encountered such opposition that he had to operate in marquees in the garden of New York's Bellevue Hospital, because his colleagues detested the carbolic fumes. He also popularized rubber gloves, introduced during the 1840s in connexion with dissection. In 1889 Miss Caroline Hampton, one of his nurses and also his fiancée, complained that the sterilizing solution was giving her hands dermatitis. Halsted got Goodyear to make thin rubber gloves which in time became standard (though Halsted himself did not wear them).

The late nineteenth-century operating environment looks in retrospect a mish-mash of old and new. Lister made a fetish of antisepsis but did not scrub his hands, merely rinsing them in carbolic; and he continued to operate in street clothes – surgical gowns and masks were developed by others. In 1897 the Polish surgeon Johannes von Mikulicz-Radecki (1850–1905), alert to the dangers of droplet infection, was probably the first to use a face mask. Others were not so fastidious. 'The surgeon arrived and threw off his jacket to avoid getting blood or pus on it,' wrote Berkeley Moynihan (1865–1936), later a distinguished surgeon, recalling his student days in Leeds in the 1880s:

> He rolled up his shirt-sleeves and, in the corridor to the operation room, took an ancient frock from a cupboard; it bore signs of a chequered past, and was utterly stiff with old blood. One of these coats was worn with special pride, indeed joy, as it had belonged to a retired member of the staff. The cuffs were rolled up to only just above the wrists, and the hands were washed in a sink. Once clean (by conventional standards), they were rinsed in carbolic-acid solution.

Moynihan developed an advanced aseptic ritual, and was the first in Britain to adopt rubber gloves.

New York hospitals were just beginning to be transformed. 'When

I first became a member of the house staff of Bellevue Hospital,' recalled the American surgeon Robert Morris (1857–1945) of the 1880s, 'the operating-room was similar to that of most other large general hospitals. The set-up consisted of a plain wooden table to carry instruments, lint or oakum dressings, unbleached muslin bandages (we had no absorbent gauze or cotton), and a large tin basin of tap water. Sometimes plaster of paris and other splint outfit was added.' Surgeons were just becoming conscious of the dangers of infections in obstetric cases:

> McLean advised us to use as many precautions in obstetric cases as were observed by us in going from one case of measles to another. Some of the leading obstetricians had become convinced that childbed fever was really contagious, although they could not at all understand why it should be. But the majority would go from such a case to their next parturition case without any sort of adequate preparation.

The carbolic spray meanwhile came under growing criticism, and in 1890 Lister abandoned it. Koch proved that chemicals were less effective than heat for sterilizing instruments. Face masks, rubber gloves, surgical gowns and the abandonment of the huge public operating theatre – all these slashed infection. What was crucial was not the carbolic but that surgeons became convinced that safe surgery was a possibility and a duty.

Anaesthesia and antiseptics expanded surgical horizons. In 1873 Sir John Erichsen (1818–96), surgeon to University College Hospital London, declared 'the abdomen, the chest and the brain [will] be for ever shut from the intrusion of the wise and human surgeon,' but all these cavities were soon wide open, and surgery was in the thick of a revolution. Lister was a transitional figure; he made operating safe but did not develop new operations. But during his later years operative improvements and the ability to control pain and prevent infection were turning surgery into an art capable of treating the cavities as well as the extremities. Formerly an emergency treatment or a last resort, surgery became a prize weapon in the therapeutic arsenal – not simply acceptable but a procedure of choice.

HOSPITALS AND NURSING

A Lady with a Lamp shall stand
In the great history of the land.

LONGFELLOW

Hospitals housed the new operative surgery, but they had many critics. Traditional Catholic establishments were condemned by medics as benighted, while urban institutions reeked of the great unwashed who filled them. Inspecting Europe's hospitals around 1780 John Howard had encountered hotbeds of infection; surgery was known to be safer at home. Surgeons estimated hospital mortality to be three to five times higher than in private cases and maternity wards were sometimes Herodian. *Pourriture d'hôpital* (hospital gangrene) was dreaded: 'It is like a plague,' despaired John Bell, 'no operation dare be performed, every cure stands still, every wound becomes a sore, and every sore is apt to run into gangrene.' At the Paris Hôtel Dieu, 'at the hearing of that ominous word, the patients gave themselves up for lost.'

Simpson coined the term 'hospitalism', later defined by Erichsen as 'a general morbid condition of the building, or of its atmosphere, productive of disease', in which patients got erysipelas and other contagions. Simpson believed hospitals needed to be periodically burnt down; a 'pyaemia-stricken' hospital should be demolished, thought Erichsen, since its walls and equipment were irremediably polluted. Believing many hospitals were gateways to death, Florence Nightingale, a staunch miasmatist who never came round to bacteria, thought temporary sheds would be safer and proposed radical redesign.

The English debate on the pros and cons of hospitals – urban or rural? large or small? – came to a head in the 1860s when old St Thomas's Hospital was demolished to make way for London Bridge railway station. Nightingale wanted it moved to the countryside but, baulking at travelling long distances to see poor patients, metropolitan consultants vetoed her suggestion. Prominent in the new St Thomas's, erected across the Thames opposite Parliament, was the pavilion ward which she advocated, a design allowing cross-ventilation – she believed stagnant air bred disease.

Fired by religious zeal and utilitarian science, reformers invested great faith in ensuring the optimal running of institutions: schools, prisons, workhouses. The hospital was criticized as a disorderly place; whether or not they deserved their reputation for being loud-mouthed, tipsy ignorant slatterns like Dickens's Sairey Gamp and Betsy Prig, English nurses certainly lacked formal training. In the event, it was better nursing that was the agent of improvement, raising the moral tone and ensuring efficiency.

Initiatives towards systematic training came from various quarters. In Catholic nations, nurses were traditionally members of religious orders, notably the Daughters of Charity founded by Vincent de Paul, and religious ideals and models remained at the fore. Indeed, new orders were founded: the Sisters of Mercy and the Irish Sisters of Charity, set up in 1831 by Catherine McAuley (1778–1841) and Mary Aikenhead (Sister Mary Augustin: 1787–1858). They sent nuns to Paris to train under the Daughters of Charity and proved energetic in providing nurses not just for Ireland but for Australia and other parts of the empire where there were concentrations of Catholics. Vowed to poverty, chastity and obedience, these sisterhoods won respect.

Among Protestants the lead was taken by the Deaconess Institute established in 1836 by Theodore Fliedner (1800–64), pastor of Kaiserswerth near Düsseldorf, and his wife Friederike (1800–42). On an early visit to England, Fliedner had been impressed by the Quaker Elizabeth Fry's (1780–1845) dedication to prison visiting. Initially the Fliedners devoted themselves to prisoner welfare, opening a hostel in 1833 for discharged female convicts. Next they turned to the sick poor. Aiming to create a corps of trained women, they opened a small hospital in 1836; two years later they took over the Elberfeld city hospital, and in 1842 they acquired a 200-bed facility at Kaiserswerth. Young women were recruited to serve as 'deaconesses', instructed by physicians, and charged to perform all tasks in rotation. Their duties embraced teaching and child management, and after a three-year course they were expected to pass public pharmacy examinations. Unlike their Catholic counterparts, Kaiserswerth deaconesses did not withdraw from the world, and they were allowed to marry.

The idea caught on; by the time of Fliedner's death the school had trained about 1600 deaconesses, and mother-houses had been set up as far afield as Milwaukee. In 1840, after visiting Kaiserswerth, Elizabeth Fry responded by founding the Institute of Nursing in London; the pious ladies who joined called themselves Protestant Sisters of Charity though, lest this smacked of Catholicism, the title was changed to 'nursing sisters'.

In England, the Crimean War (1854–56) highlighted the need for change, and produced its heroine in Florence Nightingale (1820–1910). She was from a wealthy, cultured family, born during a family sojourn in Florence, and sought in nursing an escape from the doll's house claustrophobia she suffered with her mother and sisters. Shy yet stubborn, at seventeen she had a religious vision: her mission was to serve mankind. Though her family forbade her to work in a hospital, at thirty-one she was finally allowed to go to Kaiserswerth for training. The hard discipline, however, was too much for her temperament, and she lasted only three months. After time with the Daughters of Charity in Paris, in 1853 she was appointed superintendent in London of the Establishment for Gentlewomen during Illness, before becoming superintendent of nurses at King's College Hospital. The outbreak of the Crimean War in March 1854 was her opportunity.

At the English base at Scutari, across the Bosphorus from Istanbul, hospital conditions were dreadful. Rumours of the neglect of the sick and wounded were confirmed by the anguished reports of *The Times* correspondent, William Russell: 'Not only are there not sufficient surgeons ... Not only are there no dressers and nurses ... There is not even linen to make bandages.' At least the French military hospitals had their Sisters of Charity. *The Times* demanded action; the nation took up the call; Nightingale offered her services to her friend Sidney Herbert, the Secretary at War. 'There is but one person in England that I know of,' declared Herbert, 'who would be capable of organizing and superintending such a scheme.' A party of thirty-eight nurses – ten Roman Catholic sisters, eight Anglican sisters, six St John's House nurses, and fourteen from various hospitals – was quickly despatched, over the protests of some military top-brass.

On 4 November 1854 Nightingale and her nurses arrived at Scutari, where nearly two thousand wounded and sick lay in foul rat-infested wards. Three hundred scrubbing brushes were immediately requisitioned. While the cleanliness battle was being fought, the Battle of Inkerman raged, and the hospital was soon deluged with the wounded. Nightingale organized the nursing of the sick, gaining a further eighty nurses as reinforcements. She provided meals, supplied bedding, and saw to the laundry ('I am a kind of General Dealer in socks, shirts, knives and forks, wooden spoons, tin baths, tables and forms, cabbages and carrots, operating tables, towels and soap'). Within six months, and battling against military resistance, she had transformed the place, slashing the death rate from about 40 per cent to 2 per cent. On her return to Britain in August 1856, she found herself a national heroine.*

As often, war brought change. Military medicine was given a shake-up and the Royal Army Medical Corps set up (the name dates from 1898), with a training hospital at Netley. The Royal Army Medical College for instructing officers was opened in 1902. On the outbreak of the First World War, the RAMC had a staff of 9000 – by 1918 it was 133,000. More dramatic was the Crimean War's impact on civilian nursing. An appeal was launched to start a nursing school under Nightingale's direction; £44,000 was raised, and in June 1860 the first students entered her school at Saint Thomas's. Her aim was to train 'training matrons': to produce graduates who would drill raw hospital staff. Control of hospital nursing had to be removed from men's hands and placed in the hands of the matron.

Blessed with indomitable will, Nightingale was a stern, starchy but gifted organizer. Her success in elevating nursing owed much to her insistence in her *Notes on Nursing* (1859) on the necessity for recruits to receive a thorough training in nursing theory and practice. (She was a great believer in the power of facts, calling statistics 'the most important science in the world'.) Nursing assuredly involved dedication, devotion and discipline, but it was also to be a skilled profession. 'It has been said and written scores of times, that every woman makes a good nurse. I believe, on the contrary, that the very elements of nursing are all but unknown', she insisted. Whereas it had been thought of as 'little more than the administration of medicines and the application of poultices', it should actually 'signify the proper use of fresh air, light, warmth, cleanliness, quiet, and the proper selection and administration of diet'. Nursing was a key weapon in the hygiene war – a nurse could do more good than a physician. Dirt caused disease, sickness was a warning, cleanliness a panacea, and nurses were ministers of hygiene.

---

* Nightingale's American counterpart was Dorothea Dix (1802–87), already known for her campaigns for the insane. Two months after the outbreak of the Civil War in April 1861, she was appointed superintendent to the United States Army Nurses. At first she demanded the best ('very plain-looking women . . . no curls, no jewelry, and no hoop skirts') but as the war and the nursing problems escalated, she accepted pretty women too. The most famous Civil War nurse was Clara Barton (1821–1912). Working at the front, she became known as the 'Angel of the Battlefield'; after the war she established close contacts with Nightingale.

Promoting nursing as an honourable vocation for women, the Nightingale system stressed service and subordination. There were two tiers. The well-to-do were accepted as paying pupils who were to stay two years. Probationers – that is, girls of a humbler background but of good character, got up in neat brown uniforms, with white caps and collars – would train for one year. Nightingale-trained teachers and administrators carried the system throughout Britain and the empire, and her graduates helped to set up nurses' training institutes in Sweden (1867), Australia (1867), the United States (1873), Canada (1874) and Denmark (1897).

The Red Cross was intimately involved in these developments. The battle of Solferino, fought on 24 June 1859 between Austria and the Franco-Italian forces of Napoleon III, was witnessed by a Swiss banker, Jean Henri Dunant (1828–1910). Horrified by the shocking condition of the wounded, he was spurred to found the International Red Cross (1864). Alongside its work on behalf of the war-wounded, it was to play a key role in promoting nurses' training, especially in the less advanced areas of Europe. In 1882 Clara Barton brought the Red Cross to America, introducing the 'American amendment' to the Geneva Convention which empowered the Red Cross to be active in peace as well as in war.

In many places, nursing continued to be dominated by religious orders. Out of a total nurse population of about 75,000 in early twentieth-century Germany, there were 26,000 Roman Catholic sisters and 12,000 deaconesses. Only 3000 nurses belonged to the professional Nurses' Association. Twenty-five years later there were still three Protestant nursing sisters and five Roman Catholic sisters for every lay nurse. France by contrast secularized; after the catastrophe of the Franco-Prussian War (1870–71), programmes to improve nursing were introduced by the anti-clerical Third Republic. In 1922 a state nursing diploma was created and lay nurses soon outnumbered nursing sisters nearly two to one, and only twenty-five of the eighty recognized nursing schools were in the hands of religious orders.

Nursing became a skilled profession embodying the *esprit de corps* Nightingale so valued. The British Nurses' Association was founded in 1887 by the former matron of St Bartholomew's, Mrs Bedford Fenwick (1857–1947), a woman hardly less formidable than Nightingale herself. With a thousand members in its first year, in 1892 it got its royal charter. The General Nursing Council was set up in 1919; state registered nurses came into their own with the Royal College of Nursing; and by 1960 the Register of Nurses numbered over 283,000. Mental nursing developed its own professional bodies.

The Nurses' Associated Alumnae of the United States and Canada was organized in 1896, becoming in 1901 the American Nurses' Association. By 1930 similar associations existed in thirty-five countries; elsewhere the Red Cross served as the national nurses' society. By then the typical features of modern nursing had taken shape, combining female subordination to the male medical hierarchy with a deep and quasi-religious sense of duty. This, while confirming gender divides, made the nursing staff not just indispensable but guardian angels, imparting to the modern hospital an essential aspect of its characteristic ethos.

Many developments – notably new surgical possibilities thanks to anaesthetics and Listerism and the humanizing role of nurses – were transforming the hospital from a charitable refuge for the sick poor into an all-purpose medical institution. Working people were increasingly establishing their 'right' to hospital admission. In London, the Hospital Saturday Fund, set up in the 1870s, collected donations from workmen and arranged admission tickets from the hospitals for treatment. Such insurance schemes wove hospitals into wider community health-care arrangements. More telling was the setting aside for paying patients of attractive private rooms in special wings, a development paralleling the establishment of nursing homes and clinics as small private hospitals for the affluent. Moreover, teaching and research were increasingly based on hospital sites, and everywhere the number of hospitals and beds multiplied. With a population of just over five million, America had only a couple of hospitals in 1800 – the Pennsylvania Hospital, founded in 1752 and the New York Hospital (1771). By the First World War, the number of hospitals had shot up to 5000. By then the hospital was fast becoming the headquarters of medicine. It was also becoming popular. Looking back from 1930 on fifty years of practice in America, Robert Morris reflected:

> One of the very greatest changes that I have observed in the past fifty years has been in the attitude of the public toward hospitals. Dread of them was general and well founded before the days of

antiseptic surgery. But with its widespread adoption, fear faded rapidly from the lay mind.

All over the world the very name 'hospital' suggested pestilence or insanity; few people would go voluntarily to such a place, no matter how well equipped it was for doing routine work efficiently. To-day, almost everybody with any illness at all serious wishes to go there.

SPECIALIZATION

Developments in surgery and the hospital were part of wider trends. Division of labour was one of the nineteenth century's big ideas, and it affected medicine no less than other spheres of life. It also sparked endless controversy. For centuries it had been itinerants and irregulars who had gone in for tooth-pulling, lithotomy and truss-fitting; specialization was thus tainted with quackery. Had not Hippocratic humoralism taught that disease was a constitutional not a local matter? Was not the true physician a generalist?

Other possibilities were in the air. Morgagni's pathology and Paris hospital medicine highlighted particular body parts and local sites of disease. Groups came to public attention whose afflictions were especially pitiable or posed a particular threat: those mutilated in war, crippled children, the blind, the deaf and mute, the venereally infected. Medical men convinced themselves they could improve practice, serve neglected sufferers and win fame and fortune by carving out new specialties. In Britain and the USA, initiatives were typically directed towards the founding of new hospitals fusing philanthropy and entrepreneurship. Specialization combined the scientific, the institutional and the therapeutic, and it took myriad forms. Some specialties focused on body parts, some on diseases; some on life events, some on age groups. Specialisms took paths that diverged from country to country and sparked fierce inter- and intra-professional disputes. The proper qualifications, competence and licensing of groups such as obstetricians, dentists, physiotherapists, radiographers and a host of paramedics were endlessly fought over, as were the standing and regulation of the paramedical and ancillary professions and other service groups.

Obstetrics was an early and enduring site of controversy. As discussed in Chapter 10, many countries adopted the policy of improving midwife training, but in Britain and the United States the man-midwife or accoucheur emerged, and general practitioners became involved in delivering babies as part of their family doctor role. Yet the art of obstetrics languished because, although it was a specialized skill, none of the authorized bodies wished to shoulder responsibility for it. The Royal College of Physicians considered delivering babies ungentlemanly, while the College of Surgeons, committed to sustaining an elite devoted to 'pure' surgery, was equally indifferent. The result was that obstetrics teaching and training were elbowed out. Even after the Medical Act of 1858, students could qualify without any obstetrical training – a disgrace which lasted until 1886. Even then instruction was often perfunctory, and not until 1902 was there statutory provision for the training and licensing of midwives.

In the USA obstetric practice in the nineteenth century was largely in the hands of medical practitioners, full-time obstetricians were as rare as in England, and lying-in hospitals were hazardous. Midwives were a mixed bunch, and neighbour-delivery predominated in remote parts. Bent upon eliminating the midwife, the medical profession did nothing to encourage midwifery skills, and the USA experienced some of the highest maternal death rates in the developed world.

In most European countries midwife training and state registration were introduced, and the quality and status of midwives rose. In France there was a two-tier system; the superior, being self-governing and powerful, ran the lying-in hospitals and taught students; the inferior was relegated to rural practice and closely supervised. In Sweden, Denmark and the Netherlands a high proportion of home deliveries were conducted by trained midwives. Questions of professional pecking orders, gender rivalry, and medicalization have continued to dog childbirth throughout the twentieth century.

Another new life-stage specialty was paediatrics. The Enlightenment and Romanticism gloried in childhood, teaching that the child was father to the man: the effects of child-rearing practices would be permanent. Bad baby care was responsible for later physical deformity, warned the French physician Nicholas Andry (1658–1742) in his *L'Orthopédie, ou l'art de prevenir et de corriger dans les enfants, les difformités du corps* (1741) [Orthopaedics or the Art of Preventing and Correcting Deformities of the Body in Children].

Children's complaints commanded attention. Nils Rosen von Rosenstein (1706–73) published a paediatric handbook in 1765, while in 1784 Michael Underwood (1736–1820) brought out his influential *Treatise on the Diseases of Children*, the first major English survey. Though shortlived, the London outpatient dispensary for sick children established in 1769 by George Armstrong (1720–89) heralded children's institutions elsewhere; Joseph Johann Mastalir's (1757–93) Kinderkrankeninstitut was established in Vienna in 1788. In 1816 John Bunnell Davis (1780–1824) opened a children's dispensary and published his *Cursory Inquiry into Some of the Principal Causes of Mortality Among Children* (1817), in which he blamed infant mortality on maternal ignorance – a theme of which doctors have never tired. Trained volunteers were sent out from the dispensary to instruct mothers. By 1850 Davis's dispensary had became the Royal Waterloo Hospital for Children and Women, the headquarters of British paediatric training.

Orthopaedics also emerged, paying special attention to spinal deformities, especially among the young. Percivall Pott at St Bartholomew's Hospital published a pamphlet on palsy produced by spinal caries (to be known as Pott's disease); Jacques Delpech (1777–1832) of Montpellier noted that spinal caries was tubercular. An orthopaedic innovator, Delpech also tried to correct clubfoot by sectioning the Achilles tendon. Georg L. Stromeyer of Hanover (1804–76) followed this up, carrying out a successful tenotomy on a club-footed teenager. His advocacy of sectioning the tendon for all deformities arising from muscular defects opened up modern orthopaedic surgery. Founded in 1830, Stromeyer's hospital became a centre for study of deformities, and in 1831 attracted the young William John Little (1810–94), himself club-footed. Convinced disordered muscle action was to blame, Little endorsed Stromeyer's thinking, submitted to a subcutaneous tenotomy which proved successful, learned Stromeyer's method, and returned to London to perform tenotomy. His Orthopaedic Institution became the Royal Orthopaedic Hospital in 1843.

The improvement in bandaging made possible in 1854 by Anthonius Mathijsen's (1805–78) quick-drying Plaster of Paris was a boon to surgeons attempting to correct deformities. Another advance, the Thomas splint – an iron leg or arm support with a ring at one end to facilitate extension of an injured limb – was devised by Hugh Owen Thomas (1834–91). A gifted manipulator who devised a range of appliances, Thomas shaped the course of orthopaedics in the English-speaking world. Obdurate and oversensitive, he attacked bonesetters and surgeons alike, alienating both. While forceful in his manipulations, he insisted on absolute rest for the injured limb, tailoring his own splints, casts and bandages to ensure it. His nephew Robert Jones (1858–1933) developed his ideas and practices. Surgeon at the Stanley Hospital, Liverpool, Jones pioneered institutions for crippled children. In the United States orthopaedics owed much to Fred H. Albee's (1876–1945) work in New York on bone transplantation and the use of bone grafts in treating Pott's disease, fractures and deformities.

After World War I, orthopaedics grew rapidly as a specialty, acquiring academic underpinning as medical schools developed orthopaedic departments and specialized surgical programmes. The establishment of the Nuffield chair of orthopaedics at Oxford in 1937 was a landmark in its rise to respectability.

Numerous specialisms laid claim to particular body parts or functions. Tooth-drawing had traditionally attracted spectacular showmen like '*le grand Thomas*' in Louis XV's Paris. By contrast, dentistry, that is, the claim to scientific expertise in the anatomy, physiology and pathology of the teeth, emerged in the eighteenth century, pioneered by the French surgeon Pierre Fauchard (1678–1761). Downplaying mere extraction, he gloried in a galaxy of expert and refined techniques including drilling, filling, filing, transplanting, dentures, cosmetic tooth straightening and the wider surgery of the gums and jaw. An agenda was set for later developments.

As with teeth, so with the ear: eighteenth-century studies were laying the foundations for the emergent specialty. The first monograph on ear diseases was the *Traité de l'organe de l'ouïe* (1683) [Treatise on the Organ of Hearing], by J. G. Duverney (1648–1730), professor of anatomy in Paris; Antonio Valsalva's (1666–1723) *Tractatus de aure humana* [Treatise on the Human Ear] was published at Bologna in 1704. The Paris surgeon Jean Itard (1775–1838) studied ear physiology and pathology. His 1821 textbook exposed many errors, particularly opening of the mastoid cavity as a deafness cure, and he involved himself in teaching the deaf. His fellow Paris surgeon Jean Antoine Saissy (1756–1822) opposed puncturing the tympanic membrane for suppuration as recommended of old, instead treating middle ear and mastoid suppuration by rinsing with a catheter.

Mastoiditis was a common and dangerous infection which attracted great attention. In 1853 Sir William Wilde of Dublin (1815–76), Oscar's father, recommended incision of the mastoid through the skin in serious cases to remove pus and purulence from the ear. Wilde established a

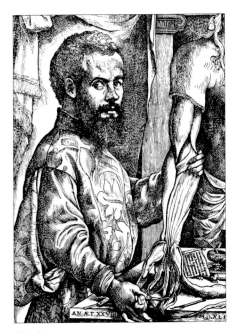

Vesalius.
Born in Brussels, Andreas Vesalius (1514–64) demonstrated anatomy at the University of Padua. Believing in the value of personal experience, he is characteristically shown in action. Woodcut, 1543 (after J. S. van Calcar). Calcar, who was a pupil of Titian, illustrated Vesalius's *De humani corporis fabrica* (1543).

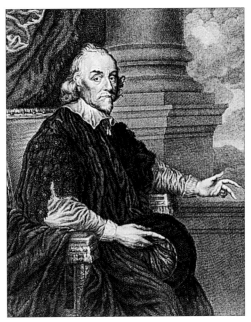

Harvey.
Through his demonstration of the circulation of the blood, William Harvey (1578–1657) epitomized the transition from the old to the new medicine. J. Hall, engraving, 1766.

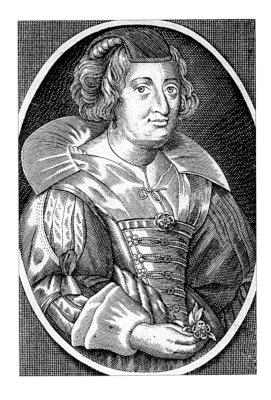

Louise Bourgeois.
Louise Bourgeois (1563–1636) was the most celebrated midwife of early modern France, serving Marie de Medici, wife to Henry IV, through six confinements and publishing books relating her experiences, one of which was translated into English as *The Compleat Midwife's Practice* (1659). Engraving, 1680.

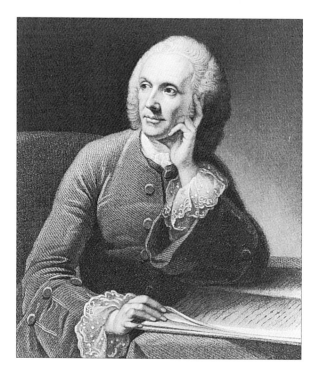

William Hunter.

William Hunter (1718–83), elder brother of John, was a Scot who settled in London and became the leading anatomy school proprietor and obstetrician of the day. As may be seen from his portrait, he prided himself on his refinement. J. Thomas, engraved portrait for Pettigrew's *Medical Portrait Gallery*, 1838–40 (after R. E. Pine).

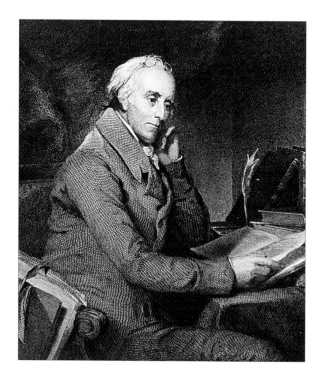

Benjamin Rush.

Benjamin Rush (1745–1813) is often known as the founding father of American medicine. He was also a signatory of the Declaration of Independence. R. W. Dodson, line engraving (after T. Sully).

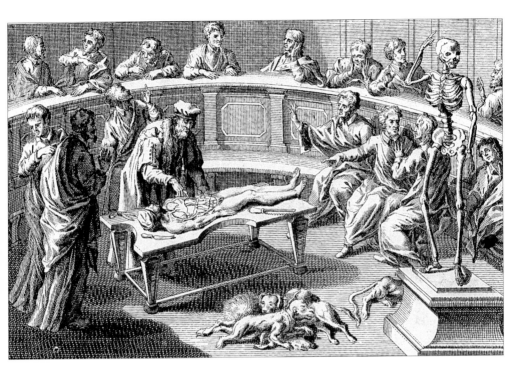

Dissection.

Bartholomaeus Eustachius (1520–1574) performing an anatomical dissection before several observers in an anatomy theatre decorated with an articulated skeleton. In this stylized reconstruction of a sixteenth-century anatomizing, it is significant that the distinguished physician is shown performing his own dissection, while the skeleton is a reminder of the omnipresence of death. Engraving, 1722 (after P.L. Ghezzi, 1714).

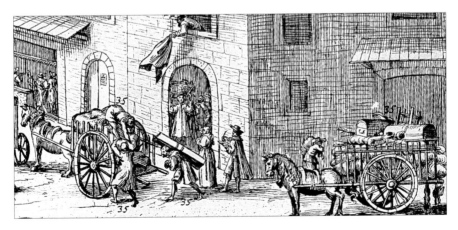

A scene from the plague in Rome of 1656.

An infected family's house being cleared and the contents loaded into carts. Aside from the personal tragedy, plague posed enormous problems of urban management, leading often to draconian ordinances and public health measures. Etching (detail).

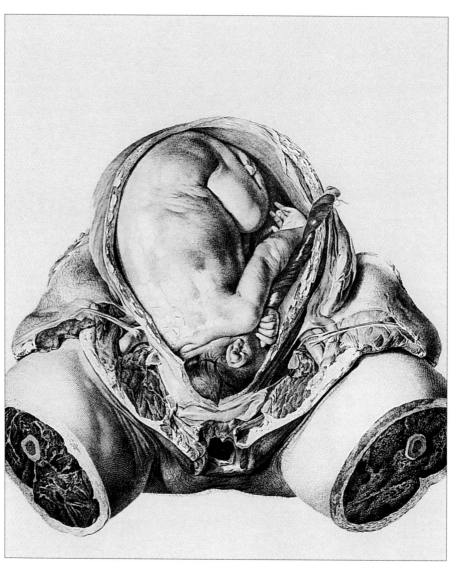

A mother and baby.

William Hunter's (1718–83) *Anatomia uteri humani gravidi* [Anatomy of the Human Gravid Uterus: 1774] was an astonishing depiction of the pregnant woman and her foetus in 34 copper plates. Its images were exceptionally lifelike, yet at the same time dehumanizing. Engraving, 1774.

Successive stages of dissection.
The successive stages of a dissection are shown here as the flesh is stripped from the musculature down to the skeleton itself. Part of a collection of 14 paintings and 1 drawing. Watercolour and pen on paper, *c.* 1807.

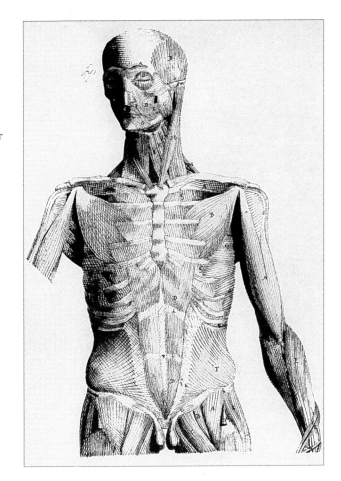

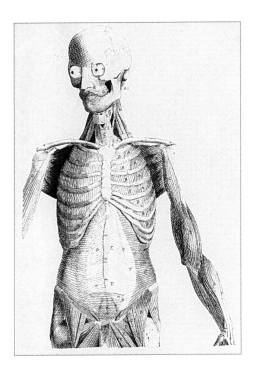

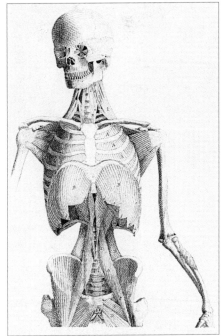

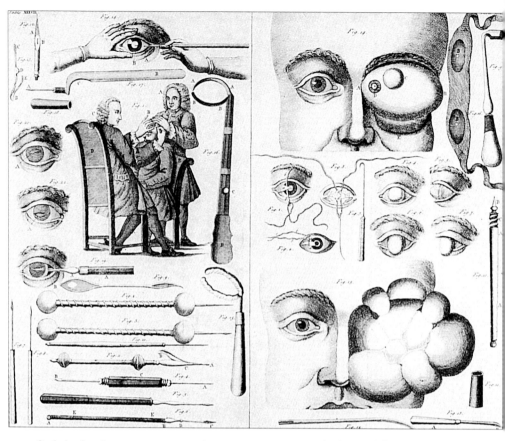

Opthalmology instruments, eye growths, a cateract operation and other eye defects.

The drawing on the left shows different ways of couching for cataracts, operations which saw considerable improvements in the early eighteenth century. R. Parr, engraving, 1743–5.

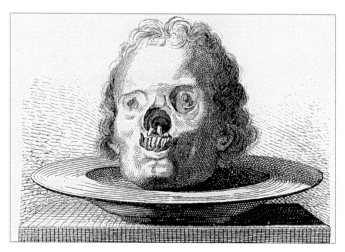

Syphilis: a preserved skull of a woman who had been suffering from syphilis and died in 1796.

German images such as these served as moral and religious reminders of the evils of unbridled sexuality, no less than as anatomical specimens. Engraving, c. 1796.

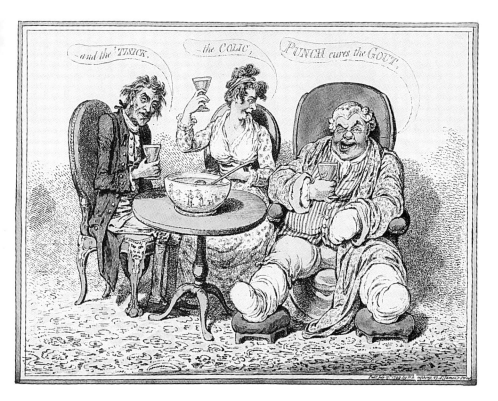

Punch Cures the Gout, the Colic, and the Tisick: An obese gouty man drinking punch with two companions.

The three diseases here represented all carried strong messages. Gout was the eligible disease of the country gentleman, and the 'tisick' (tuberculosis) the sad disorder of his poorer relation, while the colic was believed to be the consequence of corseting and tight-lacing in women. James Gillray, coloured etching, 1799.

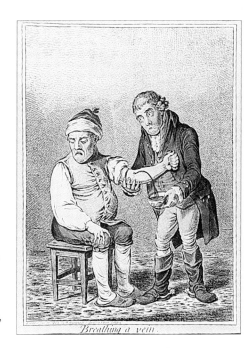

Breathing a vein: An ill man who is being bled to death by his doctor.
Blood-letting remained the commonest form of medical intervention from the time of Galen to the mid-nineteenth century. Despite the patient's expression, it was, apparently, popular with sufferers. J. Sneyd, coloured etching, 1804 (after James Gillray).

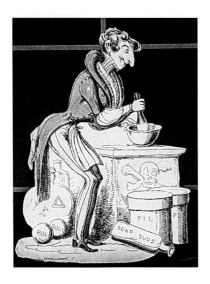

An Apothecary with a Pestle and Mortar to Make up a Prescription.

The caricature conveys the ambiguity of public feelings towards the apothecary. Despite belonging to a lowly branch of medicine, this one has pretensions to fashion; the images of death, as always, attend his efforts. A. Park, etching with watercolour, early nineteenth century.

The interior of a pharmaceutical laboratory with people at work. The shop is visible through a doorway.

In the eighteenth century, most medical laboratories were attached to the premises of manufacturing chemists. This scene conveys an alchemical flavour. Engraving, 1747.

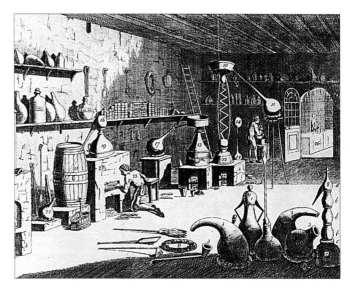

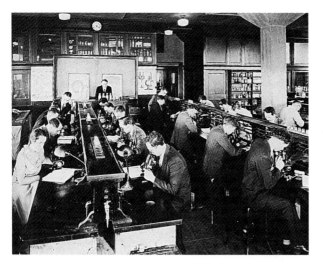

Philadelphia College of Pharmacy and Science: students looking through microscopes in a laboratory.

From the 1830s, instruction in the sciences connected with medicine was increasingly through instruction in laboratory techniques, in particular using the microscope. Photograph, *c.* 1933.

dispensary and was the first to teach otology in Britain, his *Practical Observations on Aural Surgery and the Nature and Treatment of Diseases of the Ear* (1853) distilling his teachings. Surgical interventions grew. James Hinton (1822–75), a London surgeon, and Hermann Hugo Rudolf Schwartze of Halle (1837–1910) developed mastoidectomy, removing the bony cortex overlying the mastoid air cells. By 1900 the operation had attained widespread acceptance.

The first hospital devoted to ear diseases was established in 1816 by an unqualified practitioner, John Harrison Curtis (1778–1860); this became the Royal Ear Hospital in Soho. Curtis treated all cases by syringing, using an enormous instrument. Another innovator was James Yearsley (1805–69), who recognized that deafness could arise not just from diseased ears but from the nose and throat. He founded the Metropolitan Ear and Throat Hospital in Fitzroy Square in 1838. A native of Lincolnshire and father of the Christian socialist, Arnold, Joseph Toynbee (1815–66) vowed to 'rescue aural surgery from the hands of quacks', performing over two thousand dissections, described in his *Pathological and Surgical Observations on the Diseases of the Ear* (1860). In 1851 he was appointed aural surgeon to St Mary's, the first general hospital to set beds aside for ear diseases. His death resulted from self-experimentation. Believing tinnitus (ringing in the ears) might be reduced by inhalation of chloroform and subsequent inflation of the ear, he tried it on himself – with fatal consequences.

Study of the throat also developed, owing much to the invention of the laryngoscope in 1855 by the Paris singing-master Manuel Garcia (1805–1906). A prominent British specialist was Sir Morell Mackenzie (1837–92) who in 1863 founded the Throat Hospital in Golden Square and wrote a textbook. The combined specialty of otorhinolaryngology emerged around the turn of the century, though these still met resistance. Despite his address at 19 Harley Street, Mackenzie commented, 'the truth is that we are just a little doubtful as to our position in the social scale.'

Like teeth and ears, eye troubles had long been treated by itinerants, but ophthalmology rooted itself as a specialty, with clinics and formal teaching. In 1803, Göttingen introduced it as a taught course, and Vienna established the first clinic in 1812. An unfortunate boost was given to the discipline by the scores of soldiers returning to France and England with glaucoma and other eye diseases contracted in Egypt.

As so often, the characteristic professional disease of blocked promotion played its part. Finding his career thwarted at St Thomas's Hospital, John Cunningham Saunders (1773–1810) founded the London Dispensary for Curing Diseases of the Eye and Ear (1805), which later became the London Eye Infirmary and finally the Royal Ophthalmic Hospital (Moorfields). Sister institutions were soon established, notably the Glasgow Eye Infirmary in 1824, resulting from lectures started by William Mackenzie (1791–1868). The Royal Westminster Ophthalmic Hospital was founded in 1816 by the military surgeon George James Guthrie (1785–1856), who claimed to be the first to give lectures devoted to eye surgery – but squabbles were endemic among practitioners claiming they were the first to break with quackery and set the study on a scientific basis. The Moorfields Hospital became the model for the New York Eye and Ear Infirmary (1820), the first such institution in the United States. C. J. F. Carron du Villards (1801–60) set up the first Paris eye dispensary in 1835.

Scientific understanding of the eye made great strides in mid century, thanks particularly to Frans Cornelis Donders (1818–89), professor of physiology at Utrecht, who elucidated the relations between the physics and the physiology of optics. The emergent specialty was aided by Helmholtz's ophthalmoscope (1851) and the ophthalmometer (1852), instruments permitting investigation of the interior of the eye and affording evidence of other diseases, including those of the brain. These came into regular use in the 1870s. Albrecht von Graefe (1828–70), of Berlin, the greatest of the eye specialists, expanded the clinical applications of the ophthalmoscope and initiated modern ophthalmic surgery, introducing the operation for strabismus (squint) and iridectomy (removal of a portion of the iris in glaucoma). Eye surgery was further aided by Karl Koller's (1857–1944) use of cocaine as a local anaesthetic. By the 1920s, clouding of the cornea was being treated by transplantation, and thermocautery was introduced to repair detached retinas.

Thus specialties crystallized, involving the coalescence of various elements: a localized medical problem with a definable body of knowledge and techniques, energetic boosters, and a pool of patients, patrons and donors. Specialties became identified with their institutions. By 1860 there were at least sixty-six special hospitals and dispensaries in London alone, including the Royal Hospital for Diseases of the Chest (1814), St Mark's Hospital for Diseases of the Colon and Rectum (1835), the Royal National Orthopaedic Hospital, the Brompton (1841), the

Royal Marsden Hospital (1851), the Hospital for Sick Children, Great Ormond Street (1852), the National Hospital (for nervous diseases) Queen Square (1860), St John's Hospital for Diseases of the Skin (1863), and St Peter's Hospital for urological disorders (1864). Founded by enthusiasts and supported by donations, these and dozens more were at first frowned upon by the general hospitals, but gradually elite practitioners sought posts within them, either to improve their skills or to supplement a general hospital appointment. Special hospitals became 'medicalized' early, with doctors controlling admissions, appointments and policy, and running them in an entrepreneurial, proprietorial manner.

Hospitals played a comparable role in the planting of specialization on the Continent and in North America. Children's hospitals were set up in Paris in 1802, in Berlin in 1830, St Petersburg in 1834 and Vienna in 1837. The United States looked to Britain for models. The Massachusetts Eye and Ear Infirmary, the Boston Lying-In Hospital, the New York Hospital for Diseases of the Skin, and others, all patterned themselves on British institutions. Unlike Britain, however, the special hospitals in the US which thrived were those catering for particular national immigrant groups – Germans, Italians, Jews and others. In Germany and Austria, with hospitals closely associated with universities, the tendency was for special academic departments to develop rather than separate institutions.

Certain diseases were particularly well represented in new specialist foundations, notably those routinely excluded from general hospitals, because they were contagious, 'loathsome' – like venereal conditions – or incurable. The first cancer hospital was set up in Rheims around 1750; from the 1850s they multiplied in Britain with the London Cancer Hospital and others in Leeds, Liverpool, Manchester and Glasgow, many of them set up by medical men who found their careers checked. They were often dismissed as little better than quack emporia and, with the exceptions of the London Cancer Hospital, renamed the Royal Marsden after its founder, William Marsden (1796–1867), and the Christie Hospital in Manchester, few lasted. In France, Oeuvres du Calvaire were set up to care for women with cancer in Lyon (1850), Paris (1874), Saint-Etienne (1874), Marseille (1881), Rouen (1891) and Bordeaux (1909). Inspired by a philanthropic Lyon widow, Jeanne Garnier-Chabot, the staff of the Calvary hospitals were themselves widows.

American cancer hospitals came slightly later. The first, the New York Cancer Hospital, was set up in 1884, followed by the St Rose Free House for Incurable Cancer in 1899 and others at Buffalo (1898), Philadelphia (1904) and St Louis (1905). Some embodied the new style of philanthropy which looked optimistically to science and to the laboratory for cures, rather than concentrating on care of the dying. That shift came to Britain too. Plans for Friedenheims ('homes of peace' for the dying) at the Manchester, London and Glasgow cancer hospitals were shelved in a new wave of optimism about treatment and research.

Specialties flourished when they involved a conspicuous body part or pain responsive to surgical intervention. The very idea of specialization thereby achieved legitimization, though not without continuing struggles. Looking back in an autobiography significantly called *Reminiscences of a Specialist* (1932), Greville MacDonald (1856–1944) emphasized how it had been an uphill struggle as late as the 1880s:

> Even a consulting-room in Wimpole Street could not give me a place among the really elect. The Throat Hospital, in spite of its new and irreproachable staff, was still looked upon by a carefully censorious profession as simply *not respectable*. The distrust of this newest specialty in medicine was chiefly due to the prevalent disapproval of specializing in general; for it was considered that all qualified practitioners were competent for everything.

Hostility to specialization continued. In 1900 the *General Practitioner* said of specialists, 'their minds are narrowed, judgment biased and unbalanced by disproportionate knowledge of one subject,' and the patient would suffer because the specialist 'knows nothing of the constitutional idiosyncrasies of the individual, which are essential to correct diagnosis and treatment'. By 1900, however, nothing could stop the scores of specialties taking root upon the balkanized medical map – involving hospital departments, research centres and distinctive career hierarchies. Such specialization makes it difficult to view modern medicine as a unity: rather an assemblage of elements interacting with one another in *ad hoc* ways. It brought sophisticated skills, often at the cost of the coherent vision of the patient and sickness. This in part explains why, paralleling specialization, counter-movements arose to reject much of what it stood for: these became known as alternative medicine.

ALTERNATIVE MEDICINE

The emergence of specialties shows medicine's changing configurations: growing demand (often whipped up by adroit promotion), the resourcefulness of medical men in forging careers, and the bid of the marginal to enter the mainstream. Alternative medicine also shows great diversity and the fluctuating relations of the marginal with the regulars. Continuity, change and innovation can all be seen, the whirl of consumer demand in emergent mass society and the role of charismatic individuals. Newspapers, railways and all the apparatus of nineteenth-century commercial society provided challenges to which nostrum-mongers, rejuvenators and cancer healers were quick to rise. The time-honoured rituals of the itinerant huckster continued, if generally seen as increasingly quaint and down-market. The need for miracle cures never slackens, and this produced, in a popular phrase, 'toadstool millionaires' galore, eager to purvey magnetic, electrical or chemical cures to the desperate and credulous.

New proprietary medicines won a following, memorably Lydia E. Pinkham's Vegetable Compound, sold, from 1873, by the fifty-four-year-old Lydia Pinkham of Lynn, Massachusetts, perhaps America's first millionairess. Originally marketed as a cure for 'female weaknesses', it was soon being proclaimed as 'the greatest remedy in the world', 'Lily the Pink's' kindly face appearing on the label and commemorated in song. In England James Morison (1770–1840) made a fortune with his Vegetable Pills. ('Brothers, I am sorry I have got no Morison's Pill for curing the maladies of Society', declared Thomas Carlyle.) Thomas Beecham (1820–1907) and Thomas Holloway (1800–1883) followed suit, the latter bequeathing much of his fortune to found (Royal) Holloway College, which became part of London University.

Alongside these old currents of need and greed, and stories of personal razzmatazz, rapacity or opportunism, the nineteenth century was distinctive for introducing new healing movements based on the principled rejection of orthodox medicine in favour of alternative healing philosophies. Such developments might be viewed as the reincarnation of the plain-man populism of Paracelsus, distrustful of elite faculty medicine. Many healing movements arose mirroring the myriad religious dissenting sects and socio-political groups which gained a following in an era of mass literacy and grassroots discontent, products of the 'democratic intellect'. Artisans who baulked at the power of princes and prelates might be no more disposed to swallow orthodox medicine.

Alternative healing sects were disparate – some were religious, others secular; some favoured science, others folk wisdom; some glamorized the heroic prophet, others made every man his own doctor – but typically they shared some common ground. They tended to denounce modern lifestyles as unnatural and accused regular medicine of being an oligarchic closed shop, an obscurantist racket devoted to self-aggrandizement. Fringe healers urged a return to simplicity, praising plain living and looking to nature's healthy, healing ways. They recycled venerable health advice like the non-naturals (temperance and moderation), but adapted it to the anxieties of commercial society and the aspirations of self-help common folk aiming to gain control over their lives in matters of bodily health no less than religion and politics. These doctrines gained their greatest following in America, partly because visionaries gravitated there, hoping for a better future, a fresh start, and partly because America imposed fewest restrictions on practice. Their homeland, however, was Germany.

The great inspiration and trail-blazer was homoeopathy, developed by Samuel Hahnemann (1755–1833). Hahnemann acquired his medical education at Leipzig, Vienna and Erlangen, where he graduated in 1779, imbibing that Enlightenment faith in the goodness of nature, which permeated his mature thinking. Gaining early medical experience in a variety of small Saxon towns, he developed a horror for the blunders of the medical profession, leading to his *Über die Arsenikvergiftung: ihre Hilfe und gerichtliche Ausmittelung* (1786) [On Poisoning by Arsenic – Its Treatment and Forensic Detection], a work registering his fears over the toxicity of drugs.

Moving from town to town, Hahnemann published works such as *Freund der Gesundheit* (1792–5) [The Friend of Health], which stressed that the key to well-being lay not in the costly but dangerous polypharmacy of the apothecaries but in attention to the non-naturals – above all, due attention to fresh air and exercise. He began to formulate the principles of his own method of treatment, homoeopathy; the first major statement appeared in his *Organon der rationellen Heilkunde* (1810) [Handbook of Rational Healing].

There were, Hahnemann argued, three possible approaches to healing: prevention; the allopathic method of treatment by opposites which dominated orthodox medicine but which was at best palliative and at worst harmful; and the homoeopathic method. It was common knowledge that one disease drove out another. Finding that cinchona (Peruvian bark) produced responses similar to malaria symptoms – the bark that quelled fever would induce it in a healthy person – he argued that medicine should logically be deploying drugs which produced in healthy people symptoms similar to those of the disease in question: 'In order to cure disease, we must seek medicines that can excite similar symptoms in the healthy human body.'

This became the first law of homoeopathy, the law of similars, *similia similibus curantur*: let like be cured by like (exemplified in the folk wisdom that hot compresses were good for burns, or that cowpox vaccination immunized against smallpox). This was supplemented by homoeopathy's second law, that of infinitesimals (serial dilution): the smaller the dose, the more efficacious the medicine. This seeming paradox followed from Hahnemann's lifelong preoccupations: his commitment to ascertaining the precise effects of drugs upon the individual sufferer, his contempt for the arbitrary and destructive prescribing habits of regular medicine, and his preoccupation with drug purity. The body, he held, was specially sensitive during disease and tiny quantities of pure drugs did far more good than large doses of adulterated ones.

Settling in Leipzig, Hahnemann publicized homoeopathy, giving medical lectures, gathering disciples dedicated to 'proving' (that is, testing) new medicines, and publishing his findings in such works as the *Materia medica pura* (1811–21) [Pure Materia Medica]. The outraged Leipzig faculty and apothecaries had him banned from practice, and he moved on, everywhere meeting resistance from the elite. He eventually settled in Paris and lived long enough to see widespread support for his doctrines, which struck a chord amongst patients suspicious of drugging practices. He won over a large and often fashionable clientele and captured a significant fraction of the medical profession across Europe and America. Consolidating itself as a worldwide movement (the International Congress of Homoeopathic Physicians was founded at the end of the century), homoeopathy endured while other movements rose and fell, and established its claims to recognition by licensing authorities. In Britain, for example, the homoeopathic hospitals were to be the only non-regular establishments recognized by the National Health Service in 1948. Homoeopathy's lasting appeal has stemmed from its stress on purity and the attractive idea of the body striving to cure itself.

Another movement which, like homoeopathy, stressed hygiene and purity and won support across the social spectrum was hydropathy. This variant on the old fascination with healing waters originated with Vincent Priessnitz (1799–1851), a rural prophet who, convinced of water's powers, established a spa at Gräfenberg in Austrian Silesia. Health was the body's natural condition, he maintained; sickness resulted from the introduction of foreign matter, and acute disease was the body's attempt to expel such morbid material. Regular therapies were thus misguided: drugs, purges and bleeding interfered with nature and would turn acute and functional conditions into chronic ones. Water treatment was the best way to obviate this: water would bring an acute condition to a crisis, expelling poisons from the system. Priessnitz's techniques included withdrawing all drugs and promoting sweat followed by cold baths and wet bandages. Patients had to give up alcohol and rich food, live on coarse bread and milk, and drink twelve glasses of water a day.

Gräfenberg offered a menu of water treatments: head baths – patients would lie on the floor with their heads in basins of cold water; wet stomach packs; the ascending douche, spraying water up the genitals; and the wet sheet treatment, in which patients were wrapped for hours, mummylike, in wet bandages. The cold douche was the *coup de grâce*: icy water was discharged over patients from a height of twenty feet. These were spartan measures, but they worked well on an overfed, overdrugged and stressed-out generation. Priessnitz's establishment became immensely popular; in 1839 it played host to one monarch, one duke, one duchess, 22 princes and 149 counts and countesses. Bored with Bath, the British upper classes arrived in the 1840s. Priessnitz's dictum, *man muss Gebirge haben* (people need mountains), captures the movement's links with Romanticism.

Hydrotherapy was imported into England by two medical regulars, James Gully (1808–83) and Dr James Wilson (1807–67), who became converts to Priessnitz's hydropathy, and decided to set up in the hilly town of Malvern in Worcestershire. Gully became the better known, publishing *The Water Cure in Chronic Disease* in 1848. Passing through nine editions, it helped to win him such distinguished patients as Thomas Carlyle, Alfred Tennyson, Sir Edward Bulwer Lytton and Charles Darwin. 'I am in a Hydropathy Establishment near Cheltenham (the only one in England conducted on pure Priessnitzian principles),' Tennyson explained to his fellow poet Edward FitzGerald:

I have had four crises (one larger than had been seen for two or three years in Gräfenberg – indeed I believe the largest but one that has been seen). Much poison has come out of me, which no physic ever would have brought to light . . . I have been here already upwards of two months. Of all the uncomfortable ways of living sure an hydropathical is the worst: no reading by candlelight, no going near a fire, no tea, no coffee, perpetual wet sheet and cold bath and alternation from hot to cold: however I have much faith in it.

Hydropathic establishments continued to have a following amongst those with faith in the healing powers of nature, cold water and physiological puritanism: no pain, no gain.

Equally hostile to orthodox disease theory and routine polypharmacy was the first of the indigenous American healing sects, Thomsonianism. Despising 'book doctors', Samuel A. Thomson (1769–1843) developed a people's health movement on vegetable-based therapies. Believing, as was explained in his *New Guide to Health* (1822), all ills were produced by cold and any treatment generating heat would aid recovery, his favourite herbal remedy was *Lobelia inflata*, whose seeds caused vomiting and heavy sweating; it was closely followed by cayenne pepper. The seventy plant remedies that made up the Thomsonian *materia medica* were all purportedly milder and safer than the harsh, powerful remedies favoured by allopaths.

Thomson publicized his system through the Botanico-Medical College of Ohio in Cincinnati, chartered in 1838, and its offshoots, and he recruited disciples via a network of Friendly Botanic Societies throughout New England. He claimed that some 100,000 people bought the franchise (known as Family Rights) to practise his system; between 1832 and 1838 the Family Botanic Societies staged annual conventions, gatherings blending aspects of revivalist religion and political caucuses. The Thomsonians operated infirmaries and stores where they compounded their medications and dispensed them in competition with pharmacists.

Such a commercially adroit movement was certain to trigger competitors and imitators in a society in which *laissez-faire* individualism prevailed. By 1850 the movement was riven by splinter groups, notably the so-called Neo-Thomsonians, Eclectics and the Reformed Practitioners of Medicine, all lauding nature's ways and attacking the mercenary and pernicious regulars with their calomel and other heavy-metal drugs.

The Thomsonian gospel was brought to England by 'Dr' Albert Isaiah Coffin (1800–66), who claimed, like many another American healer, to have been cured of tuberculosis by a native American woman. Arriving in 1838, he soon had a keen following among self-improving artisans and dissenters, developing his own team of agents and a chain of 'Friendly Botanico-Medical Societies'. Medical botany of various kinds appealed to artisan self-help.

Contemporary with the Thomsonians were the Grahamites who dedicated themselves to healthy living in a kind of this-worldly salvationism. Sylvester Graham (1794–1851) was a zealot who thought health too precious to be left to doctors. Inspired by the teetotal movement, he believed self-control should be extended to all domains of life. Were not men made gross, even diseased, by indulgence in food and sex? Vegetarianism and wholegrain cereals were recommended, and the 'Graham cracker' made its bow. Sexual activity was to be limited: it inflamed the passions and wasted the seminal fluid which was the essence of life.

If Paris pathology encouraged Old World medicine to stress the empire of disease and death, American alternative sects were more upbeat, taking their cue from phrenologists and other self-help groups confident that science and attention to nature's laws contained the secrets of health. Nature was benign and, if humans only heeded her, their bodies would be naturally healthy. Such was the hopeful message of the osteopathy movement, originating in 1874 with Dr Andrew Taylor Still (1828–1917), who established his college at Kirksville, Missouri. Still asserted the body's inherent capacity to resist disease and repair itself. Osteopathy also stressed the intrinsic unity of all parts of the body, attributing disease to 'structural derangements' or 'somatic components of the disease processes', also called osteopathic lesions. While he concentrated on the spine, Still's followers extended manipulation to the entire skeletal structure, enlarging the range of techniques to include electric and water treatments, massage and eventually surgery.

Somewhat similar was chiropractic, established in 1895 by Daniel David Palmer (1845–1913), after he managed to restore the hearing of a man by adjusting his backbone. An erstwhile 'magnetic doctor', Palmer based chiropractic on the hypothesis that energy flow from the brain was the essential life-giving force in the body and, rather as with mesmerism, that obstruction produced disease. The spine commonly interfered with nerve function, and manipulation by hand ('chiropractic' comes from the Greek for 'doing by hand') was the method for treating the spine.

This theory became the educational basis of the Palmer School of Chiropractic which he founded in Davenport, Iowa in 1899. His son, B. J. Palmer (1881–1961), helped spread chiropractic methods through books and the school's annual 'lyceum' of entertainment and chiropractic knowledge. Although allopathic physicians criticized chiropractic practitioners (or 'bonecrackers') for their lack of scientifically-based techniques, these healers became so widely patronized that even health insurance companies began to cover chiropractic.

The Pelagian or radical Protestant streak in many of these healing movements (universal delivery from disease) was taken to its logical extreme in the Christian Science movement. Battling against the suffocating Congregationalism of her parents, Mary Baker Eddy (1821–1910) spent much of her adolescence ill and bedridden, and regular physicians did her no good. Relieved by homoeopathy, the mesmeric treatments of Phineas Quimby (1802–66), and divine revelation after reading the Bible, she undertook a self-healing process, whose success led her to adumbrate her own system, declaring 'there is but one creation, and it is wholly spiritual.' Since all was spirit and matter a phantasm, there could be no such reality as somatic disease; all sickness was in the mind. Hence, as was explained in her *Science and Health* (1875), true 'mind healing' would dispel the 'illusions' of sickness and pain. Christian Science owed its conversions to its 'patient, heal thyself' appeal. Setting up the Massachusetts Metaphysical College, Eddy taught some 4000 students, most of whom were women excluded from regular medical education.

With rapid social change and its astonishing mix of people from every possible ethnic, religious and cultural background, orthodox medicine could seem irrelevant and stale in the United States, and many spiritual and fringe faiths shot up, targeting the individual self-help experience of the layman. Spiritualism and theosophy won followers. From their early days, both the Mormons and the Seventh Day Adventists voiced antipathy to regular medicine, Joseph Smith (1805–44) accepting only roots and herbs, and his fellow Mormons passing laws restricting the 'deadly poisons' of orthodox remedies. Mormons in particular championed the right to resist compulsory smallpox vaccination.

Growing out of earlier religious and health-reform movements, and teaching abstemiousness and vegetarianism, the Adventists proclaimed a 'gospel of health', which valued hydropathic cures. Their Health Reform Institute at Battle Creek, Michigan, was headed by John Harvey Kellogg (1852–1943), brother of the cereal manufacturer (Will Keith). Emphasizing the importance of restricting diet, alcohol and sexual activity, Kellogg's 'San' became popular with the wealthy. Medical faiths and fads went together in America, anticipating the later popularity of all manner of psychotherapy.

Alternative medicine's preoccupations highlight the ambiguities in nineteenth-century medicine. Its new scientific and professional movements generated counter-trends – a populist, anti-elitist backlash. While people wanted their diseases to be cured, they were also seeking far more from medicine: explanations of their troubles, a sense of wholeness, a key to the meaning of life. Craving reassurance from physicians, democratic generations also, paradoxically, wanted to take health into their own hands. Not least, so long as the message of orthodox medicine was pessimistic, alternative medicine instilled hope.

The nineteenth century brought medicine face to face with commercial society, with all its energies, anxieties, conflicts and contrasts. Regular medicine sought to be a profitable trade, when that suited it – how could it be otherwise? But it also had to be seen to be above all that, sometimes looking to the state as its lifeline, sometimes opting for loftier, more metaphysical supports. A commercial civilization purchased regular medicine's services but it also bought all the other therapeutic brands on offer, and the public showed little more brand loyalty than to tea or toothpowder.

Medicine strove to professionalize itself, but without some unique source of power or access to a monopoly (courtesy of the state) that remained an unrealizable struggle. The real trouble was that medicine still could do little about disease and premature death. It was only once those threats began to recede – developments which owed little to medicine *per se* – that medicine could become truly powerful.

CHAPTER XIII

PUBLIC MEDICINE

MODERNIZATION AND INDUSTRIALIZATION elicited wildly differing reactions. Optimists like the English physician Erasmus Darwin saw science, technology and industry as unbinding Prometheus, providing mankind with the tools to master nature, conquer disease and perhaps disarm death itself. The Marquis de Condorcet's *Esquisse d'un tableau historique des progrès de l'esprit humain* [Sketch for a Historical Picture of the Progress of the Human Mind], written in 1793 just before the Jacobins drove him to suicide, held out a vision of a healthy, rational future society, now that medicine had been delivered from its false theories, jargon and submission to authority. Medical modernization would bring social regeneration. 'The average length of human life will be increased and a better health and a stronger physical constitution will be ensured,' the *philosophe* predicted: 'Would it be absurd then to suppose that this perfection of the human species might be capable of indefinite progress?'

Such dreams were shattered by the Revd Thomas Malthus's *An Essay on the Principle of Population as it Affects the Future Improvement of Society* (1798). Parson Malthus didn't dispute 'the great and unlooked for discoveries that have taken place of late years in natural philosophy'. Unlike Condorcet, however, he could see only trouble ahead. Material progress would breed inexorable population growth; and with ever more mouths to feed on a limited amount of food, the consequences must be catastrophic – famine, or war, or pestilence – and the future would be plagued by worsening subsistence and health problems ('Malthusian crises'). Malthus was not ignorant of birth control, indeed the term 'Neo-Malthusian' was used by its promoters. But from his Christian viewpoint he regarded it as a 'vice', conducive to immorality. In later editions he suggested a solution in 'moral restraint' or continence.

Judgment on Malthus's merits as a prophet will depend on the consequences of population growth to come. In his own time, developments near home seemed to bear out the woeful accuracy of his forecasts. In Ireland, which had a soaring population, potato blight caused famine and thousands of deaths in 1810, 1820 and 1830, leading in the years after 1845 to the notorious Great Famine in which perhaps two million people died, some from starvation, but far more from typhus and other epidemics consequent upon malnutrition and social collapse. Mostly, however, the situation was less black and white than Malthus's reactionary doom-mongering implied – partly because (as he came to admit) personal and social action could head off many of the anticipated disasters. One such mode of prudent action was public health.

INDUSTRIAL SOCIETY

The kind of population explosion Malthus warned of brought evident health risks. In the century after 1750, Britain's population increased threefold, from around 6 to 18 million. In 1750, about 15 per cent of the population lived in towns; by 1880 a staggering 80 per cent was urban. In 1801 one in five workers was employed in manufacturing and linked occupations; by 1871 that had climbed to two in three. The largest city in the western world, London had about 800,000 inhabitants in 1801; by 1841 its population had grown by a further million, and at the death of Queen Victoria in 1901 the heart of empire contained seven million inhabitants. By 1861 six British cities had populations of over a quarter-million, and in some towns the growth rate was astounding: in the decade after 1821 Bradford's numbers rose by 78 per cent and West Bromwich's by 60 per cent; Glasgow's population of 77,000 in 1801 had rocketed to 904,000 by 1901.

The British story was repeated with a time lag throughout the industrializing world. Paris, New York, Berlin and many other cities all broke the million mark in the nineteenth century and factory towns, mining regions and ports throughout Germany, Bohemia, Belgium, France and the United States were every bit as foul as Manchester. And all the other pathogenic features of modern states and mass societies came too, not least warfare. Napoleon's wars were the first to be fought with gigantic citizen armies; the American Civil

War involved millions of fighting men, and those numbers were dwarfed by the conscript armies of the First World War. More succumbed to disease than to the new Gatling guns or howitzers. The Union army in the Civil War (1861–65) lost 186,216 men to disease, twice the number killed in action; nearly half were claimed by typhoid and dysentery. In the World War deaths through combat finally overtook deaths through disease, but even that war took a terrible disease toll.

Like the war itself, typhus began in Serbia, with 10,000 cases as early as November 1914; within six months, deaths had leapt to 150,000. With the revolution of 1917 and the civil war, typhus ran riot in Russia: between 1917 and 1921 Russia had 25 million cases with up to 3 million deaths, the worst outbreak ever known. 'If Socialism does not defeat the louse,' quipped Lenin, 'the louse will defeat Socialism.'

But at least war was temporary. For millions, entire lives – albeit often very short ones – were passed in new industrial cities of dreadful night with an all too typical socio-pathology: foul housing, often in flooded cellars, gross overcrowding, atmospheric and water-supply pollution, overflowing cesspools, contaminated pumps; poverty, hunger, fatigue and abjection everywhere. Such conditions, comparable to today's Third World shanty towns or refugee camps, bred rampant sickness of every kind. Appalling neo-natal, infant and child mortality accompanied the abomination of child labour in mines and factories; life expectations were exceedingly low – often under twenty years among the working classes – and everywhere sickness precipitated family breakdown, pauperization and social crisis. The squalor of the slums was exposed time and again by social reformers, novelists, newsmen, and clergymen appalled to find hell at the heart of civilization. Everywhere he walked, noted Friedrich Engels in his *Condition of the Working Classes in England* (1844) (Engels was a Manchester factory owner as well as Karl Marx's collaborator), he met 'pale, lank, narrow-chested, hollow-eyed ghosts', cooped up in houses that were mere 'kennels to sleep and die in':

> Passing along a rough bank, among stakes and washing lines, one penetrates into this chaos of small one-storied, one-roomed huts, in most of which there is no artificial floor; kitchen, living and sleeping-room all in one. . . . Everywhere before the doors residue and offal; that any sort of pavement lay underneath could not be seen but only felt, here and there, with the feet. This whole

collection of cattlesheds for human beings was surrounded on two
sides by houses and a factory, and on the third by the river, and
beside the narrow stair up the bank, a narrow doorway alone led
out into another almost equally ill-built, ill-kept labyrinth of
dwellings.... Everything which here arouses horror and indignation is of recent origin, belongs to the industrial epoch.

Andrew Mearns's *Bitter Cry of Outcast London* (1883) similarly asked his
readers whether they had 'any conception of what these pestilential
human rookeries are, where tens of thousands are crowded together
amidst horrors which call to mind what we have heard of the middle
passage of the slave ship'. Mearns tugged at the heart-strings:

> To get to them you have to penetrate courts reeking with poisonous
> and malodorous gases arising from accumulations of sewage and
> refuse scattered in all directions and often flowing beneath your
> feet; courts, many of them which the sun never penetrates, which
> are never visited by a breath of fresh air, and which rarely know
> the virtues of a drop of cleansing water.... You have to grope
> your way along dark and filthy passages swarming with vermin.
> Then, if you are not driven back by the intolerable stench, you
> may gain admittance to the dens in which these thousands of beings
> who belong, as much as you, to the race for whom Christ died,
> herd together.

Historians still dispute whether industrialization raised or depressed
wages and living standards – something, perhaps, impossible to measure.
But there can be no doubt that industrialism jeopardized health. Industrial injuries and disabilities were multiplied by dangerous trades. With
high speed, mechanized production, exhausting working hours and child
labour, the factory system produced a grisly crop of accidents and muti-
lations. The penalties of dangerous trades were documented. In 1775
Percivall Pott had pointed out that boy chimneysweeps developed
scrotal cancer, due to soot irritation. Pneumoconiosis afflicted coal-
miners; brown lung disease became the curse of cotton workers; 'phossy
jaw' was an occupational risk of matchworkers exposed to phosphorus;
and dust from stone, flint and sand led to silicosis and other lung disorders among miners, brick-makers, cutlers and potters. 'Some of them
gets lead poisoned soon, and some of them gets lead poisoned later:
and some but not many niver' – an old Irishwoman thus introduced
Charles Dickens to work in the lead mills.

In 1832 the Leeds physician Charles Turner Thackrah (1795–1833) published *The Effects of Arts, Trades, and Professions on Health and Longevity*, documenting the diseases and disabilities of various occupations. Apart from factory-workers, among those exposed to harmful substances were cornmillers, maltsters, coffee-roasters, snuff-makers, rag-pickers, papermakers and feather-dressers; tailors were so subject to anal fistulas they set up their own 'fistula clubs'. 'Surely this shocking and unnatural occupation ought to be abolished,' was his comment on the climbing boys. Overall, his verdict was bleak: 'Not 10 per cent of the inhabitants of large towns enjoy full health.'

Engels devoted two chapters of his *Condition of the Working Classes* to work conditions, being especially concerned with child labour:

> In the manufacture of glass . . . the hard labour, the irregularity of the hours, the frequent night-work, and especially the great heat of the working place (100 to 190 Fahrenheit), engender in children general debility and disease, stunted growth, and especially affections of the eye, bowel complaint, and rheumatic and bronchial affections. Many of the children are pale, have red eyes, often blind for weeks at a time, suffer from violent nausea, vomiting, coughs, colds, and rheumatism. . . . The glass-blowers usually die young of debility or chest infections.

Industrial towns above all proved breeding grounds of the archetypal diseases of poverty and overcrowding such as rickets, the crippling bone disease of infants, especially ominous for females who, as a result of pelvic deformities, would often suffer fatal childbirth difficulties. Though widely known as 'the English disease', Britain enjoyed no monopoly, for everywhere dinginess and deprivation provided an ideal seedbed. A 1907 survey of Paris hospitals revealed that every other child between the ages of six months and three years suffered more or less from rickets, and New York reported the same.

The single worst disease cultivated by monster cities was tuberculosis, characterized by fever, night sweats and coughing up blood (haemotysis), and called 'consumption' because victims were almost literally consumed. It was not a new disease, but it festered as population grew denser and poverty deepened. By 1800 it was said that 'no other [disease] is so common', while in 1815 Thomas Young surmised it brought a 'premature death' to one in four. The autopsies conducted at the chief Paris hospitals record tuberculosis as the cause of death in some 40 per cent of cases, while in the 1830s eastern seaboard cities in the United States had a mortality rate of around 400 per 100,000. All agreed that, Romantic poets and pianists notwithstanding, tuberculosis was a disease of the urban poor, though debate raged as to whether its cause was environmental, contagious or hereditary. Who was to blame – the 'great unwashed' or the ghastly conditions in which they lived? Whichever, there was no cure.

Industrial towns bred myriad fevers. Some were readily identifiable. With its hard cough and distinctive leathery membrane around the tonsils choking its victims, diphtheria became a major killer of the young, as did scarlet fever. Measles, chickenpox and scarlet fever all remained severe, and smallpox immunization proved ineffective in big towns. Other maladies, including what we now call typhoid and typhus, were harder to distinguish amid the ceaseless surge of fevers which, in a time of pre-bacteriology, passed under names like 'putrid fever'. Involving severe diarrhoea and dysentery, 'enteric fevers' were associated with the urban poor, but rival theories of their aetiology proliferated and, as with so many other diseases, the fact that they surfaced here, there and everywhere, and not only among the masses, muddied the waters. The Prince Consort democratically died in 1861 of what was probably typhoid. He too was a victim of overflowing cesspools, albeit those of Windsor Castle; the Prince of Wales narrowly escaped the same fate in 1871 (though his noble groom succumbed).

Fevers had always colonized the great swarming cities, but nine-teenth-century conurbations also suffered new invaders, notably cholera. Rooted in the Indian subcontinent, cholera had never gone global before the nineteenth century; the first pandemic began in 1816. Attaining epidemic proportions in Bengal, by 1820 it had spread throughout the subcontinent. Accompanying pilgrims gathering around the Ganges, or transported by soldiers and caravans along the trade routes, it had passed by 1824 through south-east Asia to the Philippines and China, toward the Russian borders and east into Japan; to the west, it followed traffic through the Persian Gulf; and northward, it moved through Persia towards the Ottoman and Russian empires. Reaching Astrakhan by the Caspian Sea, it threatened to enter Europe, but receded, and the first pandemic subsided in 1826. The second, third and fourth were not so merciful.

The second began in 1829, lasting to 1852. It spread through the Asiatic lands, broke into Egypt and North Africa, entered Russia via

Astrakhan, tracked across Europe, and familiarized a shocking way to die. Internal disturbances, nausea and dizziness led to violent vomiting and diarrhoea, with stools turning to a grey liquid (often described as 'rice water') until nothing emerged but water and fragments of intestinal membrane. Extreme muscular cramps followed, with an insatiable desire for water, followed by a 'sinking stage' during which the pulse dropped and lethargy set in. Dehydrated and nearing death, the patient displayed the classic cholera physiognomy: puckered blue lips in a cadaverous face. There was no agreement about its cause; many treatments were tried; nothing worked.

London was hit in 1832, with 7000 dying; so was Paris. 'It was as if the end of the world had come,' the poet Heinrich Heine reported from his Paris exile on the mass panic and the loathing shown towards victims:

> Like beasts, like maniacs, the people fell on them. Many saved themselves by presence of mind; others were rescued by the resolute Communal Guards who in those days patrolled everywhere; some were seriously wounded or maimed; and six were most unmercifully murdered.
>
> There is no more dreadful sight than such popular anger thirsting for blood and throttling its defenceless victims. . . . In the Rue Vaugirard, where two men were killed who had had white powders on them, I saw one of these unfortunates when he was still breathing and the old hags were just pulling the wooden shoes from their feet and beating him on the head with them till he was dead. He was quite naked and bloody and mashed; they had torn off not only his clothes but his hair, his sex, his lips and his nose, and one ruffian tied a rope to the feet of the corpse and dragged it through the streets, shouting constantly, '*Voilà le Cholera-morbus!*'

Nothing could be done, though the bourgeoisie put their faith in flannel. Heine noted: '"Today", says the *Figaro*, "Venus would wear a flannel girdle." I am up to my neck in flannel, and consider myself cholera-proof. The King, too, now wears a belly-band of the best bourgeois flannel.'

Cholera reached North America in 1832, first attacking New York and the eastern seaboard: by 1834 it had crossed the interior to the Pacific, and spread south to Mexico and South America. It re-entered the southern United States from Cuba, advanced north though New Orleans and Charleston, and eventually tracked north to Canada. The third pandemic began in 1852, and 1854 was one of the worst cholera years. Between 1847 and 1861 alone, 2,589,843 Russians contracted the disease and over a million died.

The fourth pandemic, which started in 1863 and lasted until 1875, was notable for opening a new route into Europe: Islamic pilgrims brought cholera to Alexandria, which became a transfer point by which it travelled by sea to Italy and Marseilles in France. It also brought dangerous outbreaks in central Europe in the wake of the Austro-Prussian War (1866), and a broad advance into Africa. The fifth brought death to Hamburg in 1892. Ironically it was a new water system that was to blame: in the absence of satisfactory filtration, central piping spread the polluted Elbe water more effectively.

By that time, however, most European countries had found that cholera could be controlled through public-health measures, whose rationale was reinforced by Robert Koch's isolation in 1884 of the cholera bacillus. As a consequence, the sixth pandemic (1899 to 1926) barely affected western Europe, though outbreaks occurred in the Balkans. In Russia, the disease was dreadfully severe, and it returned there during World War I and the Revolution.

Awash with people and haunted by premature death, the nineteenth-century shock towns had their evils unceasingly spotlighted. But it would be naive to assume that once the evils of industrial society were exposed they were automatically righted. Together with the question of medical efficacy, imponderable issues were raised of culpability, individual rights, the duties of government and the sanctity of private property. *Could* such evils be rectified? Or were they nobody's fault, nobody's business, all a muddle, best left to individual action or the hidden hand? And if they *could* be remedied, how and by whom? And who would foot the bill? These issues were real, even if they often served as sanctimonious excuses for inertia by those who worshipped Mammon. It had been relatively easy for Johann Peter Frank in *ancien régime* Austria to propose his medical police, but the paternalist regulation of a largely rural empire where serfs still existed was child's play by comparison with the problems posed by New York or New Orleans, Liverpool or London.

Especially in the Anglo–American world, political economy ordained freedom of trade; it was not for Parliament or Congress lightly to meddle with people's livelihoods. Government would uphold the law, and it was up to individuals to be healthy and to charity to rectify hardships. Whether to work in a deadly trade was a free and individual decision. When operatives fell sick, blame was often laid upon their faulty constitutions, regarded as the root cause of work-triggered consumption or blindness.

Nevertheless, despite the ideological attractiveness of self-help doctrines, no state could idly stand by and watch the crippling impact of mass diseases – anyone might die, Prince Consorts and all, and the social fabric was under strain with revolution in the air. Surrounded by the great unwashed and threatened by cholera, jittery members of society feared that disease might spark insurrection – or might spread to them. They began to look to urban cleansing and health reform as medicine for society, even as an opium of the people. Cleanliness was next to godliness. With disease spelling disorder and danger, public responses followed.

PUBLIC HEALTH

The nineteenth century opened on a diversity of approaches to the politics of health. German-speaking Europe embraced a health paternalism redolent of Frank's medical police; free-market England leant towards voluntarism, looking to charity to bestow health care on the poor and leaving it to locals to install pumps, provide soup kitchens and remove nuisances.

The West's two new nations seemed to be espousing very different philosophies. In the United States it was widely hoped that the health difficulties – and other problems – of the Old World would never plague the New. Thomas Jefferson expressed confidence that the right to life, liberty and the pursuit of happiness would foster a healthy nation. The great cities of Europe, warned the Virginian plantation-owner, were 'pestilential to the morals, the health, and the liberties of man'; America would be a healthy outdoors, full of sturdy freeholders. Government would have little role to play, and that was all to the good.

The French revolutionaries tried a different tack: the new state would inaugurate the reign of virtue, to which health and hygiene were integral. In 1791 the Poverty Committee of the National Assembly decreed *citoyens* had a right to health as well as to life, liberty, and property. A scheme was approved covering health inspectorates, child care, a national inoculation campaign and medical services for the young and poor. *Officiers de santé* (rural health officers) would assume responsibility for reporting on the health of communities and monitoring epidemics. Through nationalization of religious hospitals and charities, a comprehensive system of health entitlements would be established for 'citizen-patients', who would undertake the reciprocal duty of obeying the laws of hygiene to keep themselves healthy. Such hopes were scuppered by war and the Terror. Funds went to the army, not to the ailing, and most health reforms were forgotten.

The Revolutionary and Napoleonic reforms nevertheless fostered an elite, schooled in the writings of *philosophes* such as Condorcet, concerned with investigating sickness and planning public welfare. Vital statistics became the thermometer of health, providing foundations for what Adolphe Quetelet later defined as social physics or social statistics, and involving the first systematic analyses of disease patterns. 'Man is born, lives and dies according to certain laws which have never been studied as a whole nor considered in the light of their mutual reactions,' announced Quetelet's *Sur l'homme et le développement de ses facultés, essai d'une physique sociale* (1835) [On Man and the Development of His Faculties: An Essay on Social Physics]. The book was devoted to establishing vital statistics: rates of fertility and death; stature, weight and strength; the data of drunkenness, crime and insanity, and so on. Within this framework, he elaborated his most famous single concept: that of the average man (*l'homme moyen*), an individual with average mental, moral and physical characteristics which could be measured in large numbers and expressed mathematically.

French public health shared the 'gaze' of hospital medicine. Both were dedicated to detached, scientific observations, surveying the diseases of large populations – the one within institutions, the other at large. Both championed *la méthode numerique*. This led to what some historians have found a paradox. The disasters of the 1789–1815 period smothered economic development, so that the worst horrors of the industrial revolution came late to France. Nevertheless France achieved early leadership in public-health medicine, not least the appearance in 1829 of the first public-health journal, *Annales d'hygiène publique et médecine légale*.

The outstanding early figure was the ex-army surgeon René Louis Villermé (1782–1863), who addressed the relationship between disease and society, producing numerous seminal socio-medical studies as a member of the Hygiene Department of the Royal Academy of Medicine, chaired by the physiologist Jean Noël Hallé (1754–1822). The stimulus came from a massive demographic study, *Recherches statistiques sur la ville de Paris* (1821) [Statistical Researches on the City of Paris]. Villermé was then invited to examine the health implications of its findings. Analysing the differential mortality among the Paris *arrondissements*, and testing all the conventional environmental factors such as altitude, soil and climate, he found none explained the mortality patterns. Likewise with overcrowding: no clear correlations emerged.

Having exhausted the morbific environmental determinants dear to Enlightenment physicians, Villermé tried economic status. Eureka! The poorest *arrondissements* consistently showed highest mortality levels. The rue de la Mortellerie, packed like sardines with *les misérables*, had a death rate of 30.6 per 1000, while a stone's throw away the richer residents of the *quais* of the Île-Saint-Louis had one less than two thirds as high. The rich lived longest; the poor bore, and lost, most children and died young. In later studies of the textile industry, Villermé confirmed these conclusions in life-tables for the working class, correlating mortality against income. Poverty and illness went together.

What then should be done to improve matters? With his *parti d'hygiène* associates, Villermé believed the answer lay in the moral regeneration of the poor; no good would come of state intervention, doles, direct medical action or the old mercantilist economic reform. Employers should encourage their workers to live in a decent way and school them in habits of sobriety, frugality and industry; to combat socialism, Villermé suggested programmes of religious indoctrination and Christian example. Legislative reform was a non-starter, for that would undermine personal freedom, and interference with market mechanisms would be counter-productive. What was the cause of poverty? The poor themselves. If disease originated with them, the answer was to civilize them out of poverty. Such prescriptions for moralizing the masses could be seen as the political analogue of therapeutic nihilism.

Similar preferences were advanced in England, not least by Villermé's closest English equivalent, William Farr (1807–83), compiler of abstracts in the new Registrar General's Department – in 1836 registration of births, marriages and deaths had been made compulsory. Farr, who had studied medical statistics under Pierre Louis, produced a disease classification for national documentation purposes, and thereby acquired unique familiarity with the diseases of industrial society. The poor were wretched but redeemable. He opposed the traditional Poor

Laws because doles were sure to be 'expended indiscriminately upon the idle, reckless, vicious as well as the good but unfortunate', subscribing to the standard if tendentious distinction between the 'deserving' and 'undeserving' poor. But unlike his French counterparts, he gave greater credence to environmental determinants of health, and hoped action might change things: 'the aggregation of mankind in towns is not inevitably disastrous.'

Analysing mortality and salubrity, Farr used statistics to give a nudge to practical social reform through the use of life-tables as a health 'biometer', comparable to a barometer for the weather. The life-table (soon to become the instrument of every English public health officer testing the salubrity of districts, with infant mortality its key index) demonstrated how life expectations at different ages varied according to occupation, wealth and hygiene. Improvement would follow from keeping better statistics, educating the public in 'the laws of health', and making doctors more aware of their preventative responsibilities. In his *Annual Reports* for the department, Farr concluded that over-crowding was the main determinant of high mortality from what (following Liebig) he styled 'zymotic diseases'. Farr's quiet optimism that increased knowledge of sanitary problems would lead to improvement was shared by many progressive doctors, not least those who joined the Metropolitan Health of Towns Association, founded in 1844 by Thomas Southwood Smith; the National Association for the Promotion of Social Science, the Royal Statistical Society, the London Epidemiological Society and various other bodies that united reformers, policy-makers and politicians.

Social analysis of disease was undertaken in many parts of Europe in the first half of the nineteenth century, with varying political thrusts and consequences. In France little state action followed, sanitary legislation was permissive, and the introduction of amenities like piped water was slow and patchy.

The move to action was most marked in the rapidly expanding state apparatus of Victorian Britain. There was already a pre-history of voluntarism on which to build. Earlier campaigners, such as John Howard, and idealistic doctors like John Coakley Lettsom – many of whom were Quakers and Dissenters – had investigated the health of the poor, made recommendations on household hygiene, and supported dispensaries and other practical measures. The first local ginger group came into existence in 1796, when typhus among cotton-mill employees led public-spirited Manchester physicians to organize an *ad hoc* health board. Liverpool followed suit. The parish-pump nature of local politics meant that little was accomplished.

In the early nineteenth century, many different platforms – philanthropy, medicine, religion, Utilitarianism and political economy – offered nostrums for the problems of population, pauperism and the Poor Law. There was a climate of fear as economic change created class struggle and political divisions. The establishment dreaded the contagion of the French Revolution and resented the spiralling expense of the Poor Laws, which gave 'outdoor relief' (doles) to the unemployed, the old and the sick.

Cholera concentrated people's minds. As Asiatic cholera rampaged across Europe in 1830, isolation cordons, quarantines and other government and police action proved ineffective, leading to rioting from St Petersburg to Paris, with wealthy magistrates and doctors being attacked by mobs who feared conspiracies to poison or imprison them. In Britain isolation of victims in workhouse infirmaries caused riots among those accusing the medical profession of using the epidemic as a body-snatching opportunity for dissection.

Against this background, the long-mooted reform of the Poor Laws became top priority. A key figure in these initiatives was Edwin Chadwick (1800–90), formerly secretary to Jeremy Bentham (1748–1832), the philosopher of Utilitarianism. Believing social policy should be directed by experts to bring about the greatest happiness of the greatest number, Benthamites judged the old Poor Law outdoor relief system a recipe for waste and idleness. Secretary to the Poor Law Commission, Chadwick devised a new Poor Law, enacted in 1834, universalizing the workhouse solution in line with the 'less eligibility' philosophy: the workhouse must be repellent. He was confident this would make the labour market run better by deterring dependency, and convinced that workhouses would save public money.

The New Poor Law was meant to cut claimants and hence costs. Chadwick monitored its operation, and to his chagrin found that his brainchild wasn't working. Why did pauperism not decrease under this expertly designed system? He concluded it was because much poverty was due not to fecklessness but to disease. Many of those entering workhouses were the chronic sick and disabled, so much so that it was necessary to build special workhouse infirmaries at public expense. The

Poor Law medicine service inexorably expanded, and the public responsibility thereby undertaken for the sick poor became a basis for the British National Health Service.

Finding that sickness bred poverty, in 1837 Chadwick secured the appointment of three doctors sympathetic to sanitary reform: Neil Arnott (1788–1874), James Phillip Kay-Shuttleworth (1807–77) and Thomas Southwood Smith (1788–1861), to investigate the London districts with the highest typhus mortality. Kay-Shuttleworth was a Manchester physician whose familiarity with the ill health of textile workers led to his *The Moral and Physical Condition of the Working Classes Employed in the Cotton Manufacture* (2nd ed., 1832), which described the horrors of urban poverty and recommended sanitary regulation and moral education. Southwood Smith was a Unitarian and a Utilitarian; he delivered the funeral oration over Jeremy Bentham's body. Having studied medicine in Edinburgh, he settled into practice in London, where he turned himself into an expert on fevers and hygiene.

Their findings (1838) revealed the grim squalor of the London rookeries. 'The room of a fever patient, in a small and heated apartment of London, with no perflation of fresh air, is perfectly analogous to a stagnant pool in Ethiopia full of the bodies of dead locusts,' declared Southwood Smith, 'The poison generated in both cases is the same; the difference is merely in the degree of its potency.' Impressed, Chadwick broadened the study to include insanitary areas throughout Britain. Though distrusting medicine as a corrupt and inept profession, Chadwick used Poor Law medical officers' reports as the basis for his monumental *Report on the Sanitary Condition of the Labouring Population of Great Britain* (1842), charting the prevalence of disease and poverty through maps, vital statistics and descriptions of streets, dwellings, schools, refuse, privies, sewers, drainage and odours.

The report declared that unsanitary living conditions and squalor accounted largely for the poor health and truncated lifespans of the poor. In London's Bethnal Green for example, the average age of death among labourers was sixteen, whereas among the better off it was forty-five. 'More filth, worse physical suffering and moral disorder than [John] Howard describes as affecting the prisoners,' declared Chadwick, 'are to be found amongst the cellar population of the working people of Liverpool and other cities.'

The conditions exposed in London were mirrored in Birmingham, Leeds, Manchester and all other major urban centres. Twenty per cent of pauperism was due to fever, and the blame fell on overcrowding, negligent waste disposal, dirty water and bad diet. Poverty could not be abolished, but the poverty due to preventable disease could be:

> The primary and most important measures, and at the same time the most practicable, and within the recognized province of administration, are drainage, the removal of all refuse from habitations, streets and roads, and the improvement of the supplies of water.

The social costs of sickness thus converted Chadwick to the 'sanitary idea': that is, prevention. He also embraced the miasmatic theory of disease aetiology – disease was caused by gases given off by putrefying, decomposing organic matter, rotting flesh and vegetables – 'All smell is, if it be intense, immediate, acute disease.' New sewage removal systems were therefore of paramount importance, together with removal of cesspools and other nuisances. Traditional cavernous bricked sewers must be replaced by small glazed egg-shaped drains, constantly flushed by high-pressure water; liquid sewage could be lucratively recycled as fertilizer on sewage farms.

Chadwick urged the creation of a central public health authority to direct local boards of health in the provision of drainage, cleansing, paving, drinking water and the sanitary regulation of dwellings, nuisances and offensive trades. A Royal Commission on the Health of Towns was then set up (1843–5) which backed Chadwick's recommendations. Sanitary reform was given momentum by the appointment in Liverpool in 1846 of William Duncan as its medical officer of health, and by the passing of a Nuisances Removal Act, a Common Lodging House Act and an Adulteration of Food Act in 1846 and 1847.

The realization of Chadwick's agenda came in the first British Public Health Act (1848), creating a central authority, the General Board of Health, which consisted of three members, including Chadwick, with Southwood Smith as its medical adviser. A tenth of the ratepayers within any locality could petition the General Board for the adoption of the act, or it could be imposed by the board upon a local authority with an annual death rate above 23 per thousand. Whichever, the town council was then compelled by statute to set up a local board of health, responsible for sanitary supervision and inspection, drainage, water and gas supplies and empowered to raise local rates. They were to appoint local medical officers of health, whose duties were to regulate 'offensive trades' (slaughtering, tanning, dyeing, etc.), remove 'nuisances', regulate houses unfit for human habitation, provide burial grounds, and deal with water supplies, sewers, waste disposal and other environmental hazards. London alone was exempt, as it already had its own Metropolitan Commission of Sewers and to head off the General Board, the City Corporation obtained a private Sewers Act (1848) and appointed its own medical officer of health, John Simon (1816–1904).

By 1853, 103 towns had adopted the act. Others dug in their heels and robust opposition was voiced by defenders of local autonomy (or vested interests). 'We prefer to take our chance with cholera and the rest rather than be bullied into health,' proclaimed *The Times* – the same newspaper declared in 1848 that 'the Cholera is the best of all sanitary reformers'. Ratepayers resented being dictated to by a 'clean party'; for his uncompromising centralizing tendencies Chadwick was called 'Prussian' by Lord John Russell; and the General Board's unpopularity led to its discontinuation in 1854. A new professional health management succeeded, directed not by Chadwick's bureaucratic model but one based on medicine and run not by a lawyer but by a doctor. By then, however, public health was advancing on a broad front, due partly to the application of better epidemiological skills than Chadwick possessed.

A significant breakthrough against cholera was effected by John Snow. Born in York in 1813, he had become a surgeon in Newcastle upon Tyne, gaining experience of cholera during the 1831 epidemic. In 1836, he set up in London's Soho, and became established as London's leading anaesthetist. As cholera spread again in 1849, *The Times* printed the following appeal:

> Sur,
> May we be and beseach your proteckshion and power. We are Sur, as it may be, livin in a Wilderness, so far as the rest of London knows anything of us, or as the rich and great people care about. We live in muck and filth. We aint got no priviz, no dust bins, no drains, no water-splies, and no drain or suer in the hole place. The Suer Company, in Greek St., Soho Square, all great, rich powerfool men take no notice watsomdever of our complaints. The Stenche of a Gulley-hole is disgustin. We all of us suffer, and numbers are ill, and if the Cholera comes Lord help us.

Snow's first cholera investigations appeared in his *On the Mode of Communication of Cholera* in the same year, when over 50,000 people died in England of the disease. Questioning miasmatism, he argued that cholera could not be spread by a poison in the ambient air, since it affected the intestines not the lungs. He drew attention to the contamination of drinking water as a result of cholera evacuations seeping into wells or running into rivers from which drinking-water was taken. He was, sadly, soon able to put his views to the test.

In August 1854 cholera cases began to appear in Soho. A drastic increase in the week ending 2 September led him to investigate all 93 local cholera deaths. He concluded the local water supply had become contaminated, for nearly all the victims used water from the Broad Street pump. At a nearby prison, conditions were far filthier, but deaths were few – it had its own well. On 7 September he requested the parish Board of Guardians to disconnect the pump. Sceptical but desperate, they agreed; the handle was removed, the number of cases plummeted (the outbreak was already declining), and Snow had confirmation of his theory.

In 1855, he gave his views to a House of Commons Select Committee: cholera, he maintained, was not contagious nor spread by miasmata but was water-borne. He advocated massive improvements in drainage and sewage, a call that played some part in the investment by London and other major British cities in new main drainage and sewage systems. After 'the great stink' in the summer of 1858 caused Parliament to break off its proceedings, the Metropolitan Board of Works empowered its chief engineer, Joseph Bazalgette, to create an ambitious scheme for main drainage, which was completed in 1875. London's water was increasingly drawn from the higher reaches of the Thames and from the Lea Valley, and filter beds were developed. The new sanitary infrastructure was a triumph of civil engineering.

Snow won converts to his view of cholera as a specific, water-borne disease. Similar ideas were emerging with typhoid, distinguished from typhus by William Gerhard of Philadelphia and William Jenner. In 1856 the Bristol physician, William Budd, argued that the typhoid agent lay in patients' stools and thus, by implication, was due to poor hygiene and living conditions. He recommended washing, disinfection of cisterns, and boiling water during epidemics. Nevertheless, the question of the causation of urban epidemics was confused and contested. Many experts, including the influential Farr, remained committed to a more traditional and generalist model of fevers, regarding them as unspecific manifestations of insalubrity. Lumping together as 'epidemic, endemic and contagious' all those maladies 'known by experience to become epidemic in unhealthy places and among the sickly classes', Farr called them zymotic diseases, reflecting Liebig's concept of disease as analogous to fermentation: certain terrestrial and environmental circumstances would cause diseases to be released into the atmosphere. Zymosis explained how a disease suddenly became epidemic. The *materies morbi* involved 'highly organized particles of fixed matter', possibly resembling pollen, in a state of pathological molecular transformation. Non-specific decomposing organic matter was a 'predisposing' cause in a causation chain dominated by a zymotic stimulus.

With Chadwick ousted from office, in 1854 John Simon was appointed Britain's first chief medical administrator at the newly created Medical Department of the Privy Council. His powers were nominally minimal, but he proved a determined diplomat. Believing knowledge conferred power, he produced a succession of Blue Books reporting the results of scientific investigations into topics such as dangerous industries and the dwellings of the poor. He also introduced new legislation: Nuisances Acts gave local authorities wider powers to tackle street refuse, industrial waste and smoke, polluted rivers, slaughter-houses, and so on; the Local Government Act (1858) permitted compulsory purchase for sanitary purposes; the Sanitary Act of 1866 gave local authorities new powers to provide clean water supplies and regulate tenements; the 1867 Vaccination Act increased the penalties for failure to vaccinate infants.

The sanitary legislation developed since 1848 was consolidated in the codifying Public Health Act of 1875, requiring the appointment of a medical officer of health to every sanitary district in England and Wales, while Poor Law and public health administration were amalgamated in 1872 in the Local Government Board. The medical expert's role in public administration had been established, and local government had acquired extensive public health powers. In his *Eleventh Annual Report* (1868), Simon reviewed the role the state was playing in preventive medicine:

> It has interfered between parent and child, not only in imposing limitation on industrial uses of children, but also to the extent of requiring that children should not be left unvaccinated. It has interfered between employer and employed, to the extent of insisting, in the interest of the latter, that certain sanitary claims shall be fulfilled in all places of industrial occupation. It has inter-

fered between vendor and purchaser; has put restrictions on the sale and purchase of poisons, has prohibited in certain cases certain commercial supplies of water, and has made it a public offence to sell adulterated food or drink or medicine, or to offer for sale any meat unfit for human food. Its care for the treatment of disease has not been unconditionally limited to treating at the public expense such sickness as may accompany destitution: it has provided that in any sort of epidemic emergency organized medical assistance, not peculiarly for paupers, may be required of local authorities; and in the same spirit it requires that vaccination at the public cost shall be given gratuitously to every claimant.

Formerly a believer in the miasmatic theory, by the 1870s Simon had come round to the view that all contagious diseases were due to 'a specific living organism'.

PUBLIC HEALTH AND POLITICS

The transition in Britain of public health from social agitation to a professional civil service was extensive but not unique; similar developments occurred elsewhere. In many German principalities, with a strong cameralist tradition to build on, public health administration was entrenched even before political unification in 1871. When a serious typhus epidemic broke out in the winter of 1847 in Upper Silesia, a Prussian province with a suppressed Polish minority, Rudolf Virchow was sent to investigate its causes.

The epidemic, Virchow argued in a report influenced by Villermé and Chadwick, was due not to any simple aetiological factor but a socio-political nexus. 'Great warning signs on which the true statesman is able to read that the evolution of his nation has been disturbed', epidemics were symptoms of a general malaise; they mainly affected oppressed groups. The answer was thus not medicine, but 'political medicine': education, freedom and prosperity. 'The improvement of medicine would eventually prolong human life,' he proclaimed, 'but improvement of social conditions could now achieve this result more rapidly and more successfully.' Dispossessed and exploited, the Silesian Poles were sitting targets for sickness. Only democracy, he claimed, would prevent future epidemics. The physician's responsibility was to serve as an 'attorney for the poor'.

This was not what the Prussian authorities wished to hear, and Virchow fell into disfavour. By the 1860s, however, he had been elected to Berlin City Council, and for a decade he devoted much of his time to the reorganization of Berlin's sanitary and public health facilities.

In France public health administration involved much talk but little action. During the revolution of 1848 Jules Guérin called for the creation of 'social medicine', to identify the social evils producing disease, and in 1848 the Second Republic established a system of local health councils (*conseils de salubrité*). These were purely advisory, however, and the system of weak health councils remained in effect until the end of the century. Likewise, factory acts respecting health remained permissive, and health inspectors were unpaid volunteers. Edwin Chadwick was scathing. The Paris Health Council's 'representations have produced no effect', he judged, 'the labouring population of Paris is shown to be, with all the advantages of climate, in a sanitary condition even worse than the labouring population of London.' Change came slowly. Unlike Londoners, most Parisians were still getting their water in 1870 from fountains or water-sellers, and disposing of waste in court pits. Paris was a city of 85,000 cesspools; many remained until after the First World War.

On paper, the public health regulations of the Russian imperial government seemed quite advanced, and because the government was autocratic, it had the power to enforce its laws. As successive cholera epidemics revealed, however, their administration was seldom effective. The *zemstvo* reforms of 1864 created local governing councils with health responsibilities and medical staffs, but no centralized health administration appeared in Russia until after the 1917 Revolution. When it did, the People's Commissariat of Health, founded in 1918, was the most comprehensive institution of its kind in the world.

AMERICA

The trend towards the bureaucratization and centralization of public health in parts of Europe met a contrast in the United States of America. That was not surprising. The new republic was gigantic, continually expanding, and predominantly rural – in 1800 only thirty-three towns had populations over 2500. It remained a land of extreme contrasts.

The first half of the century brought industrialization, but rugged individualism prevailed; Jacksonian democracy kept government to a minimum, and many believed this a recipe for a healthy population. These hopes were not borne out. Malaria raged as far north as New England, enteric fevers were endemic and yellow fever struck again and again.

On the east coast, public health initiatives arose from philanthropists: the ideals of evangelical piety embracing sanitary reform without the political radicalism motivating many European reformers. John H. Griscom (1809–74), health inspector of New York City, physician at the New York Hospital and a founder member of the New York Academy and Medical Society, conducted a survey on *The Sanitary Condition of the Laboring Population of New York* (1845). A pious Quaker, Griscom believed cleanliness had a spiritual and a material dimension: to follow the rules of hygiene was a moral act and a religious duty, and sanitary regeneration was a crusade to improve the poor. Spreading the hygiene gospel, Griscom's philosophy was reproduced by other early health reformers, such as Lemuel Shattuck (1793–1859) in Massachusetts.

Religious moralism was prominent in the American response to cholera, which crossed the Atlantic in 1832. The effects of the 1848–9 epidemic were far more severe, however, killing five thousand in New York alone, and impacting heavily in the towns along the Mississippi, Arkansas and Tennessee rivers, as it spread upstream from New Orleans. In the absence of government action, voluntary associations organized refuse removal, street-cleaning and emergency hospital facilities – and President Zachary Taylor ordered a fast day in 1849. Believing cholera's primary predisposing cause to be sin – intemperance, atheism, vice, greed and immorality among the feckless poor – Evangelicals preached the hygiene gospel. Though prayer helped, practical measures were also needed, and from the 1870s cities and states began to establish permanent health boards. These were *ad hoc*, advisory and largely powerless; the chief function of most became the licensing of physicians.

In some places businessmen took action to clean up towns. In Newark, for instance, Asiatic cholera in 1832 and 1849 led to programmes to cleanse the city, and a final epidemic, in 1866–67, created demands for a purer water supply. Providing free vaccination against smallpox was one of the initial functions of the Newark Board of Health, founded in 1858. As smallpox worsened, compulsory vaccination became a public issue. Late in the century Newark businessmen began to play a more prominent role in promoting water and sewer systems, but there as elsewhere the business community was far from united on public health measures. Reformers were helped by the emergence of sanitary associations, civic groups whose membership included a wide range of socially conscious middle- and upper-class citizens. The local medical community showed little collective professional interest in public health, although individual physicians aided the Newark health reformers.

Another stimulus to public health was the Civil War. Costing the lives of 600,000 soldiers, it galvanized government into action, since many had perished from typhoid and dysentery in grossly insanitary encampments. A Civilian Sanitary Commission, created in 1861 and headed by New York physician Elisha Harris (1824–84) and the architect Frederick Law Olmstead (1822–1903), reported an appalling lack of hospital facilities, fresh food, medical care for the sick and wounded, and shamed the military into cleaning up. Sanitary reform in the army made its impression on the civilian population when occupying Union troops imposed new sanitary programmes upon southern towns, though these were later undermined in the chaos of reconstruction.

In the southern states, what persuaded tight-fisted legislatures to establish boards of health was epidemic yellow fever. Usually limited to coastal cities, in 1878 the epidemic extended from New Orleans to St Louis and Louisville, steamboats on the Mississippi providing excellent transportation for the exceptionally malignant strain then prevalent. In some places the mortality rate for whites exceeded 50 per cent. Health Boards accomplished little in sanitary reform, as the principal weapon in the battle against yellow fever was quarantine, which was of questionable effectiveness, deeply unpopular, and widely dodged. Fears of yellow fever did, however, prompt clean-up campaigns as well as the application of large quantities of lime, copperas, and carbolic acid in futile efforts to eradicate it.

Yellow fever led to the increasing presence of the federal government in public health because the disease readily crossed state lines and was said to be fundamentally a national problem. First with the National Board of Health, created in 1879 in response to the disastrous 1878 epidemic, and then with the Marine Hospital Service (which became the US Public Health and Marine Hospital Service in 1902), federal involvement in public health grew. But many state boards of health resisted this development, airing constitutional fears and contending that local agencies were better.

When public health initiatives prospered they provided arguments for further action. In 1901 the US military eliminated yellow fever among its troops occupying Cuba and, after the French failed, succeeded in building the Panama Canal, thanks to mosquito eradication· the lessons learned in Cuba and Panama facilitated efforts in the American south. A campaign to eliminate the 'disease of laziness' from the share-cropping community began in 1909 when the bacteriologist Charles Widdell Stiles persuaded the Rockefeller Foundation to set up a five-year Sanitary Commission for hookworm eradication.

Up to 1900 the only federal agency coordinating health activities was the Marine Hospital Service, under its director, the surgeon-general. Rejecting the setting up of a department of health, Theodore Roosevelt turned this into the United States Public Health Service in 1912. Other government departments acquired specific health responsibilities: the War Office dealt with military health and maintained a laboratory and epidemiological research; the Interior Department dealt with school hygiene, while the Department of Commerce and Trade and the Census Bureau handled health matters relating to housing and factories.

Arguing that bacteriology set new public health apart from the old, Charles Chapin (1856–1941) launched a campaign in the 1890s to eliminate diphtheria in Providence, Rhode Island, through isolation of bacteriologically tested victims and carriers, combined with compulsory antitoxin treatment, plus a comprehensive programme of disinfecting victims' dwellings. This bacteriological model was to dominate subsequent public health training. The School of Public Health at Johns Hopkins was set up to pursue prestigious biomedical research.

With the germ theory giving public health functions a plausible new rationale, the USA was active in setting up publicly supported bacteriological laboratories for disease diagnosis and control. In 1887, Joseph Kinyoun (1860–1919) of the Marine Hospital Service organized a bacteriological laboratory in Staten Island Marine Hospital. Transferred to Washington DC, this became the Hygienic Laboratory. In 1888, public health laboratories were founded in Providence, and in 1892 New York City established a division of bacteriology and disinfection in the city health department. Under Hermann M. Biggs (1859–1923) and William H. Park (1863–1939), it developed into a diagnostic laboratory where Park formulated the concept of the diphtheria carrier (1893) and developed the first diphtheria antitoxin outside Europe (1894). Becoming an important research centre for investigations into tuberculosis, dysentery, typhoid fever and scarlet fever, and on the role of milk in communicating disease, the laboratory served as a model for similar laboratories in Massachusetts (1894) and Philadelphia (1895). By 1900, diagnostic laboratories had been set up in every state and in most major cities. In Europe, the public health laboratory developed more slowly.

The bacteriological approach spearheaded the control of communicable diseases in advanced societies, but in the United States inspection and regulation of health conditions in schools, factories, and public institutions, and control over food and drugs, involved a patchwork of private associations, public laws and regulatory agencies. The creation of the Department of Health, Education and Welfare under the Eisenhower administration marked a belated effort to bring some order to the jumble of federal agencies and offices.

THE ENFORCEMENT OF HEALTH

The great spur to public health action was epidemic disease in industrial cities, associated with filth and poverty and leading to sanitary reform measures. Public authorities also intervened to control or manage health in myriad ways that were often controversial because they could involve compulsory powers which flew in the face of hallowed individualism.

Once Jenner's smallpox vaccination was broadly accepted, there were strong rationales for compelling immunization, since the unvaccinated could always spark further epidemics. In nations with strong centralizing traditions, like Sweden, compulsory vaccination was introduced rapidly; it was also made mandatory in Bavaria, Denmark, Württemberg and Prussia and, after a permissive Act of 1840, in England in 1853. An anti-vaccination backlash followed. Campaigning journals appeared, beginning with Henry Pitman's *Anti-Vaccinator* in 1869, and in 1874 the National Anti-Compulsory Vaccination League was founded, leading to civil disobedience which resulted in imprisonment for some. The campaign took a further step forward in 1880 with the London Society for the Abolition of Compulsory Vaccination, which had its moment of glory in 1909 when Parliament rescinded compulsory vaccination.

Other attempts to use coercive powers proved equally controversial. Communicable diseases created delicate problems of balancing individual rights against collective protection. In England, a string of Notifiable Diseases Acts empowered medical officers of health to quarantine those suffering from specific contagious diseases, such as smallpox, in special isolation hospitals.

One contagious condition particularly commanded political attention: sexually transmitted disease. Everywhere there was extensive state policing of sexuality, which took different forms, with a multiplicity of regulations on the age of consent, prostitution, homosexuality, abortion and so forth. In some places pre-marital medical inspection was compulsory to ensure freedom from venereal disease. In France and elsewhere, brothels had long been licensed, and prostitutes compelled to undergo regular medical check-ups.

In England, extremely high rates of sexually transmitted diseases in the army, and anxieties about their effect on combat efficiency during the Crimean War, brought the matter to a head, and led to parliamentary legislation in 1864, 1866 and 1869. The first Contagious Diseases Act (1864) specified ports and garrisons where women suspected of prostitution could be required to undergo physical examination. If found to be venereally infected, a woman would be detained for up to three months and compulsorily treated. Further acts were extended to include regular inspection of 'known prostitutes'. These amounted to a notable expansion of the state into medical supervision and control, and organizations arose to oppose them, involving an alliance of women's activists, physicians and civil libertarians. After a decade of protest, the acts were repealed.

In the United States, the 'prostitution problem' was tackled by a vigorous campaign to criminalize commercial sex. During the First World War, fears were expressed that soldiers in training would become infected and be lost to the war effort. Posters, films and educational materials warned: 'A German bullet is cleaner than a whore.' Closing down red-light districts became part of the 'hygienic gospel': 'to drain a red-light district and destroy thereby a breeding place of syphilis and gonorrhea,' explained one federal official, 'is as logical as it is to drain a swamp and thereby a breeding place of malaria and yellow fever.' A total of 110 red-light districts such as Storyville, New Orleans and Barbary Coast, San Francisco were shut, and more than 20,000 women were quarantined during the war.

In France, where American troops arrived to Make the World Safe for Democracy, the US military forbade soldiers to use the French 'regulated houses', angering French officials who feared that American demand for street-walkers ('clandestines') would jeopardize medical inspections of brothels. Nor would the military provide condoms; that would condone vice.

Tuberculosis also attracted public health legislation. A raft of treatments had been touted for the century's worst killer. Travel to warm climates was recommended for the well-off, and visits to health farms where the air was clear and clean. In 1876 a sanatorium was opened in the Taunus mountains, north of Frankfurt; another, noted for its strict discipline, was founded by Otto Walther at Nordrach in the Black Forest. In America the sanatorium was pioneered by Edward L. Trudeau (1848–1915), a wealthy doctor who discovered he was infected and relocated to Saranac Lakes in the Adirondacks, New York State. Finding his health restored in the mountains, he planned a sanatorium there, and the first 'lungers' were admitted in 1885. All such establishments were for the rich: 'TB is a good respectable disease', observed Henry Sewall (1855–1936), a Denver physician, in 1904, 'if you have money, but without it, it is a mean low-down business.'

So what was to be done about the poor, particularly once bacteriology had demonstrated that tuberculosis was an infectious air-borne disease? Campaigns were mounted to end spitting in public places, and in France and Britain in the 1890s, clamour grew for the compulsory detention of contagious cases. In the event, such drastic action did not follow, but sticks and carrots were used to persuade the consumptive poor to enter sanatoria, which often resembled custodial institutions, with perimeter walls and disciplined regimes, quasi-punitive even if justified on medical grounds.

At the end of the First World War tuberculosis accounted for about one sixth of all deaths in France and up to a quarter of mortality in some large urban centres. It became a target for public health intervention funded by the Rockefeller Foundation in 1917. The campaign used a dispensary system for tracing cases, assisting victims' families, providing disinfection and disseminating public education about reducing the risk of spreading the disease. Sanatoria were also employed to isolate patients and assist them to recover. Each *département* was required by law to establish a tuberculosis dispensary from 1916, but the state provided no funding and did not make TB a notifiable disease. By the close of 1917 there were still only twenty-three tuberculosis dispensaries.

By 1910 forty-one public sanatoria had been built in England, run mostly through the Poor Law. A degree of coercion was involved; tuberculosis was, after all, a notifiable disease. More positively, under the

National Insurance Act (1911) provision was made for financial support (sanatorium benefit) for the families of patients. Persuaded or pressurized to enter, sufferers found their lives strictly regulated; alcohol and tobacco were forbidden, and passes were required to go outside. Stringent internal discipline was enforced.

Pure air and sunshine were central to their philosophy; but in many, following Walther's Nordrach theories, these were accompanied by prolonged and systematic exposure to the elements. Windows were kept wide open, and beds wheeled onto verandahs even in snow. The sanatorium also affirmed faith in the therapeutic value of work, rationalized by some physicians, such as Marcus Paterson (1870–1932), the martinet superintendent of Frimley sanatorium (where there was no heating at all for patients), through the auto-inoculation theory – that the tubercular patient, by dint of demanding, outdoor, physical work such as chopping trees, setting concrete, planting trees in the snow, and so on, generated healing metabolic reactions. 'The patients had dug, manured, and sown over an acre of grass,' he reported proudly in 1908:

> excavated for the walls of a new reservoir to hold 500,000 gallons of rain water, mixed and laid 650 tons of concrete, made most of the paths, laid the concrete walk to the dining hall, made a concrete subway 150 yards in length from the engine room to the kitchen, cleared a 20-foot 'fire zone' round the boundary, trenched and sifted about an acre of land, fetched and sifted gravel for the paths, made the terrace and rock garden round the tennis court by the medical officer's house, made a bank around the grounds, and felled and cut into firewood about 100 trees.

Labour would build moral fibre, and return patients to the outside world with the right work ethic to prevent them from wasting their substance once again – to say nothing of taxpayers' money.

Those who returned, that is. For three quarters were dead within five years of entering the sanatorium. Nominally preventive or therapeutic, it was often terminal, a dustbin where the dying could never again infect family and workmates. Surreptitiously, the sanatorium functioned as a segregative institution, protecting society from the 'degenerates' within. Critics claimed money spent on staff and patients would have been better used to improve housing, nutrition, and domestic security.

Punitive policies thus came into force for sick people regarded as public nuisances. Meanwhile medicine was formulating new categories of 'degenerates', and teaching that drunks, syphilitics, paralytics and defectives and – worse still – the interbreeding of misfits and profligates, would lead, over the generations, to the swamping of the best by the rest. Eugenists advocated public action to contain and detain such threats (see Chapter 20).

These circumstances led the US to develop medically based immigration control. In the late nineteenth century, faced with a tidal wave of would-be immigrants – from Ireland and Italy, Poland and Russia – politicians and public health authorities instituted formal health controls. Ellis Island in New York Harbor became the chief station; there, between 1892 and 1954, over twelve million immigrants were medically inspected and interrogated. Initially, the emphasis was on infectious diseases – typhoid, smallpox, trachoma – but mental abnormality assumed growing importance, as eugenics came into fashion. In such selection processes, ethnic prejudices inevitably operated. Mediterranean types and eastern European Jews were widely regarded as inferior stock: 'Steerage passengers from a Naples boat show a distressing frequency of low foreheads, open mouths, weak chins, poor features, skew faces, small or knobby crania, and backless heads,' commented the distinguished sociologist, E. A. Ross (1866–1951), in 1914.

The great majority of immigrants, however, got through and nearly twenty-five million entered the United State between 1880 and 1924. Hardening racial prejudices resulted in the Johnson–Reed Act (1924), introducing quotas, promoted by President Calvin Coolidge, who had declared, 'America must be kept American. Biological laws show . . . that Nordics deteriorate when mixed with other races.'

The case of 'Typhoid Mary' illustrated the new perception of the immigrant threat and the powers of public health. The Irish-born Mary Mallon was a cook, who, while healthy herself, infected nearly fifty people with enteric fever in New York soon after 1900. She was apprehended and mandatorily detained in a hut in the grounds of an isolation hospital on North Brother Island, on New York's East River. Some years later, after a *habeas corpus* suit, the health department permitted her release, on condition that she worked in a laundry; but she reneged on her agreement, reverted to cooking and, under an assumed name, got a job in a maternity hospital kitchen. The result? A fresh outbreak, with two more people dying; rearrested, she was sent back to Quarantine

Island and this time detained there, alone with her dog, for life (another twenty-three years), banished 'like a leper', as she tellingly put it.

Little was then understood about being a carrier – only very recently had the phenomenon itself been discovered, thanks to the new bacteriology (see Chapter 14). The bacteriological theory behind the carrier was not well understood, but the New York health authorities had little doubt what action they needed to take: Mary Mallon's treatment was designed to set an example. She was rapidly demonized; by 1909 the press had invented the 'Typhoid Mary' label, called her a 'fiend', and produced cartoons of her cracking egg-like skulls into a frying-pan. She ended up permanently institutionalized, not because she had committed a crime but because she was deemed a threat to health.

THE BALANCE SHEET

What was the impact of industrialization? Did the workers become better off? Were they healthier? Did they live longer? And what may have been the contribution of public health to all that?

In addressing these issues, we are on shaky ground, since surviving statistics of income and illness rates are deeply defective. National censuses were only gradually becoming routine (the United Kingdom held its first in 1801) and vital statistics – height, weight, cause of death and so forth – are patchy. Among the labouring classes, life expectation remained everywhere low – little more than thirty years – and from the 1830s photographs show working people looking old by their thirties and forties, as poor nutrition, illness, bad living conditions and gross overwork took their toll. Historians of central Europe have claimed that industrial development in those territories was financed by pinching the workforce, concluding that conditions and diets worsened. But industrial Britain perhaps presents a different picture. The height of recruits to the British army was rising slowly after 1750; if height is a reliable anthropometric proxy for health, this points to better nourishment and in broad terms an improved working-class resistance to disease.

Vital statistics suggest health was generally improving towards 1900. Almost all nations (Ireland is an exception, drained by emigration) registered rapid population rise and increased longevity. One element was the decline of the old pattern of 'crisis mortality'. Traditionally, epidemics had swept through the countryside at frequent intervals and superimposed peaks of mortality on a high plateau of endemic disease deaths. By the 1850s such downward dips in life expectancy were vanishing.

Interpretations of the retreat first of epidemics and then of endemic diseases, and also of the increase in life expectancy, have been hotly debated. Some maintain the mass of the population was slowly but surely becoming less pauperized, and was enjoying better nourishment and hence improved health. Others argue that improving health was due not to rising prosperity but to better environmental salubrity due to public health measures, reducing the disease risks to which the hungry huddled masses were exposed.

Historians have distinguished between the retreat of epidemics in the eighteenth century and of endemic diseases in the nineteenth. Since plague was probably halted by the *cordon sanitaire* along the Habsburg border with the Ottoman empire, public health measures ('medical police') probably contributed to the reduction of epidemics. Smallpox vaccination from the early nineteenth century served to make epidemics less severe and frequent. The decline of plague and smallpox would thus have nothing to do with nutrition standards but some link with public health action. Endemic diseases such as tuberculosis and infant diarrhoea, by contrast, do seem to be made more severe by under-nutrition. The reduction in such diseases might be linked to wage improvements. In either case little that personal physicians did was reflected in improved survival.

Did public health measures actually do any good? The distinguished epidemiologist Thomas McKeown (1912–1988) maintained that reductions in deaths associated with infectious diseases (air-, water- and food-borne diseases) cannot have been brought about by medical advances, since such diseases were declining long before effective means were available to combat them. Applying much the same argument to sanitary measures, McKeown concluded that resistance to infectious disease must have increased through improvement in nutrition. Overall he mapped out three phases: a rising standard of living from about 1770; sanitary measures from 1870; and better therapy during the twentieth century.

McKeown, however, underestimated the effectiveness of the public health movement. Changing public opinion, the labours of medical officers of health, the creation of filtered water supplies and sewage systems, slum clearance, the work of activists promoting the gospel of cleanliness, and myriad other often minor changes – for example the provision of dustbins with lids, to repel flies – combined to create an improving urban environment.

Figures lend their support: in 1869 there were 716 deaths from typhus in London; by 1885 this had been reduced to 28; and at the beginning of the twentieth century there was none. Similar declines could be given for other infectious diseases. Tuberculosis began a remarkable disappearing act. Killing perhaps 500 out of every 100,000 Europeans in 1845, consumption sank slowly but continuously to 50 per 100,000 by 1950. Curative medicine played little part in that transition. The disappearance began before Koch discovered the tubercle bacillus. By the time antibiotics entered the picture, TB in cities such as New York had fallen to eleventh place in the death list. And the mortality graphs for most of Europe's fatal crowd diseases all dived before antibiotics had been marketed. Whooping cough killed 1400 children out of every million in 1850, but one hundred years later whooping deaths were less than 10 per million. Scarlet fever behaved in the same way. Measles, typhus, pneumonia, dysentery and polio all share similar histories. Their retreat had a dramatic impact on the European population. By 1900 civilization had lost its biological population check: infectious disease. After centuries of hostile encounters, humans and microbes found a new adjustment with little interference from drugs or vaccines. In some cases the microbe became less virulent (measles and diphtheria) or the human host more resistant (tuberculosis).

The nineteenth century brought a closer rapport between medicine and the public. Virchow was not alone in seeing the physician as a new 'saviour of humanity', and medical reformers everywhere echoed this plea. In the 1870s the chief medical spokesman in Parliament, the chemist and MP for Edinburgh University, Lyon Playfair (1818–98), predicted that society would eventually become a well-behaved patient and public health 'a great field open to growing medical men'. It was the twentieth century that saw the ambiguous realization of these views.

CHAPTER XIV

FROM PASTEUR TO PENICILLIN

> Just think of it. A hundred years ago there were no bacilli,
> no ptomaine poisoning, no diphtheria, and no appendicitis.
> Rabies was but little known, and these we owe to medical
> science. Even such things as psoriasis and parotitis and
> trypanosomiasis, which are now household names, were
> known only to the few, and were quite beyond the reach
> of the great mass of the people.
>
> STEPHEN B. LEACOCK, *Literary Lapses* (1910)

MICRO-ORGANISMS

A PATCHWORK OF IDEAS AND INSTITUTIONS, theory and practice,
craft and science, involving divided and vying professional factions,
medicine has a generally muddled history, infinitely less clear-cut than,
say, theoretical physics. But the latter part of the nineteenth century
brought one of medicine's few true revolutions: bacteriology. Seemingly
resolving age-old controversies over pathogenesis, a new and immensely
powerful aetiological doctrine rapidly established itself – one that its
apostles prized as the master-key to disease, even to life itself. Moreover,
most unusually for medicine, the new disease theories led directly and
rapidly to genuinely effective preventive measures and remedies, saving
lives on a dramatic scale.

The general thinking behind bacteriology (that disease is due to
tiny invasive beings) was far from new; theories of contagion, long
proposed for maladies like smallpox and syphilis, maintained that disease
entities were passed from the infected party to others; in the case of
the pox, sexual intercourse offered the obvious transmission mode.
Developing some hints in Galen, Girolamo Fracastoro had written in
1546 of disease seeds (*seminaria contagiosa*) carried by the wind or com-

municated by contact with infected objects (fomites); and the microscope confirmed the reality of wriggling, squirming 'animalcules'. Yet what grounds did anyone have for thinking that such 'little animals' caused disease?

Similar problems attended the putrefaction problem. What made substances go bad, decompose and stink? Why did grubs and mites appear on decaying meat and fruit? Did decay produce the insects (by spontaneous generation) or insects the decay?

By boiling up broth, sealing it in containers and showing that nothing happened, Francesco Redi (1626–98) believed he had proved that maggots did not appear on meat protected against flies, thereby discrediting the theory of spontaneous generation; in *De la génération des vers dans le corps de l'homme* (1699) [On the Generation of Worms in the Human Body], Nicholas Andry also argued that the seeds 'entered the body from without'. But, as so often, there were counter-findings. In 1748 John Needham (1713–81) repeated Redi's experiments; he boiled a meat infusion, corked it, reheated it and, on cooling, identified 'animalcules' in the broth which, he concluded, had appeared spontaneously. Convinced Needham had failed to protect his infusion from the air, Lazzaro Spallanzani maintained that broth, if boiled and hermetically sealed, would keep indefinitely without generating life. With no agreement as to where these 'little animals' came from, their alleged role in disease causation was a mare's nest.

The crucial issues raised were what such 'demonstrations' actually demonstrated (experiments are always open to multiple explanations), and whose experiments should be trusted. There were also metaphysical puzzles. For some, the very idea of 'spontaneous generation' smelt of scandal. It contravened the doctrine that God alone could create life and mocked the natural order, opening the door for whimsy and weirdness in the generation of 'monsters'. Nature, reason taught, was constant and lawlike; hence, was not spontaneous generation as preposterous as centaurs or six-headed cows? Yet certain *philosophes* of materialist leanings, like Diderot, had a soft spot for spontaneous generation precisely for that reason, since it rendered God the Creator otiose while proving that Mother Nature was fertile, creating novel forms as she went along. Spontaneous generation therefore remained a bone of contention, both experimentally and philosophically. The debate had immediate implications for disease aetiology.

Belief in specificity gained ground in nineteenth-century medicine, thanks to the rise of patho-anatomy. So might not specific animalcules (parasites and bacteria) be responsible for particular diseases? There was no clear-cut evidence for this, partly because of the common assumption that all bacteria were much of a muchness. But that began to be challenged. In 1835, Agostino Bassi (1773–1856), an estate manager from Piedmont who was faced with the devastating silkworm disease, muscarine, argued that the fungus found on dead silkworms contained the cause of the disease; by inoculating healthy silkworms with it he could induce the sickness. Bassi's conclusions inspired Johann Schoenlein of Zürich (1793–1864) to investigate ringworm. He, too, found a fungus in ringworm pustules, concluding in 1839 that it was the cause of the condition.

Putrescence was also being hotly debated, thanks to Liebig's fermentation theories and to cell pathology. Working in Müller's Berlin laboratory, Schwann maintained that yeast cells caused fermentations and showed that heat would destroy the 'infusoria' responsible for putrefaction. Persuaded by Bassi, Jacob Henle (1809–85) claimed in *Pathologische Untersuchungen* (1840) [Pathological Investigations] that infectious diseases were caused by a living agent, probably of a vegetable nature, which acted as a parasite on entering the body: 'the substance of contagion is not only organic but living, and endowed with a life of its own, which has a parasitic relation to the sick body.' Broadly anticipating Koch's postulates, he theorized criteria for testing the pathogenic role of parasites: constant presence of the parasite in the sick, its isolation from foreign admixtures, and reproduction of the specific disease in other animals through the transmission of an isolated parasite.

Splicing together various strands of evidence – clinical, veterinary, epidemiological and zoological – Henle challenged spontaneous generation and miasmatism. A political liberal who, like Virchow, supported the revolutions of 1848, he regarded his findings as a ray of hope, presaging an end to the despairing therapeutic nihilism bedevilling Paris and Vienna; once the causal organisms were found, cures would follow. But his conclusions were slighted as speculative. Liebig's reading of fermentation and putrefaction as chemical not biological processes carried greater weight and chimed with dominant miasmatism and environmentalism. From 1857, however, the controversy was transformed by Louis Pasteur (1822–96).

PASTEUR

Born in the Jura, the son of a tanner who was a veteran of Napoleon's *grande armée*, Pasteur, like all ambitious French lads, went to Paris, getting his education at the École Normale Supérieure. Chemistry was his first love, and from the beginning he displayed the dazzling dexterity that became his trademark, selecting big problems which galvanized his energies, and becoming confident all problems could be solved in the laboratory.

Chemistry led him to biology, through experimentation on tartrates. It was known that tartaric acid (a waste product of wine-making) and racemic acid had identical chemical compositions but different physical properties. The crystals of tartrate compounds were asymmetric; solutions could be produced that rotated polarized light both to the left and the right. Pasteur concluded that such molecular asymmetry fundamentally distinguished living from inanimate things. Thereafter it was the properties of the living that fascinated him. Moving from crystals to life, he began to probe the meanings of micro-organisms, thereby laying the foundations for his abiding 'vitalism': a commitment to the irreducible divide between merely chemical and truly living phenomena. Thereafter his mission was to reveal the workings of biology.

Appointment in 1854 to a university chair at the manufacturing centre of Lille led him to study fermentation: the souring of milk, the alcoholic fermentation of wine and beer, the forming of vinegar. Liebig had stated that fermentation was a chemical process, regarding ferments as unstable chemical products. Pasteur promoted the notion of their specificity: fermentation, he held, was the result of the action of particular living micro-organisms. His new inquiries, continued after his return to Paris to take up a chair, centred on the souring of milk (lactic acid) and on the fermentation of sugar into alcohol; by 1860 he had established the biological (rather than chemical) character of fermentation, showing it required such micro-organisms as brewer's yeast. These organisms could in some cases even live without oxygen, in an atmosphere of carbon dioxide; they were thus 'anaerobic'.

This research programme, probing the specific actions of micro-organisms, blossomed into some of Pasteur's most spectacular demonstrations, designed to refute Félix Pouchet's claim to have established spontaneous generation by means of critical experiments. The biologist Pouchet (1800–72) was himself no mean experimenter, and his doctrine of spontaneous generation, set out in his *Hétérogénie* (1854) [Heterogenesis], chimed with the reductionist scientific naturalism championed by anticlericals attempting to free science from the supernatural. On grounds both scientific and spiritual, Pasteur, however, discounted the possibility of life arising out of mere matter: *apparent* proofs, such as Pouchet's, merely betrayed shoddy lab techniques, and he devised ingenious counter-experiments to prove the essential role of micro-organisms.

As everyone knew, broth in a flask would go 'bad' and organisms would appear. Were these, as Pouchet claimed, spontaneously generated? Convinced they came from living agents in the atmosphere, Pasteur devised an elegant sequence of experiments. He passed air through a plug of gun-cotton inserted into a glass tube open to the atmosphere outside his laboratory. The gun-cotton was then dissolved and microscopic organisms identical to those present in fermenting liquids were found in the sediment. Evidently the air contained the relevant organisms. Further experiments showed air could be introduced without infecting a sterile infusion, if the air had previously been sufficiently heated. Thus the organisms present in air were alive and could produce putrefaction, but heating killed them. He next showed that an infusion could be sterilized and left indefinitely open to the air provided the flask's neck had a convexity pointing upwards: the *air* could pass up over this swan-neck but the *organisms* were impeded by gravity. Finally, he showed that micro-organisms were not uniformly distributed in the air. Taking numerous sealed flasks containing a sterile infusion, he broke and resealed the neck of each at a range of different altitudes; unlike in Paris, in calm, high mountain air very few of the flasks showed growth.

No fact is theory-free and incontrovertible. All the same, Pasteur's experiments were exceedingly impressive and persuasive, and when, in characteristically French manner, the lab war between Pouchet and Pasteur was officially adjudicated by the Académie des Sciences, the ruling came down decisively on Pasteur's side. (It surely helped that he was a Parisian establishment figure who could play upon conservative and Catholic anxieties that Pouchet's spontaneous generation was the creed of materialists and anticlericals.)

Developing a sense of duty and destiny, Pasteur marched majestically on to tackle the murky relations between micro-organisms, putrefaction and disease, showing that particular ferments were living forms. Continuing his work for the wine industry, he proved that the micro-organism *Mycoderma aceti* was responsible for souring wine and that heating it to 55°C eliminated the problem. Later, he applied the same principle to beer and milk: 'pasteurization' marked a major step towards the purifying of foods. Since it had been argued by Henle and others that fermentation, putrefaction and infection were related, it required no drastic leap for Pasteur to conclude that disease was a vital process, once he was sure the air was teeming with germs. The first disease he attributed to a living organism was *pébrine*, which was devastating the French silkworm industry. He showed it was caused by a communicable living organism (a protozoan), and laid bare its life cycle from moth through egg to chrysalis.

On 19 February 1878 before the French Academy of Medicine, Pasteur argued the case for the germ theory of infection. Later that year, in a joint paper with Jules Joubert (1834–1910) and Charles Chamberland (1851–1908), he spelt out his conviction that micro-organisms were responsible for disease, putrefaction and fermentation; that only particular organisms could produce specific conditions; and that once those organisms were known, prevention would be possible by developing vaccines.

In 1879 he put these ideas to the test in investigations of chicken cholera and anthrax, two diseases extremely destructive to French agri-culture. He infected healthy birds with 'stale' cholera-causing microbes, two weeks or more old, and was intrigued to discover that no serious disease followed. Next he injected these same birds, and some others, with a new culture. Whereas the additional birds fell ill, those previously injected remained healthy. Here was the way to protect chickens against cholera – he had succeeded in immunizing the chickens with the weak, old bacteria culture, which afforded protection when he later gave them fresh, strong samples. Pasteur's hunch had paid off, but it was he who said that chance favours the prepared mind.

He then applied the same principle to anthrax, a highly contagious condition commonly affecting cattle and sometimes humans. It was a disease of the lungs, which often afflicted woolsorters, and was conven-tionally attributed to rural miasmas. Livestock losses were immense, and anthrax was particularly ruinous because it continued to develop in fields from which infected animals had long been excluded.

Fortunately, the groundwork had already been laid. Franz Aloys

Pollender (1800–79) and Casimir Joseph Davaine (1812–82) had observed microscopic bacilli in the blood of cattle which had died of anthrax. Robert Koch (1843–1910), soon to emerge as Pasteur's titanic rival, had also been investigating the disease. Koch had studied medicine at Göttingen under Wöhler and Henle; after serving as a surgeon in the Franco-Prussian War, he took a post as district medical officer (*Kreisphysikus*) in Wollstein, a small town in Posen (modern Poland), avidly pursuing microbiological researches in his backyard laboratory. Anthrax was severe in Posen. Koch found that under certain conditions the rod-shaped anthrax bacilli (*Bacillus anthracis*) formed exceedingly heat-resistant spores (small encysted bodies) in the blood. Neither putrefaction nor heat killed them, and they could later develop into bacilli. The persistence of the disease in fields was thus explained: it was through the spore. Koch's early laboratory work was technically adroit and systematic – the virtues which earned his later fame.

Using Koch's anthrax bacillus, Pasteur experimented with different time periods to find the way to attenuate its effect, and finally succeeded in producing a vaccine. He then staged a characteristically stunning public demonstration. On 5 May 1881 at Pouilly-le-Fort near Melun, he injected 24 sheep, 1 goat and 6 cows with living attenuated vaccine, leaving a similar number of animals uninjected. He gave the test animals a further and stronger injection on 17 May, and then on 31 May all the animals received a virulent anthrax culture. By 2 June, the control sheep and the goat were all dead and the cattle ill, but the vaccinated animals were fine. The experiment was a striking success, suggesting the possibility of preparing vaccines against diseases by attenuating the infective agent. Such demonstrations gave the germ theory a boost, though Pasteur was concerned less with basic microbiological theory than with concrete investigations, solving problems and contributing to prevention and cures.

Aided by Chamberland and Pierre Emile Roux (1853–1933), in 1880 Pasteur moved on to rabies, a disease dreaded since antiquity because its hydrophobic symptoms were so gruesome and death inescapable. His attempt to find the causative microbe was to no avail – not surprisingly, since the virus can be seen only with an electron microscope. Undeterred, he began his search for a vaccine by injecting rabies-riddled spinal cord tissue into rabbits' brains. When rabbit after rabbit had been injected with the same virus, a consistent incubation period of about six days was produced. The virus acting in this way was called a *virus fixe*. He then injected this fixed virus into the spinal cord, and after death dried them. A cord dried for two weeks became almost non-virulent. In 1884 he made a series of 14 graduated vaccines and set up an experiment with 42 dogs: 23 received 14 injections each, one injection a day, starting with the weakest vaccine and ending with the strongest; the remaining 19 dogs were the controls, receiving no injections. At the end of two weeks, all the dogs were exposed to the rabies virus. None of the 23 immunized got the disease, whereas 13 of the control dogs did. A way had been found to give dogs immunity to rabies; Pasteur later showed that, because the incubation period was lengthy, vaccination worked even if the dogs had been infected for some time.

The moment of truth came on 6 July 1885, when Joseph Meister was brought to his doorstep. Two days before, this nine-year-old boy had been bitten fifteen times by a dog thought to be rabid, and a doctor had told the boy's mother to try Pasteur. He took the risk: he ordered a fourteen-day series of increasingly virulent (and painful) injections, and the boy stayed well. So did a second case treated three months later, a fourteen-year-old shepherd lad, Jean-Baptiste Jupille, from Pasteur's home-district of the Jura, who had been severely bitten as he tried to protect other children from a rabid dog.

These dramatic human interest events, expertly handled by Pasteur who had a flair for publicity and a way of presenting his experiments as more successful and conclusive than they were, captured the world's imagination and vindicated the role of experimental biology. Over the next fifteen months, the vaccine was given to well over two thousand people, and his rabies procedure became standard, with about 20,000 people worldwide being treated during the next decade. Though Pasteur won lavish praise, criticism was levelled as well, on the grounds that he was injecting perhaps perfectly healthy people (not all those bitten by rabid animals develop rabies) with what might prove an unsafe virus. His confidence was posthumously vindicated in 1915, however, when a ten-year study revealed that, of 6000 people bitten by rabid animals, only 0.6 per cent of those vaccinated had died, compared with 16 per cent of the rest.

On a wave of national enthusiasm created by rabies immunization, the Institut Pasteur was set up in 1888, and donations flooded in; appropriately Joseph Meister became the gatekeeper. When Pasteur died eight years later, he was buried in his Institute, consecrated as a shrine to medical science.

KOCH

Pasteur was a wizard, both within the lab and beyond, but bacteriology's consolidation into a scientific discipline was due mainly to Robert Koch (1843–1910) and his team and pupils, whose painstaking microscopic work definitively established the germ concept of disease and systematically developed its potential.

By formalizing the procedures for identifying micro-organisms with particular diseases, and by his insistence upon pure cultures, Koch elevated bacteriology into a regular science, rather as Liebig had normalized organic chemistry and Müller and Ludwig, physiology. Koch's paper on the aetiology of infectious diseases (1879) – a testament to his method and orderliness – launched upon the daunting task of discriminating among bacteria, connecting micro-organisms with particular effects, and settling the old question of whether bacteria were the cause of infection or simply background noise. It also offered an early formulation of what came to be known as Koch's Postulates. Formalized in 1882, these stated that to prove an organism was the cause of any disease, it was necessary to demonstrate

1 That the organism could be discoverable in every instance of the disease;
2 That, extracted from the body, the germ could be produced in a pure culture, maintainable over several microbial generations;
3 That the disease could be reproduced in experimental animals through a pure culture removed by numerous generations from the organisms initially isolated;
4 That the organism could be retrieved from the inoculated animal and cultured anew.

These conditions were mostly able to be fulfilled, though some pathogenic entities, notably viruses, had to be accepted without meeting all the conditions. The thinking behind these rigorous postulates, and their applicability, boosted the dogma of specific aetiology – the idea that a disease has a specific causative agent, with the implication that once this agent has been isolated, it will be possible to control the disease.

In isolating specific bacterial strains, artificial cultivation in liquid media had served Pasteur perfectly well. As superior microscopic techniques revealed the distortions these produced, Koch looked for solid culturing media, beginning by growing bacteria colonies on a potato slice and later solidifying the standard broth by adding gelatin. This liquefied at body temperature, but that problem was solved by using agar-agar, an extract of Japanese seaweed, to solidify the culture medium on a special dish devised by Richard Julius Petri (1852–1921).

Koch scored his first great triumph on 24 March 1882, in revealing before the Berlin Physiological Society the bacillus causing tuberculosis, *Mycobacterium tuberculosis*, and thus at last settling the vexed question of its aetiology. In the following year, with another cholera pandemic heading Europe's way, he was sent to Egypt to investigate, arriving hard on the heels of a French team headed by Pasteur's colleague, Roux. The latter used the classic Pasteurian method, which was to reproduce the disease in animals and then look for the organism; but the method failed, because cholera affects only humans. Working directly on cholera victims, Koch isolated and identified *Vibrio cholerae* (the comma bacillus) in Alexandria in 1883 and more convincingly the next year in India, showing the bacillus lived in the human intestine and was communicated mainly by polluted water – thus vindicating fully the work of John Snow. He then went on to Calcutta, where he confirmed his findings, and in February 1884 reported his success to the German government, amid tremendous jubilation: first tuberculosis, then cholera!*

Koch became burdened with success, his research declined, and to offset that he turned oracle. The methods he had pioneered proved their worth, however, leading to the rapid discovery, largely by his own pupils, of the micro-organisms responsible for diphtheria, typhoid, pneumonia, gonorrhoea, cerebrospinal meningitis, undulant fever, leprosy, plague, tetanus, syphilis, whooping cough and various other streptococcal and staphylococcal infections.

---

* Koch's germ theory of cholera was disputed by the Munich hygienist Max von Petten-kofer (1818–1901), who upheld a version of the miasmatic theory and denied the bacillus was the *vera causa* of cholera. He got Koch to send him his cholera vibrios and put them to the test:

> Herr Doctor Pettenkofer presents his compliments to Herr Doctor Professor Koch and thanks him for the flask containing the so-called cholera vibrios, which he was kind enough to send. Herr Doctor Pettenkofer has now drunk the entire contents and is happy to be able to inform Herr Doctor Professor Koch that he remains in his usual good health.

Pettenkofer must have been fortunate enough to possess the high stomach acidity which sometimes neutralizes the vibrios.

Pasteur's dramatic success with the anthrax and rabies vaccines had fuelled expectations of instant therapeutic breakthroughs. All that was needed, it seemed, was that the relevant micro-organism had to be isolated in the laboratory, and an appropriate vaccine would follow as the night the day. In the event, success proved mixed and often completely elusive. Two early developments provided, respectively, a dazzling victory and a dramatic setback.

The triumph was diphtheria, a disease spread through droplet infection and producing fever, sore throat and a hard cough. A leathery membrane forms on the tonsils and palate, blocking the airways and often causing death. Especially in great cities, diphtheria assumed pandemic proportions after 1850. The death rate was high, occasionally being the principal cause of death among children. In New York in the 1870s, over 2000 children a year were dying of it.

In his *Des inflammations spéciales du tissu mugueux* (1826) [Special Inflammations of the Mucous Tissue], Pierre-Fidèle Bretonneau (1778–1862), an early advocate of germ theory, had distinguished it as a specific disease, coining the word *diphtérie* from the Greek for leather (*diphthera*), alluding to the choking tissue produced in the throat. In 1883 Theodor Albrecht Edwin Klebs (1834–1913), a pupil of Virchow, isolated and described its specific organism, the diphtheria bacillus (*Corynebacterium diphtheriae*), a rod-shaped bacterium. Friedrich Loeffler, one of Koch's assistants, then succeeded in cultivating it. (He also discovered the rod-shaped bacillus in healthy children, one of the observations that led to the concept of the carrier.)

Once the cause was known, the bacillus's action in the human system had to be established. Between 1888 and 1890, brilliant laboratory investigations in France by Roux and Alexandre Yersin (1863–1943), and in Germany by Karl Fraenkel (1861–1901), Emil Behring (1854–1917) and his Japanese colleague Shibasaburo Kitasato (1852–1931) resolved the problems. Roux and Yersin showed that the diphtheria bacterium produced a poison which, when inhaled, lodged in the throat or windpipe, generating a poisonous toxin in the blood-stream. This permitted definitive diagnosis.

In December 1890 Fraenkel showed that attenuated cultures of diphtheria bacilli, injected into guinea pigs, produced immunity. Working with Kitasato in Koch's Institute, Behring announced that the blood or serum of an animal rendered immune to diphtheria through the injection of the relevant toxin could be used to treat another animal exposed to the disease. Immune animals could be prepared by challenging them with gradually increasing doses of either bacillus or toxin.

Such a diphtheria antitoxin (a toxin-resisting substance) was first used on a child in a Berlin clinic on 25 December 1891. This dramatic Christmas rescue, outpasteuring Pasteur (how the modern media would have loved it!), proved a success. Serum production began, and its introduction in 1894 into Berlin hospitals brought an instant plunge in diphtheria mortality. Meanwhile in Paris, Roux and Yersin made large-scale serum production possible by using horses as sources of antitoxin. The French serum was introduced into England by Joseph Lister; diphtheria antitoxin came into general use about 1895, and within ten years the mortality rate had dropped to less than half (the epidemic was in any case spontaneously waning).

Especially once the Hungarian Béla Schick (1877–1967) developed the test bearing his name to identify the presence of immunity, large-scale immunization programmes were undertaken. In New York, the death rate had peaked at 785 per 100,000 in 1894; by 1920, it had dipped to under 100. By 1940, with 60 per cent of pre-school children immunized, diphtheria deaths had become a thing of the past.

The campaign brought a famous victory and, because, like rabies, it also involved children, it provided further superb publicity for the new bacteriology. New scientific possibilities had been opened up since – in contrast to Pasteur's live vaccines – it had now been shown that the cell-free serum of immunized animals could kill virulent bacteria, and protection could be transferred via serum from animal to animal. (This suggested that it was not simply the bacterial cell itself that caused disease, but a toxin it yielded.) On this putatively safer basis serum therapy was launched, with the production of antitoxins not just for diphtheria but also for tetanus, plague, cholera and snake bites. Yet serum therapy encountered problems of its own, for antitoxin production was impossible to control, and supplies varied in strength and purity. Occasional deaths of patients receiving antitoxin proved shocking, and serum sickness (fever, rash and joint pains) was a common side-effect. Apart from such practical troubles, profound questions were surfacing about the nature of the body's reactions to micro-organisms and chemicals.

If diphtheria was the dramatic therapeutic success, the dispiriting failure was tuberculosis, potentially the gold medal for the new science. Consumption had become the single largest cause of adult deaths in the West. Thanks to the Paris school, cases could reliably be clinically diagnosed. Laennec and Bayle had unified the disease, and in 1839 J. L. Schoenlein, professor of medicine at Zürich, named the whole complex 'tuberculosis', since the tubercle seemed to be its anatomical root.

But its cause remained obscure and hotly disputed – was it hereditary, constitutional, environmental, or contagious? The received wisdom was that an 'innate susceptibility' or a 'diathesis' was to blame. Despite an army of 'cures', ranging from blistering to living in cowsheds to inhale the breath of cattle, and the new faith in the sanatorium on the magic mountain, tuberculosis seemed a good justification for therapeutic nihilism: 'I know the colour of that blood! It is arterial blood. I cannot be deceived in that colour. That drop of blood is my death warrant. I must die,' cried John Keats, on first coughing up blood – and how right he was. Some survived for a long time, and some recovered spontaneously; but no realist thought medicine cured the disease.

The idea that tuberculosis was communicable, though mainly rejected, had its advocates. William Budd (1811–80), best known for his work on typhoid fever, argued for contagiousness on the basis of epidemiological studies, and the French physician Jean Antoine Villemin (1827–92) attempted to confirm this by inoculating rabbits and guinea pigs with sufferers' blood, sputum, and secretions – work paralleled in Germany by Virchow's pupil Julius Cohnheim (1839–84). Villemin also argued for cross-contagiousness between humans and cattle, but his work had little immediate impact; attempts to repeat his rabbit experiments were inconclusive, and many mysteries remained. Rebutting Laennec, Virchow maintained that pulmonary and miliary tuberculosis were quite different diseases, though here he perhaps betrayed a chauvinism that killed three birds with one stone: denigrating both Paris and Pasteur, and voicing his perennial scepticism towards bacteriology.

Koch made the dramatic breakthrough. Having cultured a specific microbe apparently associated with tuberculosis, in 1882 he provided solid evidence from animal experiments, conformable with his 'postulates', that the tubercle bacillus was the specific cause of the disease. Then, after years of travelling and official duties connected with his prestigious Institute for the Study of Infectious Diseases, he began to work in the laboratory again, with great intensity and secrecy, perhaps feeling the need to eclipse Pasteur with one great therapeutic coup. In August 1890 all was revealed in a speech before the Tenth International Congress of Medicine in Berlin: Koch had found a substance which arrested the growth of the tubercle bacillus in the test-tube and in living bodies, referring to his agent, which he called 'tuberculin', as a 'remedy' and thus leading the world to believe he had a TB cure.

Dazzling publicity followed, and Koch was fêted. Before tuberculin's efficacy and safety had been evaluated, the Kaiser personally conferred upon him the medal of the Grand Cross of the Red Eagle, and he received the freedom of the city of Berlin. Despite Germany's law prohibiting 'secret medicines', Koch avoided disclosing the nature of tuberculin. Sent to Berlin to report for the press, Arthur Conan Doyle (1859–1930) paid a call on Koch's son-in-law and found his office knee-deep in letters begging for the miraculous remedy; the whole business was like Lourdes.

Within a year thousands had received tuberculin treatment, without system or controls. It seemed to help some patients in the first stages of lupus (tuberculosis of the skin), but experience quickly showed that tuberculin was useless or even dangerous for patients with pulmonary tuberculosis. The fiasco brought a violent backlash, with denunciations of Koch and his secret remedy. A study prepared for the German government found little evidence to justify the claims made for tuberculin. Koch was rumoured to have sold his 'secret' to a drug company for a million marks, to help finance his divorce and remarriage.

In a paper published in January 1891, Koch at last revealed the nature of his remedy: tuberculin was nothing but a glycerine extract of tubercle bacilli. He was accused of divulging the great secret only when it had become obvious that tuberculin was financially worthless. He disappeared to Egypt with his young bride, leaving his underlings to cope with the débâcle.

To the end of his life, he continued to express the hope that an improved form of tuberculin would serve as an immunizing agent or cure. He was mistaken, though it did prove to have a use – not as a cure but as a diagnostic aid in the detection of early, presymptomatic tuberculosis. In the heroic tradition of the time, Koch had tested tuberculin on himself: his strong reaction indicated that, like most of his contemporaries, he had not escaped a 'touch of tuberculosis'; and what he had stumbled upon was the complex immunological phenomenon now called delayed-type hypersensitivity. The tuberculin test was put into service, and microbiology laboratories were able to help the physician monitor the patient's status by analysing throat cultures or sputum samples.

Koch made a further blunder: he wielded his authority to scotch Villemin's case that bovine and human tuberculosis were very similar. Human tuberculosis, Koch insisted, could not be transmitted to cattle, nor could bovine tuberculosis be communicated to humans. In this he was wrong, and only when his mistake was undone could it be recognized that transmission of tuberculosis from cattle to humans was a serious problem. This led to measures to purify milk through pasteurization and tuberculin tests. His latest biographer has concluded that Koch 'ended his career as an imperious and authoritarian father figure whose influence on bacteriology and medicine was so strong as to be downright dangerous'.

Despite the tuberculin débâcle, the search continued for ways of immunizing against tuberculosis. Attempts to protect individuals by injecting them with tubercle bacilli, killed or treated, had no success until a new method was developed by Albert Calmette (1863–1933), of the Pasteur Institute, and his collaborator Jean Marie Guérin (1872–1961). From 1906 they used living bacilli from a bovine strain of the tubercle bacillus so attenuated as to have lost their disease-producing properties while retaining their protective reaction. The vaccine was given the name BCG (Bacilli-Calmette-Guérin); it was first used for inoculating calves and then, from 1924, after delays caused by the First World War, was extended to humans. By 1928 it had been successfully given to 116,000 French children, though its efficacy remained controversial. With medicine thoroughly tainted with nationalism, Germany declined to approve BCG, as did the USA; in Britain its uptake was dilatory, but it was used successfully in Scandinavia, where it markedly reduced the death rate. After the Second World War, the BCG vaccine was central to a huge Danish Red Cross vaccination programme in war-devastated Europe.

The great infectious diseases were targeted by the new bacteriology with mixed success: discovery of the infective agent by no means always led to effective therapies. Nevertheless, in the twenty-one golden years between 1879 and 1900 the micro-organisms responsible for major diseases were being discovered at the phenomenal rate of one a year. Typhoid was one.

By 1837 the distinction between typhoid fever and typhus fever had been established, and the typhoid micro-organism was isolated in 1884 by Koch's pupil, Georg Gaffky (1850–1918). Immunization against typhoid was introduced by Almroth Wright (1861–1947) in 1897, but its efficacy was disputed by the statistician Karl Pearson (1857–1936) and only a fraction of the British troops received it during the Boer War; in South Africa 13,000 men were lost to typhoid as against 8000 battle deaths. Controversy raged until a special anti-typhoid commission reported favourably in 1913; the army then adopted a policy of vaccinating all soldiers sent abroad. The results were dramatic: whereas in the Boer War typhoid incidence was around 10 per cent with a mortality of 14.6 per 1000, in the Great War incidence was down to 2 per cent, with a minuscule death rate. Because of the presence of paratyphoid fever on the eastern fronts, killed cultures of paratyphoid bacilli A and B were added to the vaccine, so that it became known as T.A.B.

Another success, proved by the First World War, came with tetanus. This extremely dangerous disease (the death-rate is above 40 per cent) is caused by tetanospasmin, a toxin secreted by the bacterium *Clostridium tetani* which lives in the soil. The bacillus enters the body through agricultural cuts and battlefield wounds, and the toxin travels along nerve fibres towards the spinal cord. Sweating and headaches are followed by increasingly severe muscular spasms in the head and neck (lockjaw). Though known to Hippocrates, nothing could be done until the bacteriological era. The tetanus bacillus was discovered, like so many others, in the 1880s. Arthur Nicolaier (1862–1942) produced it in mice by inoculating them with garden earth; Kitasato grew it in a pure culture in Koch's laboratory in 1889, leading to the production of antitoxin. (He also found it grew when deprived of oxygen, an early example of the anaerobic bacteria group, discovered in 1861 by Pasteur.) Tetanus became a serious problem at the outset of the 1914–18 war, when the bacillus entered the body through gaping shell wounds. From 1915 practically every wounded soldier received antitoxin, and tetanus was dramatically reduced.

Some progress was also made with plague. The bacillus was discovered independently by Kitasato and Yersin during the Hong Kong epidemic in 1894. The Swiss-born Yersin had studied in Paris, becoming Roux's assistant and publishing papers with him on diphtheria before leaving to satisfy his wanderlust in the Far East. He returned to bacteriology, but in the colonial context, going to Hong Kong to investigate the plague epidemic spreading from China.

In June 1894, more or less simultaneously with Kitasato, Yersin isolated the plague bacillus now known as *Yersinia pestis*, reproducing the disease experimentally in healthy rats and transmitting it from rat to rat. 'The plague', he wrote dryly, 'is contagious and inoculable. The rat probably is the principal vector and one of the most promising prophylactic measures would be extermination of rats.' It had long been observed that outbreaks of a deadly disease among vermin preceded outbreaks of plague in humans; these epizootics which preceded epidemics finally became recognized as being due to the plague bacillus, conveyed via the *Xenopsylla cheopis* flea.

Exploiting this discovery, however, posed further problems. Bacteriologically, plague differs from diphtheria in that the organisms, instead of remaining localized, multiply rapidly throughout the body. The filtrate of a culture of plague bacilli was not very toxic and so conferred no immunity. The first vaccine made from killed cultures of plague bacilli came from the Russian, Waldemar Haffkine (1860–1930), an ex-pupil of Pasteur working in British government service in India, one of the world's plague centres. Its success was rather limited, and nothing helped much before antibiotics.

A significant breakthrough in understanding and management also followed with undulant fever, a disease involving fever, with muscle and joint pains. Many of the British sick and wounded in the Crimean War, shipped to Malta to recover, had contracted this condition. In 1887 Major David Bruce (1855–1931) isolated the causative organism in 'Malta fever'. The organism was of the spherical or coccus type, being called *Micrococcus melitensis* (from *Melita*, Latin for Malta). Goats were found to be highly susceptible, excreting the organism in their milk, and a ban on drinking goats' milk produced a dramatic fall in the disease. Ten years later the Norwegian Bernhard Bang (1848–1932) independently described a very small bacillus found to cause contagious abortion in cattle. This *Bacillus abortus* also caused an obscure and persistent condition in humans; named undulant fever, it was common in the Mediterranean. In 1918 it was concluded that Bruce's *Micrococcus melitensis* and Bang's *Bacillus abortus* were identical. A new name *Brucella abortus* was coined in Bruce's honour, and the diseases caused by them became *Brucellosis* – another triumph for British terminological imperialism. The health gains following this discovery were limited; the British garrison on Malta was protected from contaminated milk, but no efforts were made to reduce the incidence of *Brucellosis* among the local population.

Though by any criteria bacteriology had a dazzling string of successes to its credit, certain diseases proved refractory. One was scarlet fever, a dreadful killer of infants throughout the nineteenth century. Streptococci were first isolated from the blood of scarlet fever patients by Edward Klein (1844–1925) in 1887, but he was unable to reproduce the disease in animals. And while streptococci could be recovered from the throats of scarlet-fever patients, the next steps – showing, following Koch's postulates, that the bacterium was the true cause of the disease and then producing a vaccine – were stymied. The streptococcus was found to be pathogenic for various laboratory animals, but on injection it hardly ever produced typical scarlet fever.

In 1924, George (1881–1967) and Gladys Dick (1881–1963), at the University of Chicago, identified haemolytic streptococcus as the causal agent and succeeded in infecting volunteers after swabbing their throats with a culture obtained from scarlet fever patients; they also established a test for immunity (the Dick test). But, as with many other communicable diseases, what brought its decline was not a therapeutic breakthrough but a healthier environment and improving patient resistance.

DEBATES OVER IMMUNITY

Whereas Pasteur developed attenuated live vaccines, German researchers pioneered serum therapy. They turned their attention from cellular to so-called 'humoral' immunity once it was shown that animals could be made immune to the toxins produced by diphtheria and tetanus bacilli, thanks to injections of immune serum. Opposing their view that a bactericidal property resided in the serum, a counter-theory was developed by Élie [Ilya Ilyich] Metchnikoff (1845–1916), the Russian pathologist appointed in 1887 as sub-director of the Pasteur Institute. This dispute became the scientific expression of Franco–German and Russo–Japanese rivalries.

How did the body develop immunity to protect itself against organisms? Recognition had been growing from the mid nineteenth century that normal blood could destroy bacteria, but little was understood of how that happened: Pasteur preferred vaccines to theories. In 1884 Metchnikoff observed a phenomenon which suggested a cellular theory of immunity and resistance. He saw amoeba-like cells in water fleas and other lower organisms 'ingesting' foreign substances like fungi. These cells, he concluded, might be similar to the pus cells in the inflammatory response of higher organisms. Microscopic observations on animals infected with various micro-organisms, including the anthrax bacillus, revealed white blood cells attacking and appearing to digest these disease germs, 'fighting infection' like soldiers. Pasteur gave Metchnikoff's ideas his nod, while Koch and most German bacteriologists demurred; Koch even suggested that white blood cells might be more like a fifth column through which germs spread into the organism. Metchnikoff's cellular immunity theories became connected with the French school, and chemical theories with the German view that germ wars were waged less by the blood cells than by the serum.

Metchnikoff styled the cells which ingested micro-organisms 'phagocytes' (from the Greek *phagein*, to eat, and *kutos*, cell). Macrophages was his name for the large mononuclear cells of the blood and tissues which ingested foreign particles; microphages were the leucocytes of the blood, active in ingesting micro-organisms. In what became the cellular (phagocytic) theory of immunity, he showed that one special kind of macrophage, the white cell (granulocyte), ate bacteria, and also that the body's supply of such cells multiplied when infection struck. His views constitute perhaps the first model of immune response.

The alternative serum or humoral theory viewed infections as caused by bacilli-produced toxins; filtrates of these, containing no organisms, caused disease when injected into animals, the bacillus producing its effects through exotoxins in the filtrate. But the serum of treated animals equally acquired the property of neutralizing toxin: Behring and Kitasato called this property 'antitoxic'.

By 1890 scientists had thus identified both a cellular and a serum system. Koch's tuberculin work pointed to a third – a group of smaller, light-staining white cells different from Metchnikoff's larger, dark-staining white granulocytes. These became known as lymphocytes. The body thus appeared to have an immune system made up of various elements which worked by combining forces. This possibility was strengthened in 1895 when two Belgian biologists, Joseph Denys and Joseph Leclef, modified Metchnikoff's views. The Russian held that the leucocytes from an animal immunized against a certain organism actively engulfed that organism (phagocytosis). Working with streptococci, they showed that, if the leucocytes from a treated animal were placed in immune serum, the resultant phagocytosis was exceptionally active.

These ideas were developed further by Almroth Wright, director of the Institute of Pathology at St Mary's Hospital in London, a larger-than-life figure caricatured on stage as Sir Colenso Ridgeon in George Bernard Shaw's *The Doctor's Dilemma*. Wright held that the action of both normal and immune serum was due to the presence of certain substances which promoted phagocytosis. Likening these to a sauce making the bacteria more tasty for the leucoctyes, he called them opsonins (Greek, *opsonein*, to prepare food), these being antibodies facilitating phagocytosis. The level of opsonic activity could be seen as a measure of a patient's defences against bacterial infection – hence the slogan Shaw put into Ridgeon's mouth: 'Stimulate the phagocytes!' The Englishman's work on opsonins appeared to marry the chemical (German) and cellular (French) theories of immunity, though his limitless faith in immunization ('the physician of the future will be an immunizer' he predicted) proved unjustified.

All such antigen-antibody reactions (as they were later called) had certain features in common, protecting the individual against bacterial poisons. But it was found that comparable reactions could occur which were harmful rather than preservative. With diphtheria antitoxin treatment, some patients developed serum sickness (drowsiness, sweating and rashes), something first studied in Vienna by Clemens von Pirquet (1874–1929), and his assistant Béla Schick. Examining reactions to substances such as pollen, von Pirquet decided they were due to antigen-antibody reactions and coined the term 'allergy' to indicate the hypersensitive state producing abnormal reactions to certain foreign substances. Allergic reactions had been known since the Greeks; John Bostock (1773–1846) had coined the term 'summer catarrh' (hay fever), and John Elliotson (1791–1868) identified pollen as the agent; but the cause of such reactions had remained mysterious.

Bacteriological investigations of resistance and immunity also brought to light the baffling question of the carrier. Experience showed that the diphtheria bacillus sometimes persisted in the throats of convalescent patients; in 1900 a case was reported of a healthy individual passing typhoid bacillus in his urine, and some persons convalescing from enteric fever still excreted the organism, forming a worrying source of further infection. It was soon realized that some carriers could excrete it for many years, the most notorious being the Irish-born 'Typhoid Mary' who, though well herself, infected many people in New York with enteric fever between 1900 and 1907. The mechanisms of immunity were evidently more complicated than anyone had surmised, and early military images of gunning down 'invading' micro-organic pathogens obviously needed refinement.

CHEMOTHERAPY

Chemical theories of response were systematized by Paul Ehrlich (1854–1915), from 1899 director of the Royal Prussian Institute for Experimental Therapy in Frankfurt-am-Main. A truly seminal thinker, Ehrlich had a personal interest in these matters, since he had discovered tubercle bacilli in his sputum, had tried Koch's tuberculin therapy and had spent a year in Egypt convalescing. He drove immunity investigations one stage further by developing chemotherapy, pinning his faith on the creation of artificial antibodies.

Treatment by natural drugs, above all herbs, goes back to the dawn of medicine; experience showed that certain substances had therapeutic properties. Paracelsus had proclaimed specific remedies for specific diseases, and Sydenham had hoped that one day every disease would have its own remedy, on the model of the Peruvian bark for malaria. From time to time new medications had been hit upon, as with the Revd Edmund Stone's discovery of willow bark, which was the first stage on the road to aspirin.*

As shown in Chapter 11, the study of *materia medica* developed during the nineteenth century into laboratory-based pharmacology. Meanwhile drugs research and manufacturing became inseparably linked. The booming chemical industry developed pharmaceutical

---

* That road was long. In 1826 two Italians found that willow bark's active ingredient was salicin, and three years later a French chemist obtained it in pure form. Meanwhile the Swiss pharmacist Johann S. F. Pagenstecher began extracting a substance from meadowsweet (*Spirea ulmaria*, a pain reliever well-known to folk medicine), which led to the German chemist Karl Jacob Löwig (1803–90) obtaining the acid later known as salicylic acid. Its molecular structure was ascertained in 1853 by Karl Friedrich Gerhardt (1816–56), a Montpellier chemistry professor, who tried to eliminate its severe side-effect: the painful irritation of the stomach-lining. In time Felix Hoffman (1868–1946) came up with acetylsalicylic acid, found to be not only a painkiller but anti-inflammatory and anti-pyretic. In 1899, a new name was invented for the drug: aspirin. The following year, the German Bayer drug company took out patents on it and it became their best-selling product, indeed the most popular drug of all time; in the United States, over 10,000 tons of aspirin are used annually.

divisions, often as a sideline of the thriving dyestuffs business. In Britain W. H. Perkin (1838–1907) isolated mauve (aniline purple) from coal tar in 1856, but it was German entrepreneurs who excelled in exploiting dyes and organic chemistry.

Drug production became industrialized, with many of the companies appearing that later dominated the field. In 1858 E. R. Squibb opened a laboratory to supply medicines to the US army. Benefiting from the Civil War, his firm expanded rapidly, producing pure ether and chloroform, and using steam power for pulverizing drugs. The Eli Lilly Company was founded in Indianapolis in 1876; Merck and Company, a branch of a leading German chemical firm, opened in the United States in 1891; Parke, Davis & Company, formed in 1867, established one of the earliest research institutes in 1902.

Technological advances helped the drugs firms. Mass-production of sugar-coated pills started in France, being refined in 1866 by William R. Warner, a Philadelphia manufacturer who also began production of small pills (parvules). The gelatin capsule was developed, being brought into general use about 1875 by Parke, Davis. Capsules not only made medicine easier to swallow, they ensured a precise dose. Mechanization also made the tablet possible. A tablet-compression machine was introduced in England by William Brockedon in 1843 and in the USA by Jacob Denton in 1864.

Henry Wellcome (1853–1936) was born in Wisconsin, the son of a travelling Second Adventist minister. Inspired by a doctor uncle, he went into pharmacy, sweated as a travelling salesman (peddling pills, not salvation), and hitched up in his mid twenties with Silas Burroughs (1846–1895), who had the capital Wellcome lacked. Burroughs was the first American to bring medicines to Britain in mass-produced, machine-made tablets. Setting up in Holborn, Burroughs, Wellcome and Co. procured the British patent for the process, inventing 'Tabloid' as their trade-mark (the term's application to newspapers came much later).

Developing its research side, the pharmaceutical industry joined hands with academic pharmacology, whose institutional development followed the familiar German path. Institutes, notably those at Dorpat and Bonn, produced research schools employing chemists and physiologists. By 1900, pharmaceutical manufacturers were turning discoveries made in university laboratories to profit. Such cooperation between science and commerce was not always plain-sailing: industrial patenting and profit-seeking potentially clashed with the ideals of open scientific inquiry. When John Jacob Abel (1857–1938) and some academic colleagues established the American Society for Pharmacology and Experimental Therapeutics (1908), they excluded anyone in the permanent employ of a drug firm.

Wellcome ran into similar problems in Britain when he sought registration for animal experimentation at his Wellcome Physiological Research Laboratories, set up in 1894. Although he maintained his laboratories were independent of his drug firm, they were financed out of company profits and in practice linked with the manufacturing side. With the backing of key members of the British medical establishment, however, he obtained the necessary Home Office authority for animal experiments, and other British pharmaceutical firms followed, as animals were used to raise antitoxins and test products.

The symbiosis between science and industry was closest in Germany: Ehrlich's Frankfurt Institute research laboratories had ties with the Hoechst and Farbwerke Cassella companies. In his quest for chemical cures, Ehrlich thus had a long tradition of pharmaceutical developments and microbiological investigations to draw on. His vision lay squarely within the framework of the new bacteriology, taking the idea of natural antibodies and transferring it to synthetic drugs. The idea had been already present in his doctoral thesis, which held that specific chemicals could interact with particular tissues, cells or microbial agents. Systematically exploring the range of dyes manufactured by the German chemical industry – dyes were evidently promising because, as histological staining made clear, their action was specific, staining some tissues and not others – Ehrlich was intrigued by the molecular (stereochemical) aspects of physiological and pharmacological events. Above all, he believed chemical structures were crucial to the actions of biologically active compounds, and that they could not affect a cell without being attached to it: *corpora non agunt nisi fixata* (substances do not react unless they become fixed) was one of his adages. A 'receptor' was a structure that received a dye. If there were dye receptors, why not drug receptors? Ehrlich began looking for substances fixed by microbes but not by the human host.

His first contributions to immunity theory came in the 1890s. Pondering how tetanus antitoxin actually worked, he advanced a series of significant hypotheses. Each molecule of toxin combined with a particular, invariant amount of antitoxin; the toxin-antitoxin connection involved groups of atoms fitting together like a key in a lock; tetanus toxin became bound to the cells of the central nervous system, attaching itself to the chemical 'side-chains' on the cell protoplasm, thereby blocking their physiological function. This blockage led the cell to produce fresh side-chains to compensate for what was blocked. These were the antibodies produced by toxin action.

Ehrlich's side-chain, or chemical affinity, theory was based on the assumption that the union of toxin and antitoxin was chemical in nature, involving agents specifically toxic for particular bacteria, which would have no effect on the host. An antibody in the blood, produced in response to a certain micro-organism, was specific for that organism and highly effective in killing it, but harmless to the host. Antibodies (nature's remedies) were magic bullets which flew straight to their mark and injured nothing else. The challenge was thus to find chemical equivalents tailormade for a particular organism and non-injurious to its host. Chemotherapy would be the discovery of synthetic chemical substances acting specifically on disease-producing micro-organisms.

Guided by this model of antigen-antibody reactions, Ehrlich set out to find agents specifically bound to and toxic for particular bacteria. In 1891, with quinine's action in mind, he treated malaria with methylene blue, one of the aniline dyes – the first instance of Ehrlichian chemotherapy; the results, he thought, were promising. The next targets for his new chemotherapy were the trypanosomes, the causative agents of sleeping sickness. For this he tried a drug called atoxyl and similar arsenical compounds. This was quite effective, but caused neurological damage and blindness by way of side-effects.

Next he turned to syphilis. That disease had seemingly become more virulent again in the nineteenth century; certainly it was a disease of the famous, including Baudelaire and Nietzsche, the myth being popular among the *avant garde* that it contributed to genius, providing drive and restless energy. Many writers were positively exalted at getting poxed (or were good at putting a brave face on it). 'For five weeks I have been taking mercury and potassium iodine and I feel very well on it,' boasted Guy de Maupassant in 1877:

> My hair is beginning to grow again and the hair on my arse is sprouting. I've got the pox! At last! Not the contemptible clap . . . no – no – the great pox, the one Francis I died of. The majestic pox . . . and I'm proud of it, by thunder. I don't have to worry about catching it any more, and I screw the street whores and trollops, and afterwards I say to them, 'I've got the pox'.

The natural history of syphilis had been clarified. In 1837 Philippe Ricord (1800–1889) established the specificity of syphilis and gonorrhoea through a series of experimental inoculations from syphilitic chancres. He also differentiated primary, secondary and late syphilis, the three stages of infection. In 1879 the German bacteriologist Albert Neisser (1855–1916) identified the gonococcus causing gonorrhoea, and in 1905, the protozoan parasite causing syphilis was discovered by Fritz Schaudinn (1871–1906) and Erich Hoffman (1868–1959); found in chancres, this spiralling threadlike single-celled organism was named the *Spirochaeta pallida* (since renamed the *Treponema pallidum*). Diagnostic screening was made possible in 1906 when August von Wassermann (1866–1925) developed a specific blood test. Despite these substantial advances in knowledge, no therapeutic advances had been made upon the wretched mercury, in use since the sixteenth century. Arsenical compounds such as atoxyl were mildly effective but injurious.

Seeking a chemical cure, by 1907 Ehrlich had synthesized and tested over 600 arsenical compounds. He took out a patent on Number 606, but went no further. In 1909 the Japanese bacteriologist Sahachiro Hata (1873–1938) began work as his assistant and retested the whole series of synthetic preparations for their action on the *Treponema*. It became clear that 606 was very active. After two physicians had volunteered as guineapigs, Ehrlich's collaborators began intramuscular injections of 606 on some of their most hopeless patients, and were surprised at the improvements engendered by a single injection. By September 1910 about 10,000 syphilitics had been treated with Preparation 606, by then named Salvarsan. It transformed syphilis treatment, especially once it was used in the modified form of Neo-Salvarsan (1914), now called neoarsphenamine. This represented a considerable advance, but it was toxic and still required many painful injections into the bloodstream over a long period before a cure was complete – the 'magic bullet' didn't cure syphilis 'like magic'.

Once Salvarsan was discovered, would not other chemical magic bullets follow rapidly? Though plausible, that hope proved wrong. Many compounds, including some new synthetic dyes, were tried against the common bacterial diseases (the cocci and bacilli), but without success. Chemotherapy came to seem, after all, an impossible dream. Well into the twentieth century, for most infections there were no effective therapies; ancient and useless remedies like emetics were still prescribed; as late as the 1920s, the professor of applied pharmacology at Harvard,

H. W. Haggard (1891–1959), confessed that medicine could 'do little to repair damage from diseases'. The only effective chemotherapeutic substances, as distinct from painkilling drugs like morphia, were mercury, and Salvarsan and its variants, antimony for schistosomiasis, and quinine. Quinine's action was still little understood; it was thought to have a selective affinity for malaria parasites in the blood, but in laboratory experiments it was hardly active in killing the malaria parasite. This suggested that the action was not a direct destruction of the parasites but a change produced in the body tissues inhibiting further parasite development. The situation changed, however, in 1935, when Gerhard Domagk (1895–1964) published his experiments with Prontosil.

Searching, like Ehrlich, for chemical remedies, Domagk devoted his early years to testing the therapeutic potential of metal-based compounds – gold, tin, antimony and arsenic. None worked: their antibacterial actions were too weak or their toxic side-effects too strong. In 1927 he was appointed research director of I. G. Farbenindustrie, the chemical company which had absorbed such familiar names as Bayer and Hoechst. Since his firm's main products were azo dyes used for colouring textiles, he decided, like Ehrlich, to see whether they had any negative effect on streptococci, organisms that produce infections including erysipelas, tonsillitis, scarlet fever and rheumatism. In 1932 he found that one azo compound, Prontosil red, a brilliant red dye, cured mice injected with a lethal dose of haemolytic streptococci. Domagk successfully treated his own daughter with it for a streptococcal infection.

Scientists at the Pasteur Institute in Paris obtained Prontosil samples for investigation. Synthesizing the drug, they verified Domagk's results, and found it worked when the compound split into two parts within the body, and that one of the two parts, later called sulphanilamide, was largely responsible for Prontosil's 'bacteriostatic' action – that is, it did not *kill* bacteria but prevented them from multiplying in the host, thus allowing the host's immune system to destroy them.

Domagk went into production with his new drug. As it could not be patented (Prontosil was basically sulphonamide, which had been synthesized back in 1907), it became readily available. At Queen Charlotte's Maternity Hospital in London, Leonard Colebrook (1883–1967) used it to treat puerperal fever and found it was a 'miracle drug', slashing mortality from 20 to 4.7 per cent – and at last realizing Semmelweis's dream.

Though effective against streptococci, Prontosil was little use against pneumococcal infections, and scientists began to look for comparable drugs. In 1938, a British team, led by A. J. Ewins (1882–1958) of May and Baker, developed M & B 693 (sulfadiazine 693, later called sulphapyridine), which worked well against pneumococci and was even better than sulphanilamide against streptococci. M & B achieved fame when it saved the life of Winston Churchill, seriously ill with pneumonia at a critical stage of the Second World War.

All these compounds were bacteriostatic, affecting the bacterial metabolism and preventing its multiplication in the host, thereby permitting natural body defences to succeed against the invader. As well as puerperal fever, the new drugs checked the pathogens in erysipelas, mastoiditis, meningitis, and some urinary diseases, including gonorrhoea: sulphanilamide could dispose of a case of gonorrhoea in just five days. Domagk was awarded the Nobel Prize in 1939, but Hitler disapproved of such things and had Domagk detained by the Gestapo to prevent his going to receive it (he received it in 1947).

These new 'sulpha drugs' began to be prescribed in vast quantities: by 1941, 1700 tons were given to ten million Americans. However, deaths were reported, and strains of sulpha-resistant streptococci appeared. Controls over pharmaceuticals were then minimal, and experience showed that the sulphonamides had their dangers and could also become ineffectual. They nevertheless represented a major step towards the control of bacterial diseases, and their development spurred research into other anti-microbial agents.

ANTIBIOTICS AND THE DRUGS REVOLUTION

Pasteurian bacteriology opened up the vision of biological (as distinct from chemical) agents being deployed to destroy bacteria. But what sort of biological agents might prove effective? Folklore suggested that fungi might be antibacterial: popular medicine widely recommended mould for treating wounds or cuts. But the first clear observation of antibacterial action was made in 1877 by Pasteur: while anthrax bacilli rapidly multiplied in sterile urine, the addition of 'common bacteria' halted their development. In 1885, the Italian Arnaldo Cantani (1837–93) painted the throat of a tubercular child with bacterial strains and reported that the bacteria in his mixture displaced tubercle bacilli while reducing fever. He stated the principle of bacterial antagonism: one infective pathogen would drive out another, a notion chiming with popular Darwinian notions of the struggle for existence.

The condition in which 'one creature destroys the life of another to preserve his own' was called 'antibiosis' by Paul Vuillemin (1861–1932). He termed the killer or active agent the 'antibiote'. In due course the word antibiotic (meaning destructive of life) was brought in by Selman Waksman (1888–1973). The first antibiotic to be described was penicillin, a natural by-product from moulds of the genus *Penicillium*. It was brought to light through the work of Alexander Fleming (1888–1955), a Scottish bacteriologist at St Mary's Hospital, London.

During the First World War, Fleming had been working on wounds and resistance to infection, demonstrating that the harsh chemical antiseptics used to cleanse wounds damaged natural defences and failed to destroy the bacteria responsible for infection. He was therefore receptive to the phenomenon of lysis, then under investigation. Exploring staphylococci in 1915, Frederick Twort (1877–1950) noticed that in some cultures the microbial colonies tended to disappear. He filtered some of these, and found a few drops poured over a staphylococcus culture produced degeneration. In 1917, working with cultures obtained from dysenteric patients, Felix d'Hérelle (1873–1949) found that the diluted filtrate produced lysis (dissolving) of the organisms in a broth-culture of the dysentery bacillus. He called the lytic agent the *bacteriophage* (or simply *phage*, meaning eater). Such experiments tended to suggest that lytic agents, generally found in the intestinal tract, were most active against one particular bacterial species or related types, having no effect on others.

Aware of these developments, Fleming's mind was receptive to the first of his discoveries, made in November 1921, when he identified the enzyme lysozyme, a component of tears and mucous fluids. This arose from accidental contamination of a culture of nasal mucus by a previously undescribed organism; it happened to be uniquely sensitive to the lytic action of the enzyme in the mucus, and Fleming observed its colonies being dissolved. The enzyme, which he called 'lysozyme', while it did not kill harmful bacteria, was clearly part of the body's defence system. Sceptical about chemotherapy – once infection entered the body, he believed, it was the body which would have to contain it – Fleming regarded lysozyme in a different light, belonging as it did to that class of substances which bodies themselves produced against outside intrusions.

Fleming's identification of penicillin came six years after the lyso-zyme discovery, in August 1928. He had been working on staphylococci, the pathogens responsible for boils, carbuncles, abscesses, pneumonia and septicaemia. Returning from holiday, he found that a mould which had appeared on a staphyloccus culture left in a petri dish in his St Mary's lab seemed to have destroyed the staphylococcus colonies. In a paper published in 1929 he identified the mould as *Penicillium rubrum* (actually it was *Penicillium notatum*). While the penicillin strongly affected such Gram-positive* bacteria as staphylococci, streptococci, gonococci, men-ingococci, diphtheria bacillus and pneumococci, it had no toxic effect on healthy tissues and did not impede leucocytic (white cell) defence functions. This weighed heavily with Fleming in view of his general opinions on wound treatment; penicillin appeared not just strong but safe. Yet it had no effect on Gram-negative bacteria, including those responsible for cholera and bubonic plague; it was hard to produce and very unstable, and thus did not seem clinically promising. Fleming did nothing, and the scientific community paid little heed.

Ten years later, however, a team of young Oxford scientists, led by the Australian Howard Florey (1898–1968), head of the Dunn School of Pathology, and including the ebullient biochemist Ernst Chain (1906–79), a refugee from Nazi Germany, launched a research project on microbial antagonisms. Combing the scientific literature for antibac-terial substances, Chain found Fleming's report, and the team began to grow *P. notatum*, soon encountering the difficulties involved in isolating the active ingredient from the liquid the mould produced – only one part in two million was pure penicillin. Another biochemist in the team, Norman Heatley (b. 1911), devised improved production techniques. They continued purifying the drug and began testing. On 25 May 1940 they inoculated eight mice with fatal streptococci doses, and four were then given penicillin. By next morning, all had died except the four treated mice.

Florey seized upon the drug's potential; his department went into production, using, in best Heath-Robinson manner, milk churns, lemon-ade bottles, bedpans and a bath tub until they thought they had enough to try it on a patient – a policeman near death from staphylococcal septicaemia following a scratch while pruning his roses. There was, in

* The bacteriologist J. M. C. Gram (1853–1938) devised a method for differentiating different sorts of micro-organisms, using a stain.

fact, so little available that his urine was collected to recycle as much of the drug as possible. By the fourth day, he had improved remarkably, but then the penicillin ran out and he died.

Recognizing that his laboratory could not produce enough, Florey approached British pharmaceutical companies, but they were too busy supplying wartime needs; so in July 1941 he went to the United States, enlisting aid at the Northern Regional Research Laboratory in Peoria, Illinois. There Heatley, working with Andrew J. Moyer (1899–1959), increased the penicillin yield thirty-four-fold (they made it in beer vats), and three American pharmaceutical companies went into production.

By 1943, British drug companies too had begun to mass-produce penicillin and, in May, Florey travelled to North Africa to perform tests on war wounds. The success was extraordinary. By D-Day in June 1944, enough was available to allow unlimited treatment of allied servicemen. In 1945, Fleming, Florey and Chain shared the Nobel Prize – Heatley received nothing. He was made to wait until 1990 for his reward: an honorary MD from Oxford University.

Penicillin proved highly effective against most types of pus-forming cocci, and against the pneumococcus, gonococcus, meningococcus and diphtheria bacillus, the bacilli of anthrax and tetanus and syphilis. Pre-penicillin, the pneumonia fatality rate was around 30 per cent; it dropped to around 6 per cent, and pneumonia, once the old man's friend, ceased to be a major source of death.

Research continued on the antagonism between fungi and moulds and harmful bacteria, but with sporadic success. In 1927 René Dubos (1901–81) had gone to the Rockefeller Institute Hospital in New York to conduct research on antibacterial agents in the soil. In 1939, with Rollin Hotchkiss, he isolated a crystalline antibiotic, tyrothricin, from a culture media of the soil organism *Bacillus brevis*. Tyrothricin proved active against a range of important bacteria but too toxic for the treatment of infection in humans. These observations, however, were suggestive, and they gave a major impetus to the development of more effective antibiotics.

In 1940 Selman Waksman (1888–1973), a Russian who had migrated to the United States and become a distinguished soil microbiologist, isolated an antibiotic called actinomycin. Though impressively lethal to bacteria, it proved so toxic that it was not tried clinically; however, it convinced Waksman that he was on the right trail. In 1944 he discovered another species of this fungus, to which the name *Streptomyces griseus* was later given. From this he isolated the antibiotic streptomycin, which proved active against the tubercle bacillus, and its toxicity was relatively low. Use of streptomycin rapidly led, however, to resistant strains and it was found more effective when used in combination with para-amino-salycylic acid (PAS).

In 1950 testing began on a third anti-tuberculous agent, developed by Squibb and Hoffman-La Roche in the United States. This was isonicotinic acid hydrazide, or isoniazid. Like streptomycin, it was prone to resistance, but the shortcomings of these anti-tuberculosis drugs were minimized after 1953 by combination into a single long-term chemotherapy. Tuberculosis had been steadily declining over the previous century; antibiotics delivered the final blow.

The long anticipated therapeutic revolution had eventually arrived. A flow of new drugs of many kinds followed from the 1950s, including the first effective psychopharmacological substances. Some proved extremely valuable, others marginal, and a few positively dangerous. One of the most successful, or at least adaptable to many purposes, has been cortisone, isolated in the Mayo Clinic in the 1930s and put to use with spectacular success after the war, initially for rheumatoid arthritis and other inflammatory conditions. 'If the word "miraculous" may ever be used in referring to the effects of a remedy,' claimed Lord Horder (1871–1955), 'it could surely be excused here.' Arthritis sufferers, long bedridden, were able to get up and walk. Yet it had strong side-effects: ugly skin disorders, heart disease and stomach ulcers sometimes occurred; patients became obese and highly susceptible to certain infections. Clearly, hormonal treatments could disturb the body's homeostatic balance.

Drugs finally began to appear against viral conditions. For centuries the term 'virus' (from the Latin for 'slime' or 'poisonous juice') had signified a poison produced by living beings and causing infectious disease. But viruses understood as specific entities emerged as great enigmas out of bacteriological experimentation. Isolation of them became much easier from 1884, when Chamberland made a filter with pores small enough to hold back bacteria but large enough to allow viruses to pass through.

In 1886 Adolf Eduard Mayer (1843–1942) discovered that tobacco mosaic disease could be transmitted to healthy plants by inoculating them with extracts of sap from the leaves of diseased plants. Mayer filtered the sap and demonstrated that the filtrate was still infectious. In 1897 Martinus Willem Beijerinck (1851–1931), seeking the micro-organism responsible for tobacco mosaic disease, discovered that the disease was apparently transmitted by a fluid after it had passed through a 'bacteria-tight' filter. Concluding that the toxin was in the form of an infectious fluid, he introduced the term 'filterable virus' to refer to a cell-free filtrate as a cause of disease. Although few bacteriologists gave much credence to his notion of life in a fluid form, the discovery of the filterable virus attracted considerable attention. In 1901 James Carroll (1854–1907) reported that filterable virus caused yellow fever in humans, shifting the study from botany to virology, and freeing biology from the dogma of the cell.

Viral diseases were successively identified, for instance poliomyelitis, first clinically described at the end of the eighteenth century, while Simon Flexner succeeded in producing paralysis in monkeys with virus derived from infected nasal secretion. Vaccines for viral diseases followed, a key figure being the American John Enders (1897–1985). Growing viruses in animal tissues with Thomas H. Weller (b. 1915) and Frederick C. Robbins (b. 1916) at the Children's Hospital in Boston, by March 1948 Enders had grown mumps viruses in chicken-broth cultures, and by 1949 polio virus on human tissue. Enders next turned his attention to a measles vaccine, tested in 1960 and licensed in 1963. By 1974, it was judged to have saved 2400 lives in the US alone.

While vaccines had success, drug treatments against viruses proved difficult to develop, since viruses are intracellular parasites, with an intimate association with the host chemical solution. Only since the 1970s has progress been made, first with acyclovir, potent against herpes zoster (shingles), cold sores, and other herpes infections. In cells infected with the herpes virus, acyclovir is converted to a metabolic blocking agent, thereby largely overcoming the old and plaguing problem of toxicity to the host. Other viruses have been less amenable; influenza viruses continue to be a hazard, since they mutate rapidly.

Up to the 1960s new drugs could be launched without strict safety requirements. As laws became more stringent, requiring lengthy and exacting testing, the pace of innovation slowed. That may in some measure explain why the late twentieth century brought no new drugs whose impact could compare with the sulpha drugs or penicillin. Yet in the wider perspective the twentieth-century transformation appears impressive: effective vaccines were developed against smallpox, measles, mumps, typhoid fever, rubella (German measles), diphtheria, tetanus, yellow fever, pertussis (whooping cough), and poliomyelitis, and success-ful drugs against many bacterial conditions, some viral infections, and numerous metabolic disorders.

'I will lift up mine eyes unto the pills', sang the journalist Malcolm Muggeridge in 1962, doubtless tongue in cheek. 'Almost everyone takes them, from the humble aspirin to the multi-coloured, king-sized three deckers, which put you to sleep, wake you up, stimulate and soothe you all in one. It is an age of pills.' He was right. Whereas before 1900 the physicians' pharmacy was largely a magazine of blank cartridges, many effective drugs have been introduced: antibiotics, antihypertensives, anti-arrhythmics, anti-emetics, anti-depressants and anti-convulsants; steroids against arthritis, bronchodilators, diuretics, healers of stomach and duodenal ulcers, endocrine regulators and replacements, drugs against parkinsonism and cytotoxic drugs against cancers.

Disasters happened too. Introduced as a safe sleeping tablet, Tha-lidomide was withdrawn in 1961 after causing horrendous foetal defects in over 5000 babies. Other tragedies and scandals came to light only later. For instance, beginning in the 1940s, the synthetic oestrogen diethylstilbesterol (DES) was given to women to prevent miscarriage and subsequently to prevent pregnancy. Some early studies showed that it was ineffective and, moreover, caused foetal abnormalities in animals, but these findings were ignored. Even after 1971, when it was discovered that DES caused a rare form of vaginal cancer in 'DES daughters' as well as other reproductive problems, it continued to be prescribed in the United States as a 'morning-after' pill. It was also used as a growth stimulant in livestock and, despite being known as carcinogenic from the 1960s, the influential US agricultural lobby stood behind DES.

In the century from Pasteur to penicillin one of the ancient dreams of medicine came true. Reliable knowledge was finally attained of what caused major sicknesses, on the basis of which both preventions and cures were developed. In the general euphoria created by the microbe hunters and their champions, some of the wider conditions of life con-tained within the evolutionary struggle were easily disregarded, the prospects of killing off diseases being too precious to ignore. In retro-spect, far from the bacteriological and antibiotic paradigms then adopted becoming the basis for the progress of all future medicine, the period between Pasteur and Fleming may one day be nostalgically recalled as an anomalous, if fortunate, exception to medicine's sisyphean strife.

CHAPTER XV

TROPICAL MEDICINE,
WORLD DISEASES

DISEASES OF WARM CLIMATES

IN THE MODERN EPIC OF HEALTH, a hero's part has often been assigned to tropical medicine, the branch of the microbiological revolution bearing fruit in the Third World: intrepid doctors going off to the steaming jungles and overcoming some of the most lethal diseases besetting mankind.

'Tropical diseases', however, do not constitute a single natural class of pathogens; they amount to the medley of maladies that came to be dealt with by 'tropical medicine', a discipline which took shape towards 1900 and comprised a multiplicity of skills, interests and personnel. It fed off striking developments within medicine, above all bacteriology, but the discipline came into being primarily because of the needs of imperial powers competing to enlarge their stakes in Africa, Asia, the Americas and Oceania – for better medical protection for their nationals and control over the peoples and environments they were mastering.

Contemporaries frankly recognized, indeed gloried in, the intimate relationship between colonization and medicine. Without new medical skills, how could the imperial mission have been realized? Tropical medicine, some argued, was the true or even sole justification of empire:

> Take up the White Man's burden
> The savage wars of peace –
> Fill full the mouth of famine
> And bid the sickness cease.

urged Rudyard Kipling. For Cecil Rhodes, empire meant civilization, and tropical medicine was high among its crowning glories. Joseph Chamberlain (1836–1914), who became Britain's colonial secretary in

1895, viewed disease control as integral to imperialism. Hubert Lyautey (1854–1934), one of the architects of the French colonial medical service, declared 'La seule excuse de la colonisation, c'est la médecine.'

The problems of the tropics were nothing new to European nations. Long before germ theory, Spanish and Portuguese, Dutch, French and British officers and sea captains had tried to create sanitary encampments for their troops, developing a rule-of-thumb military hygiene based upon the miasmatic view that diseases came out of the earth. During the nineteenth century the British applied their public health notions to the administration of India: as well as threats from the climate and the physical environment, the Raj was moved by the dangers to health supposedly posed by Indians and their strange ways. Smallpox vaccination was introduced, but there was little success in dealing with cholera. Anti-plague activities involved the medical surveillance of populations at risk, the isolation of sufferers in hospitals, the rapid disposal of corpses and the destruction of personal property, all of which prompted Indian resistance to what were condemned as draconian measures.

The diseases beneath the umbrella of what in time became organized, taught and practised as tropical medicine formed a miscellany. They included long-familiar conditions like malaria. 'Marsh fever' or the 'ague' was still endemic in low-lying, swampy and estuarial parts of Europe as well as the wider world. From early modern times, fen drainage and capitalist agriculture brought a retreat of the disease from northwest Europe, but it remained severe around the Mediterranean littoral. Colonists encountered it in many parts of Africa and Asia, notably India; 'fever' was also something settlers spread, wherever destruction of forests by slash-and-burn clearance techniques, irrigation schemes and other environmental disturbances produced the myriad pools and sheets of standing water which formed mosquitoes' breeding grounds.

Diseases deemed 'tropical' also included conditions like bubonic plague, which had decimated Europe before retreating, but still occasionally flared out beyond Africa and Asia. Plague disappeared from Europe (final devastation: Marseilles, 1720) and declined in the Ottoman empire (the last great Egyptian outbreaks occurred around 1850), but still remained devastating in south-east Asia. The 'third plague wave' originated in China between 1856 and 1866 and took its severest toll in east Asia and north Africa. Late in the century it spread northwards to Hong Kong and Manchuria, and west to Bombay, killing a million Indians in 1903, while also invading Java, Asia Minor, South

Africa and even the Pacific shores of the Americas. San Francisco was struck, and plague became permanently established among wild rodent populations in California, to this day producing occasional human fatalities.

Many parts of Asia were plagued throughout the twentieth century. There were grave pneumonic plague outbreaks in 1910–11 and 1920–21 in northern Manchuria, and India remained a victim, suffering over twelve million deaths in the first half of the twentieth century. As recently as 1994 a serious outbreak of what was possibly pneumonic plague occurred around Delhi.

Overseas trade and colonial expansion exposed Europeans to deadly diseases unknown or little known in Europe. Amongst these, one that struck repeatedly and ruthlessly was yellow fever, an explosive disorder, causing haemorrhaging and intense jaundice, followed by coma and often death, first experienced along the west coast of Africa, and then carried by European traders and conquerors to the New World, together with their slave cargoes. By 1700, it was infecting ports in the Caribbean and Latin America; it spread along the Atlantic coasts of the New World as far north as Boston, later also becoming a regular visitor to Colombia, Peru and Ecuador. Between 1800 and 1850 it devastated the port cities of the southern USA, visiting Savannah with fifteen epidemics, Charleston with twenty-two and New Orleans, the necropolis of the America south, with at least thirty-three. As late as the 1870s it was still rippling up the Mississippi from New Orleans to Memphis.

Early control measures relied on quarantines. Infected ships were isolated, flying a flag called the yellow jack, which became a term for the disease itself. Quarantining assumed that the fever was contagious, but a growing body of miasmatist medical opinion, encouraged by commercial lobbies fretting at the trade standstills quarantines brought, claimed the true source of the infection was filth; heat acting on rotting animal and vegetable matter caused putrid exhalations.

Unlike cholera, yellow jack never seriously threatened Europe, though once in a while it found its way to ports like Bordeaux, Nantes or even Swansea, bringing deaths and panic. But in the colonies it caused extensive fatalities among settlers; in that respect it differed from other conditions exposed by colonization which were viewed primarily as 'native diseases'. Disorders like sleeping sickness rarely afflicted whites but impeded colonization, as well as being affronts to medicine and civilization.

In many villages and clearings where the white man took his wares and weapons, he encountered ghastly unknown conditions: *kala-azar*, with its leprosy-like symptoms, in India and Africa, 'big belly' (bilharzia) in the Nile Valley, sleeping sickness on the savannas. Though this was little recognized at the time, such diseases were not features waiting to be discovered, like the source of the Nile; they had often been aggravated or even created by imperialism. Bringing war, the flight of peoples, clearings, settlements, encampments, roads and railways and other ecological disruptions, and the reduction of native populations to wage-labour or to marginal lands, colonization spread disease. 'When the Europeans came,' reflected the medical missionary Albert Schweitzer (1875–1965),

> the natives who served them as boats' crews, or as carriers in their caravans, moved with them from one district to another, and if any of them had the sleeping sickness they took it to fresh places. In the early days it was unknown on the Ogowe, and it was introduced about thirty years ago by carriers from Loango.

Colonial powers, however, would see disease in one light only: an evil, an enemy, a challenge, it had to be conquered in the name of progress. 'Malarial fever . . . haunts more especially the fertile, well-watered and luxuriant tracts,' explained Ronald Ross:

> There it strikes down not only the indigenous barbaric population but, with still greater certainty, the pioneers of civilization – the planter, the trader, the missionary and the soldier. It is therefore the principal and gigantic ally of Barbarism. . . . It has withheld an entire continent from humanity – the immense and fertile tracts of Africa.

Fortunately it was possible to point to progress being made, partly thanks to quinine: its success, particularly as used by Dr William Baikie (1825–64) on the 1854 Niger expedition, has been viewed as the prime reason why Africa ceased to be the white man's grave. In 1874 for instance 2500 quinine-dosed British troops were marched from the Atlantic to the far reaches of the Asante empire in west Africa without serious loss of life; armed with quinine, the French began settling in Algeria in large numbers.

The efficacy of quinine and the later war on mosquitoes gave colonists fresh opportunities to swarm into the Gold Coast, Nigeria and other parts of west Africa and seize fertile agricultural lands, introduce new livestock and crops, build roads and railways, drive natives into mines, and introduce all the disruptions to traditional lifestyles that cash economies brought. The ecological transformation and social proletarianization created by Ross's 'pioneers of civilization' triggered massive epidemics, in particular sleeping sickness, while the planting of coffee, cocoa, rubber and other cash-crop monocultures led to decline in the nutritional status and general well-being of natives in Africa, Asia, America and the Pacific.

Moreover, as with the earlier *conquistadores*, colonists imported new diseases to which natives had no resistance. Tuberculosis proved especially severe, being introduced by whites and then spread by African labourers to sub-Saharan Africa. Before the advent of Europeans, the inhabitants of Pacific islands had suffered from their own diseases, from *Filariasis* and tropical skin afflictions, but these horticulturalists, isolated for thousands of years, were easy game for foreign infections. The Hawaiian islands had remained 'undiscovered' until Captain Cook's landing in 1778; his crew introduced syphilis. Within a century, venereal diseases, together with smallpox and other epidemics, reportedly reduced the indigenous population by 90 per cent. When measles first struck Fiji and Samoa in the 1870s, it slaughtered 20–30 per cent of the natives.

A similar headlong decline set in among aborigines after English settlement of Australia began in 1788. Smallpox erupted almost immediately and destroyed half those who had contact with Port Arthur (Sydney). 'Wherever the European has trod, death seems to pursue the aboriginal,' mused the sensitive young Charles Darwin (1809–82) in his *Beagle* journal. Shortly afterwards the Tasmanian aborigines became totally extinct.

Initially at least, colonial medicine was aimed at preserving colonists. In due course, medical missionaries were also sent out, supplementing their religious brethren, to save the bodies as well as the souls of the natives. They were the acceptable face of colonialism. 'The foreign doctor is *persona grata*,' one missionary noted in 1899. However dedicated, they proved a mixed blessing. Their medical work was sometimes subordinated to evangelizing while, set up in the name of health, leper colonies broke up families, forcibly removed sufferers and imposed alien western values and living patterns; and, as has happened more recently with AIDS, hospitals and mission posts inadvertently served as centres for disease *communication* no less than *control*. In any case, what magic bullets did nineteenth-century western medicine have for sleeping sickness or bilharzia?

TROPICAL MEDICINE

The hazards facing white men abroad – trading, fighting, preaching, planting – had long attracted medical attention. The fevers endemic to warm climates were rationalized by humoral theory. Sailors and settlers were advised to avoid 'hot' food and strong liquor and to drink 'cooling' fluids. Europeans arriving in the Caribbean or East Indies were known to be at high risk from local diseases, and experience counselled a gradual acclimatization process. Being costly commodities, slaves too were 'seasoned'.

Supplanting this traditional 'medicine of warm climates', a distinctive tropical medicine arose in the last third of the nineteenth century. The timing was no accident, for it was then that imperial rivalries climaxed, as Britain, France and other European nations scrambled for Africa and other bits of the globe that were still there for the taking. Millions of Europeans were crossing the oceans to aid in the work of conquest, conversion, and civilization – more Britons migrated to the empire in the decade before the First World War than were killed in the war itself. Among them were doctors.

The great epidemiological breakthrough came with Patrick Manson's recognition that the diseases of warm climates could involve parasites and vectors. A bank manager's son from Aberdeen, where he studied medicine, Manson (1844–1922) moved to the Far East in 1866, spending a dozen years in the Chinese Imperial Maritime Customs Service in Formosa (Taiwan) and Amoy (now Hsaimen). There he encountered *elephantiasis*, the chronic disfiguring disease which, through lymph-flow blockage, produces grotesque swelling of the limbs and genitalia. He determined it was caused by a nematode worm, *Filaria*, and in 1877 traced the role played by bites from the gnat *Culex fatigans* in spreading filarial parasites to the human bloodstream: the first time an insect had been shown to be part of the natural history cycle of a disease. The membranes in the gnat stomachs broke down, releasing the worms that tunnelled into the thoracic muscles, where they metamorphosed in preparation for their entry into humans. This discovery that insects acted as hosts to a disease attracted little immediate notice, but was to have profound consequences once it became accepted that mosquitoes and other insects were the vectors of other deadly conditions.

Six years after helping to found a medical school in Hong Kong, Manson returned to London in 1889, successfully specializing in diseases contracted overseas and becoming physician to the Seaman's Hospital on the Thames, which was to serve as the clinical facility to the School of Tropical Medicine which he established in 1899. An avid natural historian of disease, Manson stamped his model of tropical medicine on the specialism he shaped, partly through his *Tropical Diseases: A Manual of the Diseases of Warm Climates* (1898), a textbook which popularized the new parasitology.

Building on bacteriology, the new tropical medicine then proceeded to lay bare, alongside the by then well-known bacilli, the pathogenic role of other classes of micro-organisms: in dysentery, an amoeba; in *Schistosomiasis*, a class of worms, the trematodes; in sleeping sickness, a *Trypanosome*, a protozoan, and in malaria, another protozoan, the *Plasmodium*. The infection chains were typically more complicated than with the familiar European water or air-borne diseases.

MALARIA

The world's most serious endemic disease was malaria, with its hot and cold fever, commonly leading to death. Perception of its gravity was sharpened when the French entrepreneur Ferdinand de Lesseps' bid to add the Panama Canal to the Suez came to grief because of the fever – in the 1880s over 5000 workmen died on the project. The first breakthrough came in 1880, when Alphonse Laveran (1845–1922), a French army surgeon working in Algeria, observed the malaria plasmodium in its first stage of sexual reproduction. This squared with Manson's finding that *Filariasis* grew in mosquito stomachs, but how was it transmitted?

Anticipating the mosquito to be both the malaria host and vector, Manson shared his thoughts in 1894 with a young Indian-born British army surgeon, Ronald Ross (1857–1932), who, though preferring poetry to medicine, had studied at St Bartholomew's Hospital and entered the Indian Medical Service, becoming involved from 1892 in the malaria problem. Inspired by Manson's hunch that it was transmitted through mosquitoes, Ross returned to India, determined to prove the hypothesis.

His brief was clear: he would find patients suffering from malaria, allow mosquitoes to feed on their blood, kill the insects and dissect them to see what became of Laveran's organism. 'The Frenchies and Italians will pooh-pooh it, then adopt it, and then claim it as their own,' Manson warned his disciple.

Many problems became clarified in due course: the complex interaction between the *Plasmodium*'s life cycle and the disease; the existence of several forms of the organism capable of causing the different types of malaria (tertian, quartan, etc.); and the recognition that not all mosquito species acted as vectors.

Confirming Laveran's work, Ross discovered the *Plasmodium* in the stomachs of *Anopheles* mosquitos which had bitten malaria sufferers. The great breakthrough was made in his laboratory in Secunderabad on 'Mosquito Day', 20 August 1897:

At about 1 p.m. I determined to sacrifice the seventh *Anopheles*. . . of the batch fed on the 16th, Mosquito 38, although my eyesight was already fatigued. Only one more of the batch remained.

The dissection was excellent, and I went carefully through the tissues, now so familiar to me, searching every micron with the same passion and care as one would search some vast ruined palace for a little hidden treasure. Nothing. No, these new mosquitoes also were going to be a failure: there was something wrong with the theory. But the stomach tissues still remained to be examined – lying there, empty and flaccid, before me on the glass slide, a great white expanse of cells like a great courtyard of flagstones, each of which must be scrutinized – half an hour's labour at least. I was tired, and what was the use? I must have examined the stomachs of a thousand mosquitoes by this time. But the Angel of Fate fortunately laid his hand on my head; and I had scarcely commenced the search again when I saw a clear and almost perfectly circular outline before me of about 12 microns in diameter. The outline was much too sharp, the cell too small to be an ordinary stomach-cell of a mosquito. I looked a little further. Here was another, and another exactly similar cell.

The afternoon was very hot and overcast; and I remember opening the diaphragm of the sub-stage condenser of the microscope to admit more light and then changing the focus. *In each of these cells there was a cluster of small granules, black as jet* and exactly like the black pigment granules of the *Plasmodium* crescents. As with that pigment, the granules numbered about twelve to sixteen in each cell and became blacker and more visible when more light was admitted through the diaphragm. I laughed, and shouted for the Hospital Assistant – he was away having his siesta. 'No, no', I said; 'Dame Nature, you are a sorceress, but you don't trick me so easily. The malarial pigment cannot get into the walls of the mosquito's stomach; the flagella have no pigment; you are playing another trick upon me!' I counted twelve of the cells, all of the same size and appearance and all containing exactly the same granules. Then I made rough drawings of nine of the cells on page 107 of my notebook, scribbled my notes, sealed my specimen, went home to tea (about 3 p.m.), and slept solidly for an hour. . . . When I awoke with mind refreshed my first thought was: Eureka! the problem is solved!

Ross had found in the stomach wall of an *Anopheles* mosquito the oocysts (eggs) which are the intermediate stage of the *Plasmodium* life cycle. Assured of the parasite's presence, he was then able to outline its history within the mosquito: first, as a zygote in the stomach; then as an oocyst in the stomach wall; and finally as a mature sporozoite that reaches first the proboscis and then a human host when the insect bites and squirts its saliva prior to sucking blood. Ross thus demonstrated the mosquito's role in malaria transmission, working out, through experiments with birds, the detailed relationship between the *Plasmodium* life cycle and the disease. Still the poet, he celebrated his triumph in doggerel:

> I know this little thing
> A myriad men will save
> O Death, where is thy sting?
> Thy Victory, O Grave?

Meanwhile, working with his fellow Italian, Amico Bignami (1862–1929), Giovanni Grassi (1854–1925) had independently linked human malaria to the *Anopheles* mosquito and showed how the insect becomes infected through feeding off the blood of a person with the *Plasmodium* parasite in the bloodstream. Deeply fascinated by parasites, in 1891 Grassi discovered the malaria parasite of birds, *Protosoma praecox*, which looked very similar to *Plasmodium vivax*, and inoculated malaria parasites from one bird to another. Broadening his study, he became convinced that whenever malaria occurred, mosquitoes were present, but not all mosquito-infected areas were malarial. Hence particular species had to be responsible. In August 1898 he discovered that the female of *Anopheles* was the carrier of malaria; in an experiment, a healthy volunteer was bitten by *Anopheles*, developing a malarial fever, and in the next year he proved that *Anopheles* became infected on biting a diseased person.

When Ross claimed priority over Grassi, a sharp and chauvinistic controversy followed (the Englishman denounced the 'Italian pirates'). In 1902 Ross was awarded the Nobel Prize, leaving the Italians outraged and Grassi embittered. Certainly Ross reached the conclusion before Grassi that mosquitoes transmitted malaria, but Grassi first identified *Anopheles* as the agent of transmission and elucidated the complete sequence of steps in the life cycle of the parasite. The Nobel Committee made amends to Laveran in 1907 by awarding him the prize for the discovery of the *Plasmodium* parasite, but Grassi, who by 1898 had worked out the entire *Plasmodium* life cycle, was left empty-handed.

This parasitological model opened up an astonishing new vision of disease aetiology. While it yielded no cures, it afforded a prospect of malaria control, through eradicating mosquitoes. Measures attempted included using copper sulphate, spreading kerosene on ponds to prevent hatching, screening windows and sleeping under nets. Control programmes were launched. With the support of the Rockefeller Foundation, the US Public Health Service began an anti-malaria assault in the south, starting in Arkansas. The results were amazing: malaria incidence dropped 50 per cent in three years at a cost of under a dollar per capita, Paris green dust (copper arsenic) proving a cheap and effective method for killing mosquito larvae. By 1927 the disease had essentially been eliminated from American towns.

At the end of the Great War, Italy still had some two million cases a year. An American-style anti-mosquito campaign was established, and between 1924 and 1929 a marked reduction in infections was achieved in a test area. During the 1930s operations were extended; within ten years the worst malarial regions in Italy were under control and, in the previously uninhabitable Pontine marshes, 200,000 acres of new farmland had been brought under cultivation.

Success encouraged similar ventures in Africa, Asia, and Brazil. The introduction of DDT (dichloro-diphenyl-trichloroethane) made control procedures more effective. Synthesized in 1874 from chlorine, alcohol and sulphuric acid, DDT's insecticidal powers were discovered in the mid 1930s. The fact that it remained active for weeks obviated repeated respraying. By 1945, though malaria was still annually infecting 300 million people globally, eradication was being touted as a practical possibility; in 1957 the World Health Organization judged its conquest an attainable goal, and the US Congress voted large sums for a worldwide campaign to eradicate malaria through spraying with insecticide and immunizing with chloroquine. The plan was to wipe malaria out by 1963.

Hopes were dashed, however. Mosquitoes quickly became DDT-resistant, and the insecticide was found to enter the food chain, creating grave health and environmental dangers, including bizarre genetic mutants. The *Plasmodium* also became resistant to drugs, including quinine and chloroquine. The tide turned adversely; in 1963 Congress cut off funds, and that encouraged the disease to return with renewed strength. Sri Lanka had one million cases in 1955, hardly any in 1964, but half a million again by 1969. Malaria in India climbed from its 1961 low point of under 100,000 cases to 350,000 in 1969, and 2.5 million by 1974. By 1977, incidence in India was thought to have soared above six million cases. In Brazil malaria cases have similarly shot up, partly as a result of deforestation, logging and open-cast mining. In sub-Saharan Africa, malaria is now annually responsible for the death of nearly a million children. Globally, as wonderdrugs produced superbugs, there were three times as many cases of malaria in the 1990s as there had been in 1961.

YELLOW FEVER

Early investigations of malaria shed light on the yellow fever problem. In 1807 John Crawford of Baltimore (1746–1813) had suggested links between mosquitoes and yellow fever; Josiah Nott (1804–73) of Mobile, Alabama, and Louis Beauperthuy (1807–71), a native of Guadeloupe, suggested around 1850 that the mosquito was a possible vector, though without firm evidence. In 1881 Carlos Finlay (1833–1915), a Havana physician of Anglo-French descent, repeated the suggestion.

Finlay's attention was drawn to the possibility of mosquito transmission by noticing that in the haemorrhages of yellow fever red blood globules were discharged unbroken. He hypothesized that this was akin to smallpox and vaccination in general, the implication being that if one wanted to transfer yellow fever from a sufferer to a healthy person, the inoculable material had to be extracted from within the former's blood vessels and introduced into those of the latter. That was something that could certainly be achieved by mosquitoes. Finlay then conjectured a chain of events: a yellow fever patient whose capillaries the mosquito could bite; survival of the mosquito until it could bite another person;

those bitten by the same mosquito contracting the disease. In 1881 he singled out the *Aedes aegypti* mosquito as the agent – an early ascription of disease transmission to insects.

In the mid 1880s Finlay studied the natural history of the mosquito. The stinging mosquitoes were fecundated females, he concluded, which would lay eggs within a few days on suitable water. Finding that the blood of the sick person, when transferred to the mosquito, underwent some modifications, he speculated that the microbes multiplied in the mosquito's mouth, though he had not yet arrived at his later views suspecting the salivary glands. Between 1881 and 1898 he conducted over a hundred experiments, inoculating with yellow fever, but these did not convince his colleagues. Meanwhile in 1897 Guiseppi Sanarelli, an Italian bacteriologist working in Uruguay, announced he had identified a bacillus (*Bacillus icteroides*) in yellow fever patients which might be the causal agent.

Following appalling disease mortality in the 1898 Spanish–American War and a yellow fever outbreak among American troops based in Cuba, a US Army Yellow Fever Commission was appointed in 1900, headed by Walter Reed (1851–1902) from Johns Hopkins University and James Carroll (1854–1907) of the US Army Medical Corps. Their reasoning pointed to a vector. Ross's recent identification of the mosquito's role in malaria and the cumulative evidence for insect involvement in other diseases, including sleeping sickness, led the commission to conduct a trial of Finlay's hypothesis.

Because no animals were then known to suffer from yellow fever, the researchers became their own experimental subjects. Using *Aedes aegypti* mosquitoes raised by Finlay, three researchers attempted the experiment. Jesse Lazear (1866–1900) allowed some mosquitoes to bite yellow fever patients and then his own arm. Nothing happened. Carroll repeated the exercise and within four days fell severely sick, but, because he could have picked up the disease elsewhere in Havana, this proved nothing. Then a soldier who had had no contact with yellow fever volunteered to be bitten by the same mosquito. He went down with a mild attack: the first clear proof that mosquitoes spread the disease. (Lazear was meanwhile bitten accidentally while working in a yellow fever ward, developed fever and died.)

The researchers set up a properly controlled experiment. Soldier volunteers were divided into two groups. The first lived among the clothing and bedding of yellow fever victims to see if it contained anything contagious; the second were put in isolation and then bitten by mosquitoes infected by yellow fever patients. Not one of the former sample contracted yellow fever; 80 per cent of those bitten by the infected mosquitoes fell sick (all survived).

Once the mechanism was understood – yellow fever must follow the bite of an infected mosquito – the commission was in a position to conclude that it was caused by an unknown microscopic agent, indeed one which passed through a filter that would retain the smallest known bacteria – the first time a filterable virus was implicated as the cause of a human disease.

The findings of the Reed Commission led to a programme in Cuba, launched in 1901 by William C. Gorgas (1845–1920), an American military doctor from Mobile, Alabama, to control yellow fever by destroying mosquitoes. Every barrel in Havana where water might collect was targeted. Kerosene was spread on ponds; wells and tanks were screened, and yellow fever patients isolated. The infective chain was disrupted; within three months the disease had vanished from Havana.

Success spurred the American authorities to tackle yellow fever and malaria mosquitoes in Panama. A few years earlier the French had abandoned construction of the Panama Canal primarily because of fever: in October 1884 alone, no fewer than 654 workers had died of yellow fever. In 1904 the Americans took over the operation, with Gorgas in charge of the medical department. Despite scepticism from the Canal Zone's governor, General G. W. Davis ('spending a dollar on sanitation', he snapped, 'is as good as throwing it into the Bay'), Gorgas was given the go-ahead for a sanitation plan. Pumped water was installed and all domestic storage receptacles withdrawn; mosquito traps were set; undergrowth scorched and insects hunted down. This too proved a success; by September 1906 the last yellow fever victim had died in the Canal Zone; it became a quarter where Europeans could work! When the canal was finally opened in 1913, the zone was said to be twice as healthy as the United States, a dramatic vindication of the new power of medical science to aid civilization. Subsequent programmes were carried out in Guatemala, Peru, Honduras, El Salvador, Nicaragua, Mexico and Brazil – though in some parts, notably Brazil, mosquitoes recovered much of the ground formerly ceded, and the yellow fever threat returned.

Meanwhile, findings in Africa forced a rethink. In 1925, the Rockefeller Foundation West African Yellow Fever Commission discovered a new jungle variety of yellow fever, established that monkeys as well as people were susceptible, and decided that the virus could shuttle between men and monkeys. There being no feasible way to eradicate arboreal mosquitoes, immunization became the only possible protection in the jungles. Fortunately by 1937 an effective vaccine had become available, and vaccination programmes were launched; but yellow fever remains a severe problem wherever breeding grounds for the *Aedes* mosquito are provided by road ruts, old tyres, and anything else that serves as a water trap.

SLEEPING SICKNESS

Many other diseases were to be elucidated through the parasitological model, leading to prospects of control if not cure. Amongst these was dengue, a haemorrhagic fever, prevalent in the Caribbean and the hot zones of the East. Classic dengue involves a fever that comes on rapidly after an initial mosquito bite, striking children in particular. The temperature rises to 104°F, a severe headache develops, with prostration and excruciating joint pains ('breakbone fever' was its popular name). Though an insect vector was suspected, the epidemiology long remained a mystery.

In Beirut in 1905, under the direction of T. L. Bancroft (1860–1933), volunteers were infected using the *Aedes* mosquito; researchers injected filtered blood from a patient into a healthy volunteer and brought on an attack: the transmission agent was clearly the mosquito. In the 1940s Albert Sabin (1906–1993) managed to cultivate the virus in the laboratory, and it is now known that there are four distinct types of virus which cause dengue and at least three other arbo viruses producing dengue-like diseases. The last major New World epidemic occurred in Trinidad in 1954, but it has returned sporadically in Latin America, for instance in Costa Rica in 1993 and Puerto Rico in 1994, when it also struck US soldiers in Haiti. A severe outbreak hit New Delhi in 1982; and dengue remains endemic in Africa, China, south-east Asia and Australia.

Another condition cracked was Chagas' Disease, named after Carlos Chagas (1879–1934), scion of a wealthy Brazilian coffee-planting family. In early work on malaria and yellow fever, Chagas noticed that some insects were hosts to a trypanosome, naming it *Schizotrypanum cruzi* (later *Trypanosoma cruzi*), and concluding that it affected monkeys, cats and dogs. He then detected it in human blood, and linked it to a local disease whose acute symptoms were fever and generalized oedema. He discovered that its animal reservoir was the armadillo, an animal common in those regions. It has been suggested that Charles Darwin's lifelong ailments might have been the long-term consequences of Chagas' disease, contracted while in South America during the voyage of the *Beagle*.

Among the gravest diseases facing colonial medicine was sleeping sickness, found widely in sub-Saharan Africa, to which both animals and humans are susceptible. There are now known to be two main types, producing distinctive conditions. The chronic form – the Gambian or west African version, *Trypanosomoa brucie gambiense* – develops very slowly; the acute form caused by *Trypanosoma brucei rhodiense*, has a short incubation period of 5–7 days and is found in eastern and southern Africa. Once bitten by an infected fly, swelling begins, with discolouration and a rash; headache, irritability and insomnia develop, and general lymph-node swelling. The parasites multiply in blood, lymph, tissue fluids and eventually the cerebrospinal fluid. Consequences include male impotence, spontaneous abortion in females, tachycardia and hypotension. Once the disease enters the central nervous system, deterioration leads to death.

Symptoms of what was known as 'African lethargy' or 'Negro lethargy' were known to Arabs and Europeans in Africa from the fourteenth century. John Atkins (1685–1757), an English naval surgeon who had visited the Guinea coast, discussed the 'sleeping distemper' in *The Naval Surgeon* (1734), noting it was prevalent among natives in western Africa and extremely dangerous. Sufferers who did not die, he reported, have an irresistible tendency to sleep, 'lose the little reason they have and turn idiots'. A century later Robert Clarke described 'narcotic dropsy' in Sierra Leone, commenting that it appeared more prevalent in the interior. In 1876, a French naval surgeon found sleeping sickness common in Senegal, with whole villages being abandoned.

This was a clear sign that the disease was spreading, mainly due to the disruptions caused by colonization. Henry Stanley, the explorer who found Dr Livingstone, became economic development director for Belgium's King Leopold II, and his success in opening up the Congo to commerce flushed the disease into the central areas. Missionaries reported emptied villages, while conveying the sick to mission stations inadvertently triggered infection of previously uninfected zones. Fatalities soared; between 1896 and 1906 devastating epidemics killed over a quarter of a million Africans around the shores of Lake Victoria, and double that number died in the Congo. The horrors of sleeping sickness seized the public imagination.

In 1894 Major David Bruce was sent to Zululand to investigate the cattle disease, nagana. He found the sinuous long-tailed *Trypanosoma* protozoan in cattle blood and deemed the tsetse fly, two centimetres long, brownish and blood-sucking, responsible for its transmission (its bite, Livingstone had noted, 'is certain death to the ox, horse, and dog').*

While Bruce was uncovering the transmission of what came to be known as animal trypanosomiasis, its human form continued to spread. In 1901 a severe epidemic in Uganda claimed more than 20,000 victims. In response, Sir Patrick Manson's First Sleeping Sickness Commission, which included young Count Aldo Castellani (1875–1971), was sent out from the London School of Tropical Medicine. It sought the cause of sleeping sickness by studying the action of *Filaria pustans*, thought to play a role in elephantiasis. This got nowhere, but Castellani stayed on to pursue his researches.

In the meantime, Robert Mitchell Forde (1861–1948), a hospital surgeon in Bathurst, Gambia, and Joseph Dutton (1876–1905), from the Liverpool School of Tropical Medicine, isolated a trypanosome from the blood of an English shipmaster suffering from 'Gambia fever'. Dutton named it *T. gambiense*. Trypanosomes were also found in a fever patient, leading to speculation that the tsetse fly was responsible.

Working at Entebbe in Uganda, Castellani identified a streptococcus in sleeping sickness victims which he thought was the causal agent. He also found trypanosomes in the cerebrospinal fluid of dying patients. Piecing together the jigsaw, it was becoming recognized that sleeping sickness took two forms, depending on the body part in which the

---

* A sometime Glasgow millhand, David Livingstone (1813–73) decided to become a medical missionary, qualified in 1840 and offered his services to the London Missionary Society. His exploration of the Zambesi, discovery of the Victoria Falls, efforts to find the source of the Nile, disappearance in the heart of Africa, and meeting with Stanley formed one of the great Victorian adventure stories. His *Missionary Travels and Researches in South Africa* (1857), included an account of the tsetse fly, and of the horse and cattle diseases resulting from its bite, although the trypanosome carried by the fly was as yet undiscovered. He administered arsenic to horses as a nagana remedy.

infection was active. When the parasite circulated freely in the blood, a chronic, episodic fever ('Gambia fever') resulted; but when it established itself in brain tissue, lethargy and loss of function – sleeping sickness proper – developed. On Bruce's arrival in 1903 to head the Second Sleeping Sickness Commission, Castellani reported these conclusions, and, building on his nagana work, Bruce targeted the trypanosome. Together they found trypanosomes in the spinal fluid of sleeping sickness cases. Another Anglo-Italian priority controversy resulted; Bruce credited Castellani for finding the trypanosomes, but claimed he had recognized that they were the causal agent in the disease.

The aetiology of sleeping sickness had been unravelled, but how was it to be prevented or treated? Paul Ehrlich and other chemists were experimenting with arsenical compounds such as atoxyl which were moderately effective if applied at the earliest stages. In Africa Dr Schweitzer and Dr Eugene Jamot (1879–1937) both relied on chemotherapy, the former operating from his hospital centre at Lambaréné in Gabon, the latter going in search of his cases. Preventive strategies were to include forcible removal of natives from areas like the shores of Lake Victoria, where the disease was endemic. It was, however, a disease destined to suffer from neglect; most of the victims were poor Africans, so there was little incentive for pharmaceutical companies to devote research dollars to its eradication.

Through these and other studies, tropical medicine established a role for itself and put down roots. Within a few years of the foundation of the London School in 1899 by Manson and of its Liverpool cousin, under Ross, funded by merchants persuaded that better control of disease would facilitate imperial commerce, similar institutions were established in France, Germany, Italy, Belgium and the United States. In its first half century, tropical medicine scored many successes: 'I now firmly believe', Manson declared, 'in the possibility of tropical colonization by the white races.' In the process, medicine's tasks in the tropics were to change. Though the protection of European soldiers, administrators and settlers remained the top priority, it came to be understood that the health of whites could not be wholly separated from that of natives. Founded in 1714, the Indian Medical Service broadened its concerns, and in Africa a Colonial Medical Service for the British colonies was started in 1927. Natives were mainly catered for, however, not by governments but by missions. In Africa, medical missionary work had begun in 1799 with John Vanderkemp (1748–1811), a Dutch physician sponsored by the London Missionary Society. Different denominations – Anglican, Baptist, Methodist, etc. – carved up particular territories, though there was often competition between Protestant and Catholic missions.

Such missions were not merely set up among 'savages'. From the seventeenth century, western medicine had been introduced into China and Japan by Jesuit missionaries. The Japanese doctor Narabayashi Chinzan (1643–1711) produced a book called *Koi geka soden* [Surgery Handed Down] in 1706, which drew upon the writings of Ambroise Paré he had obtained from the Dutch physician, Willem Hoffman, operating at Deshima from 1671 to 1675. Missionary work by physicians started at Canton around 1840. Evangelical physicians subsequently took western medical education to imperial China, in due course introducing bacteriology and pathology. Western medical schools were founded, leading to the Peking Union Medical College, set up in 1917 with Rockefeller Foundation support, the idea being that 'secular philanthropy' would expose China to western science. By 1937 the Peking Union Medical College had graduated 166 practitioners, skilled in western theories and therapies. After 1949 under the communist government, western religious missions were discontinued, but the PUMC was kept going as a high-level medical school.

As this suggests, in the twentieth century religious missions were supplemented by intervention from philanthropic bodies, notably the Rockefeller Foundation. Set up in 1913, the Rockefeller International Health Division promoted health activities in Latin America and Asia involving basic research, training personnel and model health programmes. A notable example of Rockefeller 'missionary activity' (on its own patch) was the campaign to eradicate hookworm from the American south. This 'disease of laziness' affected many poor southerners, black and white, producing chronic anaemia, fatigue and lethargy. Essentially a disease of poverty spread through poor sanitation and going barefoot over infested ground, it was both treatable and preventable. The Rockefeller Sanitary Commission, headed by Wickliffe Rose (1862–1931), was charged with investigating the prevalence of hookworm and educating the public about prevention. Rose's sanitary inspectors treated some 700,000 individuals, held more than 25,000 public meetings, and distributed more than two million booklets between 1910 and 1915, when the campaign ended and the commission was absorbed into Rockefeller's International Health Board (IHB).

The IHB extended the hookworm campaign into tropical areas, added malaria and yellow fever eradication to its agenda, and invested money in schools and institutes of public health and tropical medicine in many countries in Europe, Asia and Latin America. Success was mixed. A hookworm campaign in China in the early 1920s foundered on the age-old practice of fertilizing mulberry trees with human faeces, often infested with hookworm eggs.

The inter-war years brought the gradual rapprochement of tropical medicine with epidemiology at large, as researchers viewed their subject in terms of a wider medical ecology. The influential policy-maker, Simon Flexner (1863–1946), at the Rockefeller Institute for Medical Research, and Wade Hampton Frost (1880–1938), at the Johns Hopkins School of Hygiene and Public Health, moved from narrow pursuit of infectious agents to broader views of disease and its environments.

Tropical medicine was fraught with ambiguities. Based in the metropolitan centres of colonial or neocolonial powers rather than in the infected countries themselves, the specialty inevitably reflected white priorities and attitudes. Funds were channelled into high-profile laboratory research, though critics claimed problems could better be managed by investing in things of little interest to scientists – drinking water, sanitation, food. Not least, tropical medicine was vulnerable to characterization as the tool of colonial powers or post-colonial multinationals, mopping up the mess created by the 'development' (or perhaps 'undevelopment') which imperialism and capitalism produced.

Medicine also seemingly set itself at the service of empire by providing justifications for racial dominance. Colonial doctors often portrayed 'savages' as ignorant, filthy, childlike and stupid, sometimes out of real contempt, sometimes prompted by 'rescue' motives, or to raise money in the mother country for hospitals and education.

MEDICAL ANTHROPOLOGY

Medicine played its part in the construction of racist anatomy and physical anthropology. Studies of skulls and skeletons allegedly proved white superiority, while with the triumph of Darwinism from the 1860s natives could be stigmatized as evolutionarily 'primitive' and destined to be defeated in the struggle for existence.

Such issues provoked controversy, and medical authors figured on both sides. In Britain, James Cowles Prichard (1786–1848), brought up a Quaker, and the Quaker Thomas Hodgkin (1798–1866), seeing 'God in everyone', were committed to the biblical doctrine of monogenesis and the unity of the human race. Prichard's *Researches into the Physical History of Mankind*, first published in 1813 and going through many later editions, held that all humans shared a single physical origin and mentality, dwelling on similarities between different peoples in terms of physical type, language, customs, political organization and religion. This view of the 'psychic unity of man' was countered by the Scottish anatomist, Robert Knox (1791–1862), whose *The Races of Man* (1850) developed polygenism. Race, Knox believed, explained all, and in the 1862 edition he held that only certain races fell within the human species. The debate between mono- and poly-genists expressed conflicting attitudes to colonial expansion. Hodgkin's Aborigines Protection Society (1835) aimed to collect 'authentic information concerning the character, habits and wants of uncivilized tribes' so as to ameliorate colonial practice. The argument became reflected in competing learned societies, the Ethnological Society of London being liberal and the Anthropological Society of London (1872) racist.

The science of anthropology was largely promoted by medically trained travellers. One of the first major British field trips, the Torres Straits expedition, was organized by Alfred Haddon (1855–1940), a protégé of Michael Foster's Cambridge school of physiology. The expedition included two scientists trained in neurophysiology and experimental psychology, C. S. Myers (1873–1946) and W. H. R. Rivers (1864–1922). Rivers' *Medicine, Magic and Religion* (1924) viewed indigenous medical systems as social institutions to be studied in the same way as kinship, politics or other institutions, seeing native medical practices as following rationally from the culture at large. Such views were further developed in E. E. Evans-Pritchard's (1902–73) *Witchcraft, Oracles and Magic among the Azande* (1937). Asked why Africans explained disease in terms of witchcraft, he responded, 'Is Zande thought so different from ours that we can only describe their speech and actions without comprehending them, or is it essentially like our own though expressed in an idiom to which we are unaccustomed?'.

Like anthropology at large, medical anthropology initially set about explaining the aberrations of the native or primitive mind, with a view to governing it better and perhaps educating it. In time such medical systems came to be studied in less ethnocentric ways, and some of the insights of medical anthropology were later applied to western societies and western medicine themselves.

The bonds between medicine and empire were many-faceted. Disease and medicine played a part in the establishment of European empires overseas. Epidemics devastated and demoralized indigenous populations in the New World in the sixteenth century, and later in Africa, Australia, New Zealand and the Pacific islands, clearing the way for European conquest. Without disease, European intruders would not have met with such success or found indigenes so feeble in their resistance. Yet endemic diseases also held back European expansion into Africa. Imported from Africa, yellow fever and malaria shaped the ethnic composition and distinctive history of colonization and slave labour in the Caribbean.

Colonialism was hardly good for the health of the Third World. Epidemiological link-ups between previously isolated regions, the movements of fleets and armies, of millions of slaves and indentured labourers, the spread of disease by ecological change and social dislocation, the misery bred by shanty-towns – all have been implicated in the hail of death that European rule brought. The good that western medicine did was marginal and incidental. It formed, however, an integral part of the ideological baggage of empire. With colonialism equated with civilization, a prominent place was claimed for medicine among the benefits the West could bestow. White man's medicine excluded others, and Christianity's 'healing' doctrine was a challenge to the rival power of local 'witchdoctors'. The imperialism latent in western medicine was obvious in its attitudes towards indigenous healing: it aimed to establish rights over the bodies of the colonized. The vigorous denunciation of the 'witchdoctors' of Africa and other indigenous healing specialists was supported by claims that their practices were grounded in dangerous superstition. As western medicine became more convinced of its uniquely scientific basis, colonial authorities intervened to ban practices and cults which they saw as medically or politically objectionable, hence the prohibition against witchcraft in Britain's African colonies in the 1920s and 1930s.

INTERNATIONAL MEDICINE

Mirroring changes in world politics and economics, medicine's orientations shifted in the century after 1850. International capitalism, war and new technologies challenged national barriers. Before the twentieth century, the health problems of the industrial world were largely distinct and independent from those of the colonized: in many respects, the 'West' and the 'Rest' were still just making contact. During the twentieth century all grew interlocked, through the transformation of empires, gigantic population migrations, the changes brought by multinational capitalism, communications revolutions, world war and global politics.

As if to signal the consequences for world health, the early twentieth century brought the most mobile and lethal pandemic the world has ever seen, the influenza pandemic which swept the globe from 1918, killing over twenty-five million people in six months (about three times as many as died in the First World War), followed by an epidemic of encephalitis lethargica (an inflammation of the brain and spinal cord) and another wave of killer influenza in 1920. Perhaps a mutant of swine flu, it went global due to the massive movements of peoples associated with the war. It showed, were any proof needed, that the globe had shrunk.

The influenza epidemic appeared in three waves, the first being mild and unimportant. Beginning in August 1918, the second turned rapidly to pneumonia, against which medicine had no defence. It exploded in centres separated by thousands of miles: Freetown, Sierra Leone, Brest – the French port for American expeditionary forces – and Boston, Massachusetts. Two-thirds of Sierra Leone's population contracted flu, and more than 1000 died in Freetown alone. In Boston 10 per cent of the population was affected, and over 60 per cent of the sufferers died.

At San Francisco Hospital in California, 3509 pneumonia cases were admitted, with 25 per cent mortality. Throughout the US public gatherings were banned; schools, churches, cinemas and businesses were closed, and face masks worn – but nothing helped.

Influenza spread rapidly among American soldiers in the United States and abroad. At Camp Devens, Massachusetts, the first diagnosis was made on 12 September 1918; in less than a fortnight, the tally had reached 12,604. By October, some 20 per cent of the US army was ill: 24,000 soldiers died of flu; battle deaths were 34,000. In all, the United States lost over 500,000, England and Wales, 200,000; a quarter of the population of Samoa perished. Frantic efforts were made to culture it, discover its aetiology and devise treatments – with little success. The influenza disappeared as quickly and mysteriously as it had arrived. It was the greatest single demographic shock mankind has ever experienced, the most deadly pestilence since the Black Death.

Nothing since has struck on such a scale. Is that luck? Or a mark of the effectiveness of the better nutrition, public health measures, vaccines, chemotherapy and antibiotics since developed? It is hard to be sure. After the flu, the international health community grew more confident that the risk of great pandemics was dwindling. Hopes were pinned on a medical internationalism encouraged since the mid nineteenth century. Against the backdrop of the cholera pandemics a meeting had been held in Paris in 1851, involving twelve nations (including the Ottoman empire) and designated an International Sanitary Conference. It directed its attention to disputes that remained unresolved as to whether plague, yellow fever and cholera were contagious, miasmatic or resulted from an 'epidemic constitution'. Most delegates voted for cholera to be subject to quarantine regulations, but none of the participating governments ratified the regulations.

Setbacks like this constantly dogged medical internationalism. A second International Sanitary Conference was held in Paris in 1859. After five months, it adjourned with no resolution of the dispute between contagionists and miasmatists. A third was held in Constantinople in 1866, a fourth in Vienna in 1874, another in Washington in 1881 and a sixth in Rome in 1885. Still no agreement could be reached; that was left for the International Sanitary Conference in Venice (1892). Forty-one years of discussion had been needed to reach a limited accord on the quarantining of westbound ships with cholera on board – and by then the cholera problem had largely gone away!

In 1907 twenty-three European countries established a permanent establishment, the Office International d'Hygiène Publique (OIHP), located in Paris. It was to collect and disseminate knowledge on infectious diseases, with a view to its being embodied in international quarantine regulations. Eventually the OIHP included nearly sixty countries, including Persia/Iran, India, Pakistan and the United States.

The OIHP's initial focus was on cholera, plague and yellow fever, but it broadened to other communicable diseases, such as malaria, tuberculosis, typhoid fever, meningitis and sleeping sickness. It also provided an international forum for discussion of sanitation, inoculation, notification of tuberculosis cases and the isolation of leprosy cases.

The Versailles settlement following the First World War brought the League of Nations into being, and this established a subdivision, the Health Organization of the League of Nations. The United States was not a member of the League and, as a member of OIHP, it vetoed a proposal to integrate that body into the League. By consequence, in 1921 there were two parallel international agencies: the OIHP and the League's Health Organization. There was also the Pan-American Sanitary Bureau.

With typhus raging in Russia and the influenza pandemic, an International Health Conference met in London in 1919, but it was attended by only five countries: Great Britain, France, Italy, Japan and the United States. Eventually cooperation improved between the Health Organization and the Office International d'Hygiène Publique. Several new international health activities were initiated by the League, including a Malaria Commission (1923), and a Cancer Commission. These bodies reported on drugs standardization and the unification of pharmacopoeias, malnutrition, typhus, leprosy, medical and public health education.

With the German invasion of Poland in 1939, the League of Nations collapsed and, with it, the Health Organization. In view of this, those who established the World Health Organization (WHO) following the Second World War were insistent that it should not depend on the survival of its parent body, the United Nations. By June 1948, WHO had fifty-five national signatories, and a secretariat in Geneva. In ringing and idealistic tones WHO declared that its goal was 'a state of complete physical, mental and social well-being and not merely the absence of disease or infirmity'.

WHO launched campaigns for immunization of the world's children against six diseases: diphtheria, tetanus, whooping cough, measles, poliomyelitis and tuberculosis (with BCG vaccine). After deep political dissensions, it promoted the training of auxiliary health personnel, such as China's 'barefoot doctors' and India's traditional birth attendants. In 1946 the United Nations General Assembly had also established an International Children's Emergency Fund (UNICEF), which worked in close cooperation with WHO, directing funds for the provision of food and drugs supplies and equipment. UNICEF came under the general supervision of UNESCO (United Nations Educational, Scientific and Cultural Organization). The World Health Organization has attempted in many ways to monitor international disease developments – collecting statistics, improving cooperation, intervening in health crises, and developing plans for Third World health improvements. Other agencies like the International Red Cross have spearheaded famine relief and epidemic interventions.

A further type of international initiative developed: bilateral foreign aid to developing countries, involving investment, agricultural and industrial development, educational programmes and medical schemes. By 1980, bilateral expenditures by most industrialized countries had outstripped multilateral programmes. The United States, for example, was providing health assistance to sixty countries in 1980.

The world health movement scored some signal triumphs, notably the worldwide eradication of smallpox – the first time a disease has been entirely eliminated by human intervention. In 1966, when 10–15 million people in 33 countries still caught smallpox every year and 2 million died, WHO voted for a ten-year mass vaccination campaign to eradicate it once and for all. The multinational WHO team comprised 50 full-time and 600 temporary medical workers, led by an American, Dr Donald Henderson (b. 1928). Gradually, the disease vanished from the Americas, Africa and the Middle East, but remained in India and Pakistan. In November 1974, a famous victory was celebrated, when Bangladesh's freedom from smallpox made world headlines. The last smallpox fatality was, ironically, in Birmingham. In 1978, Janet Parker, a British photographer, was working above a research laboratory when the virus escaped through the ventilation system; she caught the disease and died. Today, the virus officially exists in only two laboratories, in Atlanta and Moscow. The rest of the world's stocks have been destroyed, unless (as is widely suspected) samples are being held in reserve as biological weapons among other biological and chemical weapons stockpiled by the great and would-be great powers.

With smallpox eradication accomplished, the World Health Organization developed programmes to eradicate other major childhood diseases – measles, whooping cough, diphtheria, polio – responsible for the deaths of millions every year. The prospects, however, are less propitious than with smallpox; a combination of features set that apart from most other infectious illnesses, in that it was not especially contagious, had no animal reservoir, was easily recognized and diagnosed, and there was a very effective vaccine.

Measles and polio also have no animal reservoir, but the prospects of success in the short term remain slim. In central Africa few countries achieve a 50 per cent immunization rate of children under one year of age. With twenty-two million children born each year, India immunizes little more than half, though China has succeeded in reaching over 90 per cent of its susceptible population.

Recognition has grown that the application of western medicine, though well-meaning, has often been inappropriate, ineffective, selective or even counter-productive. The West neglected bilharzia until US personnel began to acquire it in the Philippines during the Second World War. Critics of subsequent bilharzia campaigns have condemned the over-reliance on science and on single interventions such as molluscicides to kill the snail vectors, maintaining that the 'commando' approach – going in and striking the vectors with disease-specific magic bullets – fails to deal with the deep problems and is at best a temporary expedient.

Others have greater faith in scientific advances directed against specific diseases, preferring these to mass-participatory, broad-scale interventions against afflictions associated with poverty. In the case of schistosomiasis, currently infecting some 150,000 million people, research on molluscicides continues; the techniques of molecular biology are being used to seek vaccines, and praziquantel has transformed therapy. Supporters of high-tech medicine believe it may prove more practical to attack diseases one by one with vaccines and drugs than to raise living standards sufficiently to reduce the tragic burden of ill health on a broad front.

NEW DISEASES

National and international instability, especially war in Africa and Asia, has disrupted health administration and created the poverty, famines and refugee problems that foment disease: at least twenty million people round the world live in refugee camps. Economic crises, political upheavals, and mass population migrations have militated against the high levels of financial investment, administrative support, organizational infrastructure and international cooperation required to sustain campaigns against world diseases. One outcome was that hopes that malaria might be eradicated by pesticides and drugs were abandoned in the 1980s.

By 1970 malaria had been eradicated from most of Europe and the USSR, North America, several Middle Eastern countries, and much of the Mediterranean littoral. That was a fine public health achievement, but not enough. Seasonal or endemic transmission continued in many tropical countries, and difficulties dogged the implementation of eradication programmes. More worryingly, the parasite steadily became seriously drug-resistant. Resistance to cheap drugs like chloroquine began in south-east Asia, and by the 1980s most malarial parasites in that region were completely resistant. By 1990 chloroquine resistance was common throughout Africa. The parasite changes its genetic makeup more rapidly than the pharmaceutical industry can produce new and tested drugs. Moreover, some of the newer drugs, like Mefloquine, produce severe side-effects.

In many nations it has grown more difficult to implement control programmes because, with population growth, the numbers at risk are increasing dramatically. Not least, air travel has provided a perfect means of speeding infected mosquitoes around the globe, while global warming is extending the habitats suitable for them. At the close of the twentieth century, malaria is still afflicting over 300 million people – far more than in 1960 – and causing between two million and three and a half million deaths a year.

Improvement in some countries balances deterioration in others. Hopes have been held out for the vaccine developed by a Colombian physician, Manuel Patarroyo, which has been chemically synthesized rather than made using a biological process. Others are less sanguine. 'It is folly for anyone to tell you', Dr Thomas Eisner (b. 1929) of Cornell University has commented, 'that we can cope with spreading insect populations. I'm anxious about that kind of technological optimism. We tried to wipe out malaria, and what have we got? DDT-resistant insects, drug-resistant *Plasmodium* and a vaccine that's not working.'

With other diseases, too, 'progress' proved counter-productive; in Egypt schistosomiasis was worsened by the construction of the Aswan dam, causing a backing-up of stagnant waters. Many factors make the worldwide epidemiological situation more ominous: political and economic destabilization, rocketing population growth, mass migrations, especially of refugees, and the intensification of poverty. In such circumstances, recent decades have brought the resurgence, among rich and poor nations alike, of diseases once believed to be decisively in retreat. Tuberculosis is once more becoming common in the First World and rampant in the Third, multiplying in inner city areas of the USA and to a lesser degree in Europe.

There are several reasons. One is the vulnerability of the immuno-suppressed: TB may be the first sign that a person is HIV positive. Another is low-grade health care for the poor and powerless. In the United States tuberculosis began to appear most visibly among drug addicts and the homeless, many of whom had little access to health care. Such sufferers commonly abandoned treatment before it was complete, creating ideal circumstances for the emergence of drug-resistant strands. By 1984, half of those people with active tuberculosis had a strain of the germ that resisted at least one antibiotic. Ten years later many strains were resisting several of the drugs for treating TB; some resist them all.

Between 1985 and 1991, when tuberculosis increased 12 per cent in the United States and 30 per cent in Europe, it rose 300 per cent in the parts of Africa where TB and HIV frequently go together. Approximately 10 million people have active tuberculosis; it kills 3 million each year, 95 per cent of them in the Third World.

Diphtheria has returned to the former Soviet Union and parts of the old eastern bloc. A development symptomatic of decaying sanitary and public health standards, it also marks the emergence of new strains of micro-organisms until recently believed vanquished by vaccines and antibiotics. Such 'superbugs' were to be predicted in the light of evolu-tionary and adaptational pressures upon bacilli and viruses. This Darwinian process has been hastened by the overuse and misuse of pharmaceuticals.

Cholera is another disease, thought to have been eradicated, which has returned. The Americas had long been free of cholera – the United States had suffered no major outbreak since 1866, South America none since 1895. In 1961, however, the seventh pandemic erupted, initially in Indonesia. Its source was the new El Tor strain of *V. cholerae*. El Tor spread through Asia and hit Africa in 1970, attacking twenty-nine countries in two years. By 1991, after thirty years, the El Tor outbreak was the longest cholera pandemic ever. It reached Peru in January 1991, probably in water flushed from the ballast tanks of a ship from Asia, in the same way that vibrios briefly infected Mobile Bay in the Gulf of Mexico that year. The epidemic in Lima began after inhabitants ate a local delicacy made from tainted raw fish. The wastes of infected people then entered Lima's antiquated sewer systems, and within three months 150,000 cholera cases had been reported. The disease reached a new country almost every month during 1991, racing through Chile, Colombia, Ecuador, Bolivia, Brazil, Argentina, and Guatemala. By early 1992, it had affected 400,000 Latin Americans, killing 4000.

In 1993 a new strain of *V. cholerae* erupted in India and Bangladesh, killing 5000 people. Called strain 0139 (it was the 139th to be discovered), it soon spread to south-east Asia and may herald the eighth pandemic. Cholera's resurgence shows the fragility of barriers against epidemics in a world that has shrunk. The demands of international capitalism for migrant workforces, the opening up of borders, the ebb and flow of peoples due to war and persecution, the increased mobility of affluent air-travelling populations – all these factors mean that formerly contained diseases now have no fixed abode.

These are among the key factors in the new diseases, notably AIDS, spreading since the 1970s. Seemingly originating in sub-Saharan Africa, the transmission of AIDS has been through sexual fluids and blood. It first came to the attention of physicians in the USA in 1981, when it was found that young homosexual men were dying from rare conditions associated with the breakdown of the immune system. A period marked by moralizing and victim-blaming, wild recriminations, political squirming and intensive medical research led by 1983 to the discovery of the virus (HIV), generally held responsible for the condition.

Early hopes for a cure or a vaccine have been frustrated, partly because the human immunodeficiency virus (HIV) mutates even more rapidly than the viral agents of influenza, thwarting development of both vaccines and drugs. Moreover, because HIV breaks down the immune system, sufferers often fall victim to illnesses such as pneumocystis pneumonia, tuberculosis and other opportunistic infections. It was widely predicted in the mid eighties that a global total of ten million cases would be reached by 1996. Though AIDS continues to spread as a pandemic, some of the more apocalyptic projections have been scaled down: the total as of 1996 appeared to be about 1,393,000. However, it remains out of control, exceedingly dangerous (being initially asymptomatic and hence unwittingly transmissible), and at its most severe in those nations of central Africa which are poorest and have the fewest medical services.

It is unlikely that AIDS is a new disease; it probably long possessed its own niche in the African rain-forests. The opening up of hitherto isolated areas to economic exploitation, travel and tourism, and the ceaseless migration of peoples, have probably flushed it out and unleashed it onto a defenceless world. It may also not be a coincidence that AIDS appeared in Africa at the same time that the World Health Organization was eradicating smallpox. During the 1970s members of the WHO were vaccinating young people in central Africa with live smallpox vaccine, re-using needles forty to sixty times. Live vaccines directly provoke the immune system, and can awaken sleeping giants such as viruses.

Other comparably dangerous viral diseases have emerged. These include Lassa, Marburg, and Rift Valley fevers in Africa, and others in South America such as Bolivian haemorrhagic fever. Most, it is supposed, are transferred from animal reservoirs. In 1976, a hitherto unknown virus even more frightening than Marburg and Lassa appeared. Ebola haemorrhagic fever broke out suddenly in Nzara, a town in southern Sudan. The illness began with fever and joint pains; then came haemorrhagic rash, black vomit, kidney and liver failure, seizures, bleeding from all orifices, shock and death. The virus spread to a hospital in a nearby town, where it killed many patients and staff. Of almost 300 victims, more than half died. Two months later, it broke out 500 miles away, in the Ebola River region of Zaire, killing 13 of 17 staff at a mission hospital and spreading to patients, who carried it to more than 50 villages. One nurse was taken for treatment to the country's capital, Kinshasa, a poor, crowded city of two million with direct air links to Europe – an event which might have triggered a disaster in Zaire or beyond.

The epidemic had run its course by November 1976; in 1979 a smaller outbreak occurred in southern Sudan, and in 1979 another hospital-centred outbreak occurred in Tandala, Zaire. Thirty-three patients were diagnosed, of whom 22 died: Until now, such outbreaks have remained restricted. But it is conceivable that, like AIDS, these or similar viruses could pounce, and spread throughout the world. As more traditional habitats are invaded, risks exist of major catastrophes from such diseases.

In 1969, the US surgeon general, Dr William H. Stewart, told the American nation that the book of infectious disease was now closed. The West seemed to have conquered epidemics, and epidemiology seemed destined to become a scientific backwater. The manifest shortsightedness of that view is a measure of the medical optimism prevalent a generation ago.

Could there ever be solid grounds for the return of that optimism? There seems little reason to believe that western scientific medicine can single-handedly overcome pathogenic agents. And that must be all the truer as so many medical problems are the product of environmental and social disruptions caused by western economies and nation-states. Fertilizers, hormones, herbicides and pesticides introduce fresh hazards into the food chain; global warming is producing changes in atmospheric gases and affecting the balance of land and sea; the greenhouse effect is enhanced; as a result of the use of chlorofluorocarbons (CFCs), the ozone layer continues to be eroded. Such developments bring new disease threats: radiation and cancer, the spread of malaria and other 'tropical' diseases to new habitats, and the migration of microbes.

CHAPTER XVI

PSYCHIATRY

BEFORE THE NINETEENTH CENTURY the treatment of the mad hardly constituted a specialized branch of medicine. General physicians would handle the insane as part of their regular caseload, and a few acquired a reputation for it; but when doctors wrote about madness it was essentially as part of wider discussions of humoral imbalances or fevers. In late eighteenth-century England, the emergent 'trade in lunacy', focusing on private madhouses, lay only partly in doctors' hands. At the onset of his madness in 1788, George III was first treated by regular court physicians and then by a mad-doctor, Francis Willis, who was a clergyman of the Church of England as well as a doctor of medicine.

On both sides of the Atlantic, it was the community that had traditionally judged individuals to be out of their minds, and the community that principally coped with them. Mad people were a family responsibility; failing that, the parish or town would provide a carer or custodian, or have a maniac put into safe-keeping in a jail, dungeon or house of correction (the German *Zuchthaus* or the *hôpital général* in France) or would simply send them packing. In Catholic countries, certain monasteries and religious houses had a tradition of caring for mad people; exorcism was occasionally used and assorted individuals – priests and healers as well as doctors – were reputed to have special personal powers over madness. Until the close of the eighteenth century, madhouses were not primarily medical institutions; most, like Bethlem in London, had their origin as religious or municipal charities. They might have an honorary physician who paid visits, and patients would occasionally be 'physicked' – mainly purging and bleeding – with the violent under restraint with manacles and straitjackets.

THE RISE OF THE ASYLUM

All this changed in the nineteenth century, as the development of psychiatric medicine made it first common, then routine, and finally almost inescapable, for the mentally ill to be treated in what were successively called madhouses, lunatic asylums and then psychiatric hospitals, where they increasingly fell under the charge of specialists.

The madhouse was an ambiguous institution. It was long criticized as a gothic horror, all cruelty and neglect, whips and chains. William Hogarth and many other satirists exposed London's Bethlem Hospital (Bedlam). Yet by the nineteenth century the 'new' asylum had become the object of praise as a progressive institution, indeed the one truly effective site for the treatment of insanity, the place, the eminent British psychiatrist John Conolly (1794–1866) maintained, 'where humanity, if anywhere on earth, shall reign supreme'. In 1837 Dr W. A. F. Browne (1806–85), soon to be head of the Montrose Royal Lunatic Asylum in Scotland, pronounced on *What Asylums Were, Are, and Ought to Be.* Traditional institutions had been abominations, he told his readers; present ones were better, and the asylum of the future would be positively idyllic:

> Conceive a spacious building resembling the palace of a peer, airy, and elevated, and elegant, surrounded by extensive and swelling grounds and gardens. The interior is fitted up with galleries, and workshops, and music-rooms. The sun and the air are allowed to enter at every window, the view of the shrubberies and fields, and groups of labourers, is unobstructed by shutters or bars; all is clean, quiet and attractive. The inmates all seem to be actuated by the common impulse of enjoyment, all are busy, and delighted by being so. The house and all around appears a hive of industry. . . . There is in this community no compulsion, no chains, no whips, no corporal chastisement, simply because these are proved to be less effectual means of carrying any point than persuasion, emulation, and the desire of obtaining gratification . . .
>
> Such is a faithful picture of what may be seen in many institutions, and of what might be seen in all, were asylums conducted as they ought to be.

The nineteenth century, in other words, brought the 'discovery of the asylum' – growing faith in the institution, with ceaseless attempts to rectify, refine and perfect it.

For progressives reform meant freeing the insane from chains and other benighted cruelties. In France the physician Philippe Pinel (1745–1826), a devout Roman Catholic who had thought of becoming a priest, was given responsibility for the insane at the Bicêtre in 1793 at the height of the Revolution. Believing the mad behaved like animals because that was how they were treated, he experimented with reducing mechanical restraints – though the dramatic image of Pinel 'striking the chains off the mad', once beloved of historians, belongs to legend. This was a huge success, and ultimately most of his mental patients were freed from their irons.

Pinel had picked up some of his ideas about madness from folk wisdom; he was far from being a specialist psychiatrist. A supporter of the dominant Paris patho-anatomical approach, in his own day he was more famous for his *Nosographie* (1798) [Nosography] and *La médecine clinique* (1804) [Clinical Medicine] than his *Traité médico-philosophique sur l'aliénation mentale* (1801) [Medico-philosophical Treatise on Mental Alienation]. His writings reflected the concerns of mainstream medicine: an intense admiration for Hippocrates and an emphasis on hard clinical observations, combined with aversion to speculation.

As to the aetiology of insanity, Pinel stressed mental over physical causes: 'Derangement of the understanding', he reflected, 'is generally considered as an effect of an organic lesion of the brain,' consequently as incurable, but that supposition was, 'in a great number of instances, contrary to anatomical fact'. A devotee of Locke and Condillac, and committed to Enlightenment optimism, he made much of psychological factors. Yet, unlike Locke's emphasis on the role of delusion, and the association of ideas, Pinel's preferred *traitement moral* ('moral treatment') was directed at the emotions no less than the intellectual faculties. And, while retaining the traditional division of insanity into melancholia, mania, idiocy and dementia, he developed new disease categories, especially partial and affective insanity. His idea of *manie sans délire*, later called *folie raisonnante*, involved a partial insanity (patients who were mad on one subject) in which the personality was warped but the understanding remained sound. Viewing passions as the primary source of this condition, he held that such patients were under the 'domination of instinctive and abstract fury'. When, in 1835, James Cowles Prichard put affective disorders of this kind into the category of 'moral insanity', he acknowledged his debt to Pinel.

What did moral treatment involve, as envisaged by Pinel? The alienist, he maintained, was to prefer the 'ways of gentleness'. This strategy of hope assumed that insanity did not entail a descent into animality or a total and permanent obliteration of the patient's sane self; some humanity remained to be worked upon. Humanity was effective, but the alienist might also be obliged to call upon 'repression', and his physical presence would radiate authority. Pinel's contemporary, Francis Willis, was renowned for a piercing stare which imposed mastery, and many mad doctors at this time learned a trick or two from actors and Mesmerists.

During the Reign of Terror, a Parisian tailor expressed reservations about Louis XVI's execution, a confession which aroused the suspicion of his peers. Misconstruing a conversation he later overheard, the tailor became persuaded that his own death at the guillotine was approaching. Soon this delusion grew into a fixation which haunted him, necessitating his confinement in a lunatic asylum, where he was treated by Pinel. He arranged a kind of occupational therapy: the tailor would patch the other patients' clothing for a small payment. The patient seemed to recover, but the improvement proved temporary, and he suffered a relapse. This time Pinel opted for a more inventive approach which involved staging a complicated demonstration; he arranged for three doctors, dressed as magistrates, to appear before the tailor. Pretending to represent the revolutionary legislature, the panel pronounced his patriotism beyond reproach, 'acquitting' him of any misdeeds. As a consequence of the *faux* trial, Pinel noted, the man's symptoms disappeared at once (although, he confessed, they later returned).

More broadly, moral treatment also proposed to end the faulty thinking, which, according to the prevalent Lockean sensationalist psychology, was implicated in insanity. The alienist could attempt to distract the patient from his 'deluded imagination', perhaps by diverting his mind, perhaps by engaging him in useful labour; or he could subject him to shock. Similarly, in a tradition loaded with Renaissance precedents, contemporary English asylum-keepers such as Joseph Mason Cox (1762–1822) suggested hiring performers to act out patients' delusions. The management of disordered passions was to be achieved through face-to-face authority.

Pinel's impact at the Bicêtre (for men) and its sister institution the Salpêtrière (for women) was signal, and the *Traité* was quickly translated into English, Spanish and German, spreading his ideas on the moral causation and treatment of insanity, and arguing the case for a reformed asylum milieu and for innovative management techniques. His message was optimistic: organic brain disease might indeed be incurable, but melancholy and mania without delirium would typically respond to moral methods.

Minimizing restraint and replacing cruelty with kindness were also advocated in Florence by Vincenzo Chiarugi (1759–1820), while moral therapy developed independently in Britain, where the York Retreat, opened in 1796, achieved celebrity as the symbol of progress. The Retreat was set up after the mysterious death of a Quaker patient in the York Asylum, a subscription hospital milked and mismanaged by two successive physicians. Outraged, the local Quaker community decided to establish its own charitable asylum. Partly by religious conviction, partly by practical trial and error, it evolved a distinctive therapeutics grounded on quiet, comfort and a supportive family atmosphere, in which the insane were treated like ill-disciplined children. Its success was publicized by Samuel Tuke's (1784–1857) *Description of the Retreat* (1813) and later by the testimony which he and his grandfather, William (1732–1822), gave to a Parliamentary Committee on Madhouses (1815): 'neither chains nor corporal punishment are tolerated,' it was claimed.

If the York Retreat was presented to the MPs as a kind of heaven, or at least a haven, old Bedlam appeared as hell. At Bethlem, the committee was informed, one patient, James Norris, had been restrained in a shocking manner:

> a stout iron ring was riveted round his neck, from which a short chain passed through a ring made to slide upwards and downwards on an upright massive iron bar, more than six feet high, inserted into the wall. Round his body a strong iron bar about two inches wide was riveted; on each side of the bar was a circular projection; which being fashioned to and enclosing each of his arms, pinioned them close to his sides.

Bethlem's physician, Thomas Monro (1759–1833), somewhat lamely reassured the committee that chains and fetters were 'fit only for the pauper lunatics: if a gentleman was put in irons he would not like it.' The hearings revealed comprehensive mismanagement at Bethlem;

Monro was a supine absentee. George Wallet, the steward, was asked: 'How often does Dr Monro attend?' He replied, 'I believe but seldom . . . I hear he has not been round the house but once these three months.' The late surgeon had been an alcoholic (for ten years 'generally insane and mostly drunk. He was so insane as to have a strait-waistcoat'). Thus the staff ratted on one another and Bethlem was exposed.

Tuke's *Description* offered, by contrast, a shining model for early nineteenth-century reformers. As with Pinel, moral therapy was justified in England on the twin grounds of humanity and efficacy. The Retreat was modelled on the ideal of family life, and restraint was negligible. Patients and staff lived, worked and dined together in an environment where recovery was encouraged through praise and blame, rewards and punishment, the goal being the restoration of self-control. The root cause of insanity, physical or mental, mattered little. Though far from hostile to doctors, the Tukes, who were tea merchants by profession, stated that experience showed nothing medicine had to offer did any good.

Medical men, however, grew increasingly involved in psychological medicine and in treating the mad – a response, among other things, to the wider nineteenth-century trend towards specialization and the division of labour in an overstocked medical market. The success of the Tukes' experiment at York, and its glowing repute, presented opportunities for doctors, since it legitimated the institutionalization of the mad. But it also posed a challenge: after the Tukes' assertion that medicine achieved nothing, how were doctors to demonstrate that madness was a medical condition for which they possessed special skills?

While accepting much of moral treatment, most nineteenth-century physicians maintained that insanity was ultimately rooted in the organism, particularly the brain; for that reason therapy needed to be incorporated within a medical model, and prescribed by physicians. There followed a dramatic increase in books on insanity, virtually all by doctors; and a growing body of 'mad-doctors' emerged, called 'alienists'.

In England an Act of 1808 permitted local authorities to raise ratepayers' money to build lunatic asylums for the mad poor, but the response was uneven. Following scandals, the Metropolitan Commissioners in Lunacy were established in 1828, with a brief to inspect London's lunatic asylums: that five of its fifteen members were medical indicates the still rather ambiguous status of mad-doctors in the public eye. Professional identity was consolidated in 1841 with the Association of Medical Officers of Asylums and Hospitals for the Insane, providing Victorian psychiatry with a platform. It published the *Asylum Journal* (1853), later renamed the *Journal of Mental Science* (1858), and in due course became the (Royal) Medico-Psychological Association. In 1971 it became the Royal College of Psychiatrists. The German equivalent, the Association of German Alienists, came into being in 1864; by 1900 it had 300 members, by 1914, 627.

Growing public preoccupation with insanity – the disorder seemed to be worsening, yet high hopes were initially held out for its curability – led to an Act of 1845 compelling each county to erect, at public expense, an asylum for the pauper insane. The development and reputation of English psychiatry became strongly identified with these public asylums; the private 'trade in lunacy' had always been suspect, and 'office psychiatry' was slow to develop. In these circumstances the leaders of the profession cut their teeth and made their names in the large new public asylums which offered challenges to the ambitious, energetic and talented.

The outstanding early Victorian British psychiatrist was John Conolly (1794–1866), who served as superintendent between 1839 and 1844 at the large public asylum at Hanwell in Middlesex, and was noted for his introduction of non-restraint, though in that he had been anticipated by Robert Gardiner Hill (1811–78) at the Lincoln Asylum. Conolly's *Treatment of the Insane without Mechanical Restraints* (1856) advanced the ideal of moral therapy in an institutional context under a presiding physician. His case histories show his awareness of psychological and social factors; he was sensitive to the dangers of improper confinement, and a humane optimism marked his repudiation of the bad old practices of the past.

While stressing moral therapy, Conolly upheld the physical basis of insanity, drawing on the controversial phrenological doctrines developed by the Austrian, Franz Joseph Gall (1758–1828), and J. C. Spurzheim (1776–1832). Phrenology held that the brain was the organ of thought and will, that it determined character, and that its configurations revealed personality. The brain was a jigsaw of separate 'organs' (amativeness, acquisitiveness and so forth) occupying specific cortical areas and shaping the personality. An organ's size governed the exercise of its functions; the contours of the skull signalled the brain configurations beneath, while the overall balance of the 'bumps' determined personality. Gall initially identified twenty-seven faculties, and more were added later. A talented anatomist, Gall was in 1805 hounded out of Vienna on the grounds that his doctrines were materialistic.

At bottom, phrenology was organic, but it could be used to underpin moral therapy: while basic psychological traits were held to be innate, the phrenological concept of human nature was flexible enough to allow a role for education in developing the faculties and hence the mind. Phrenology could thus serve as a flexible resource within psychiatry, endowing it with a somatic foundation yet affording therapeutic promise. It captured a wide public following, appearing to be a means to self-understanding and self-improvement; it appealed to many alienists too. Treatments nevertheless remained a rag-bag. Together with moral therapy's emphasis on socialization and labour, inmates might be subjected to cold baths and showers, isolation, electric shocks and rotating chairs, or they might be purged and bled. Every superintendent had his favourite cocktail of cures, blending the physical and the moral, while in reality most patients spent their time in idleness, inside or outside their cells, or were left to the dubious ministrations of untrained and often thuggish attendants.

American psychiatry developed along comparable lines. The York Retreat provided a model for the Hartford Retreat in Connecticut, founded in 1824, the Friends' Asylum near Philadelphia (1817), the McClean Hospital in Boston (1818) and the Bloomingdale Asylum in New York (1821). The New World also had its heroes. In 1812 that founding-father of American medicine Benjamin Rush published his *Medical Inquiries and Observations upon the Diseases of the Mind*; like Pinel, he elaborated notions of partial and affective insanity. Rush's style of moral therapy employed physical restraint and fear as psychotherapeutic agents, and his zeal for venesection extended from yellow fever to his psychiatric practice. 'The first remedy under this head should be bloodletting,' was his advice for mania: 'It should be copious on the first attack . . . From 20 to 40 ounces of blood may be taken at once . . . The effects of this early and copious bleeding are wonderful in calming mad people.'

The early asylum era in America was marked by Samuel B. Woodward (1787–1850) at the Worcester State Hospital, and Pliny Earle (1809–92) at the Bloomingdale Asylum, both of whom incorporated moral therapy within a medical approach. They were among the founders of the Association of Medical Superintendents of American Institutions for the Insane (AMSAII), set up in 1844, the year that Amariah

Brigham (1798–1849) established the *American Journal of Insanity*, later the *American Journal of Psychiatry*, which became identified with the AMSAII.

A sign of psychiatry's coming of age as a medical specialty was forensic psychiatry. It had long been accepted that the insane should not be punished for criminal acts. In 1799 James Hadfield tried to assassinate George III, but the trial was halted when his defence lawyer convinced the judge that Hadfield was labouring under an insane delusion. Thereafter juries in England brought in special verdicts of 'not guilty by reason of insanity'. Distinguishing criminality from insanity was not traditionally considered a matter of medical expertise. From the early decades of the nineteenth century, however, the insanity defence was increasingly likely to involve medical testimony. Certain mad-doctors, including John Haslam (1764–1844), once of Bethlem, and Forbes Winslow (1810–74), became celebrated for their court-room testimony and their treatises on forensic psychiatry. Expert psychiatric witnesses staked out claims to be able to detect 'partial' insanity, particularly monomania, imperceptible to the public. The implication was that only psychiatrists could tell who was really sane – only they could plumb the criminal mind.

During the 1840s, the insanity plea became a matter of dispute. The trial in 1843 of Daniel M'Naghten for the murder of Edward Drummond, Sir Robert Peel's private secretary, was stopped on the grounds of insanity. After the controversial acquittal, the Law Lords were asked to draw up guidelines to form the legal basis for criminal insanity and responsibility. The resulting M'Naghten Rules (1844) established the insanity defence as the criminal's inability to distinguish right from wrong. This legalistic formula ('the nature and quality of the act') scotched the claim being advanced by post-Pinelian psychological medicine for the recognition of disorders of emotion and volition ('irresistible impulse') without disorder of the understanding, since the jurists saw in the psychiatrists' notion of partial insanity a threat to the idea of free will, which forms the sheet anchor of concepts of guilt and punishment. Debates over the insanity defence thus expressed conflicts between legal and psychiatric models of consciousness and conduct. The boundaries between the bad and the mad remained contested, as did the public role of psychiatry.

By mid century the rise of professional bodies, journals and legislation concerning the insane marked the high point of asylum psychiatry in Britain and America. Progressive alienists pinned therapeutic faith on the architecture and atmosphere of their asylums, trusting to order and organization, discipline and design, and their leadership qualities. Asylums were prized as scientific, humane, cost-effective, curative institutions.

Similar optimism prevailed in France, where from 1838 each *département* was required to erect a public asylum for the pauper insane. Provision was to be made for the segregation of noisy from quiet patients, dirty from clean, violent from peaceful, and acute from chronic; patients would be removed from their 'pathological' home environment; and 'moral measures' (work, re-education and self-discipline) would be prominent. The 1838 code spelling out these requirements incorporated the recommendations of Pinel's pupil, Jean-Etienne Dominique Esquirol (1772–1840), who had travelled extensively observing psychiatric institutions, campaigning for improvement, and had begun formal psychiatric lectures in 1817. His *Des maladies mentales* (1838) [Mental Maladies] was the outstanding psychiatric statement of the age. Experience led Esquirol to a remodelling of psychiatric thinking. While asserting the ultimately organic nature of psychiatric disorders, he documented their social and psychological triggers, developing the concept of 'monomania' to describe a partial insanity identified with affective disorders, especially those involving paranoia, and framing conditions like kleptomania, nymphomania, pyromania and other forms of compulsion. Advocating the asylum as a 'therapeutic instrument', he became an authority on its construction, and planned the National Asylum of Charenton, of which he became director.

Esquirol had pet ideas about the asylum's therapeutic efficacy. He advanced the theory of isolation, 'removing the lunatic from all his habitual pastimes, distancing him from his place of residence, separating him from his family, his friends, his servants, surrounding him with strangers, altering his whole way of life'. As with other forms of moral treatment, this was grounded in sensationalist psychology. A radical change in environment supposedly shook up the pathological ideas entrenched in the disturbed person, leaving the psychiatrist in a position to provide new stimuli to establish sane ideas.

With their psychopathological doctrines and influential accounts of illusion, hallucination and moral insanity, all based on impressive case experience, Esquirol and his pupils exercised dominance over French psychiatry, mirroring French hospital medicine's emphasis on close clinical observation and routine autopsy. His main students were E. E. Georget (1795–1828), who wrote on cerebral localization; Jean-Pierre Falret (1794–1870), author of a classic description of circular insanity; Louis Calmeil (1798–1895), who described dementia paralytica; J. J. Moreau de Tours (1804–84), one of the pioneers of degenerationism; and Jules Baillarger (1809–90), who worked on general paresis and is best remembered for his account (1854) of the manic depressive cycle (*folie à double forme*), characterized by a succession of attacks of mania and depression. Baillarger's claim to its discovery was hotly disputed by Falret who called the disease *folie circulaire* and held that a lucid period interrupted the two pathological states. The Esquirolians radically transformed contemporary classification and diagnosis of mental disorder.

THE ASYLUM UNDER FIRE

The asylum movement in Europe and the US established a lasting scheme of care, but other models were also tried. Communities were advocated along the lines of the long-established Belgian therapeutic village of Geel, providing a family and domestic setting for the mentally disturbed; and a greater diversity of mental institutions sprang up after 1850, including polyclinics and private 'rest homes' and 'nerve clinics' for the affluent, which sought to avoid the stigmatizing connotations of madness. Despite governmental licensing and regular inspections, abuses remained. In England the Alleged Lunatics' Friend Society, founded by the ex-patient John Perceval (1803–76) aimed to expose and rectify these.

Also vigilant in this field was the crusading American Dorothea Dix (1802–87). The daughter of a fanatical Christian, she took up philanthropic activities, and in 1841, finding several insane prisoners dumped in an unheated room at the East Cambridge (Massachusetts) House of Correction, she took the issue to court. She then spent two years investigating the condition of the insane in jails, almshouses and houses of correction, while urging the founding of proper asylums for the insane. Subsequently she extended her campaign to other states, visiting institutions, exposing evils, and soliciting the support of sympathetic politicians. By 1852, seventeen states had founded or enlarged hospitals for the insane. Visiting Europe, her exposure of abuses helped to prompt the setting up of a royal commission to examine the treatment of the insane in Scotland.

Asylum abuse proved an endemic disorder. In England a series of Madhouse Acts passed from 1774 onwards was intended to put an end to such iniquities through certification procedures, but scandals throughout the nineteenth century leave no doubt that confinement of those protesting sanity or malicious imprisonment remained common, sometimes coming to a head in *causes célèbres*, like that of Louisa Lowe – a case which underlines the vulnerability of women. Married in 1842 to the Revd George Lowe, in 1870 she moved out. Her husband demanded she return home, she refused; he had her kidnapped and taken to Brislington House asylum in Bristol. Though the certificates authorizing her admittance were found to be invalid, the proprietor Dr Fox detained her for a further two months. She brought an action against him for false imprisonment, but the lord chief justice ruled it was not a criminal offence to incarcerate a sane individual, provided the intent was not malicious.

There she remained until February 1871, when she was moved to Lawn House, Hanwell, the private asylum of the distinguished Dr Henry Maudsley, who diagnosed her as 'suffering from delusions'. During a visit by the commissioners in lunacy in March, she demanded to be set free, but on her request that a jury be convened to decide her fate, the commissioner, Dr Lutwidge, retorted, 'It is very possible but very undesirable.' In October the commissioners again visited Lawn House. Mrs Lowe again begged to be released, but they replied that it would be 'contrary to all etiquette', as a suit had been brought by her husband to gain control of her property, then yielding £500 p.a. Overall, she was detained for eighteen months. Warning 'that many sane, and still more merely eccentric and quite harmless persons, are languishing in the mad houses', she founded the Lunacy Law Reform Association to protect future family victims, and documented her plight in *Quis Custodiet Ipsos Custodes?* (1872).

Further asylum evils were exposed around 1900 by Clifford W. Beers (1876–1943), a young Yale graduate and businessman, after a severe mental breakdown led to his being institutionalized first at a private hospital and later in a public institution. 'I left the state hospital in September, 1903', he wrote in his immensely influential *A Mind That Found Itself* (1908), 'firmly determined to . . . organize a movement that would help to do away with existing evils in the care of the mentally ill, and whenever possible to prevent mental illness itself'. Beers claimed to have been neglected and tyrannized by a regime which was positively vicious. The Mental Hygiene Society, which he established in 1909, turned into the National Committee for Mental Hygiene, a campaigning force for mental health, first in the United States and then more widely, pledged to improve the standard of care available for the mentally ill, raise the level of professional psychiatric training, and promote mental hygiene through public education.

Meantime, other voices had been criticizing the asylums, not for their lapses into cruelty but on the grounds that they were misconceived and counter-productive. Around 1840 the American physician, Edward Jarvis (1803–1884), visiting Conolly's Hanwell Asylum, just outside London, had this to say on how the ideals of that asylum were being undermined by size and economy:

> This is a huge establishment. . . . Here hundreds are gathered and crowded. The rulers prefer such large asylums. They think them economical. They save the pay of more superintendents, physicians, and other upper officers; but they diminish the healing powers of the hospital. . . . The economy is not wise, or successful.

The National Association for the Promotion of Social Science, founded in 1856 by philanthropists, statisticians and reformers, pondered as early as 1869 whether

> we cannot recur, in some degree, to the system of home care and home treatment; whether, in fact, the same care, interest, and money which are now employed upon the inmates of our lunatic asylums, might not produce even more successful and beneficial results if made to support the efforts of parents and relations in their humble dwelling.

At roughly the same time, the asylum superintendent, John Arlidge (1822–99), concluded, 'a giant asylum is a giant evil.'

Asylums provided a mountain of information to support new models and classifications of mental diseases, enabling diagnosticians to build up clearly defined pictures of psychiatric diseases, capable of being recognized symptomatically. General paresis was described in 1822 by Antoine Laurent Bayle (1799–1858). Although the causative micro-organism of syphilis remained unknown, the neurological and psycho-logical features of general paresis (euphoria and expansiveness), combined with its distinctive organic changes as revealed by autopsy, strengthened the hand of those who believed that psychiatric diseases could be described using the techniques employed by Laennec and Louis with tuberculosis. Early volumes of the *Annales médico-psychologiques* reflect this clinico-pathological orientation.

The confinement and isolation of the mentally ill created opportunities for the accumulation of observations on patient behaviour and symptoms, leading to new descriptions and illness classifications. Epileptics, for instance, began to be segregated from the insane, and in 1815 Esquirol organized a special hospital for them, fearing they would worsen the mentally disturbed. By 1860, special epileptic hospitals had been founded in France, Britain and Germany, and in 1891 the first American hospital was established in Gallipolis, Ohio. Esquirol produced an improved description of *petit mal*; Calmeil described 'absence', distinguishing between passing mental confusion and the onset of a *grand mal* attack, and W. R. Gowers (1845–1915) clarified the 'aura'. A major therapeutic step dates from 1912, when phenobarbital was found effective in suppressing epileptic seizures.

There were comparable developments in asylums for so-called 'idiots'. Idiotism had long been accepted as hopeless: 'absolute idiocy admits of no cure,' noted the nineteenth-century psychiatrist George Man Burrows (1771–1846). But Enlightenment optimism led some physicians to believe that much could be done with the mentally deficient. Inspired by Condillac's utilitarian psychology and by experiments with blind, deaf and feral children, special schools were set up, first of all in France. The great pioneer was the physician and educator Edouard Séguin (1812–80), who, like so many others, migrated to the New World to realize his utopian dreams. He was confident that colonies of defectives, headed by valiant paternalistic pedagogues, could be disciplined into normalcy, ultimately rejoining society as productive workers.

Training also became the keynote in the major idiots' asylums established in mid Victorian England. Five rural colonies were created around the middle of the century, most famously Earlswood near Redhill in Surrey. By herding together large numbers of 'abnormal' people, these in turn prompted the framing of new medical categories. The mongoloid type, or Down's Syndrome, was first identified at Earlswood by Dr John Langdon Down (1828–96). Hopes were expressed that stimulating institutional environments would lead to mental improvement, but in due course such colonies became essentially segregative, isolating 'defectives' to stop them from breeding. In a notorious American legal ruling of 1927, Justice Oliver Wendell Holmes (1841–1935) ruled that 'three generations of imbeciles are enough'.

GERMAN PSYCHIATRY

Germany also developed prominent lunatic asylums, notably Illenau in Baden-Baden, where Richard von Krafft-Ebing (1840–1902) gained early clinical experience. But, unlike Britain or France, German psychiatry was chiefly associated with the universities and their research-oriented medicine. Perhaps for this reason, it became embroiled in sharper debates between rival organic and psychological traditions. At the beginning of the century, Johann Christian Reil (1759–1813) developed a holistic approach, somatically based yet indebted to Romanticism, and with an emphasis on psychodynamics. His *Rhapsodien über die Anwendung der psychischen Curmethode auf Geisteszerrütingen* (1803) [Rhapsodies on the Use of Psychological Treatment Methods in Mental Breakdown] offered a version of moral treatment: the charismatic alienist with a powerful personality commanding the patient's imagination; a staff trained in play-acting to further the alienist's efforts to expel the patient's fixed ideas – all this combined with salutary doses of therapeutic terror (sealing-wax dropped onto the palms, whipping with nettles, submersion in a tub of eels) to overwhelm the patient. His *Magazin für die psychische Heilkunde* (1805) [Journal for Psychological Therapy] helped put German psychiatry on the map.

The psychological approach to madness was developed with J. C. A. Heinroth (1773–1843) and Karl Ideler (1795–1860). This also drew heavily on Romanticism, with its speculative metaphysics and empathetic exploration of the inner consciousness. A pious Catholic who taught psychiatric medicine at Leipzig University, Heinroth viewed mental disorder in religious terms, and the aetiological explanations offered in his *Lehrbuch der Störungen des Seelenlebens* (1818) [Textbook of Mental Disturbances] disparaged physical causes. He compared insanity and sin; both were voluntary and hence transgressive renunciations of the rational free will which was God's gift. Moral treatment must expose the madman to the healthy and religious personality of the alienist. 'In the great majority of cases,' he insisted, 'it is not the body but the soul itself from which mental disturbances directly and primarily originate.' He proposed a combination of gentle therapies with severe methods (shock, restraint and punishments) for intractable conditions. Each case required individual diagnosis and prescription, for which detailed case histories were essential.

Other German psychiatrists deplored the speculative fantasies of such 'psychicists', which they associated with the anti-scientific tendencies of Romanticism, cultivating instead an organic orientation which looked for its model to the prestigious science of physics. In this Maximilian Jacobi (1775–1858) was the key early figure, but the main aetiological assumptions were laid down in J. B. Friedreich's (1796–1862) *Versuch einer Literärgeschichte der Pathologie und Therapie der Psychischen Krankenheiten* (1830) [Attempt at a History of the Literature of the Pathology and Therapy of Psychic Illnesses]. Rebutting Heinroth, Friedreich stressed material causes. The Viennese physician Ernst von Feuchtersleben (1806–49) aimed to weave psychic and somatic strands into a personality-based psychiatry, aiming for an ambitious synthesis of neurophysiology, psychology and psychotherapeutics. To Feuchtersleben, developing something akin to the modern concept of 'psychosis', 'psychopathy' meant a disease of the whole personality.

The core tradition of German university psychiatry was founded by Wilhelm Griesinger (1817–68). Sympathetic to the new materialistic currents emerging in the physiology of Helmholtz and du Bois-Reymond, Griesinger boldly asserted that 'mental illnesses are brain diseases'. His insistence that 'every mental disease is rooted in brain disease' encouraged brain pathology research aimed at finding the physical location of mental disorders. Yet even Griesinger conceded in *Pathologie und Therapie der psychischen Krankheiten* (1845) [Pathology and Therapy of Psychiatric Diseases] that not all pathological states were accompanied by detectable cerebral lesions. Mental disease, in his view, was typically progressive, moving from depressive states to more behaviourally and cognitively disruptive conditions. The underlying somatic abnormality would begin with excessive cerebral irritation, leading to chronic, irreversible patho-anatomical brain degeneration, and ending in the disintegration of the ego, common in chronic mania and dementia.

Griesinger's pronouncements defining mental disorder as brain disease ('Psychological diseases are diseases of the brain'; 'insanity itself . . . is only a symptom') had a dogmatic ring. But he qualified them, and his aetiology was multifactorial. Among predisposing and precipitating causes of mental disease, he mentioned heredity, brain inflammation, anaemia, head injury and acute febrile disease; however, he also discussed 'psychical causes'. His stress upon the transition from normal to pathological psychic processes, and on the progressive course of psychiatric illnesses was later taken up by Kraepelin. For Griesinger, belief in the somatic origin of such disorders was meant to give hope to science and restore dignity to patients traditionally stigmatized by a diagnosis of lunacy.

Griesinger set academic psychiatry on course, pressing for the congruence of psychiatry and neurology and for the establishment of neuropsychiatric clinics – campaigns conducted in the *Archiv für Psychiatrie*, which he established in 1868. His Berlin successor, Carl Westphal (1833–90), continued in his tradition of brain psychiatry, publishing monographs on diseases of the brain and spinal cord. After 1850, this kind of university psychiatry prospered in German-speaking Europe, supported by the twin pillars of German medical education, the polyclinic and the research institute. Unlike asylum superintendents in England, the top university psychiatrists did not share their patients' lives night and day, and their orientation was hardly therapeutic. The goal of university psychiatry was more the scientific understanding of psychiatric disorders through systematic observation, experimentation and dissection.

Following Griesinger, Theodor Meynert, Carl Wernicke and other scions of this academic tradition sought to create a rigorous psychiatry wedded to neurology and neuropathology and rooted in scientific materialism. A product of the illustrious Vienna medical school, Meynert (1833–92) spent his entire career there, first as assistant to Rokitansky, and from 1870 as professor of psychiatry. Essentially a neuropathologist and more dogmatically somaticist than Griesinger, he subtitled his textbook, *Klinik der Erkrankungen des Vorderhirns* (1884) [A Clinical Treatise on the Diseases of the Forebrain], in protest against what he condemned as the wishy-washy mentalistic connotations of 'psychiatry'. He conducted distinguished research in neuroanatomy, and his laboratory established his reputation and attracted students including Forel and Wernicke. In practice, however, his organic programme ran into grave problems, and he was reduced to concocting various vague entities, such as the primary and secondary ego, to describe his patients' behavioural and thought disorders.

Wernicke (1848–1905) represents the apogee of German neuro-psychiatry. His lifelong pursuit of cerebral localization centred around a consuming interest in aphasia. He helped establish the concept of cerebral dominance and delineated the symptoms following various sorts of brain damage in two extremely influential texts: his three-volume *Lehrbuch der Gehirnkrankheiten* (1881–3) [Manual of Brain Diseases], and his *Grundriss der Psychiatrie* (2nd ed., 1906) [Foundations of Psychiatry].

DEGENERATION

While claiming their science could provide explanations of the patho-physiological and neurological mechanisms of psychiatric disorders, organicists were far from sanguine about cures. This pessimism, reflected elsewhere, was in part a product of their patient populations; asylums everywhere were filling with patients with intractable and seemingly irreversible organic disease, notably tertiary syphilitics. Therapeutic pessimism bred a new hereditarianism. Advocates of moral therapy and asylum reform had expressed confidence in early treatment and environmental manipulation; by mid century, however, the accumulation of long-stay cases eroded hopes, and attention to family backgrounds suggested inherited psychopathic traits. These observations were systematized into a degenerationist model by two French psychiatrists, Esquirol's pupil J. Moreau de Tours (1804–84) and Benedict Augustin Morel (1809–73), and in England by Henry Maudsley.

Physician to large asylums in Mareville and Saint-Yon, Morel turned degeneration into an influential explanatory principle in his *Traité des dégénérescences physiques et morales* (1857) [Treatise on Physical and Moral Degeneration]. Produced by both organic and social factors, hereditary degeneration was seen by him as cumulative over the generations, descending into imbecility and finally sterility. A typical generational family history might pass from neurasthenia or nervous hysteria, through alcoholism and narcotics addiction, prostitution and criminality, to insanity proper – and finally utter idiocy. Once a family was on the downhill slope the outcome was hopeless. Alcoholism – a concept coined in 1852 by the Swede Magnus Huss (1807–90) – provided a model for a degenerative disease, since it combined the physical and the moral, was widespread among pauper lunatics, and supposedly led to character disintegration. Valentin Magnan (1835–1916) set Morel's theories into the mould of evolutionary and reflex biology with his idea of 'progress or perish'; his opinions were dramatized in Emile Zola's novels, particularly *L'Assommoir* (1877), in which Magnan appears as an asylum doctor.

These French attitudes caught the mood of the times, echoing bourgeois fears in a mass society marked by proletarian unrest and socialist threats. Griesinger acknowledged his debt to Morel, and Meynert, Wernicke and other brain psychiatrists documented the hereditarian dimensions of insanity. Meynert's Viennese successor, Richard von Krafft-Ebing was an exponent of degenerationist thinking. Best known for his *Psychopathia Sexualis* (1866) [Sexual Psychopathology], a study of sexual 'perversion' and 'inversion' (that is, homosexuality), he classified various disorders as *psychische Entartungen*, constitutional degeneration.

Paul Möbius (1854–1907) and Max Nordau (1849–1923) helped to popularize degenerationist thought. Exploring the presumed connexions between genius and insanity, Möbius was intrigued by hypnosis, hysteria and the relations between sexual pathology and madness, publishing widely on sexuality and gender differences. Women were slaves to their bodies: 'Instinct makes the female animal-like.' High intelligence in women was so unusual as to be positively a sign of degeneration. Producing a classification of psychiatric disorders admired by Emil Kraepelin (1856–1926), Möbius endorsed the notion of hereditary degeneration, though his particular fascination was with those called '*dégénérés supérieurs*', i.e. individuals of abnormally high intelligence. He produced 'pathographies' which examined the relationships between genius and insanity through the lives of men such as Rousseau and Goethe.

Morel's ideas were taken up in Italy by the psychiatrist and criminologist Cesare Lombroso (1836–1909), who viewed criminals and psychiatric patients as degenerates, evolutionary throwbacks often identifiable by physical stigmata: low brows, jutting jaws and so forth. Comparable physical evidence of degenerative taints could be found in non-European races, in apes and in children.

A more optimistic reading of tendencies towards degeneration was predictably taken in America. There George M. Beard (1839–83) popularized the concept of 'neurasthenia', regarded as a kind of nervous weakness produced by the frantic pressures of advanced civilization and diagnosed as an early stage of progressive hereditary degeneration, all of which proved a drain on the individual's finite reserve of 'nerve force'. Beard's ideas were developed further by Silas Weir Mitchell of Philadelphia (1829–1914), who introduced the 'Weir Mitchell treatment' (bed rest and strict isolation) as a way of overcoming such tendencies. But American thinking had its darker side too; the filling up of asylums brought fears that insanity was epidemic. The trial in 1881 of Charles Guiteau, the murderer of President Garfield, spotlighted issues of heredity, criminality and moral insanity, since psychiatrists based defence testimonies on their conviction that the assassin was a degenerate. By 1900 lobbies were urging compulsory confinement, sterilization and other eugenic measures, as well as the use of psychiatry for immigration control.

Late nineteenth-century psychiatry also came under other scientific influences. The neurologist John Hughlings Jackson (1834–1911) used the evolutionary philosophy of Herbert Spencer (1820–1903) as the basis for his accounts of nervous function and dysfunction, and Henry Maudsley (1835–1918) developed an outlook heavily influenced by neurology and evolutionary biology. Inspired by the institutional achievements of Kraepelin, and finding asylum psychiatry hamstrung by routine cures, Maudsley laid the foundations for the Maudsley Hospital in his will. It opened in London in 1922. Its medical school, which became the Institute of Psychiatry, was intended as a site where graduate psychiatric training and research could be pursued in conjunction with a large psychiatric hospital.

Kraepelin's work was the culmination of a century of descriptive clinical psychiatry and psychiatric nosology. Building on Karl Kahlbaum's (1828–99) conception of the disease entity as distinct from the patient's psychopathological state, Kraepelin approached his patients as symptom carriers, and his case histories concentrated on the core signs of each disorder. Combining earlier descriptions by Kahlbaum (*catatonia*), Morel (*démence précoce*) and Ewald Hecker (1843–1909) (*hebephrenia*) into a single category, he formulated the idea of *dementia praecox*, a degenerative condition, which was the forerunner of schizophrenia, distinguishing it from manic-depressive psychoses (Falret's old 'circular insanity'). Kraepelin's classification remains the framework for much modern psychiatry – indeed, his textbook can be seen as the forerunner of today's *Diagnostic and Statistical Manuals*. His interest in the natural history of mental disorders involved him in the entire life histories of his patients in a longitudinal perspective which privileged prognosis.

A follower of the great experimental psychologist Wilhelm Wundt (1832–1920), Kraepelin also pioneered psychological testing in psychiatric patients and made quantitative correlations between bodily state and mental disorders. Fostering research, his Munich clinic became an international attraction and the inspiration for similar establishments elsewhere. Among his colleagues was Alois Alzheimer (1864–1915), whose researches into dementia led to the formulation of Alzheimer's disease.

Heredity played a part in his conceptual framework, but Kraepelin was critical of the wider theory of degenerationism – one point he had in common with Freud, though in general they viewed each other warily. With only nominal expectations about the efficacy of treatment, Kraepelin was gloomy about the outcome of major psychiatric disorders, especially *dementia praecox*. By 1900 the optimism for curability with which the nineteenth century had opened had almost entirely run into the sands; the asylums had filled up with patients for whom cures were no longer expected. 'We know a lot and can do little,' commented Georg Dobrick, a German asylum doctor, in 1910.

It is not surprising that psychiatry seemed to many to turn into society's policeman or gate-keeper, designed to police the boundaries between the sane and the insane, the normal and the pathological. When such attitudes linked up with degenerationism and eugenics, it could lead to psychiatric politics in which it would be decided that the lives of the mentally ill were not 'worth living' and were a threat to society; from the 1930s, Nazi psychiatry decided that schizophrenics as well as Jews had to be eliminated.

To some degree in reaction against the hopelessness of asylum psychiatry and the dogmatism of the somaticists, a new dynamic psychiatry appeared in the late nineteenth century. Its historical roots include Mesmer's therapeutic use of 'animal magnetism', later called hypnotism by the Manchester surgeon James Braid (1795–1860). With its dissociations and apparent automatism of behaviour, hypnotism unveiled hitherto hidden dimensions and layers of the personality and raised new issues about the will, unconscious thinking and the unity of the self.

Linked to scientific exploration of mediums and spiritualism, the dynamic aspects of the psyche were investigated by physicians such as A. A. Lièbault (1823–1904) and H. M. Bernheim (1840–1919) in Nancy, while Jean-Martin Charcot (1825–93) made hypnotism central to his hysteria studies. At his clinic at the Salpêtrière, the giant public hospital in Paris, Charcot demonstrated the diagnostic potential of hypnotism and developed ideas of the aetiology of hysteria and related neuroses. Addressing its manifestations, he undertook a massive clinical scrutiny of hysterical pathology, exploring motor and sensory symptoms, bizarre visual abnormalities, tics, migraine, epileptiform seizures, somnambulism, hallucinations, word blindness, alexia, aphasia, mutism, contractures, hyperaesthesias, and numerous other deficits – and had some measure of success in mapping hysteria onto the body. He was delighted, for instance, to discover hysterogenic points, zones of hypersensitivity which, when fingered, provoked an attack; it confirmed his conviction of the reality of 'latent hysteria'. Yet his early faith that scientific investigation into hysteria would systematically reveal demonstrable neurological substrates proved a forlorn hope.

Charcot made extensive use of hypnosis as a diagnostic device to uncover hysteria. What he failed to realize was that the hypnotic and hysterical behaviours of his 'star' hysterical performers were artefacts produced by his own personality and expectations within the theatrical and highly charged atmosphere of the Salpêtrière, not objective phenomena waiting to be scientifically observed. He deceived himself into thinking his patients' behaviours were real rather than the products of suggestion. The months Sigmund Freud spent in Paris in 1885 were crucial to his development, and psychoanalysis has never been able to escape the charge that, as with Charcot, its 'cures' are largely the product of suggestion.

FREUD

Trained in Vienna in medicine and physiology, Freud (1856–1939) received his MD in 1881, specializing in clinical neurology. Working with the Viennese physician Josef Breuer (1842–1925), he became alerted to the affinities between hypnosis, hysteria and neuroses. Breuer told Freud about a patient, 'Anna O.', whose bizarre hysterical symptoms he treated from 1880 by inducing hypnotic states during periods of 'absence' (dissociation), systematically leading her back to the onset of each symptom, one by one. On re-experiencing the precipitating traumas, the relevant hysterical symptom vanished. The time Freud spent with Charcot gave him a theoretical framework for understanding

Breuer's experiences – not least a hint of the sexual origin of hysteria ('*c'est toujours la chose génitale,*' Charcot confided to him). When he returned to Vienna, Freud and Breuer began a close collaboration that resulted in 1895 in the publication of their joint *Studien über Hysterie* [Studies on Hysteria].

In the early 1890s Freud developed his theory that neurosis stemmed from early sexual traumas. His hysterical female patients, he then maintained, had been subjected to pre-pubescent 'seduction' – that is, sexual abuse by the father; repressed memories of such assaults were the triggers of their trouble. He spelt out this 'seduction theory' to his friend Wilhelm Fliess in May 1893, and during the next three years his enthusiasm for his shocking hypothesis mounted until, on 21 April 1896, he went public in a lecture in Vienna on the aetiology of hysteria.

The next year, however, on 21 September 1897, he confessed to Fliess, 'I no longer believe in my *neurotica*' – that is, the seduction theory. Freud had convinced himself that his patients' seduction stories were fantasies, originating not in the perverse deeds of adults but in the erotic wishes of infants. The collapse of the seduction theory brought the birth of the idea of infantile sexuality and the Oedipus complex – first disclosed to Fliess a month later:

> I have found love of the mother and jealousy of the father in my own case too, and now believe it to be a general phenomenon of early childhood . . . if that is the case, the gripping power of *Oedipus Rex*, in spite of all the rational objections to the inexorable fate that the story presupposes, becomes intelligible. . . . Every member of the audience was once a budding Oedipus in phantasy . . .

Up to his very last publication in 1939 Freud held to its importance: 'If psycho-analysis could boast of no other achievement than the discovery of the repressed Oedipus complex, that alone would give a claim to be included among the precious new acquisitions of mankind.' The twin pillars of orthodox psychoanalytic theory – the unconscious and infantile sexuality – thus emerged from Freud's *volte face*; had the seduction theory not been abandoned, psychoanalysis would not exist.*

---

* In his *The Assault on Truth* (1983), Jeffrey Masson has argued that Freud got it right first time; it was the abandonment of the seduction theory that was the error, a betrayal of the truth and of his patients. This betrayal was in part due to the death of Freud's father in October 1896: thenceforth Papa Sigmund stood in the father's shoes; psychoanalysis was a cover-up.

In due course, tensions separated Freud from Breuer, who favoured physiological hypotheses and the use of hypnotic techniques. Freud moved more in the direction of psychological mechanisms, abandoning hypnosis and developing psychoanalysis. He advanced challenging theoretical concepts such as unconscious mental states and their repression, infantile sexuality and the symbolic meaning of dreams and hysterical symptoms, and he prized the investigative techniques of free association and dream interpretation, two methods for overcoming resistance and uncovering hidden unconscious wishes.

In his *Introductory Lectures* (1916–17), Freud promoted the notion of conversion as a 'puzzling leap from the mental to the physical', and continued to describe hysterical symptoms as symbolic representations of unconscious conflicts. During the First World War, his ideas about the psychogenesis of hysterical symptoms were applied to shellshock and other war neuroses: soldiers displaying paralysis, muscular contracture, and loss of sight, speech and hearing with no apparent organic basis were regarded as suffering from conversion hysteria. Though in principle still committed to scientific biology, in reality Freud explained psycho-dynamics without reference to neurology.

His ideas became central to the twentieth-century understanding of the self – among them the dynamic unconscious and the insights into it afforded by free association; the meaning of dreams; repression and defence mechanisms; infantile sexuality; the sexual foundations of neurosis and the therapeutic potential of transference.

In his later years, while continuing to elaborate his theories of individual psychology – for example, developmental phases, the death instinct, the ego, superego and id – Freud extended his insights into the social, historical, cultural and anthropological spheres, including psychohistorical studies of Leonardo da Vinci, the origins of incest taboos, patriarchy and monotheism. He saw himself as a natural scientist, but his ideas enjoyed their main impact in other fields. With its new view of the personality, Freudian psychoanalysis changed the self-image of the western mind.

PSYCHOANALYSIS

Freud visited the New World in 1909, and psychoanalysis proved particularly influential in the United States, with a number of pioneer analysts emigrating there, notably Alfred Adler (1870–1937) and Helene Deutsch (1884–1982).

Adler is remembered largely for his theory of inferiority: a neurotic individual would over-compensate by manifesting aggression. After participating in the psychoanalytic circle of Sigmund Freud in its early years, he broke with orthodox Freudianism and elaborated his own theory in *Über den nervösen Charackter* (1912) [The Nervous Character]. Later, he directed his psychological theories to exploring the social relations between individual and environment, stressing the need for social harmony as the way to avoid neurosis. His views became part of an American commitment to social stability based on individual adjustment and adaptation to healthy social forms.

There was a strong Swiss tradition in psychiatry. Eugen Bleuler (1857–1939) at Burghölzli, the Zürich psychiatric hospital, deployed psychoanalytic theories in his descriptions of schizophrenia, a term he coined for the illness idea he developed from Kraepelin's *dementia praecox*. But it was Carl Jung's (1875–1961) influence which was predominant, especially after he broke with Freud in 1912 and developed 'analytical psychology', a less sexual vision of the unconscious psyche. A pastor's son, Jung trained in medicine in his native Basel before specializing in psychiatry. After meeting Freud in 1907, he was for a few years the master's favourite son. Schisms developed, however, worsened in 1912 when Jung's *Wandlungen und Symbole der Libido* [The Psychology of the Unconscious] repudiated many of Freud's key theories (e.g., the sexual origin of the neuroses), and by 1914 the rift was complete.

Jungian analytic psychology claimed to offer a more balanced view than Freud of the psyche and its different personality types, developing the concepts of the extravert and introvert in his *Psychologische Typen* (1921) [Psychological Types]. He prized a healthy balance of opposites (animus and anima, the male and female sides of the personality), and was fascinated by the symbiosis of thought, feeling and intuition. He maintained the existence of a 'collective unconscious', stocked with latent memories from mankind's ancestral past. Studies of dreams, of art and anthropology led to a fascination with archetypes and myths (e.g., the earth mother), which he believed filled the collective unconscious, shaping experience, and, as stressed in his final book, *Mensch und Seine Symbole* (1964) [Man and His Symbols] forming the springs of creativity. With its vision of the self finding realization in the integrated personality, Jung's analytic psychiatry remains inspirational on 'new age' thinking as a personal philosophy of life.

In France Pierre Janet (1859–1947) elaborated theories of personality development and mental disorders which long dominated French dynamic psychiatry. Exploring the unconscious, Janet has left sensitive clinical descriptions of hysteria, anorexia, amnesia and obsessional neuroses, and of their treatment with hypnosis, suggestion and other psychodynamic techniques. He proposed a general theory to account for mental phenomena, correlating hysteria with what he called 'subconscious fixed ideas' and proposing to treat it with 'psychological analysis'. There were many similarities between Janet's views and early Freudian psychoanalysis.

Psychoanalysis spread rather slowly to the United Kingdom. There was, perhaps, a deep-rooted Anglo-Saxon distrust of depth psychiatry. Mental disturbances and other personal crosses were viewed as private tragedies, to be coped with domestically, with the aid of a discreet family doctor and trusty retainers. An early British Freudian, David Eder (1866–1936), recalled addressing a paper in 1911 to the Neurological Section of the British Medical Association on a case of hysteria treated by Freud's method. At the end of his talk, the entire audience, including the chairman, rose and walked out in icy silence. The distinguished psychiatrist, Charles Mercier (1852–1919), a one-time colleague of Hughlings Jackson, gloated in 1916 that 'psychoanalysis is past its perihelion, and is rapidly retreating in to the dark and silent depths from which it emerged. It is well that it should be systematically described before it goes to join pounded toads and sour milk in the limbo of discarded remedies.'

Nevertheless inroads were made, aided by the crisis in explanations produced by shellshock during the First World War. The main pioneering individual in spreading the gospel was Ernest Jones (1879–1958). A founder of the London Society of Psychoanalysis (1913) (reborn in 1919 as the British Society for Psychoanalysis), the Welshman Jones became a close friend of Freud and later his biographer. In 1912, he brought out the first book published in England in this field: *Papers on Psycho-Analysis*. His ebullient personality, vanity and extraordinary energies made him a born proselytizer. Later, Melanie Klein (1882–1960) and Anna Freud (1895–1982) enriched the scene, Anna having fled to England with her father in 1938. Freudians and Kleinians crossed swords over the interpretation of the infant unconscious; in London the Tavistock Clinic promoted the cause of psychotherapy, especially for children and families.

Perhaps shocked into modernity by the horrors of the war, the lay public became increasingly receptive. In the 1910s the number of publications noting psychoanalytical matters was increasing. In 1919, it was reported that interest in psychoanalysis was 'now growing by leaps and bounds'; Freud's books, grumbled *The Saturday Review*, were now 'discussed over the soup with the latest play or novel', while 'every moderately well-informed person now knows something about Jung and Freud.' On the whole, the press preferred Jung's theories to Freud's, finding the latter's sexual views 'repugnant to our moral sense'.

In due course, the spread of Freudian notions led to his ideas gaining ground – it became reputable in the inter-war years and conventional by the 1950s that ordinary people might have 'complexes', and that neuroses ran like a watermark through the population at large: juvenile delinquency, housewife blues, family conflicts, alcoholism, adjustment problems, generational tensions and so forth. By the 1950s, popular psychological culture had created new and exciting images like the 'crazy mixed-up kid' – the more modern and down-market version of the melancholy poet or Romantic genius.

The psychiatrization of everything occurred first in the United States. It was a trend deliciously mocked in some of Stephen Sondheim's lyrics to *West Side Story* (1956), in which the crazy mixed-up young New Yorkers taunt the police officer on the warpath:

> Officer Krupke, you're really a square;
> This boy don't need a judge, he needs an analyst's care!
> It's just his neurosis that oughta be curbed,
> He's psychologic'ly disturbed.
> We're disturbed, we're disturbed, we're the most disturbed,
> Like we're psychologic'ly disturbed.

DESPERATE REMEDIES

The phenomenal growth of psychoanalysis overshadowed developments in the medical treatment of mental problems. The consequences of bacterial infections for brain function were identified, beginning with syphilis, and Julius Wagner-Jauregg (1857–1940) discovered that counter-infection with malaria was effective against general paresis of the insane. Medicine developed a variety of techniques for treating neurosis or psychoses – some successful, others dangerous failures. Insulin was employed against schizophrenia. Though hazardous, insulin shock brought some positive results. While working with epileptics, Ladislaus Joseph Meduna (1896–1965) developed a shock treatment in which camphor was the convulsive agent, producing convulsions so violent that patients suffered broken bones. In 1938, working at a neuropsychiatric clinic in Genoa, Ugo Cerletti (1877–1963), began to use electric shocks (ECT) for alleviating symptoms in severe depression. Psychosurgery too enjoyed popularity in the 1930s and 1940s. At Lisbon University, Egas Moniz (1874–1955) claimed that obsessive and melancholic cases could be improved by frontal leucotomy, surgical severance of the connections of the frontal lobes with the rest of the brain. Although he received universal acclaim and a Nobel Prize in 1949, Moniz was attacked for altering the mental states of individuals.

Such developments – violent, invasive and frankly experimental – signal the desperation of well-meaning psychiatrists to do something for the masses of forgotten patients in asylums. Equally, they reflect the powerlessness of those patients in the face of reckless doctors, and the ease with which they become experimental fodder.

MODERN DEVELOPMENTS

From the mid twentieth century expectations rose for psychopharmacology. The first psychotropic drug, lithium, was used to manage manic depression in 1949. Antipsychotic and antidepressant compounds, notably the phenothiazines (Largactil – referred to by its critics as the 'liquid cosh') and imipramine, were developed in the early 1950s. The prominent British psychiatrist William Sargant (1907–88) saw in the new drugs a release from the shadowland of the asylum and the folly of Freudianism. Drugs, he said, would enable doctors to 'cut the cackle', predicting that the new psychotropic drugs would eliminate the problem of mental illness by the 1990s. Psychopharmacology certainly brought a new self-confidence and therapeutic optimism to the psychiatric profession. It promised a relatively safe, cost-effective method of alleviating mental suffering without recourse to lengthy hospital stays, psychoanalysis or irreversible surgery. It also restored psychiatry's wishful identity as a 'hard' science.

Growing reliance on psychotropic drugs seemed one solution to the problem of the asylum. The more forward-looking psychiatrists of the inter-war years in Europe and America had grown critical of the old mental hospitals which haunted the landscape. Not least, their putatively clear segregation of the sane from the mad no longer seemed to make epidemiological sense. Psychiatrists increasingly voiced the view that the bulk of mental disorders were to be found not among asylum populations but in the community at large. The emphasis was falling upon neuroses not severe enough to warrant hospitalization or certification but considered to be endemic. 'During the last 30 years,' Willy Mayer-Gross tellingly noted, 'the interest of psychiatry has shifted from the major psychoses, statistically relatively rare occurrences, to the milder and borderline cases, the minor deviations from the normal average.' Psychiatry needed to become properly informed about apparently new patterns of morbidity.

Psychiatric attention was thereby being extended to 'milder' and 'borderline' cases, and mental abnormality began to be seen as part of normal variability. A new social psychiatry was being formulated, whose purview extended over an entire populace. The implied blurring of the polar distinction between sane and insane was to have momentous practical consequences for custody and care. As emphasis tilted from institutional provision *per se* to the clinical needs of the patient, it pointed in the direction of the 'unlocked door', prompting a growth in outpatients' clinics, psychiatric day hospitals and regular visiting, and encouraging treatments which emphasized discharge. These developments presaged the waning of the asylum era.

Yet that passage was not smooth. Some hoped to effect a modernization of the mental hospital from within, and from the late 1940s a few English mental hospitals unlocked their doors. 'Therapeutic communities' were set up – distinct units of up to a hundred patients within the larger hospitals – in which physicians and patients cooperated to create more positive therapeutic environments, eroding authoritarian hierarchies between staff and inmates. A therapeutic community designed for the rehabilitation of those with personality disorders was established at Belmont Hospital by Maxwell Jones (1907–1990), ushering in ideas of shared decision-making and an increasingly relaxed atmosphere.

Others insisted on far more drastic measures. This led to the 1960s' antipsychiatry movement, with three main beliefs: mental illness was not an objective behavioural or biochemical phenomenon but a label; madness had a truth of its own; and, under the right circumstances, psychotic madness could be a healing process and should not be pharmacologically suppressed.

The most charismatic proponent of antipsychiatry was Ronald Laing (1927–89), a Scottish psychiatrist influenced by existential philosophers. In 1965 Laing established an antipsychiatric community ('hospital' was deliberately avoided) at Kingsley Hall in a working-class London neighbourhood, where patients and psychiatrists lived under the same roof. Psychiatrists were said to 'assist' patients in living through the full-scale regression entailed by schizophrenia. An attractive writer, Laing in particular won a following among liberal intelligentsia at the time of the counter-culture and student protests against the Vietnam War. Films like *Family Life* (1971) and *One Flew Over the Cuckoo's Nest* (1975) mobilized public feeling against the policing role of psychiatry and the ageing asylums.

The movement had many centres. Its chief American spokesman was Thomas Szasz (b. 1920); in France Michel Foucault (1926–84) lent his support. Antipsychiatry gave impetus to the deinstitutionalization of the insane in the late 1970s and the 1980s. At the same time, and from a different angle, politicians took up the cause of community care, keen to reduce costly psychiatric beds and to phase out mental hospitals. Enoch Powell, British minister of health, announced in 1961 that the old mental hospitals ('isolated, majestic, imperious, brooded over by the gigantic watertower and chimney combined, rising unmistakable and daunting out of the countryside') should be scaled down or closed down, and that those requiring in-patient treatment should be treated by local hospitals.

The question of the reality of psychiatric diseases continues problematic. With each new edition of the *Diagnostic and Statistical Manual* of the American Psychiatric Association, some disorders disappear and others appear, including 'post-traumatic stress disorder' and 'attention deficit disorder'. There are now tens of thousands of people in the United States claiming that parental abuse in childhood has produced major psychological trauma, the repressed memory of which is being recovered thanks to the ministrations of their psychoanalysts. Sceptics claim that such 'recovered memories' memories are false and pure arte-facts created by the suggestion of psychotherapists, and licensed by fashionable diagnostics.

The antipsychiatry movement has now largely spent its force. But as the end of the twentieth century approaches, psychiatry lacks unity and remains hostage to the mind-body problem, buffeted back and forth between psychological and physical definitions of its object and its techniques. Drug treatments have become entrenched. During the 1960s, the tranquillizer Valium (1963: diazepam) became the most widely prescribed drug in the world; also important were Miltown (1955) and Librium (1960). For a decade and more, central nervous system drugs have been the leading class of drugs sold domestically by American manufacturers, usually accounting for about one fourth of all sales. Such preparations, developed in the last three decades, have permitted treatment of the mentally disturbed on an outpatient basis and substan-tially reduced the numbers of institutionalized mental patients. The most explosive growth, however, has been in psychotherapy, where techniques involving group sessions, family therapy, sensitivity training, consciousness-raising, game- and role-playing, and behaviour modifi-cation through stimulus and reinforcement have transformed treatment of mental problems.

During the last twenty years, growing cynicism, patients' rights lobbies, the exposure of administrative abuses and similar scandals, feminism, and other critical currents have questioned and undermined dramatically the standing of orthodox professional psychiatric services and Freudian psychoanalysis. The psychiatric profession has become a sitting target for the press and politicians.

At the beginning of the twentieth century the *British Medical Journal* was upbeat: 'In no department of medicine, perhaps, is the contrast between the knowledge and practice in 1800 and the knowledge and practice in 1900 so great as in the department that deals with insanity.' Not so the *Journal of Mental Science*. Pointing in the same year to the 'apparent inefficacy of medicine in the cure of insanity', it took the gloomy view: 'Though medical science has made great advances during the nineteenth century, our knowledge of the *mental* functions of the brain is still comparatively obscure.' The *Lancet* managed to look in both directions at once, editorializing in 1913 that only then and belatedly was 'British psychiatry beginning to awake from its lethargy'.

The close of the twentieth century may bring the same variety of diagnoses on developments within psychiatry. For some, it has been the century when the true dynamics of the mind have been revealed by Freud; for others, psychoanalysis was a huge sideshow, and at last the organic understanding of the brain is resulting in effective drugs, including, most recently, the anti-depressant Prozac. Within five years of its introduction, eight million people had taken Prozac, which was supposed to make people feel 'better than well'.

The trump card of a new science of the brain has often enough been played, unsuccessfully, in the history of the discipline, and the claims of brain scientists to understand consciousness and its terrors have been shown to be shallow, indeed deluded. Whether civilization's treatment of the mentally ill has become more humane in a century which gassed to death tens of thousands of schizophrenics is a question which permits no comforting answers about rationality and sanity.

CHAPTER XVII

MEDICAL RESEARCH

LAUNCHING A RESEARCH TRADITION

DURING THE SEVENTEENTH-CENTURY SCIENTIFIC REVOLUTION, controversies flared about the proper relations between theory and practice, science and craft, and pure and applied knowledge. The Baconian tradition stressed the marriage of thought and action through experimentation; the scientific society, the private laboratory and other institutions formal and informal put the programme into practice. All these were to have lasting significance for medicine, alongside a further bone of contention: the ethics of the links between the advancement of knowledge and the relief of suffering.

Yet, for long, debates about the methodology of natural philosophy touched medicine only obliquely. Medicine continued to rely upon its own canonical texts, and had its own procedures and sites for pursuing knowledge: the bedside and the anatomy theatre. Most doctors swore by the tacit knowledge at their fingers' ends, and in their heads, which they acquired in going about the quotidian business of tending the sick. Even those anxious to make a name for themselves through authorship tended to operate within conventional frameworks. In his London practice, Thomas Sydenham observed the natural history of seasonal fevers like a good Hippocratic, and Morgagni cut up bodies much as anatomists had been doing for a couple of hundred years. Being guided by practice and case-oriented, medicine was slow to change. The microscope had been in existence for two hundred years before it became part of everyday medical practice and transformed understanding.

Nineteenth-century observers noted that in many theatres of life what had once been personal and subjective was becoming formalized. 'It is the Age of Machinery', declared Thomas Carlyle, 'in every outward and inward sense of that word; the age which, with its whole undivided might, forwards, teaches and practises the great art of adapting means to ends. Nothing is now done directly, or by hand; all is by rule and calculated contrivance.' Teaching, administration, organization, licensing, certification, the dissemination of knowledge – all changed in line with Carlyle's dictum; scholarly journals proliferated, and soon there were international conferences. The first was held in Paris in 1867; the seventh, in London in 1881, attracted more than 3000 participants from seventy countries. Increasing specialization can be seen from the growing list of topics covered: hygiene (from 1852), ophthalmology (1857), otology (1876), tuberculosis (1888), dermatology (1889), physiology (1889) and psychology (1890).

Medicine too was mechanized in the wider, Carlylean sense, and the pursuit of medical knowledge was increasingly carried out by teams in institutions, in a planned and organized way which obeyed the division of scientific labour, whether following the model of Paris hospital medicine or of Liebig's chemist-breeding laboratory. The virtues of the new order were thoroughness and efficiency; the methods of discovery had been discovered, innovativeness made routine. 'The future belongs to science', declared William Osler (1849–1919).

These developments threw up thorny problems. Could any single individual now know all, in the manner of Galen or the polymath Haller? Was specialization to be welcomed or resisted – was it even quackery in new guise? Must the good clinician be a generalist (given that the sick person was a whole, a union of the mental and the physical) or should he be the master of a single organ, one particular body system, one investigatory technique? More difficult perhaps, how was medicine to relate to the wider sciences of nature and living systems? How was it to interact with the rapidly expanding domains of physiology, chemistry, zoology and botany, physics, and (more broadly still) with the philosophy of science? Paris patho-anatomy had assumed the autonomy and sovereignty of medicine as a discipline: it would fathom disease, the whole disease and nothing but the disease. But all subsequent nineteenth-century developments were implicit demonstrations that pure pathology couldn't operate in isolation; the physician or medical scientist needed to assimilate other bodies of knowledge: physiology, biology, histology, cytology, neurology, chemistry, physics, statistics, sociology and so on.

How, then, should this knowledge be mastered? How should the young medical student best be instructed? Should research and specializ-ation be encouraged to instil the severe discipline of science? Or was clinical acumen paramount? Not least, was there a gold standard in medical knowledge? Were mechanical or molecular models uniquely compelling, because physics and chemistry were exact sciences, objective and numerical? Or were they misleading because they were reductionist, hence blind to the power of organization and the spark of life? For similar reasons, might it be misleading to make inferences to life itself from the phenomena of dead bodies and to disease in the living? And what of vivisection experiments? Could one draw reliable inferences from animals to humans? Or did artificial experimental conditions produce only misleading findings, inapplicable to the daily realities of sickness and recovery among humans with minds and emotions?

Many debated these issues and their wider ramifications for philo-sophy, ethics and truth, and reflections like Claude Bernard's *Introduction à l'étude de la médecine expérimentale* (1865) [Introduction to the Study of Experimental Medicine] attained classic status. As already seen, the debates between Pasteur and Pouchet over spontaneous generation were about metaphysics no less than sound laboratory technique. But medicine never deliberately stopped to resolve the fundamental issues of truth and methods, or questions of the relations between knowledge and healing, basic research, clinical research and bedside practice. These were tackled as they arose, when they were tackled at all. Neither a monarchy nor even a parliament, medicine was a contested field occupied by rivals; it pro-ceeded by opportunities and emergencies, lucky breakthroughs, fortu-itous alliances, national traditions, the alchemy of individuals.

Nothing better describes the modern medical environment than the vision of the struggle for survival conjured up by Darwin's *Origin of Species* (1859): a competitive arena in which adaptation produces niches in which some flourish, develop, innovate or adapt while other thinkers and practices fall by the wayside; nothing is pre-ordained in fulfilment of some overriding transcendental scheme. As with Darwin's vision of nature, the panorama of medicine is an arena of waste, pain, death and imperfect mechanisms – but also remarkable developments.

The nineteenth century brought specialization, bifurcation and frag-mentation in medical research and practice. Anatomy was already established, and human physiology leapt forward in certain directions, including rapid advances in understanding the functions of the lungs and digestive tract and in investigating the composition and functions of the blood. Neurophysiology grappled with the reflex activity of the spinal cord, the electrical properties of nerve fibres and the functions of the brain. By 1900 organic chemistry was making great strides with the study of proteins, enzymes, and nucleic acids, and elucidating the mechanisms of energy production and nutrition. The newly christened biochemistry proceeded to show how cells were regulated by different chemical catalysts (enzymes). Sub-branches of physiology went on to explore how the functions of groups of cells and organs were governed by hormones or reflex pathways in the nervous system. The principle that all living processes could and should be understood in terms of the methods and models of chemistry and physics led to the emergence of a new science: molecular biology.

There was a geography to these developments. After 1850, the main site of medical science moved from France to Germany – 'As regards scientific medicine', remarked the American John Shaw Billings in 1881, 'we are at present going to school in Germany.' 'When I was a student,' wrote his countryman Carl Binger (1889–1976), referring to the first decades of the twentieth century,

> a shift in emphasis had already occurred. The autopsy room, where so many of our predecessors had spent hours of concentrated labor, was giving way to the physiological laboratory, and correspondingly, in the clinic a brilliant and correct diagnosis (sometimes, to be sure, only corroborated at post-mortem examination) was no longer the supreme intellectual achievement. Insight and understanding of mechanisms and processes became increasingly important. The dynamic view was ascendant. No longer were anatomists content with describing bones, muscles, and nerves, or pathologists with describing the gross and microscopic appearances of tissues. Experiment entered all these domains as it did the domain of medicine and surgery, and before long it became difficult to tell from the nature of the problem and the equipment in use what department you were in. The ancient, fixed, traditional academic borders were breaking down.

Bigger and better laboratories were developed to promote research in the blossoming basic sciences: microanatomy, physiology and organic chemistry. In Germany the universities provided its main base, with associated or independent institutes as well. Robert Koch headed four special centres in Berlin, the Institut für Infectionskrankenheiten [Institute for Infectious Diseases], erected in 1891 amid the hoopla over his apparent tuberculosis cure, being especially palatial, doubtless with a view to eclipsing the Institut Pasteur, opened in 1888. Financed by benefactions independent of the state and privately run, it was followed by the seeding of the Instituts Pasteur d'Outre-Mer in Saigon, Nhatrang, Algeria and Tunis, which concentrated on research into plague, cholera and malaria and other diseases afflicting Europeans in hot climates.

A comparable research establishment was set up in London, the British Institute for Preventive Medicine (1891), subsequently renamed, after national heroes, first the Jenner Institute of Preventive Medicine (1899) and then the Lister Institute (1903). While hospital charities prospered in Britain, medical research elicited little generosity, partly because of the intensity of anti-vivisectionism. When the Jenner Institute staged an appeal, less than 6 per cent of its target was attained in two years. Partly for this reason, the British scientific-medical lobby appealed to the state. The case for the endowment of research was recognized in the creation of a Medical Research Committee (later Medical Research Council: MRC), with a budget derived from income collected through the 1911 National Health Insurance scheme, and initially earmarked for investigating tuberculosis. The MRC was to prove influential not just through its role in funding research but as a coordinator of British energies. For example, at a later date it was responsible for the introduction of the randomized controlled clinical trial.

On the initiative of Austin Bradford Hill (1897–1991), professor of medical statistics and epidemiology at the London School of Tropical Medicine and Hygiene, the MRC set up in 1946 a trial of the efficacy against tuberculosis of the new drug streptomycin. Since the drug was in short supply it was considered ethically justifiable to carry out a test in which one group of patients received streptomycin and a control group was treated by traditional methods. The design of the trial followed the recommendations of R. A. Fisher (1890–1962) in his *The Design of Experiments* (1935). The *British Medical Journal (BMJ)* pointed out that this was the first randomized controlled trial reported in human subjects. The test offered 'the clearest possible proof' that acute tuberculosis 'could be halted by streptomycin'. The randomized controlled clinical trial has since become the gold standard for all such studies.

From the early twentieth century, scientific medicine made strides in the United States. The federal bacteriological laboratory attached to the Marine Hospital, Staten Island, New York (1866), grew in significance, becoming in 1930 the National Institutes of Health and relocating to Bethesda (Maryland). The NIH became a major research centre, especially with respect to cancer. Initially, however, medical research was mainly privately financed by 'robber baron' industrialists, notably Andrew Carnegie (1835–1918), John D. Rockefeller (1839–1937), and his son, John Jr (1874–1960), laundering their stupendous business profits. Scottish-born Carnegie made his fortune in iron and steel. Dedicated to the 'survival of the fittest', he upheld the gospel of wealth but believed that a man who *dies* rich 'dies disgraced' – hence his passionate commitment to philanthropy. He was committed to education, and sponsored the investigations into American medical education conducted by Abraham Flexner (1866–1959).

American medical schools had grown up in a competitive market. From the early nineteenth century 'proprietary' (profit-making) medical colleges were set up, attractive to students because they were practically oriented and did not require a long general education. Sixty-two were established between 1802 and 1876, in addition to eleven homoeopathic and four eclectic schools. Quality had been sacrificed to quantity, judged Flexner's *Medical Education in the United States and Canada* (1910). A good medical education, he believed, could be obtained only by reducing their number and improving their standards. Educated at Johns Hopkins and the University of Berlin, he strongly believed that medical schools should be university departments on the German model, situated in big cities where there was abundant clinical material. Of all American medical schools, only five produced research: Harvard and Johns Hopkins, and the Universities of Pennsylvania, Michigan and Chicago.

Flexner was convinced that the key to medical progress and medical education was science. Critical of the French system (too clinical), the British system (decentralized and too clinical in its focus), and of most existing American schools (grossly commercial), Flexner wanted the medical school to be part of a university, with medical students receiving a sound grounding in natural sciences. The medical school of the future should have its own biomedical departments to encourage research; it had to have a teaching hospital and stiff entrance requirements and end with the doctoral degree; and, finding existing lab provision 'wretched',

Flexner insisted that new medical schools must have good scientific facilities. Committed to raising medical standards, he recommended a reduction in the numbers of colleges to thirty-one; students should have at least two years of college education prior to entry, and teachers should be full time, not practising physicians.

The majority of medical schools failed his gold standard test and within ten years forty-six colleges had closed, including most of the colleges for women and blacks (only two colleges for blacks remained). The number of homoeopathic and eclectic schools also declined rapidly. In 1910, 4400 doctors had graduated; by 1920, this had dropped to 3047, indirectly boosting physicians' status and income. The schools that survived and thrived felt compelled to discontinue their proprietary character, to reinforce their links with hospitals and universities, and generally to raise their standards. In return for this, many received substantial financial assistance from the new philanthropic foundations, notably Rockefeller.

A devout Baptist who made his millions through oil, John D. Rockefeller channelled his early giving into religion but later made vast donations to medicine. Here the stimulus came from Frederick T. Gates, the Baptist minister who was his chief adviser. Reading William Osler's textbook, *The Principles and Practice of Medicine* (1892), Gates was shocked to learn how few diseases medicine could treat; he convinced his patron that attempting to change this through investing in scientific medicine would be a worthy cause.

Established in New York in 1901, the Rockefeller Institute for Medical Research was envisaged along Germanic lines – its goal was research, and private practice was strictly forbidden. Abraham Flexner's brother Simon (1863–1946) was appointed director of laboratories. A protégé of William Welch, who had also studied in Europe, Simon Flexner was a fine laboratory scientist in his own right, isolating the *Shigella* organism, a cause of dysentery. At first the institute was devoted entirely to biomedical studies but in 1910 a small hospital, given over to clinical research, was opened. The Rockefeller Institute quickly established itself both as a training ground and as a research site.

Aided by foundations and better schools, medical scientists and clinical investigators began to flourish. The American Society of Clinical Investigation was established in 1907, its membership being restricted to those under the age of forty-five. Its *Journal of Clinical Investigation* (1924) became the world's leading journal of clinical research.

Swayed by the recommendations of the Flexner report, the Rockefeller Foundation made funds available to Johns Hopkins University for the creation of full-time chairs in clinical specialties such as cardiology. Developments of this kind spread in subsequent years – mainly with Rockefeller support – throughout the United States, and many medical schools sprouted their Rockefeller laboratory, building or chair.*

Clinical departments in the medical schools were increasingly staffed by full-time workers, with a view to encouraging research, and this gained further support with the foundation of the National Institutes of Health. What Germany had been in the nineteenth century for medical research, the United States became in the twentieth.

In these matters the United Kingdom lagged. True, physiological research had been put on the map: in 1878 Michael Foster had founded the *Journal of Physiology*, and by 1900 both the British Medical Association (BMA) and the British Association for the Advancement of Science (BAAS) offered specialist physiological sections. But on moving in 1905 from Baltimore to the Regius chair of medicine at Oxford, Sir William Osler was depressed at the educational desert he encountered. The London medical schools were mainly venerable, isolated, self-governing institutions founded before the University of London, with which they had little formal contact. Individual consultants had their fiefdoms but there was no collective encouragement of clinical research; Samuel Gee (1839–1911), a distinguished physician at St Bartholomew's Hospital, had insisted that medicine was in essence an art not a science. Osler had more Flexnerian ideas, favouring 'an active invasion of the hospitals by the universities'.

A Royal Commission on University Education in London under Lord Haldane (1856–1928) initiated change. In his evidence, Abraham Flexner extolled the virtues of German medical education as developed in America, in particular at Johns Hopkins; Osler was stinging in his condemnation of the state of affairs in Britain. The commission recommended in 1913 that academic clinical units, led by full-time professors,

---

* It was not only American institutions that benefited from Rockefeller money. In the UK and elsewhere in Europe, Rockefeller invested vast sums of money in projects, building and posts. When, for example, Medical Research Council funds dwindled, Howard Florey's laboratory in Oxford was supported by Rockefeller money in its researches into penicillin. In return very strict guidelines were specified on the kind of scientific medicine to be pursued.

should be developed in the London medical schools. These were shelved during the war, but in 1919 St Bartholomew's Hospital appointed its first full-time professor of medicine, and by 1925 there were five chairs of medicine among the twelve medical schools in London, with stirrings in the provinces. A long battle followed between full-time academics and part-time consultants, over who was to control medical education and research in England, but the move towards academically controlled medical schools made headway.

Further developments followed. The Athlone Committee (1921) recommended the setting up of a specific school for postgraduate medical education, attached to a hospital dedicated to this purpose. When the existing London teaching hospitals declined to act, it was agreed that the school should be sited at Hammersmith Hospital in west London, a London County Council institution which did not belong to the gilded elite. Hammersmith was opened, finally, in 1935, and proved an important development in British academic medicine, playing a role comparable to that of the Rockefeller Institute Hospital in New York in training clinical research specialists.

Universities and medical schools provided little research money. Finance came from the MRC, and from charities such as the British Heart Foundation, the Imperial Cancer Research Fund and the Wellcome Trust. The MRC gave long-term support to the work of (Sir) Thomas Lewis, pioneer of British cardiology and energetic advocate of full-time clinical research posts, to investigate what he called 'clinical science'. By the early 1930s, Lewis's department at University College Hospital was the Mecca for aspiring clinical research workers.

Not all approved of these developments to give medicine a more scientific edge. Some grieved that the old clinical skills were being edged out. In 1933 the pathologist Sir Andrew Macphail (1864–1938) reflected:

> I am well aware that in these days, when a student must be converted into a physiologist, a physicist, a chemist, a biologist, a pharmacologist, and an electrician, there is no time to make a physician of him. This consummation can only come after he has gone out into the world of sickness and suffering, unless indeed his mind is so bemused by the long process of education in those sciences, that he is forever excluded from the art of medicine. . . .
> In that case he is destined for the laboratory, the professor's chair, or the consultant's office. What would have happened to Sydenham

had he been put through this machinery is a problem in infinity
which no human intelligence is competent to solve.

The remainder of this chapter and Chapter 18 examine some of the
investigations pursued within these frameworks. They are but a bare
sample, for modern medicine is extremely heterogeneous and sub-
divided, with numerous islands of knowledge linked by an erratic network of often temporary bridges. The picture is one of competition
and cooperation, rivalry and symbiosis – universities, hospitals, research
units, government funding agencies and schools of researchers interacting in *ad hoc* and unpredictable combinations. Fields which were
prima facie developing independently have uncovered hidden affinities;
for example, neurology and biochemistry, which usually plough their
own furrows, combined in explanations of the homeostatic mechanisms
of the metabolism or the workings of the brain.

In addressing some of the mainstreams of modern biomedical
research, the links between basic science, clinical research and medical
practice are highlighted. A number of different fields are examined,
beginning with neurology, a discipline with strong foundations in basic
science, since experimentation could be performed upon animals in
laboratories – though for long the therapeutic pay-offs were small. The
tour leads eventually, in the next chapter, to two areas – cancer and
cardiology – where the practical constraints, combating lethal and prevalent diseases, have been paramount.

NEUROLOGY

Neurology took shape within the traditions constructed in the nineteenth century. It thrived on research techniques pioneered in laboratories, drawing on the model of cell tissues that microscopy made
possible, on animal experiments designed to verify nerve pathways, and
on human pathological cases. Investigation of the micro-anatomy of the
nervous system, however, dated back to the seventeenth century, when
nerve endings had been observed in animals by the indefatigable Malpighi. It was greatly forwarded in the nineteenth century by Remak
and Purkinje. Robert Remak (1815–65) revealed how much could be
discovered about the nerves through the microscope. He found sympathetic nerve fibres were grey because they were non-medullated, and

nerve axons were continuous with nerve cells in the spinal cord; he observed the neurolemma (myelin sheath of nerve fibres) and delineated the six cortical cell layers of the cerebrum.

His contemporary, Johannes Purkinje (1787–1869), professor at Prague, conducted analogous research into the microscopic features of the human brain. He too described myelinated nerve fibres and the large flask-like 'cells of Purkinje' characteristic of the cerebellar cortex. Most importantly, he demonstrated that nerve cells had a protoplasm-filled main body (the nucleus) and a fibrous 'tail' (the process) extending from the main body. Soon it was recognized that the long tails were actual nerve fibres, and that every such fibre had a parent cell body, even though this might be several feet distant, as with the nerves of the toes. The nature of the tail was not clear, nor were the nerve cell's role in electrical action and the related question of whether or how the nerve cells were connected.

Another outstanding histologist, Rudolf Albert von Kölliker (1817–1905), author of the first comprehensive histology treatise (1852), showed that nerve fibres were secondary to nerve cells, and that at least some of them were the processes of nerve cells. Augustus Volney Waller (1816–70) discovered that if a bundle of nerve fibres were cut, the parts separated from their cells rapidly degenerated. Wilhelm His (1831–1904), who occupied the anatomy chairs at Basel and Leipzig for forty-seven years, showed in 1887 that axons were outgrowths of primitive nerve cells. All such work yielded information which formed a basis for the neuron theory, formulated in 1891 by Wilhelm Waldeyer (1836–1921).

Understanding of nerve cell function was helped from the 1850s by improvements in methods for sectioning, preserving and staining tissue. It remained very difficult, however, to observe nerve connections micro-scopically, though it had become clear that nerve cells had one main process and that 'nerves' were bundles of these processes. There agree-ment ended. One school of thought argued that the cells were connected by a network of fibres conducting impulses from cell to cell: this was known as the reticular theory. Criticizing this, His suggested that nerve cells had 'free endings' in the central nervous system's grey matter.

Microscopic findings remained contested, and the reticular theory gained support from research by Camillo Golgi (1843–1926), who introduced a new stain for central nervous system tissue using silver chromate, which made the nerve elements appear black when microscopically examined. The Golgi stain revealed the nerve cell clearly, showed its process, and for the first time a large number of shorter processes (dendrites) could be seen. Golgi believed his observations of how axons and dendrites were intricately intermingled supported the reticular position. The function of the axons consisted in conducting the nervous impulse; the role of the dendrites was mainly trophic (nutritional). There were two types of nerve cell, he believed, each characterized by its own type of axonal extension: those with an axon maintaining their individuality and rooted into the medullary fibres; and those whose axon subdivided soon after its origin. He suggested that the former had a motor function and the latter a sensory one.

Golgi was challenged by the Spanish histologist Santiago Ramon y Cajal (1853–1934), a master microscopist whose ambition was to elucidate the brain cell so as to 'know the material course of thought and will'. Ramon y Cajal's theory became the basis for what Waldeyer named the neuron doctrine. This held that each nerve cell was a self-contained unit with an axon reaching towards but not continuous with another cell. Nerve fibres were composed of these processes, but it was the cell that formed the communicating links in nerve tissues. The axons were insulated against one another except for delicate endings, which made contact with the next cell. Nerve circuits were thus valved, with the valves 'where one nerve cell meets the next one'. It was Charles Sherrington (1857–1952) who named that valvular connection (later found to be a gap) the synapse. The neuron theory resolved the question of the direction of nerve currents; histology thus helped to lay bare a structural vision of neuroanatomy. But how did the system work? How did the nerves fulfil the body's purposes?

Beginning with Charles Bell's *Idea of a New Anatomy of the Brain* (1811) and François Magendie's contemporaneous experiments, neurophysiology carved out and ploughed three main fields: reflex action, cerebral localization, and nervous integration. Each had ramifications for understanding disease – for instance, it was known that in certain nervous diseases reflexes of the limbs were diminished or lost; hence, a grasp of reflex action was clinically important.

The basic reflex concept had been formulated by Descartes: a stimulus was transmitted along nerve fibres (afferent) to the central nervous system, where it triggered a fresh impulse which passed along outgoing (efferent) nerve fibres to produce activity in an organ or muscle. To explain nervous activity, Descartes postulated the presence of spirits in

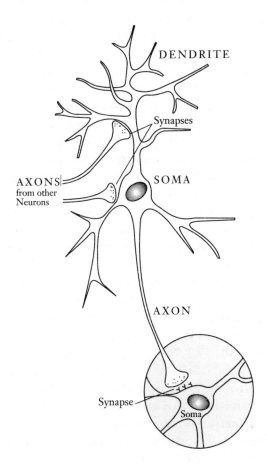

The modern understanding of neurotransmission. Axons from near or distant neurons carry electrical activity which triggers the release of a neurotransmitter at the point of a synapse with another neuron.

the nerves, and hypothesized that the pineal gland, a pea-sized, unitary organ towards the back of the brain, was the seat of the soul, controlling brain function.

Practical investigations into reflex action were pioneered by Stephen Hales, who around 1730 decapitated frogs and found that reflex movements in the legs could still be produced by pricking the skin. These reflex movements ceased, however, if the spinal cord were destroyed.

The Edinburgh professor Robert Whytt (1714–66) confirmed Hales's experiments and established that the spinal cord was essential to the reflex. Whytt believed that the reflex was due to a stimulus acting according to an unconscious sentient principle situated in the brain and cord, relaying the stimulus back to the muscles. Reflex action did not require the integrity of the cord as a whole, because stimulation of the skin would produce a reflex even if only a small segment remained intact. The reason why reflexes like blinking were not perceived by the individual was that they were performed without the involvement of the higher brain centres or consciousness. The associations between reflexes and conscious actions were explored in the nineteenth century by investigators such as W. B. Carpenter (1813–85) and Thomas Laycock (1812–76), who developed the idea of 'cerebral reflexes'.

George Prochaska of Vienna (1749–1820) championed the concept of the *sensorium commune*: the brain functioned as a single unit without particular zones for specific functions. But this view was strongly countered: Charles Bell's *Idea of a New Anatomy of the Brain* had outlined an anatomically-based theory of localization, maintaining that the brain's anatomical complexity indicated functional specialization. His experiments showed that there were two kinds of nerve, sensory and motor, each serving a distinctive function.

Of the two nerve roots emerging from each level of the spinal cord on each side, the front was motor in function, initiating muscle action, and the rear sensory. Bell concluded that the anterior root fibres derived from the cerebrum and were both motor and sensory, whereas the posterior fibres came from the cerebellum, carrying 'secret' and 'vital' messages – that is, governing reflex and autonomic function. When François Magendie also demonstrated how the anterior root was motor and the posterior sensory, an acrimonious priority dispute followed and the 'law' is still known as the Bell-Magendie Law.

The notion of brain localization received a boost from the teachings of phrenology. Franz Josef Gall of the University of Vienna, who began lecturing on the faculties of the brain in 1796, postulated the localization of mental faculties, and tried to demonstrate their manifestations from the indentations of the skull. Working with Johann Caspar Spurzheim, he won considerable attention for phrenology (or organology); their *Anatomie et physiologie du système nerveux en général, et du cerveau en particulier* (1810–19) [Anatomy and Physiology of the Nervous System in General, and of the Brain in Particular] taught that character could be read by correlating bumps on a subject's head with those on a phreno-logical chart. Each of over thirty human faculties – acquisitiveness, amativeness, combativeness, holiness, liberality, love of glory, and so forth – was governed by a particular, localized part of the brain.

Other research strategies attempted to open up the brain in different ways. In a series of experiments on pigeon brains, the French anatomist Marie Jean-Pierre Flourens (1794–1867) cut connecting tracts and fibres and observed the progressive deterioration of function. His *Recherches expérimentales sur les propriétés et les fonctions du système nerveux dans les animaux vertébrés* (1824) [Experimental Researches on the Properties and Functions of the Nervous System in Vertebrates] told of how a pigeon from which he had removed both cerebral hemispheres became blind. When only one hemisphere was removed, the bird lost sight in the eye on the opposite side. A pigeon with its cerebellum removed could see and hear well, but its balance was destroyed. Flourens concluded that the cer-ebrum was the organ of thought, sensation and will, whereas the cerebel-lum was concerned with muscular coordination. He made no attempt to stimulate or remove particular localized areas of the cerebral hemispheres, and his *Examen de la phrénologie* (1842) [Examination of Phrenology] cast the phrenologists' doctrines into question, upholding in a holistic manner the unity of the brain. All the parts of the nervous system, he declared, 'concur, conspire and consent'. He countered the materialistic tendencies of phrenology with a Cartesian dualism.

Serving to confirm ablation experiments on animals, accidental dam-age in diseased and injured human patients afforded further opportunities for the elucidation of nerve pathways. In 1811 the French surgeon Jean Legallois noted respiratory difficulties in a person with a damaged medulla oblongata (the hindpart of the brain), and concluded that it must be part of the brain responsible for breathing control. Other functions could be traced at autopsy by correlating disease symptoms with evident brain damage; for example, a patient with left-sided paralysis associated with apoplexy or stroke might be found to have had right hemisphere cerebral haemorrhage. Quite astonishing phenomena came to light, notably in the case of Phineas Gage, a Connecticut quarryman who, in an explosion in 1848, had a three-foot crowbar pass right through his head and out the other side. Although a doctor could poke fingers inside his brain, Gage recovered and lived for another twelve years, his only disability being personality change – it would now be said that he was the inadvertent recipient of a frontal lobotomy. Investigation of the relationship between movement or sensation loss and physical damage led in a piecemeal way to the filling in of a sketch of functional localization.

Simultaneously other experiments refined understanding of the reflex system. Of key importance was the work of Marshall Hall (1790–1857), who practised in his native Nottingham before moving to London in 1826. In a sequence of adroit experiments, Hall showed that, if the spinal cord of a frog were severed between the front and the back legs, that part of the body anterior to the injury could still be moved voluntarily; the back legs, however were drawn up and motionless. But if a stimulus were applied to them, they twitched violently, though only once per stimulus; pain stimuli applied to them were not felt by the animal.

From these facts, disclosing how reflex actions occurred even when the spinal cord had been severed from the brain, Hall deduced that the nervous system must be made up of a series of segmental reflex arcs. In the intact spinal cord, stimuli passing through these arcs were co-ordinated by the ascending and descending pathways in the cord to form movement patterns. The spinal cord was thus more than a great nerve conduit – it had a life of its own, like the cerebrum. It was a spinal brain with its own initiating role, 'superior', Hall reflected, 'to the real brain, for the spinal one is always awake and alert while the brain needs sleep'. Reflex action explained involuntary acts like blinking, coughing, movement when threatened, and the first breath of a new-born child. The knee-jerk, that classic reflex, was described independently in 1875 by Wilhelm Heinrich Erb (1840–1921) and by Carl Friedrich Otto Westphal (1833–90).

One growth point of neurophysiological research after Bell lay in measurement of electrical impulses in nerve fibres, pioneered by du Bois-Reymond. Another of Müller's pupils, von Helmholtz, succeeded in measuring the conduction speed of the nerve impulse (between twenty-five and forty metres per second), and electrical methods for brain-mapping were developed by Gustav Theodor Fritsch (1838–91) and Eduard Hitzig (1838–1907). Working with wounded soldiers who had had portions of their skull destroyed, Hitzig, a military surgeon from Berlin, availed himself of the opportunity to apply wires from a battery to the cortex and observe what happened. Eye movements and other reactions could, he found, be stimulated by the electric current. With Fritsch, he performed similar experiments on animals to locate the areas of the brain controlling muscle movement. In a dog, electrical stimulation of certain points of the cerebral cortex anterior to the central sulcus resulted in movements on the opposite side of the body. The area which could be stimulated artificially was known as the motor area. Electrical stimulation of the brain became central to the work of the English neurologist David Ferrier, who began systematic mapping in 1873.

Electrical stimulation techniques worked on impulses passing from the brain to the muscles, but the reverse process – sensations received through the nerve endings and transmitted to the brain – were harder to study. Using an improved galvanometer on exposed rabbit and monkey brains, a Liverpool physician Richard Caton (1842–1926) showed alterations in brain electricity when external stimuli were applied or when an animal moved or ate. He also recorded currents in the optical area of the brain cortex when a bright light was shone into the eye: the first example of the direct detection of sensory input to the brain. Putting his galvanometer wires on the skull instead of the exposed brain, he still picked up currents, paving the way for the electroencephalogram (EEG), later a key diagnostic tool. Inspired by Sechenov's work on electricity in the brain and spinal column in epileptics, Abraham Adolph Beck (1863–1942) extended Caton's investigation of electrical activity in the brain. In 1891 he showed how it had a continuous low-level activity, which peaked during sensory stimulus.

In Britain the major theorist of modern neurology was a Yorkshireman, John Hughlings Jackson (1835–1911). After studying medicine in London, he turned his attention to neurology, and when the National Hospital for the Paralysed and Epileptic (later the National Hospital, Queen Square) was founded, he joined the staff. Building on the reflex arc as the basic functional unit at all levels of the nervous system, his first researches were concerned with speech defects associated with lesions of the brain. He confirmed the findings of the Frenchman Paul Broca (1824–80), by showing how right-handedness was governed by the left cerebral hemisphere. Tackling the localized epileptic movements now known as Jacksonian epilepsy, he correlated such motions with lesions in the motor area of the cerebral cortex. Jackson did not, however, believe individual muscles were represented in the cortex: 'the cerebral cortex knows nothing of muscles, it knows only of movements.'

The work of Fritsch, Hitzig and Jackson on the localization of speech and motor functions in the cerebral cortex was taken further by the superb experimentalist David Ferrier (1843–1928), who worked at

King's College Medical School in London, and also at the National Hospital, Queen Square. Operating on monkeys, Ferrier delineated the 'motor region', the part of the cerebral cortex in which motor functions are located. Like Hitzig and Fritsch, he cut away specific areas and thereby induced negative features (paralysis); he also used stimulation. Locating motor and sensory functions in the cerebral cortex, he concluded that vision was governed by the angular gyrus, though evidence was to accumulate in favour of its location in the occipital lobes. His *The Functions of the Brain* (1876) became the classic discussion of electro-stimulation of various cortex areas and the results of removing portions of the cerebral cortex.

At the International Medical Congress in 1881 Ferrier showed one of his paralysed monkeys; so remarkable was its behaviour that the French neurologist Charcot exclaimed: '*C'est un malade*' (It's a patient). Animal experiments were in this respect highly pertinent to clinical issues concerning neurological damage, brain disease and likely prognoses. If functions were strictly localized, could the brain and the central nervous system adapt to and overcome damage? In early work on monkeys Charles Sherrington showed that, when paralysis of a chimpanzee's arm had been produced by destruction of the arm area in the motor cortex, complete recovery of function took place within four and a half months though, as later shown, the destroyed area of the brain was not regenerated. Clearly the brain possessed a certain adaptive flexibility.

A distinct and new field of neurological investigation was the internal regulation of the body by the autonomic nervous system. Earlier centuries had brought isolated observations; it was known, for instance, that paralysis was often followed by alterations in the temperature of the paralysed parts, but coherent investigations began in the 1850s. Charles Édouard Brown-Séquard (1817–94) determined that the cervical sympathetic nerve was a vasoconstrictor, its stimulation producing contraction of the capillaries. In 1857 Claude Bernard discovered there were also vasodilator fibres in the nerve supply to the submaxillary gland, stimulation of which produced capillary dilation. Taken together, the vasomotor nerves (constrictor and dilator) were thus shown to be responsible for blood-flow control (and particular phenomena like blushing) via the governing action of the nervous system.

Knowledge of the autonomic nervous system was further advanced by two Cambridge physiologists, Gaskell and Langley. Walter Gaskell

(1847–1914) studied the vasomotor nerves of striated muscle (1874), and published studies of the innervation of the heart. He later worked on the central sympathetic nerves. Succeeding Foster at Cambridge, John Newport Langley (1852–1925) in 1898 applied the name autonomic nervous system (replacing involuntary nervous system) to the nervous system of the glands and involuntary muscles, including the sympathetic system. This work was described in Gaskell's *The Involuntary Nervous System* (1916) and Langley's *The Autonomic Nervous System* (1921).

Understanding of neuro-physiology was synthesized by Charles Scott Sherrington, professor of physiology at Liverpool and later at Oxford. His marathon career had three phases, the second of which culminated in his masterpiece, *The Integrative Action of the Nervous System* (1906). Embarking upon reflex studies, he decerebrated animals, removing the upper parts of their brains so that only the primitive brain stems and spinal cords were left, experimenting on these 'brainless beasts' to discover the workings of the central nervous system without the interference of consciousness.

Sherrington also developed the concept of inhibition. If, when a reflex was about to operate, the extensors of the limb were in a state of tension, flexion would be produced only with difficulty. Descartes and later observers had been of the view that the extensor muscles were either relaxed or remained dormant, but Sherrington showed that there was an active relaxation of the antagonistic muscles, produced by reciprocal inhibition, thus making possible the first quantitative estimate of inhibition as an active neuronal process. For instance, in the case of the knee-jerk, two simultaneous processes are involved: the active excitation of the muscle which executes the movement, and the equally active inhibition of the muscle which would otherwise oppose it. All movement involves a balance of give and take.

In *Integrative Action*, Sherrington synthesized his reflex experiments into a far-reaching conception of neuronal system activity. Examining the nature of the conduction of nerve impulses between cells, he concluded that there was a barrier between one cell and the next, permitting the impulse to pass with varying ease under different conditions. He named this physiological barrier between two neurones the synapse. He also developed the theory of the final common path for efferent impulses. The impulse from any receptor point in the skin followed a path of its own, but if it connected through a reflex arc with any muscle, it did so through the motor nerve to that muscle. As numerous receptor points would thus be connected with that muscle, impulses from all must converge and reach it by a common motor nerve.

Overall, the reflex was the elementary expression of an integrative action of the nervous system, Sherrington maintained, enabling the body to function with one single purpose at a time. Similar reflexes, arriving at the same time at the common path, were allowed to pass and reinforce each other; dissimilar reflexes had successive (rather than simultaneous) use of the common path. This co-ordination principle was applicable to the nervous system as a whole, resulting in unity of action, despite the multifarious conflicting sensory impulses which might be received by the surface receptors at the same time. In stressing integrative action, Sherrington was rescuing neurology from an excessive concentration on localization or 'specialization'.

The reflexes which he studied and upon which he built his theory of nervous integration were inborn, hereditary and characteristic of the central nervous system. His contemporary, the Russian physiologist Ivan Pavlov (1849–1936), worked on the conditional reflex. Pavlov revered Ivan Sechenov (1829–1905), whose *Reflexes of the Brain* (1866) argued that physical life was shaped by the environment and that reflexes controlled both unconscious and conscious action. The environment shaped action through the nervous system, and so all actions from the most simple to the most exalted were, according to Sechenov, 'mere results of a greater or lesser contraction of definite groups of muscles'. The czarist authorities denounced this as materialism, turning the neurologist into a symbol of political resistance. A great admirer of Sechenov, Pavlov brought together neurology and psychology in his work on conditional or learned reflexes; his materialist orientation placed him among the progressive intelligentsia and, after 1917, made his research ideologically congenial to the ruling Bolsheviks.

Pavlov's most famous experiments centred on gastric-juice secretion. This was controlled by a nervous mechanism. If food were placed in a dog's mouth, its stomach secreted juice: this (a simple reflex, like those which Sherrington studied) Pavlov styled unconditional. But the dog's stomach would secrete juice if it were allowed merely to sniff the food. Here the reflexes involved were different, conditioned by the animal's previous experience, acquired not innate. Pavlov next showed that, if a bell were rung every time the dog was given food, the stomach would secrete juice, even if this was not actually followed by food.

He thus distinguished two types of reflex: inborn and learned. The former, studied by Sherrington, was located in the spinal cord and brain stem, functioned even when the brain was removed, and was stable. The conditional reflex had to be learned, was highly unstable, and was located in the cerebral cortex. Study of reflexes would reveal the way the brain dealt with stimuli and thus lead to a general theory of human function.

Pavlov formulated a theory in which the brain, composed of millions of active cells, was every moment receiving countless stimuli, to each of which there was a conditional response. All such stimuli and responses 'meet, come together, interact, and they must, finally, become systematized, equilibrated, and form so to speak, a dynamic stereotype'. Brain action was to be understood in terms of a constantly shifting centre of action within the cerebral cortex.

NEUROPATHOLOGY

Much of the neurological research just described was conducted on experimental animals and had only an oblique relation to human disease. At the same time, however, information accumulated about clinical conditions familiarly associated with pathological conditions which would be associated with the models of the brain and nervous system outlined.

In 1658, the pioneering pathologist Johann Jakob Wepfer (1620–95) of Basel had shown that apoplexy or stroke was due to haemorrhage from the cerebral vessels, and in 1686 Thomas Sydenham described chorea, separating it from the old descriptions of dancing mania and the supernaturalist connotations of what had been called St Vitus's Dance. In 1817 James Parkinson (1755–1824) published *An Essay on the Shaking Palsy*, the first description of *paralysis agitans*, delineating what he termed the 'pathognomonic symptoms' (*tremor coactus* and *scelotyrbe festinans*). By the nineteenth century, particular clinical conditions were beginning to be traced to specific nerves. Charles Bell showed that lesions of the seventh cranial nerve produced the facial paralysis later known as Bell's palsy.

The most dedicated explorer of neuropathology in the first half of the nineteenth century was Moritz Romberg (1795–1873), who devoted his career to sorting out the jungle of clinical and pathological facts associated with neurological disorders. Becoming director of the Berlin

University clinic in 1840, he set beds aside for the study of a wide variety of nervous conditions. He studied mainly diseases of the peripheral nerves, together with apoplexy, epilepsy and chorea, which had long been known. He also gave attention to *tabes dorsalis* (locomotor ataxia or a type of syphilis of the nervous system), establishing 'Romberg's sign' – a sufferer would sway and fall to the ground if made to stand with his/her eyes closed. Only later was its syphilitic aetiology established, but, as Romberg recognized, its main lesion was wasting of the spinal cord.

Romberg's *Lehrbuch der Nervenkrankheiten des Menschen* (1840–6) [Textbook of Human Nervous Diseases] was a pioneering attempt to produce a nosology which drew upon Cullen's taxonomy of the 'neuroses', disorders of the nervous system. Following the work of Magendie and Bell, he divided neurological disorders into two groups: those due to motor and those due to sensory dysfunction. His symptom-based nosology would soon be discarded as old-fashioned and replaced by distinct neurological and neuromuscular disease entities, each with specific morbid anatomical changes, but, in attempting to bring order to a tangled part of clinical medicine, he was setting the agenda for his successors.

Discussed by Romberg, Cruveilhier and others, *tabes dorsalis* became a focus of clinical and pathological research, especially with growing awareness of its syphilitic source. It was the subject of a masterly account published in 1858 by Guillaume Duchenne (1806–75). A Boulogne sea captain's son, Duchenne studied medicine in Paris and was the first to describe many conditions, including progressive muscular atrophy, locomotor ataxia and bulbar paralysis. His description of tabes was so complete that the condition was named 'Duchenne's disease'. He located the lesion in the posterior columns of the spinal cord, and established its syphilitic origin.

Duchenne's contemporary, Jean-Martin Charcot, clinical professor of the nervous system at the Salpêtrière, ranks as one of the most famous teachers of the time and his clinic became the neurologists' Mecca. Charcot praised Duchenne's work on tabes, and gave the first description of sclerosis and the peroneal type of muscular atrophy. Investigating the clinical aspects of cerebral localization, his *Leçons sur les maladies du système nerveux faites à la Salpêtrière* [Lectures on Nervous Diseases Delivered at the Salpêtrière] brought order to their classification. Despite a common misconception, Charcot was never an alienist or psychiatrist in the tradition of Pinel and Esquirol, nor was he exclusively preoccupied with hysteria. He was an ardent neurologist, committed to deploying patho-anatomical techniques to reduce to order the chaos of fiendishly complex neurological symptom-clusters. Conditions like 'epilepsy, hysteria, even the most inveterate cases, chorea, and many other morbid states', he granted in his *Leçons*, 'come to us like so many sphinxes,' defying 'the most penetrating anatomical investigations'.

The 'Napoleon of the neuroses' nevertheless aimed to trace nervous phenomena to organic lesions, and thereby to normalize general paralysis, neuralgias, seizures, epileptiform fits, spastic symptoms, tabes dorsalis, and – probably his special favourite – hysteria. This, he hoped to show, partook of the general characteristics of neurological disorders. He undertook massive clinical neuropathological scrutiny, examining motor and sensory symptoms, bizarre visual abnormalities, tics, migraine, epileptiform seizures, aphasia, somnambulism, hallucinations, word blindness, alexia, mutism, contractures, hyperaesthesias and numerous other deficits. Clinical observation, he was confident, would expose the natural histories of families of related neurological deficits: hemilateral anaesthesias, pharyngeal anaesthesias, *grands paroxysmes*, palpitations, chorea, St Vitus's Dance, tertiary neurosyphilitic infections and temporal lobe epilepsy. 'These diseases', he insisted, 'do not form, in pathology, a class apart, governed by other physiological laws than the common ones.' Backed by his colleagues and students and with unlimited access to clinical material, Charcot mobilized a research industry.

Among other things, he followed up Parkinson's work on the shaking palsy (it was he who coined the term Parkinson's disease). His masterly depiction of *paralysis agitans* gave, for instance, a particularly good account of the quirky parkinsonian hand tremor whereby the thumb moves over the fingers 'as when a pencil or paper ball is rolled between them . . . [or] in crumbling a piece of bread'. In his Salpêtrière lectures, he attended closely to the nuances of tremors, distinguishing case types in which 'tremor is only shown when an intensive movement is made' from other clusters in which 'tremor is a constant symptom, from whom it rarely departs except during sleep.'

A younger contemporary was Jules Dejerine (1849–1917), who went to Paris in 1871 and for many years worked on diseases of the peripheral nervous system, in 1883 describing peripheral neuritis (later recognized as due to vitamin B deficiency). In 1886 he described muscular dystrophy, a slowly progressive disease which produces wasting of the facial and shoulder-girdle muscles, later spreading to the pelvic girdle. He was also fascinated by the role of heredity in nervous disease.

Multiple sclerosis was studied, its lesions being illustrated by Jean Cruveilhier in his great *Anatomie pathologique du corps humain* (1829–42) [Pathological Anatomy of the Human Body]. He related the clinical symptoms (numbness, falling, disordered voluntary movements of the limbs) to 'grey degeneration' in the spinal cord, brain stem, cerebellum and even the cerebrum. An extended clinical study was made in 1849 by Friedrich Theodor von Frerichs (1819–85), who also investigated other grave nervous conditions characterized by rigidity and contractures. Charcot later gave the classical picture of inco-ordination, tremor and nystagmus. Its most typical form was delineated by Samuel Kinnier Wilson (1878–1937), who named it progressive lenticular degeneration (it is now called Kinnier Wilson's disease).

Aphasia also attracted attention. Postmortem examinations of aphasia cases connected loss of capacity to speak with damage to specific cortical areas, especially on the left side, and Paul Broca began to map those areas of the brain. In 1861, he held that the third frontal convolution of the left cerebral hemisphere (Broca's convolution) was more developed than that on the right side, and that this was the centre for articulate speech. Soon afterwards Hughlings Jackson published the first of his aphasia papers. In 1869 H. C. Bastian described the speech impairment known as sensory aphasia, and five years later it was redescribed by Carl Wernicke (1848–1905), after whom it is now known.

Benefiting from the key new developments of the nineteenth century – the clinical gaze, pathological anatomy, reflex theory – the development of neurology may be measured by its leading textbooks. Romberg placed the emphasis on individual sensory and motor characters. He gave detailed accounts of symptoms, but did not group these localized, specific disease concepts; practically the only nervous diseases he mentioned were apoplexy, paralysis, epilepsy, chorea and *tabes dorsalis*. Charcot's textbook (1872), by contrast, contained descriptions of many more named diseases, and symptoms and signs were fully integrated in the classic patho-anatomical manner. Clinicians were thus identifying nervous diseases as such. In 1882 Byrom Bramwell's (1847–1931) work on diseases of the spinal cord was arranged by lesion sites and not by symptoms at all. The next edition, which appeared thirteen years later, had almost doubled in size. The *Manual of Diseases of the Nervous System*

(1886–8) by Sir William Gowers was in the same mould. The journal *Brain*, co-founded in 1878 by Crichton-Browne, Hughlings Jackson and Ferrier, helped to reinforce the links between psychiatric and neurological sciences, as did much late nineteenth-century investigation which came out of Kraepelin's stable and other German centres.

Kraepelin became involved in a major controversy over the relations between depression, degeneration and senile dementia. He did not dispute that depression could be an early stage of senile dementia; but it was not an invariable symptom. When melancholy in an elderly patient was attended by inability to 'retain impressions', senile dementia should be suspected. But he disputed belief that depression inescapably degenerated into dementia. Kraepelin was thus open to the possibility that dementia was not a life stage but a definite disease: the idea advanced by his younger colleague, Alois Alzheimer (1864–1915).

The son of a small-town Bavarian notary, Alzheimer received his medical training at the universities of Berlin, Würzburg, and Tübingen, and trained in neuropathology at the Städische Irrenanstalt in Frankfurt, before joining Kraepelin at Heidelberg. There, and later at Munich, he offered classical descriptions of various kinds of neuropathology, including Huntington's chorea and general paresis of the insane.

Alzheimer's views challenged the degenerationist ideas of senility popular among the French. In 1906, he spelt out the clinical and neuropathological evidence for the origins of what we now know as Alzheimer's disease, showing the now familiar senile plaques and neurofibrillary tangles in the brain of a fifty-one-year-old demented woman. Alzheimer contended that the dementia common among the old was not intrinsic to ageing; it was not growing old *per se* that produced the organic alterations which constituted the pathological state of senescence. He also dismissed the idea that dementia was a general condition: it was a specific disease.

THE TWENTIETH CENTURY

Neurology has seen stunning developments in the twentieth century which go far beyond the scope of this book. Building on du Bois-Reymond's demonstration of the resisting current in nerves, major work followed on nervous impulses. Electro-physiology was advanced by Francis Gotch (1853–1913) in Oxford and Keith Lucas (1879–1916) in Cambridge, and especially by his pupil, Edgar Douglas Adrian (1889–1977).

The study of brain waves, impulses emanating from the cerebral cortex which reflect states of consciousness, external stimuli and mental operations, provided an important diagnostic tool, especially in epilepsy. Using a capillary electrometer for sensitive detection of nervous impulses, Adrian found that a stimulus of constant intensity applied to the skin caused immediate excitation of an end-organ. Though the stimulus continued, the excitation diminished. He thus gave an account of a mechanism that enables us to sense our environment without being constantly inundated by millions of signals. Work on brain waves proved medically useful, stimulating studies of brain function, sleep research, diagnosis of psychiatric disorders and new approaches to migraine and blood pressure.

Recent developments in scanning technology are at long last affording a picture of the brain and the rest of the central nervous system at work, as, for example, the damage done by strokes or progressive neurological disorders like Alzheimer's. It is also being recognized that the brain is more plastic in its functions than once thought. Nineteenth- and early twentieth-century images of the brain were derived largely from railway systems or a telephone switchboard, and suggested a rigid framework. Computer analogies have also tended to be rather mechanistic. Nowadays the emphasis is upon the adaptability of the brain to meet particular needs. Damage in one area will result in compensatory activity in another. The most challenging recent view has been put forward by Gerald Maurice Edelman (b. 1929). An immunologist who won the Nobel Prize for his structural analysis of the gamma globulin molecule, Edelman switched his attention to neuroscience. Investigating the emergence of brain activity, he has theorized that a selective process occurs among neurons comparable to the selection mechanism occurring when species compete in nature. 'The brain, in its workings,' Edelman holds, 'is a selective system, more like evolution than computation.' Rather than genetic 'predestination', it is adaptation and an accumulation of mental activity which determine the development of the mind.

Neurology thus developed a well-defined image of the functions of the central nervous system, leading to more effective measures for identifying and treating dysfunction. In modern medicine, it explains and guides the treatment of a wide range of nervous, psychiatric, behavioural and personality problems. Neurology also remains a field in which diagnosis of pathology continues to outrun ability to cure or even to relieve. Neurological conditions remain amongst the most intractable, especially with an ageing population.

BIOCHEMISTRY AND NUTRITION

Chemistry became a powerful tool in the nineteenth century for explaining the phenomena of life. The new study of enzymes and proteins was essential, for instance, for the development of modern genetics and genetic disease theories (see Chapter 18). In this section the focus is on the part played by chemical concepts, as well as clinical observations, in the creation of a new category and model of diseases: deficiency diseases.

Organic chemistry was premised upon a distinct predictive model for understanding the functioning of metabolism. Liebigian chemistry posited a purely quantitative and reductionist theory of nutrition and energy. Its practical implication was that it would be possible to construct an artificial diet to satisfy bodily needs on the basis of carbohydrates, fats, proteins and mineral salts alone. Clinical evidence accumulated, however, to challenge this assumption. In Paris (then under siege during the 1871 Commune), J. B. H. Dumas (1800–84) proved, through an enforced and harrowing experiment, that the Liebigian dietary constituents failed to sustain life when synthesized artificially. Having to feed a nursery of starving infants and short of natural food, Dumas mixed a formula by emulsifying fat in a sweetened albuminous solution. Though it contained the requisite proteins, carbohydrates and fats, the paste failed to nourish the children. Laboratory tests confirmed his suspicions: mice would thrive on milk, but they could not survive on milk-like artificial compounds of fats, proteins and carbohydrates. Feeding mice on a synthetic mixture of the constituents of milk (proteins, fats, carbohydrates, and salts), Nicolai Ivanovitch Lunin (1853–1937) found that they died; his conclusion that milk must contain small quantities of as yet unknown substances proved prescient.

Findings like these suggested the possibility that various pathological conditions should be viewed as deficiency diseases, arising from lack of vital dietary elements. That notion – that disease was due to a *lack* – involved a new paradigm. 'Disease is so generally associated with positive agents – the parasite, the toxin, the *materies morbi*', noted a report in 1919, 'that the thought of the pathologist turns naturally to such positive associations and seems to believe with difficulty in causation prefixed by a *minus* sign.' Among the disorders to which this novel conception seemed applicable was marasmus, afflicting young babies in impoverished areas and characterized by muscle-wasting, fat loss and low body weight. Another was kwashiorkor, found in tropical Africa, typified by oedema and muscle-wasting, enlarged liver, diarrhoea and lassitude.

In 1755 the French physician Gaspar Casal (1680–1759) published an account of pellagra, then a new disease in Spain. Characterized by dermatitis ('a horrible crust, dry, scabby ... crossed with cracks') but also causing diarrhoea, dementia and premature death, it flared up each spring. Casal noted that its victims were poor; maize meal was their staple food, and they had very little meat or milk. The same was true in Italy, where the disease grew serious after 1800. Various theories were offered about its cause; the main one pointed a vague finger of blame at the staple maize diet. A New World plant, maize had been brought back by the *conquistadores* and adopted in Mediterranean Europe. A French physician writing in 1845 suggested that the 'predisposing cause' was a diet with too few animal products and that the 'efficient cause' was bad maize. Yet in 1865 a Mexican doctor pointed out that pellagra was not a problem in his country despite maize being the staple food. Why? He thought the secret was in the habit of soaking maize in lime water before cooking, which had a disinfectant effect, whereas the European-style baking of corn mush to polenta left it contaminated with moulds and toxins.

Bacteriology brought new theories to bear on the problem. Since malaria and yellow fever were being shown by the new tropical medicine to result from insect-borne infections, might not this hold for pellagra too? Some suggested flies were transferring infectious material from the faeces of pellagrins to the food of future victims. Hungarian-born Joseph Goldberger (1874–1929), of the US Public Health Service, noticed, by contrast, that at orphanages and mental asylums where the inmates developed pellagra, the staff (naturally on better rations) escaped. If eggs and milk were added to the inmates' diet, the disease diminished. After dermatitis appeared in convict volunteers put on a maize-meal diet, Goldberger concluded that the disease was due to lack of (as then unknown) dietary factors. The diarrhoea, dermatitis, dementia and premature death associated with pellagra were also widespread among poor people in southern Europe and the Middle East. In the early twentieth century, it spread in the southern states of the USA, peaking around 1930, when it was estimated that there were 20,000 cases in Georgia alone among people eating maize meal and little animal food except pork 'fat back' (all lard, no lean).

Beriberi was common in the rice cultures of Asia. Sinhalese for 'I cannot', beriberi is characterized by weakness in the legs, hands and arms. Weakening of the cardiac muscles leads to water-logged dropsical limbs and heart failure. In infants suckling from afflicted mothers, sudden death from heart failure is common. Hindsight shows that beriberi became especially severe in late nineteenth-century south-east Asia because the large populations labouring on rubber plantations and in the tin mines survived largely on milled rice, produced by new steam-driven plant.

In 1882 a Japanese naval vessel was sent on a long training cruise. Of the 275 crew, over 60 per cent developed beriberi and 25 died. Dr Takaki (1849–1915), a German-trained naval surgeon, noted the protein content of their diet was far below the German standard, and proposed increasing the protein. On a voyage the following year, the diet was modified by replacing part of the rice with barley, while beef, milk and tofu (soybean curd) were added. No deaths occurred. Takaki believed he had shown that beriberi was due to protein deficiency.

In the 1890s Christiaan Eijkman (1858–1930), director of the research laboratory at Batavia (Jakarta), also confronted beriberi. As with pellagra, there was a hunch that it was due to a bacterial infection, and so bacteriologists were sent from the Netherlands to try to identify the micro-organism. Eijkman happened to find that the hospital chickens developed polyneuritis when they were fed the white rice given to patients, rather than their normal brown rice chicken-feed. Given whole rice once again, they recovered; from this he deduced that there was a toxin in the polished rice, and an antidote in the husk. His colleague, Gerrit Grijns (1865–1944), disagreed, believing that some essential substance in the food was being destroyed by heat. He suggested that both diseases – fowl polyneuritis and beriberi – were due to absence from the diet of some factor present in rice polishings.

Eijkman meanwhile distributed a questionnaire to all the prisons in Java, inquiring about the incidence of beriberi, the physical environment, and the diet. The returns showed no relation between environment and beriberi, but the disease was a serious problem in 71 per cent of the prisons using white rice and in only 3 per cent of those using 'rough' rice. Following up such work in 1905, William Fletcher (1874–1938) experimented on asylum inmates in Kuala Lumpur, showing that nearly a quarter of those who received polished rice alone developed beriberi, while only two out of 123 patients who received unpolished rice fell victim.

In 1906, Axel Holst (1860–1931), an Oslo bacteriologist, set out to study beriberi which had broken out among crews on Norwegian sailing vessels, following changes in their rations. In an experiment he fed guineapigs on different kinds of flour. The animals all died after approximately one month, but this could be prevented, he found, by giving cabbage leaves or lemon juice supplements. Explanations were thus beginning to take shape: all pointed to the likelihood that scurvy, beriberi, pellagra and rickets could be caused by dietary deficiencies.

This was also the view of Frederick Gowland Hopkins (1861–1947) in Cambridge. In a series of experiments from 1906, he fed young rats on casein, lard, starch, sugar and salts (supposedly everything essential to health), and gave some of them milk additionally. Only those receiving the milk thrived. 'Astonishingly small amounts' of certain substances in food – his term was 'accessory food factors' – were essential, he concluded, for the body to utilize protein and energy for growth. Animals were adjusted to live on vegetables or meat containing a variety of substances other than the standard nutritional components: if these were lacking, deficiency diseases would develop. The key to nutrition, therefore, lay in these missing links.

In 1912, working at the Lister Institute in London, the Polish-born biochemist Casimir Funk (1884–1967) took this thinking a stage further by isolating the active substances in rice husks which were preventing beriberi. He named such dietary missing links 'vitamines' (= 'vital amines') in the belief that they were amines, compounds derived from ammonia. (The final 'e' was dropped in 1920, when it became clear that not all vitamins were amines.) Funk linked vitamin deficiency with such diseases as beriberi, scurvy, pellagra and rickets. Deficiency syndromes had thus been isolated in the laboratory, and the nutritional roles of various foods – vegetable products (leaves, stems, seeds), milk, egg yolk and meat – were in the process of being elucidated. A theoretical basis for nutrition had been established.

Attention turned to elucidating vitamins themselves. In 1913 Thomas Burr Osborne (1859–1929) and Lafayette Benedict Mendel

(1872–1935) showed in rat experiments conducted at Yale that butter contained a growth-promoting factor necessary for development. Soon known as fat-soluble vitamin A, its chemical character was established in 1933, and it was finally synthesized in 1947. Elmer Verner McCollum (1879–1967), a former Kansas farm lad, and Marguerite Davis of Wisconsin (1888–1967) showed a similar growth factor in egg-yolk and cod-liver oil (absent from lard and olive oil). Cows' milk was found to contain another growth-promoting factor, soluble in water, later also found in foods such as wheat embryo, rice polishings and yeast. This was given the name vitamin B; isolated in pure form in 1926, it was synthesized ten years later.

Rickets, meanwhile, was under scrutiny. An ancient disease described by Francis Glisson in the seventeenth century, it had become widespread in industrial cities. 'It is in the narrow alleys, the haunts and playgrounds of the children of the poor,' wrote Theobald A. Palm in 1890, 'that the victims of rickets are to be found in abundance.' Extremely common among young children in northern industrial cities on both sides of the Atlantic, there were signs of rickets, it was estimated in 1900, in 80 per cent of those under two in Boston, and a quarter of infants from low-income families lacked sturdy leg bones. What caused it? Was it dietary? Was it a chronic infectious disease? Or was it, as suggested by David Paul von Hansemann (1858–1920) of Berlin, due to lack of fresh air, sunlight and exercise? In Glasgow research was carried out during the First World War by Leonard Findlay (1878–1947), who investigated the role of social and economic factors, while the preventive value of sunshine was emphasized by Palm.

Meanwhile Edward Mellanby (1884–1955) induced rickets in puppies by feeding them diets lacking a factor found in some animal fats; giving it in the form of cod-liver oil restored them. Having demonstrated that it was a deficiency disease, Mellanby attributed it to lack of fat-soluble vitamin A. Researchers had shown that rickets could be cured by sunlight or by cod-liver oil. From 1922 it was established that vitamin A consisted of two separate factors. For one the old term vitamin A was retained; the other, the anti-rachitic factor, was renamed vitamin D. In the US the enrichment of milk with vitamin D was extremely effective against rickets.

When experiments showed that rats reared on whole milk grew normally but were usually sterile, the absence of a factor basic to reproduction was surmised. In 1922 Herbert McLean Evans (1905–83), of the University of California, and Katherine Scott Bishop (1889–1976) showed it was abundant in green leaves and wheat germ. Fat-soluble, but not identical with any known vitamin, it became known as vitamin E.

Another problem came into focus. It had been recognized at least since the work of Lind in the eighteenth century that many foods could cure and prevent scurvy. The nineteenth-century pathologist August Hirsch (1817–94) identified potatoes as antiscorbutic, and doctors in London hospitals who suspected scurvy in children treated them with diets of meat, milk, potatoes and citrus juices. Scurvy was accidentally introduced in guineapigs in 1906 by Axel Holst and Theodor Christian Brun Frölich (1870–1947) while attempting to produce beriberi by restricting their diets. Funk suggested a vitamin must be responsible, and attempts followed to isolate it. In the process it was found that while several foods seemed to ward off scurvy, some such as apples, lemon juice and cabbage lost the antiscorbutic effects when heated.

During the First World War, scientists at the Lister Institute in London, led by Harriet Chick (1875–1977), began a series of painstaking investigations into the antiscorbutic qualities of different foods. Ultimately, Arthur Harden (1865–1940), of the Lister Institute, separated citric and other acids from lemon juice, leaving a residue with a high antiscorbutic effect which the acids themselves lacked. By 1919, the antiscorbutic factor had been recognized as an essential nutrient. Albert Szent-Györgyi (1893–1986) meanwhile isolated from the adrenals a substance he called hexuronic acid, and in 1932 W. A. Waugh and Charles Glen King (1896–1988) isolated the lemon vitamin and showed it identical with the hexuronic acid. In 1932 this vitamin (vitamin C) was the first to be synthesized in a laboratory, by Szent-Györgyi, and in 1933 its name was changed to ascorbic acid. When this was found to be easily destroyed by heat and by contact with metals, an explanation was finally provided of why James Lind's concentrated syrup, prepared by evaporating lemon juice, had lost its potency.

Research continued into vitamin B. The original assumption that it was a single substance was disproved in 1926, when Morris Smith (1887–1951) and E. G. Hendrick showed that it consisted of two distinct substances: the anti-neuritic factor came to be called vitamin B_1, and the growth-promoting factor vitamin B_2. Vitamin B_1 was isolated from rice husks in 1926 and from yeast in 1932; its chemical structure was worked out and the name thiamin adopted; it was commercially marketed by Merck. By the 1930s, vitamin sales were making large profits for big pharmaceutical companies.

These researches into deficiency diseases caught the attention of workers in cognate fields, who pondered whether other conditions could be due to a deficiency of factors in the diet. Might this provide the clue, for example, to anaemia?

In 1849 Thomas Addison had described a fatal anaemia, later known as pernicious anaemia, involving the production of too few red blood cells. For long its cause was unclear and there was no known cure. First in California and then in Rochester (New York), George Whipple (1878–1976), experimenting on dogs which he had made anaemic by persistent blood-letting, found he could cure the condition by feeding them beef liver, beef muscle or spinach, rich in iron. After reading Whipple's work, in 1925 George R. Minot (1885–1950) and William P. Murphy (1892–1936), puzzled by anaemia and other blood disorders, set about feeding pernicious anaemia patients on large quantities (a pound a day) of raw or lightly cooked liver. The results were spectacular: there was a rapid increase in production of red blood cells and the patients' anaemia disappeared. An effective treatment had been found for a potentially fatal condition.

But the scientific problem remained to be solved: why did patients with pernicious anaemia not absorb the factor from their diet unless they were fed enormous quantities? This was investigated by William Castle (1897–1990), a young resident physician in Boston City Hospital. He knew of the work of Whipple and Minot and also that there was something unusual about the gastric juice of patients with pernicious anaemia. Evidence had accumulated over the years that, unlike normal gastric juice, the stomach secretions of these patients were almost completely lacking in hydrochloric acid. Was it that the stomach of normal persons derived something from food which was the equivalent of eating pounds of liver?

To test his hypothesis, Castle carried out a simple but clever series of experiments involving patients with pernicious anaemia. For ten days he fed them rare steak minced up from lean beef muscle. Their blood showed no sign of improvement. At the same time he fed ordinary men the same amount of steak, and recovered their gastric contents through a stomach tube. These were liquefied and fed through a stomach tube to the patients with pernicious anaemia. After about six days the patients' blood showed clear signs of regeneration.

He then asked whether the response was due to the stomach contents alone or due to its action on the beef muscle diet. He found that stomach juices alone were ineffective: there was no response unless the stomach juice and the beef muscle were given together. There had to be an interaction between an unknown 'intrinsic factor' in the gastric juice and an 'extrinsic factor' in the beef. The extrinsic factor turned out to be vitamin B_{12}, and the intrinsic factor was later found to be a substance secreted in normal stomachs and involved in transporting vitamin B_{12} across the wall of the lower bowel. Since pernicious anaemia is caused, it is now known, by a deficiency of gastric intrinsic factor, the vitamin B_{12} in the patients' food is unavailable unless present in enormous quantities.

One problem led to another. Although Castle had identified the basic defect in pernicious anaemia and found a way to counter it, it remained a mystery why some individuals destroyed the lining of their stomach and were unable to produce hydrochloric acid and intrinsic factor. This was not resolved until many years later, when scientists in Denmark and England found that – rather as in the insulin-dependent form of diabetes (marked by self-destruction of the pancreatic islet cells) – pernicious anaemia occurs because of the production of antibodies against the stomach lining. It thus became included on the long list of what are styled autoimmune diseases – which also includes thyroid disease, rheumatoid arthritis, other diseases of endocrine glands, some blood diseases, and chronic diseases of the nervous system. The explanation of this pathology still largely remains to be resolved. What is clear, however, is that a monthly injection of vitamin B_{12} will control the symptoms of pernicious anaemia and restore patients to complete health.

Study of nutrition attained particular salience during the inter-war period, bringing together laboratory scientists, clinicians and advocates of the importance of diet in positive health. Over the generations innumerable diet fanatics had offered everything from pure beef to strict vegetarianism and water-drinking as the secret of health and long life. Adequate roughage and fibre had become a nostrum of the early twentieth century. Now it seemed the dietary contribution to health had been put on a scientific basis, and some thought it would unlock the secret of all diseases. Economic depression in the West ('the hungry thirties') and growing awareness of famine and starvation in the Third World concentrated idealists' minds. Of those perhaps the most prominent was John Boyd Orr (1880–1971), who spent his career fighting world hunger and malnutrition, working with institutions such as the United Nations to bring about worldwide changes in public health. A Scot, Boyd Orr founded the Rowett Research Institute in Aberdeen in 1922 and served as director until 1945, editing a journal, *Nutrition Abstracts and Reviews*, which drew attention to the universal problem of malnutrition. He found that in the UK only the top two (out of six) social groups ate a satisfactory diet.

Boyd Orr statistically correlated poverty, improper nutrition and poor health. While presenting a frightening picture of malnutrition and suggesting that much was due to poverty, inequality and market forces, he recommended ways of reconciling the interests of agriculture and public health. Proposing a number of programmes for increasing world food production, he championed science as crucial to solving the problem of world hunger. Under his influence, the League of Nations established its Committee on Nutrition, and he became the first director of the United Nations Food and Agriculture Organization. Convinced that an adequate world food supply was essential to peace, he advocated a system of world government in works such as *Food: Foundation of World Unity* (1948).

Through activists like Boyd Orr, a vision of health, immunity and resistance, which was largely nutrition-oriented and squared with a humanistic commitment to the abolition of hunger, became entrenched. It was no accident that the Beveridge Report isolated 'want' as one of the evil giants. The science of nutrition of course developed in many directions, broadcast different messages and served many masters. Practical advice pamphlets and films to housewives, issued by government propaganda agencies, may be interpreted either as aiming to raise nutritional standards or to blame bad housekeeping, while the involvement of food science with the food processing industry has been, to say the least, a mixed blessing. As a result of increased food processing the average consumption of sugar doubled between 1860 and 1960 (leading to more tooth decay and diabetes), fat consumption rose by around 40 per cent and there was a 90 per cent decline in fibre in British diets (partly because of the growing consumption of milled white bread).

Modern junk foods worsen this situation. Since the 1960s diet has increasingly been implicated in all manner of diseases, from allergies and cancers to the well-documented associations of fat-rich diets with cardiovascular conditions (discussed in the next chapter). Inappropriate foodstuffs have been sent to starving Third World nations while in the

West the preoccupation with food has in part been responsible for a epidemic of anorexia nervosa. No more than there is a free lunch is there such a thing as an unalloyed medical breakthrough.

CHAPTER XVIII

CLINICAL SCIENCE

CLINICAL SCIENCE IS a useful name for modern traditions of medical investigation which aim to identify, record and analyse symptoms presented in sickness; determine deviations from the norms demonstrated by physiological research; and on those bases develop valuable therapeutic interventions.

Various streams have fed into it. The Paris school had laid down the goals of the anatomical approach: to identify pathological conditions in the corpse in terms of organ changes, and to recognize signs in the living patient revealing the presence of such pathological conditions. Physiology as promoted by Virchow, Ludwig and Bernard was to make functions more significant than structures. Changes in temperature, blood pressure and breathing rates assumed greater significance in revealing the basic indications of illness. 'The subjects of therapy are not diseases but conditions,' Virchow characteristically maintained. Along these lines German experimental physiology, studying what Virchow called 'life under altered conditions', sought to develop techniques for measuring and recording organ functions, while establishing norms to determine deviations and hence pathological conditions.

By 1900 clinical medicine was assimilating the physiological or functional approach. This chapter surveys aspects of these developments, in which the dialogue of scientific research and clinical medicine has had particularly dramatic implications for human health and the public standing of medicine: investigations into hormones, genes and the immune system, and the struggles against cancer and heart disease, which by the inter-war years had become far and away the diseases with the worst death rates in the western world.

ENDOCRINOLOGY

Claude Bernard's explorations of the *milieu intérieur* created a paradigm for future studies of the workings of the metabolism. An influential thinker in this tradition was Walter Cannon (1871–1945), at Harvard. Fascinated by the effects of strong emotions in modifying gastro-intestinal function, he systematically investigated the mechanisms and functioning of the autonomic nervous system, examining the effects on it of pain, fear and rage. Triggering dilation of pupils, constriction of blood vessels and increase in heart rate, the sympathetic nerves prepare the body (as he put it) for 'fright, fight or flight'. Confronting the phenomenon of traumatic shock during the First World War, he showed that the stimulation of the sympathetic nerves released a substance subsequently shown to be nor-adrenaline – thereby pointing towards the chemical transmission of nerve impulses.

In his *The Wisdom of the Body* (1932), Cannon coined the term 'homeostasis' to describe the capacity of animals to maintain physiological equilibrium through the autonomic nervous system's ability to adjust salt, sugar, oxygen and temperature levels within the narrow range in which life could be sustained within the body. Continual internal readjustment to maintain a stable internal environment was accomplished primarily by the regulation of hormones. Through such concepts Cannon synthesized research in the new field of endocrinology, and provided a 'scientific' basis for his own conservative political philosophy, which valued social stability.

Bernard's physiology had raised fundamental questions about the body's capacity for internal regulation, drawing attention to the hitherto enigmatic tube-like ducts carrying off the secretions of such organs as the liver. These had been described in the great burst of anatomical exploration in the seventeenth century: the pancreatic duct by Johann Georg Wirsung (1600–43) in 1642, the submaxillary duct by Thomas Wharton (1614–73) in 1656, the parotid duct by Nils Stensen (1638–86) in 1662.

The functions of these structures had long remained conjectural. The Dutch anatomist Frederik Ruysch (1638–1731) supposed that the thyroid discharged substances into the bloodstream; Théophile de Bordeu speculated in 1775 that various organs gave off emanations affecting other parts; while in 1849 Arnold Berthold (1803–61) gave experimental evidence of such an internal secretion. It had long been known that castrating a cock led its comb to atrophy; Berthold showed that if the testes were then transplanted to another part of the creature's body, this did not occur.

In 1855, Bernard had shown that whereas the external secretion of the liver formed bile, its internal secretion (*sécrétion interne*) made blood sugar. In the next year Brown-Séquard, noting that Addison's disease involved the failure of the adrenal (or suprarenal) glands near the kidneys, removed them in experimental animals, and thus proved they were necessary for life – they must, he decided, be adding something essential to the bloodstream. This line of inquiry, and the practice of experimental excision, bore rich fruit.

The English physiologists William Bayliss (1860–1924) and Ernest Starling (1866–1927) shed fresh light on the biochemistry of gland secretions. On 16 January 1902, they conducted an experiment which involved introducing hydrochloric acid into a dog's duodenum. Finding its pancreas began secreting pancreatic juice, they inferred the duodenum must be secreting a substance that passed into and travelled along the bloodstream. Calling this unknown substance 'secretin', they showed the potential dividend of the study of chemical messengers that moved from one organ (basically a ductless or 'endocrine' gland) to other body parts via the bloodstream, regulating various body systems. As a generic term for this 'secretin' and similar substances, Starling adopted the word 'hormone' (Greek *hormao*: I excite) in 1905.

The thyroid gland had been known from antiquity. Galen thought it lubricated the larynx, whereas Wharton believed it was there to beautify the female neck. Astley Cooper observed the large lymphatics passing from it into the thoracic duct and suggested they conveyed a secretion, and in 1844 John Simon deemed the thyroid a secreting gland whose product passed into the circulation. Meanwhile Moritz Schiff (1823–96) at Bern, in a typical extirpation experiment, showed thyroidectomy was fatal to dogs and guineapigs.

It was a well-known fact that the thyroid was affected in various diseases. In certain regions goitre was common: the Roman author Juvenal had casually observed the frequency of such swollen necks in the Alps, while in England 'Derbyshire neck' (goitre) was common in the Peak District. Paracelsus associated goitre with cretinism, both being endemic in mountainous districts. Superficially, of course, these conditions were very dissimilar – in goitre the main change was the neck swelling, whereas cretins showed mental retardation – but links began to be suspected. In 1850 Thomas Curling (1811–88) described two mentally deficient children with fat pads above their collar-bones; neither had goitre, but postmortem revealed absence of the thyroid.

Various treatments for goitre had been tried. It was supposedly cured, like scrofula, by the royal touch; in the Middle Ages Arnald of Villanova recommended burnt sponge ash and seaweed; in 1812 William Prout used iodine. In a characteristic development, the post-Lister era brought attempts at surgery. By 1869 Billroth had done twenty thyroid-ectomies with eight deaths, but the technique was improved by his pupil, Theodor Kocher (1841–1917) of Bern, who had ample local patients to practise on: by 1914 he had performed the operation over 2000 times, with low mortality.

In 1873 William Gull (1816–90) described five cases of 'a cretinoid condition' in adult women, associated with obesity and sluggishness; this condition came to be known as myxoedema. Jacques Louis Reverdin (1842–1929), a Geneva surgeon, then described how, after thyroidec-tomy, symptoms had appeared similar to those seen in myxoedema, and Kocher, in a follow up, found that in thirty out of his first hundred thyroidectomies the operation had been followed by similar distressing symptoms (he called it cachexia strumipriva). The obvious inference was that myxoedema, goitre and cretinism were due to thyroid failure.

If so, might it be possible to remedy this by the administration of thyroid extract? In 1891 George Redmayne Murray (1865–1939) reported the improvement of a forty-six-year-old myxoedemic woman treated with sheep's thyroid injections. Undoubtedly the thyroid played a part in the control of metabolism. When in 1895 Eugen Baumann (1846–96) found an iodine compound in the thyroid, it became clear that iodine deficiency in the diet produced overgrowth of thyroid cells; this opened the way for the control of goitre by the addition of iodine to table salt. Since slow growth and sluggish mental functions were widely associated with cretinism, a fad set in for putting retarded chil-dren on thyroid extract, and for a time it was recommended as a panacea for all manner of symptoms in adults, from obesity to depression.

Another gland, the adrenal, had been mentioned by Eustachius in the sixteenth century and called suprarenal capsules by Jean Riolan (1580–1657). In 1893 George Oliver (1841–1915) and Edward Schäfer (later Sharpey-Schäfer: 1850–1935) injected a dog with an adrenal gland extract: its blood pressure jumped, but they were unable to isolate the active ingredient responsible. Jôkichi Takamine (1854–1922) and Thomas Bell Aldrich (b. 1861) did the same independently in 1901, and three years later Friedrich Stolz (1860–1936) synthesized the substance: 'adrenaline' (epinephrine in the US) was the first 'hormone' to be synthesized.

In 1904 John Newport Langley showed that when adrenaline was injected into the circulation, it produced the same effects as stimulation of the sympathetic nervous system: constriction of the skin and digestive blood vessels and relaxation of visceral muscles. Adrenaline, it was inferred, was constantly being secreted into the bloodstream to maintain normal blood pressure, though this view was disputed by Cannon, whose *Bodily Changes in Pain, Hunger, Fear and Rage* (1919) argued that adrenaline was liberated when required in much larger doses in response to emotional stimuli.

The pituitary gland at the base of the brain had also been known since early times, but its function remained obscure. Most of the diseases now known to be caused by pituitary dysfunction had also been described, but there was no reason to connect them to the gland. Galen's view that the pituitary secreted mucus into the nose was challenged in 1655 by Conrad Viktor Schneider (1614–80) as part of the great rejection of Galenic physiology. Bonet, Wepfer and other early pathologists described enlarged pituitaries but did not associate them with any particular pathological condition.

In 1886 Pierre Marie (1853–1940) described a disease characterized by overgrowth of the jaws and facial bones, hands and feet, and curvature of the spine. Oscar Minkowski (1858–1931) noted that in fatal cases of such 'acromegaly' the pituitary was enlarged, and the American Woods Hutchinson (1862–1930) deduced from this that the pituitary was likely to be a growth centre for the body.

Growth was a disputed topic: deficient growth rate and faulty sex characteristic development had been widely observed but variously explained. The term 'infantilism' was first used by Paul Joseph Lorain (1827–75), while in 1900 Joseph Babinski (1857–1932) described a case of adiposity and arrested sex characteristics in a seventeen-year-old girl; she was found to have a tumour on the pituitary gland. The pieces were beginning to fit together.

Soon after demonstrating the similar effects of adrenaline, Oliver and Sharpey-Schäfer showed that injection of a pituitary emulsion produced a striking blood-pressure rise. In 1909, Henry Dale (1875–1968) produced an extract from the posterior lobe of the pituitary; its active hormone, oxytocin, stimulated uterine contractions during childbirth. Experiments suggested the anterior pituitary had an effect on many of the other ductless glands; it was, according to Walter Langdon-Brown (1870–1946), the 'leader of the endocrine orchestra' (another analogy was prime minister in charge of a cabinet).

The eminent Johns Hopkins neuro-surgeon Harvey Cushing finally clarified the pituitary's function. He determined that the gland secreted growth hormone and delineated the effects of under- and over-secretion. Over-secretion was part of a syndrome whose characteristic features were adiposity of the face and abdomen, hypertension, poor bones, virilism in the female and feminization in the male, all of which he attributed to abnormalities of the anterior pituitary. Cushing evolved operations for removing pituitary tumours, another novelty in brain surgery.

Investigating the hormones produced by the specific brain area called the hypothalamus, Roger Guillemin (b. 1924), Andrew Schally (b. 1926) and Rosalyn Yalow (b. 1921) showed they acted by regulating the secretions of the anterior pituitary gland. By pointing to the role of the brain as a master control centre for the complex chemical functions of the body, their research synthesized neurology and endocrinology, ushering in the hybrid discipline of neuro-endocrinology.

Investigations into secretions confirmed the importance of the physiology of normal functions. They occasionally had spectacular clinical implications, as with studies of the pancreas. Various hypothetical functions had been ascribed to that organ, but recognition of its nature as a digestive gland had begun with de Graaf's collection of pancreatic juice in the seventeenth century.

Quite independently, disorders characterized by weakness, thirst and excessive urination were known from antiquity, Aretaeus applying to them the term *diabetes*, Greek for a siphon.* Avicenna observed the characteristic urine, 'wonderfully sweet'; Thomas Willis added the Latin *mellitus* ('honey sweet') and noted that diabetics 'piss a great deal' while

---

* *Diabetes mellitus* is an extremely grave metabolic disorder in which the diabetic is unable to metabolize glucose, and sugars accumulate in the blood. Large quantities of sugar-laden urine are secreted to flush out the glucose concentrations, while to compensate for energy lack caused by the inability to utilize sugar as a food, the body consumes its fat, resulting in wasting. The sufferer becomes very hungry and thirsty, rapidly loses weight and dies.

suffering from 'persistent thirst'; Matthew Dobson found sugar in the blood, indicating diabetes was not a kidney problem but was systemic.

Links were drawn from time to time between diabetes and the pancreas. Richard Bright reported morbid changes in the pancreas in such cases in 1831, and Friedrick Theodor Frerichs (1819–85) pointed out that one diabetes case in five showed pancreatic changes. Meanwhile Bernard's glycosuria experiments – showing that sugar was produced in the liver with the aid of an enzyme – led others to construe diabetes as a liver disease.

In 1869, Paul Langerhans (1847–88) observed the special cell construction in the pancreas that now bears his name (Islets of Langerhans), but its function puzzled him. In 1889 an animal experiment provided a clue; when Oskar Minkowski and Joseph von Mering (1849–1907) removed a dog's pancreas, it developed diabetes, being unable to digest fat or proteins. Edward Sharpey-Schäfer determined that the substance necessary for carbohydrate metabolism was produced in the Islets of Langerhans, naming this new substance 'insuline' after the Latin *insula* (island). It became plain that diabetes was caused by a disorder of the endocrine portion of the pancreas. Attempts to supply pancreas extract by mouth did not relieve the disease.

After many attempts, the isolation of the active principle of the Islets was achieved in the summer of 1921 by Fred Banting (1891–1941) and Charles Best (1899–1978), working in the laboratory of John Macleod (1876–1935), professor of physiology at Toronto, who had given them the run of his lab and gone off on a fishing holiday in Scotland. They made an extract of the Islets of Langerhans from the pancreas of a specially prepared dog and injected it into a diabetic dog close to death, which soon sat up and wagged its tail.

With the help of a biochemist, J. B. Collip (1892–1965), they made more pancreatic extracts, and their diabetic dogs survived. On 11 January 1922, after some self-experimentation, they gave injections to a fourteen-year-old boy, Leonard Thompson, dying of diabetes in Toronto General Hospital. Almost immediately his blood-sugar level fell; within days, he was out of bed, and within weeks, home and well, although dependent on insulin injections. The world applauded and the Nobel Prize committee in 1923 honoured them: Banting shared the prize with Macleod the fisherman; Best (as Macleod's assistant) and Collip got nothing. Meanwhile, the Eli Lilly Company in Indianapolis, who had helped solved technical problems with producing insulin, had gone into large-scale production. It proved to be one of the century's most valuable life-savers, not least because diabetes is spreading and remains incurable.

Investigation of the sex hormones led to no less momentous consequences. Intrigued all his career by glands, Brown-Séquard sensationally reported to the world in 1889 that he had rejuvenated himself through injections of extracts of guineapig and dog testicles. As early as the third day (so he boasted to the French Academy of Sciences), 'I had recovered at least all my former vigour ... My digestion and the working of my bowels have also improved considerably ... I also find mental work easier than for years.' Such 'organotherapy' created a stir, although the medical profession was divided and his death soon afterwards dented his claims. Sharing with serum and vaccine therapy the promise of scientific miracles, testicular implants enjoyed a vogue nevertheless; the Russian Serge Voronoff (1866–1951) and others popularized monkey-gland implants in the 1920s, and in the United States John R. Brinkley (1885–1942) made a specialty of implanting goats' testicles, promising his clients not simply sexual rejuvenation but the relief of high blood pressure. A charlatan, Brinkley won fame and fortune, setting up his own radio station and running for the governorship of Kansas.

The male sex hormone was fairly easy to investigate. Androsterone was isolated in 1931 by the Berlin chemist Adolf Butenandt (1903–95) and synthesized three years later by Leopold Ruzicka (1887–1976). Soon after, an Amsterdam team led by Ernst Laqueur (1880–1947) succeeded in extracting pure hormone from ground-up bulls' testicles, calling it 'testosterone'. The female sex hormones proved more complex, there being two distinct sources: the ovary proper and the corpus luteum, the 'yellow body' remaining when the egg leaves the ovarian follicle. The role of the corpus luteum in the oestrous cycle and in pregnancy was shown in 1929 by G. W. Corner (1889–1981) and Willard Allen (1904–93) to depend on a hormone named progestin, later called progesterol. Charles Stockard (1879–1939) and George Papanicolaou (1883–1962) had already shown that the vaginal epithelium of certain mammals undergoes characteristic changes during the menstrual cycle.*

---

* Coming to the United States from his native Greece, Papanicolaou had another claim to fame. In 1927, while investigating the reproductive cycle by using vaginal smears obtained from human and animal subjects, he observed the presence of cancer cells. This led him to develop his famous test. Papanicolaou devoted the remainder of his life to campaigning for routine use of the Pap smear as a simple and effective means of early cancer detection.

Though the effect of the lack of sex organs was well known, precisely how the bodily changes involved in sexual maturation and excitation occurred remained a mystery. Again, animal experiments provided the clues. In 1923 the zoologist Edgar Allen (1892–1943) found that injecting fluid from pigs' ovaries into spayed mice brought them into heat. The fluid, he inferred, must contain a female hormone. With Edward Doisy (1893–1986), Allen heard of a discovery by two Berlin gynaecologists who, aiming to diagnose pregnancy, had hit on injecting a woman's urine into a laboratory mouse or rat. If she were pregnant, the animal would go into heat. Evidently, the urine of pregnant women contained a female hormone. In 1929, they announced that they had isolated the female sex hormone oestrin (oestrone), and, by 1933, two more had been discovered: oestriol and oestradiol (with others, these form the oestrogen family).

A year later, a further hormone – progesterone – was isolated from the corpus luteum. Associated with the onset of ovulation, progesterone is secreted in the body by the corpus luteum to prepare the womb and Fallopian tubes in the event of fertilization. Hoping to discover ways of improving the likelihood of conception for infertile couples, John Rock (1890–1984) investigated its therapeutic possibilities and experimented with synthetically produced hormones to regulate progesterone levels. Oestrogen was injected to see whether ovulation itself could be affected by hormones. Obtaining adequate quantities of hormonal substances for research was impossible, however, until the early 1940s, when Russell E. Marker (b. 1902) found that he could extract diosgenin from a wild yam growing in Mexico; this could be transformed in the lab into progesterone – or progestogen, as the synthesized variety became known.

Marker's colleagues took up his work. Carl Djerassi (b. 1923) and George Rosenkrantz synthesized, respectively, the steroid cortisone and the male sex hormone testosterone from the same Mexican yam. Then in 1951, Luis Miramontes, working under Djerassi, modified Marker's progestogen to form the compound norethisterone (norethindrone in the US), which was far more active than human progesterone. This was sent for assessment to four researchers, including Gregory Pincus (1903–67), a biologist at the Worcester Foundation for Experimental Biology in Massachusetts, who soon established that the substance did indeed inhibit ovulation. Pincus was not at first interested in producing a method of birth control, but its potential was stressed by the veteran campaigner on women's sexual issues, Margaret Sanger (1879–1966), who as early as 1916 had opened a birth control clinic in Brooklyn (she was arrested and jailed).

Sanger enlisted the help of Katharine McCormick (1875–1967), who arranged for Pincus, Rock and Dr Min-chueh Chang (1908–1991) to receive a large grant for research into effective hormonal birth control. In 1955, a major clinical trial was mounted among the poor of Rio Piedras, Puerto Rico. Results published the following year showed success. In 1957 norethynodrel was approved by the US Food and Drug Administration as a 'menstrual regulator' and, two years later, as an oral contraceptive.

The amount of oestrogen contained in 'the pill' was arbitrary and women were seriously overdosed from the first. By 1961, adverse side-effects were being reported – thrombosis, phlebitis, migraine and jaundice, and in 1969 the UK Committee on the Safety of Medicines advised doctors to prescribe oral contraceptives with no more than fifty microgrammes of oestrogen. The 'pill generation' had arrived, with its pleasures and problems.

A devout Roman Catholic, Rock began to campaign for the reform of Catholic hostility towards artificial birth control. Arguing that the operation of the pill was the same as that of the body's endocrine system, he maintained that oral contraceptives fell within the bounds of 'natural' sexual activity. In 1963 he presented his case in *The Time Has Come: A Catholic Doctor's Proposal to End the Battle for Birth Control*. The Vatican thought it hadn't.

CHEMISTRY AND THE NERVES

Running parallel with these endocrinological developments came momentous work on other aspects of the body's self-regulatory system. The pivotal figure was Henry Dale (1875–1968). After studying physiology at Cambridge, Dale worked at University College London under Starling and Bayliss, before becoming pharmacologist to the Wellcome Physiological Research Laboratories in 1904. In 1914 he became pharmacologist to the MRC's newly established National Institute for Medical Research, and was appointed its first director in 1928.

A major problem staring physiology and neurology in the face was the transmission of impulses and stimuli: how were messages transmitted from nerve fibre to nerve fibre? Descartes had suggested there were 'spirits' in the nerves, but that answer was no longer acceptable. Certain pieces in the jigsaw were available.

It was known that muscarine, a drug derived from the fungus *Amanita muscaria*, had an effect similar to that produced by stimulation of the para-sympathetic nerves. Adrenaline gave results paralleling the stimulation of para-sympathetic nerves. Nicotine, the chief alkaloid of tobacco, had a complex action on the nervous system, first stimulating and then depressing autonomic ganglia. Extracts of many tissues, when injected, produced a pronounced depressor action. Leon Popielski (1866–1920) suggested such extracts all contained a substance which he called 'vasodilatin'.

Meanwhile, the substance soon to be called histamine was chemically synthesized, George Barger (1878–1939) and Dale obtaining it from an ergot extract in 1910. They found it produced powerful contractions of the smooth muscle of a cat's uterus. Histamine had never been isolated from a living body, but it was recalled that when Bayliss and Starling had hit upon 'secretin' (secreted from the duodenum), they had found that the intestinal extracts contained a further substance with a profound depressant action. Following up this lead, Barger and Dale came upon histamine. The paradox that histamine, a potent stimulator of plain (smooth) muscle, produced a fall of blood pressure by vasodilation, was still unexplained.

The Great War necessitated close study of traumatic shock, and Edward Mellanby observed that a large dose of histamine produced effects similar to surgical shock: fall in body temperature, drowsiness, slow breathing. The striking resemblance between histamine shock and surgical shock led Thomas Lewis to demonstrate that histamine was released by the injured cells in shock. Other substances were also released by cells as a result of injury, leading to the study of allergic disorders. In 1914, Dale found an ergot extract produced activities resembling those of muscarine; the active chemical principle proved to be acetylcholine, which affected muscle response at certain nerve fibre junctions, and could thus mimic the actions of the para-sympathetic nervous system.

A further piece in the puzzle was put in place in 1921 by Otto Loewi (1873–1961), professor of pharmacology at Graz. Loewi had been carrying out a series of experiments on transmission of nerve impulses, working on the assumption that messages between nerve fibres and their organs were chemically transmitted. He had been working chiefly with an isolated frog's heart, testing the effects of drugs, including digitalis. In 1920, in dreams on two successive nights, he envisaged the design for a critical experiment.

> The night before Easter Sunday of [1921] I awoke, turned on the light, and jotted down a few notes on a tiny slip of thin paper. Then I fell asleep again. It occurred to me at six o'clock in the morning that during the night I had written down something most important, but I was unable to decipher the scrawl. The next night, at three o'clock, the idea returned. It was the design of an experiment to determine whether or not the hypothesis of chemical transmission that I had uttered seventeen years ago was correct. I got up immediately, went to the laboratory, and performed a simple experiment on a frog heart according to the nocturnal design. I have to describe briefly this experiment since its results became the foundation of the theory of chemical transmission of the nervous impulse.
>
> The hearts of two frogs were isolated, the first with its nerves, the second without. Both hearts were attached to Straub cannulas filled with a little Ringer solution. The Ringer solution of the first heart, during the stimulation of the vagus nerve, was transferred to the second heart. It slowed and its beats diminished just as if its vagus had been stimulated. Similarly, when the accelerator nerve was stimulated and the Ringer from this period transferred, the second heart speeded up and its beats increased. These results unequivocally proved that the nerves do not influence the heart directly but liberate from their terminals specific chemical substances which, in their turn, cause the well-known modifications of the function of the heart characterisitic of the stimulation of its nerves.

What was this chemical substance producing the stimulus? Loewi suspected it might be acetylcholine or a related chemical, as was proved in 1933 by Dale and his colleagues Wilhelm Feldberg (1900–93) and John Henry Gaddum (1900–65). Other chemical agents, adrenaline-like substances, were found in the sympathetic nervous system, and a nerve classification was developed according to their suspected transmitter substances: 'cholinergic' (vagus) nerves secreted acetylcholine while 'adrenergic' (sympathetic) nerves secreted adrenaline.

Elucidation of impulse transmission in the muscles and organs was a remarkable breakthrough. Far more daunting was the investigation of the central nervous system. While there was indirect evidence of chemical action there, experimentation was difficult in that area. Research at

Oxford in 1941 indicated the presence of acetylcholine, secreted by motor nerve fibres in response to electrical stimulation. Later experiments showed that acetylcholine was the chemical agent through which nerves worked on muscles – the first neurotransmitter to be identified. Evidence also grew of monoamines in the central system, including adrenaline, dopamine and serotonin.

With the principal transmitters identified as noradrenaline at sympathetic endings and acetylcholine at most other sites, it became possible to draw a picture of the actions of atropine (blocking muscarine-like actions of the acetylcholine receptor), eserine (delaying the destruction of acetylcholine and so enhancing its actions), curare (blocking acetylcholine), and a number of other drugs.

Once chemical agents in the brain and their role in the nervous system were recognized, the use of drugs to combat mental maladies and modify behaviour became feasible. In 1943, the Swiss biochemist Albert Hofmann (b. 1906) accidentally swallowed lysergic acid diethylamide (LSD). Suffering severe hallucinations and loss of emotional control, he had to be tranquillized. LSD was found to inhibit serotonin action and to block noradrenaline and adrenaline. Similar studies were done on reserpine, benzedrine (amphetamine) and tranquillizers such as chlorpromazine: all inhibited transmitter functioning. The psychotropic effects of such substances led to extensive psychiatric use for some and criminalization for others.

This burgeoning chemical understanding of the brain bore fruit in the treatment of diseases such as parkinsonism, named after the London doctor James Parkinson (1755–1824), author of the classic *Essay on the Shaking Palsy* (1817). Characterized by tremor in the limbs, stiffness of the muscles and difficulty in initiating movement, Parkinson's disease develops when a group of nerve cells in the brain fails to function normally. Their location was established in the 1950s as the *substantia nigra*, a layer of grey matter in the midbrain. Once a new neurotransmitter, dopamine, was found to be synthesized there in large amounts, the possibility of a pharmaceutical cure was glimpsed.

Scientists grasped that the new neuroleptic drugs, reserpine (also much used for lowering blood pressure) and the phenothiazines seemed to produce Parkinson-like symptoms by way of side-effects. Since they interfered with the action of dopamine at nerve endings, it was surmised that there was a direct link between dopamine and the disease: the *substantia nigra* cells of parkinsonism sufferers were producing insufficient dopamine to establish muscular movement. In 1961 trials using L-DOPA, a chemical analogue of dopamine, showed that the drug enabled the affected brain cells to make dopamine once more, alleviating symptoms of Parkinson's disease. Six years later L-DOPA therapy was officially introduced and hailed as a wonder drug: bed-ridden patients could walk; others found relief from a rigid posture.

They were not the only beneficiaries. Just after the close of the First World War, a disease called encephalitis lethargica had appeared, apparently linked to the influenza pandemic. Survivors had been left with post-encephalitic parkinsonism, a kind of sleeping sickness. Forty years later, the British neurologist Oliver Sacks (b. 1933) tried treating such patients with L-DOPA, and watched as the drug awakened them. Many began talking, walking and gradually becoming normal. It seemed a miracle cure. But the disease could be kept at bay only with ever larger doses, side-effects took the hapless patients over and eventually outweighed the advantages. The post-encephalitic patients returned to their sleeping state.

Before these advances in brain chemistry, little could be done with central nervous system failures unless they were open to surgery. Once the transmitter-inhibitor set-up was known, however, correction of brain function defects became a realistic possibility. Such understanding of chemical action in the brain and nervous system stimulated fruitful lines of research regarding the neurophysiology governing behaviour. The knowledge that specific chemicals selectively stimulate certain brain cells has led both to the new psychopharmacological 'wonder drug' Prozac, and to chemical nerve gases of extraordinary toxicity, like Sarin.

CANCER

In some modern research fields, endocrinology perhaps being one of them, the initial impulse for gigantic transformations arose from scientific curiosity put to good use in the laboratory. Other research enterprises have been driven by the desperate need to relieve a particular disease. Of these the most prominent, but problematic, has been cancer.

Cancer became the modern disease *par excellence* (one distinguished sufferer was Freud), and above all the American disease. Cancer ('the big C') became the subject of terrible taboos, seen not just as fatal but as psychogenic, the product of the so-called 'cancer personality', the self that eats itself away through frustration and repressed anger. Such myths made the disease unmentionable and created a terrible stigma.

About 1.3 million new cases occur a year in the United States and half a million die of it annually. Among males, prostate, lung and colon cancer amount to around half of all cases; for women the most common forms are cancer of the breast, colon and lung. After a century in which research has received billions of tax dollars and attracted the talents of top scientists, the situation is little less bleak than before. Lung, colon, liver, pancreas and other major cancers continue to have appalling fatality rates, with fewer than one in five alive after five years of diagnosis (survival in uterine and stomach cancer has improved).

Cancer was familiar in antiquity, Hippocrates employing the term *karcinos* (Greek for crab), presumably because the pain resembles a crab's pinching. Hippocratic medicine attributed tumours to an abnormal humoral accretion, and Galen regarded the disease as a species of inflammation. A tumour might form because there was too much blood in the veins; or a flux of black bile mixed with blood produced a scirrhus, a tumour which could transmute into cancer. Galen endorsed the Hippocratic counsel against attempting to treat deep or hidden cancers; Rhazes warned that surgery generally made matters worse unless the tumour was completely removed and the incision cauterized, and Paré confessed he had never seen cancer cured by the knife.

The old black bile theory was long held, but once the lymphatic system was delineated by Gasparo Aselli (1622), the lymph was increasingly blamed as carcinogenic. John Hunter maintained that under certain conditions coagulating lymph (the part of the blood which spontaneously clots) was the carcinogenic inflammatory factor. Metastases reached distant parts via lymphatic channels. This supported the nineteenth-century idea of 'blastema', the fluid substance supposedly carried in the blood and circulated to the tissues to provide the nutritive, generative substance for cells. Tumours were said to result from a defect in the blastema, causing cell growth to turn malignant.

The triumph of cell theory transformed the understanding of cancer, Virchow holding that neoplasms developed from immature cells. In 1867 Edwin Klebs proposed that most cancers originated in epithelial tissues,* while in the same year Wilhelm Waldeyer outlined the

---

* When a tumour originates in epithelial tissues of the breast, lungs or stomach, for example, it is called carcinoma; originating in connective tissues of bone or muscle, it is called sarcoma.

approach that formed the basis of later theories. Denying blastema theory and the possibility of outside infection, Wildeyer maintained that cancer cells developed from normal cells, multiplying by cell division. Long-distance spread (metastasis) resulted from transportation of cancer cells by blood or lymph.

It was one thing to pinpoint the cell as the locus of cancer, but quite another to identify the source of carcinogenesis. Disputes flared as to whether cancer was unitary or whether there were many different sorts with different aetiologies. The model of infectious disease made the possibility of a viral origin attractive, partly because of the implied possibility of a vaccine cure. Laboratory experiments in the 1930s showed that viruses could produce tumours in animals.

From the late 1960s research into oncogenic viruses was particularly advanced by David Baltimore (b. 1938) and Howard Temin (b. 1934), who simultaneously published a report of the discovery of an enzyme reverse transcriptase. Based on his investigations of animal cancers, Temin suggested that when a tumour-causing virus enters a cell, the RNA of the virus makes DNA copies of itself, thereby causing the host cell to become cancerous. Because the idea was widely interpreted as a violation of the 'central dogma' of genetics, it was scornfully dismissed by most of the scientific establishment, with the notable exception of David Baltimore. The theory of viruses as the cause of cancer in humans remains highly contested.

By the early twentieth century laboratory research had also shown that the disease could be experimentally produced in animals by various chemical and physical agents including coal tars; ultraviolet light and X-rays, as well as radioactive substances such as radium and uranium, also induced cancer. The dream of chemotherapy dates from the same period. With Ehrlich's discovery of salvarsan, hopes were raised that a drug would be found to destroy cancer cells. In the 1920s, hopes were pinned on variants of the mustard gas prepared as a chemical warfare agent in the First World War; it was thought that this would prove a cytotoxic agent useful in cancer. As with other chemotherapeutic agents, the problem with mustard gas was that it destroyed or inhibited healthy cells as well as cancer cells; the drug produced a temporary improvement but no long-term cure and hence only a delayed death.

No 'magic bullet' has ever been found, though chemotherapy had enjoyed substantial success with childhood leukaemia, a bone-marrow cancer resulting in proliferation of white blood cells and reduced output

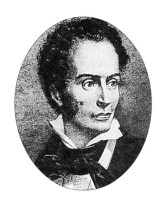

LEFT *Laennec.*
René Théophile Hyancinthe Laennec (1781–1826), inventor of the stethoscope, epitomized French medicine in the Romantic era. A pioneer investigator of tuberculosis, he himself suffered from the disease. Reproduction of a miniature on ivory, early nineteenth century.

BELOW LEFT *Pasteur.*
Louis Pasteur (1822–96) was the greatest non-doctor in the history of medicine. Trained as a chemist, his practical wizardry in developing vaccines helped establish the science of bacteriology. E. Pirou, photograph, late nineteenth century.

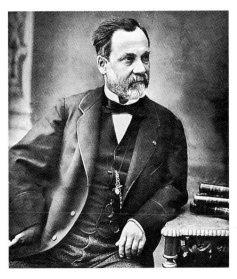

BELOW FAR RIGHT *Gorgas.*
General William Crawford Gorgas (1845–1920), a military doctor from Mobile, Alabama, played a major part in the control of yellow fever in Cuba and Panama, using the techniques of the new tropical medicine. Photograph, late nineteenth century.

RIGHT *Christiaan Barnard.*
Performing the first human heart transplant in 1967 made Christiaan Barnard (1922–) the most widely known medical figure of the second half of the twentieth century. B. Govender, photograph, *c.* 1967.

ABOVE *Lister.*
Joseph Lister (1827–1912) developed the techniques of modern antiseptic surgery in Glasgow in the 1860s. He was the first medical practitioner to be made a peer. Photograph, late nineteenth century.

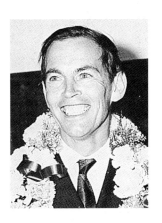

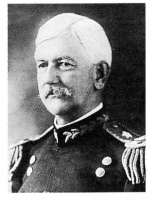

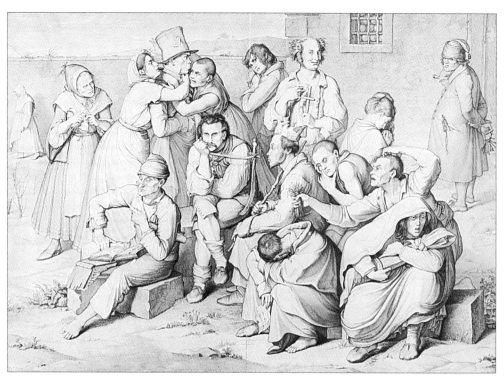

Mentally ill patients in the garden of an asylum.

Before the era of photography, the mad were usually depicted by artists according to low-life traditions of the comic and the grotesque. K. H. Merz, under the direction of S. Amsler, engraving, *c.* 1834 (after W. Kaulbach).

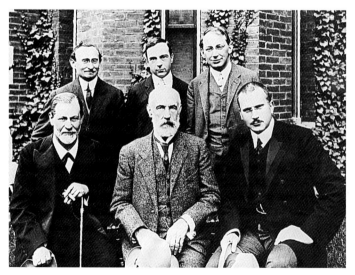

Sigmund Freud, Carl Gustav Jung, Ernest Jones, Sandor Ferenczi, Abraham Brill and G. Stanley Hall.

This picture was taken at the twentieth anniversary celebration of the founding of Clark University, Worcester, Massachusetts. Back row (left to right): Brill, Jones (1879–1958), Ferenczi (1873–1933); front row: Freud (1856–1939), Hall, Jung (1875–1961). Photograph, 1909.

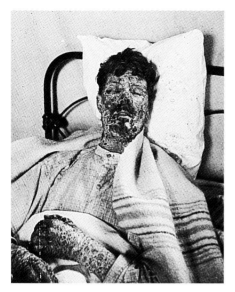 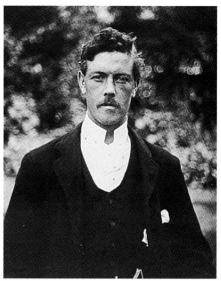

Male smallpox patient in sickness   *. . . and in health.*

The great outbreak of smallpox in Gloucester in the 1890s was one of the last serious epidemics of that disease in England. It was significant since Gloucester had been one of the major centres of resistance to vaccination. Photograph from Gloucester smallpox album, 1896.

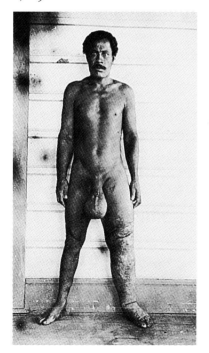 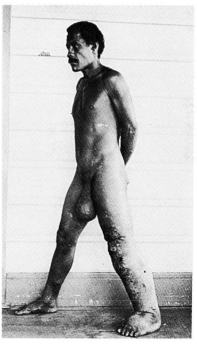

Elephantiasis: Fijian man, with elephantiasis of the left leg and scrotum.

Elephantiasis is a chronic disfiguring disease which, through lymph-flow blockage, produces grotesque swelling of the limbs and genitalia. It is caused by a nematode worm, *Filaria*. It was first seriously studied by Patrick Manson, the founder of modern tropical medicine. Photographs, 1920/21.

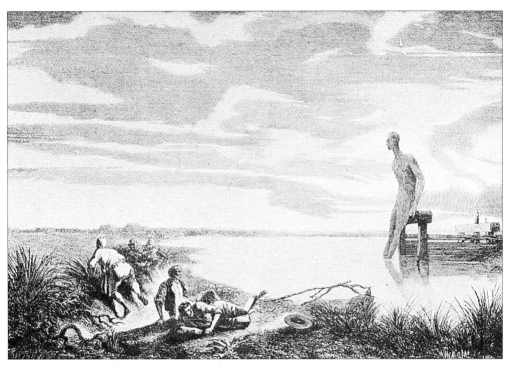

An Allegory of Malaria.

The image of malaria as a disease which left its victims pale, wan and enfeebled remained widespread until the public health campaigns of the early twentieth century and the introduction of pesticides like DDT in the 1930s. Maurice Dudevant, engraving, *c.* 1889 (after M. Sand).

A white doctor vaccinating African girls all wearing European clothes at a mission station.

Vaccinations were to become one of the major rituals of the implantation of Western medicine into colonial contexts, particularly through the work of medical missionaries. Meisenbach, process print after a photograph.

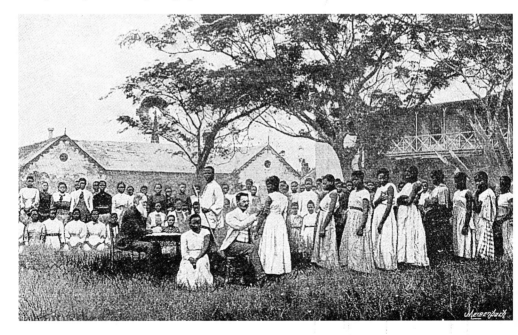

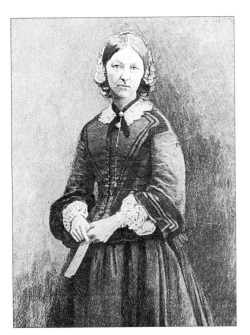

Florence Nightingale.
As well as being the 'lady with the lamp' in the Crimean War, Florence Nightingale (1830 – 1910) reformed nursing, rendering it an esteemed profession suitable for respectable women. Reproduction of wood engraving, 1872 (after Goodman, 1858).

A Nurse Checking on a Playful Child.
The sick child and the humane nurse loom large in the image of the modern hospital as the most successful institution of modern medicine. J. E. Sutcliffe, watercolour drawing, 1904.

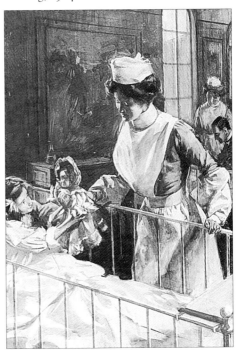

A district health centre where crowds of local children are being vaccinated.
Smallpox vaccinations were delivered to the poor through medical charities and the agency of the Poor Law. In reality, there was much popular opposition to vaccination. E. Buckman, wood engraving, 1871.

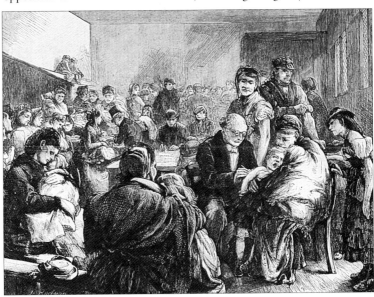

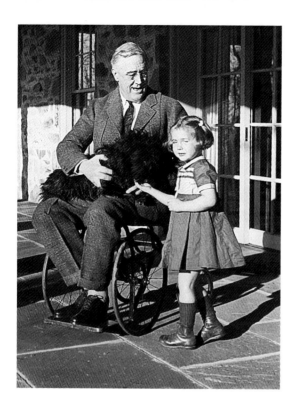

Franklin D. Roosevelt.
One of only two known
photographs of FDR in
a wheelchair. Photograph,
1941.

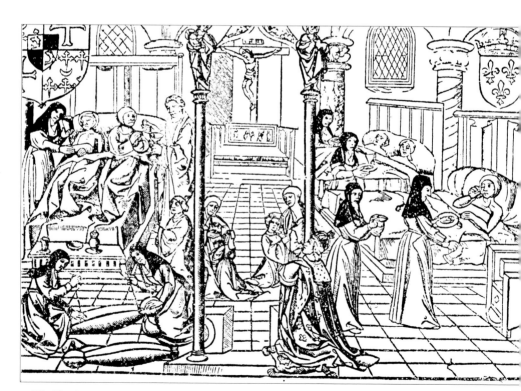

The Hôtel Dieu, Paris: interior showing patients being nursed by nuns and clergy.
Note the prominence of the crucifix: the medieval hospital might be a place to die, as well as a
scene of recovery. Woodcut, early sixteenth century.

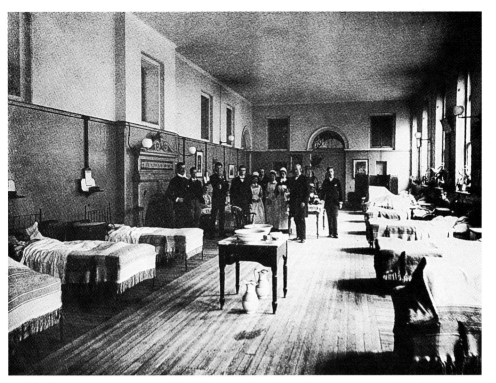

Lister and his assistants in the Victoria Ward (King's College Hospital's male surgical ward).
By the end of the nineteenth century, the homely atmosphere of the Victorian hospital ward was giving way to something more austere, in line with the new emphasis upon hygiene, cleanliness and order. Photograph, 1890.

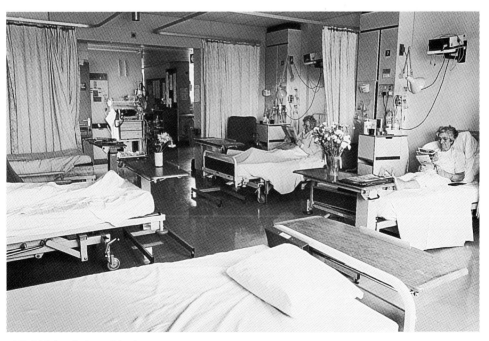

A British hospital ward in the 1990s
A ward in St George's Hospital, London. Emma Taylor, photograph, 1997.

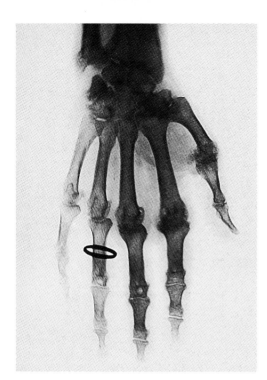

The bones of a hand, with a ring on one finger, viewed through X-ray.

The discovery of the power of X-rays at the close of the nineteenth century triggered a staggering series of advances in diagnostic devices, allowing direct access to the interior of the living body. Photoprint from radiograph (after Sir Arthur Schuster, 1896).

BELOW *A brain in a skull.*

Three-dimensional computed tomograph (CT) scan of the top of the human brain seen within the skull. The right cerebral hemisphere is seen intact (at top left) with surface convolutions. CT scanning combines the use of a computer and X-rays passed through the body to produce cross-sectional images of the body tissue. It is particularly useful for the diagnosis of abnormalities of the brain.

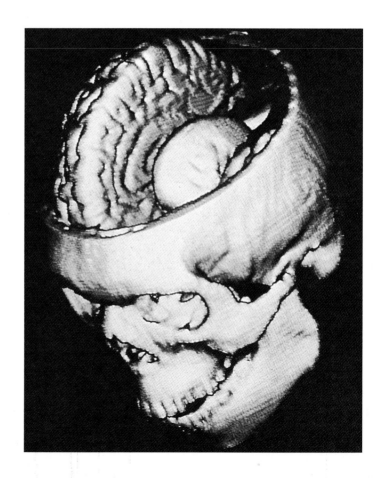

of red cells and platelets. Until the early 1960s little could be done for acute leukaemia, which was speedily fatal. The administration of cortisone-like drugs helped, and it was found that other drugs used in combination with corticosteroids could prolong remissions. Ultimately, it was possible to cure a high proportion of childhood leukaemias – one of the genuine medical successes of the postwar period.

Before the twentieth century, the main institutions dealing with cancer were hospitals to die in. The situation changed radically as public concern mounted: societies to support cancer studies proliferated. The German Central Committee for Cancer Research was organized in 1900. Two years later the Royal Colleges founded the Imperial Cancer Research Fund, and the French Association for Cancer Research followed in 1906. The American Association for Cancer Research was launched in 1907; the massive and influential Memorial Sloan–Kettering Cancer Center in New York City in the 1930s. With cancer established as the most dreaded disease, President Nixon, drawing comparisons with the Manhattan Project and the Apollo Program, secured the passing of a National Cancer Act in 1971, with an initial allocation of $500 million; by 1976 the US budget had risen to over $1 billion a year. To wage the 'Crusade Against Cancer', the act implemented a research programme, the creation of a new cancer institute independent of the National Institutes of Health (it had a 'hot-line' to the president), and an international cancer data bank.

Despite the immense investment of money and research effort, cancer remains a disease imperfectly understood, in which relief is far more common than cure, and relief generally temporary and subject to serious side-effects. All manner of therapies have been tried, leading to the now familiar combination of surgery, radiotherapy and chemotherapy. X-ray screening programmes, CAT-scans, ultrasound and MRI-scans have brought advances in early detection. Monoclonal antibodies represent another advance. Developed by Cesar Milstein (b. 1927) and Georges Köhler (b. 1946) in one of biotechnology's early triumphs, these laboratory-cloned 'designer' antibodies can be used to identify foreign material on a cell wall, attach themselves to it and destroy it, rather like a guided missile. If tagged with radioactive isotopes, they provide a radioactive profile for scanners when they track down cancer cells. In some cases, such aids to early diagnosis save lives. But diagnostic advances have continued to outrun cures.

True, there have been some victories, as with child leukaemia, but at no time this century could a sober analyst think the cancer war was being won with the routine weaponry in the arsenal: surgery, chemotherapy and radiation. Combined assaults from all three may grant extra months or years to many, but proven cures have been the exception, and, that is why the chequered history of immunotherapy is so fascinating.

In view of the shortcomings of the other interventions, it might have been expected that the claims of immunology – co-opting and stiffening the body's own resistances – would always have been to the fore. After all, by 1900, thanks to the pioneering microbiology of Pasteur and Koch, it was known that the body fought back against invasive pathogens through its cells and serum (antibodies). Pasteur's anti-anthrax and anti-rabies vaccines, and the German serum vaccines, notably diphtheria antitoxin, had shown that modern medicine could stiffen the body's innate defences. So why didn't the immunological approach come to dominate cancer research?

The answer is laced with irony. William B. Coley (1862–1928) was a young New York surgeon in the 1890s. He operated on his cancer patients as best he could but they routinely died. In those days, before aseptic surgery had become foolproof, patients still developed terrible operating-room infections, and Coley came across a cancer patient who had gone down with the often lethal erysipelas. Not only did he survive the infection – his sarcoma disappeared! Some rooting around showed Coley that these miracle recoveries were not unknown in medical folk-lore. Infections would provoke a massive immune response that might sometimes knock out cancer. Gaining a post at what became the Memorial Sloan–Kettering Cancer Center, Coley made biological vaccines against cancer his life's work.

But to little avail. For one thing, he was a surgeon not a scientist. Then his domineering colleague/rival/enemy at the hospital, James Ewing, was a passionate champion of radiation therapy. Coley's 'biological cures', Ewing would say, were probably all baloney. So lethal was cancer that Coley's occasional 'miracle' cure helped to discredit him – it sounded like quackery. Not least, his immunotherapy seemed to imply that cancer, like tuberculosis, was caused by an invasive micro-organism; that hypothesis was never substantiated.

Thereafter cancer immunotherapy was marginalized and did not reclaim the limelight until immunology itself had made further strides. Not least, the field experienced the great expectations and crashing disappointments of interferon. By the late 1950s hopes were high that this newly isolated and commercially developed anti-viral protein which stimulated the body's defences and was toxic to certain cells might be the wonder treatment for neoplasms. It proved far from that, and the interferon ballyhoo had abiding untoward consequences. It led to endless hype about the latest drug 'breakthroughs'; to personality cults among researchers who suddenly found themselves on the front cover of *Newsweek*; and to the contamination of the whole field by big money: astronomical grants thanks to President Nixon's war against cancer, and the lure of gigantic profits through patenting laboratory processes.

This modern era of glitzy research and its prima donnas is epitomized perhaps by the career of Steven Rosenberg of the National Cancer Institute, a dedicated if egotistical cancer mogul. Of Polish parentage, Rosenberg has described cancer as the biological equivalent of the Holocaust. For all Rosenberg's passion and drive, his activities are no less problematic for cancer research than Robert Gallo has proved for AIDS, a symptom of the perils of science when it operates through careerist entrepreneurship and a macho star system.

The interferon hullabaloo saved no cancer sufferers, but it did revitalise the search for comparable molecular agents produced by the body which could be modified to enhance effectiveness. The production of clonal antibodies in the 1970s constituted a breakthrough: substances which would boost the immune system could now be made *ad lib*, not just in the body but in the laboratory.

Out of this molecular milieu there followed the interleukins, discovered in the 1980s, and at last doctors began to be able to point to cases where (as with Coley much earlier) tumours shrivelled and patients at death's door began to mend. Again, the business was oversold. Around 1985, to great acclaim, Rosenberg treated some twenty-five cases with immunity-boosting LAK cells and interleukin-2. Ten years later only one of the twenty-five was still alive. Without the treatment perhaps none would be, and of course therapies inevitably have their teething problems; but, given the huge adverse side-effects which such treatments entailed, it's not clear how much those patients really benefited. Nor is it self-evident that Rosenberg was having more success than Coley, seventy years earlier.

Given the tribulations of surgical and chemical interventions, the best break we have had with cancer has come from epidemiology. Concerned with increasing mortality from lung cancer, the Medical Research Council in 1947 commissioned Austin Bradford Hill (1897–1991) and Richard

Doll (b. 1912) to analyse the possible causes. Their meticulous statistical survey (published in 1951) of patients from twenty London hospitals showed that 'smoking is a factor, and an important factor, in the production of cancer of the lung.' Studying smoking in the medical profession, they showed in 1956 that the mortality from the disease fell if individuals stopped smoking. An easy way to reduce drastically, if not to eliminate, a major form of cancer had been discovered. Nearly half a century later, one in three adult men in the UK still smokes, and the figure for women is almost as high and rising. It is, moreover, widely believed that thorough studies, comparable to those of smoking, would reveal that many cancers are environmentally produced. X-rays and ionizing radiation are thought to be the source of 3 per cent of cancers; radon gas causes lung cancer in uranium miners. Synthetic food additives and dyes, fertilizers and pesticides may all be carcinogenic. The implications of this paradox – vast investment in research, yet public indifference to practical preventive action – are discussed in Chapter 21.

CARDIOLOGY

As with cancer, heart disease became big news in the twentieth century. As late as 1892 Sir William Osler had described coronary disease as 'relatively rare', but less than two decades later one in eight of all deaths in advanced nations was attributed to heart disorders. By the 1980s that figure had risen to 30 per cent, making coronary disease the chief killer of all – and for every two people *dying* from a heart attack, three others *suffered* one. This huge increase prompted myriad medical studies, most famously the long-running Framingham Heart Study in the United States, begun in 1948.

Knowledge of cardiovascular disease was gathered from many sources. The blood was studied by John Hunter (who died from a heart attack) and his successors. The physiological understanding of hypertension was given its foundations by Bernard's and Brown-Séquard's studies of vasodilation and vasoconstriction. Other studies meantime explored the physiology of the heart muscle; in 1859 Michael Foster showed that a part of a snail's heart continued to show rhythmical contractions when separated from the rest of the organ, and Gaskell, using frogs' hearts, proved that the heartbeat was, as Haller had suggested, of myogenic origin.

By that time there was an extensive clinical record of heart disease. A major early work was the *Traité de la structure du coeur* (1749) [Treatise on the Structure of the Heart] by Jean-Baptiste Sénac, which published descriptions based on patients' symptoms. Morgagni's morbid anatomy (1761) contained much evidence of heart damage; the heart lost force, he noted, as its parts became 'tendinous' (like tendons) instead of fleshy. In 1768 William Heberden coined the term *angina pectoris* to describe a distinctive crushing chest pain:

> They who are afflicted with it, are seized while they are walking, (more especially if it be up hill, and soon after eating) with a painful and most disagreeable sensation in the breast, which seems as if it would extinguish life, if it were to increase or to continue; but the moment they stand still, all this uneasiness vanishes.

Caleb Parry's (1755–1822) *Inquiry into the Symptoms and Causes of the Syncope Anginosa, Commonly Called Angina Pectoris* (1799) discussed 'ossification' and obstruction of the coronary arteries together with pathology of the aorta, and Antonio Scarpa (1752–1832) described what was later termed arteriosclerosis. Pointing to the danger of clots in the pulmonary artery, Virchow introduced the idea of thrombosis.

Diagnostic skills were refined. Corvisart, Laennec and Bayle listened to the heart at the bedside, relating unusual murmurs to damage of the valves which they verified postmortem. Other symptoms of heart disease were noted, largely on the basis of the pulse. A very slow pulse or one with striking abnormalities became associated with syncope or intermittent loss of consciousness, later known as Stokes-Adams disease after the Dublin physicians Robert Adams and William Stokes. Julius Cohnheim (1839–84) identified 'heart aneurysm' with coronary obstructions, believing that failure of oxygen supply (ischaemia) was responsible for myocardial damage. In 1880 Carl Weigert (1845–1904) gave a classic description of the heart attack or myocardial infarction, and these descriptions grew more common (as perhaps did the phenomenon).

New diagnostic techniques led to a greater attempt to monitor the heart, notably Karl Vierordt's (1818–84) sphygmograph (1855) and Scipione Riva-Rocci's (1863–1937) sphygmomanometer (1896). In 1859 Etienne-Jules Marey (1830–1904) modified Ludwig's kymograph to produce a permanent record of the pulse on a drum of smoked paper. James Mackenzie (1853–1925) developed a polygraph by which two or three simultaneous tracings could be inked onto a roll of unsmoked paper, correlating pulses in the arteries and veins with the heart-beat, to shed light on irregularities of the heart's rhythm.

In his *Diseases of the Heart* (1908), Mackenzie, who complained about the 'utmost confusion prevailing as to the significance of the signs detected in the heart', emphasized the dangers of mechanistic, technology-driven diagnosis: what mattered in certain heart conditions was not the presence of a murmur, but the capacity of the heart muscle to compensate for disabilities caused by valvular abnormalities. He thus distinguished between harmless alterations in heart rhythm and those indicative of severe heart disease. The trouble was that it was difficult to predict which abnormalities in rhythm were harmless.

The electrocardiograph, a specialized type of galvanometer recording and photographing the minute electric currents generated by the heart's action, was invented in 1903 by Willem Einthoven (1860–1927) of Leiden. Initially it was an unwieldy and expensive contraption, requiring the patient to place both hands and both feet in buckets of water, and needing five technicians to operate it. It involved a silver-coated quartz fibre suspended between the poles of an electromagnet; electrical signals from the heart were conducted through the fibre, which bent at right angles to the electromagnetic field produced by the signals. The fibre's shadow showed up on a moving glass photographic plate; the record is known as the electrocardiogram (ECG, or EKG in America). It pointed the way to differentiating rhythmic abnormalities which posed no threat from those which did. The fact that it was mainly confined to large hospitals was instrumental in turning the hospital into the heart investigation and treatment centre which it became.

Intensive studies were carried out with it by Thomas Lewis, a great *aficionado*. It enabled him to record the waves that spread through the atria and to follow the electrical events accompanying ventricular contraction (though many of Lewis's inferences were contested). With the ECG it became possible to recognize thickening of the walls of the ventricles and diseases of the pericardium (the membrane covering the outside of the heart). The Chicago physician James Herrick (1861–1954) formulated a description of coronary thrombosis and ascertained its characteristic changes in the ECG. By the 1920s the clinical definition of acute myocardial infarction (heart attack) was becoming consolidated, though only after huge debate and negotiation over the meaning of clinical and machine-readable signs. Perhaps such events were becoming more common; certainly doctors were training themselves to perceive and identify them.

The predisposing high blood pressure or hypertension became the high-profile heart condition of the twentieth century, being diagnostic for heart attacks. Arteriosclerosis – thickening and hardening of the arteries – means that the heart must beat more strongly to perfuse the body; this produces the 'hard pulse' familiar to clinicians and brings on shortness of breath and angina pains. A sudden occlusion of the coronary artery precipitates a heart attack, sometimes with loss of heart rhythm which may prove fatal. Studies demonstrated that arteriosclerosis was caused by a build up of fatty deposits in arterial walls; stress, smoking and excessive drinking were found to exacerbate the condition.

By the inter-war years cardiology had become established as a specialty on both sides of the Atlantic. Vast ingenuity went into new methods for understanding the physiology and pathology of the heart and for making diagnoses in the individual case. Catheterization was developed in the 1930s, leading to modern angiocardiography; these advances were later augmented by the development of non-invasive methods of studying the heart: computerized axial tomography (CAT-scanning) and nuclear magnetic resonance (NMR-scanning).

More so than with most cancers, diagnostic advance was accompanied by progress in managing hypertensive heart disease. Bypass and other open-heart surgery to relieve the occluded arteries causing angina and heart attacks was introduced from the 1960s, and became immensely popular, especially in the United States. Such surgical interventions are discussed in Chapter 19.

Drug treatments for failing hearts had long been tried and were steadily improved. For long, the only drug of value for treating heart failure was digitalis, discovered by William Withering in the mid eighteenth century. Alongside a low salt diet, the first major pharmacological advance was the advent of oral diuretics to counteract fluid retention due to a failing heart. From the 1930s prostaglandin and other new drugs were introduced to lower blood pressure, in the light of a better understanding of control by the autonomic nervous system of the tone of blood vessels.

The medical treatment of angina, long assisted by amyl nitrate which dilates the vessels, has been improved by beta-blockers. Developed by the English chemist Sir James Black (b. 1924), beta-blockers block the action of the sympathetic nervous system on the heart. The sympathetic nervous system speeds the heart up, activating receptors called beta adrenergic receptors. The beta receptors may be blocked by the drug propranolol (Nethalide) and subsequent drugs, which are therefore called beta-blockers. First targeted at angina, they were subsequently prescribed for reducing blood pressure and steadying the heartbeat. They were not an unalloyed gain: by the mid 1970s, side-effects had predictably begun to appear – Eraldin, marketed in Britain, was linked with deafness, peritonitis, pleurisy and damaged sight.

Other drugs possessing blood-thinning and clot-dissolving qualities have proved useful: streptokinase, developed in the 1960s, and the faithful aspirin. Experience showed that if streptokinase were given within a few hours of a heart attack and followed by aspirin, deaths were reduced by 40 per cent. It is currently believed that small quantities of aspirin taken regularly may substantially reduce the risk of heart attack. Similar anticoagulants which interfere with blood-clotting have been developed (a clot moving and lodging in the lungs may prove fatal). From the 1960s, the physician was faced with a choice of a large array of anti-hypertensives, anti-arrhythmics, anti-anginals, vasodilators, hypolipedmics (cholesterol-reducing), and other drugs.

Apart from surgical and pharmacological treatments, there have been other major developments, notably in managing abnormalities of the heart rhythm resulting from disease of its electrical conduction system. Heart block is a common disorder in the elderly and in patients who have had a heart attack. It involves a failure of the electric circuitry, leading to a slowing of the pulse, unconsciousness and a risk of death. Its management has been transformed by the development of artificial pacemakers. Procedures have also been developed for previously fatal abnormalities of the heart rhythm, especially tachycardia (very rapid heartbeat) and ventricular fibrillation, a complication involving a state of electrical chaos in the heart muscle, resulting in the failure of the heart to pump in a regular way. From the 1950s defibrillators were designed to rectify this condition. Electrodes are placed on the chest and a shock delivered; techniques of cardiac massage have been developed for cardiac resuscitation, frequently used by paramedics and ambulance teams.

From the 1950s, especially in the US, it became normal to deal with serious heart conditions (and above all heart-attack survivors in special coronary care) with batteries of sophisticated monitoring equipment. These are extremely costly and skill-intensive. Since the critical time with most heart attacks is the brief period of the seizure itself, it has been questioned whether it is sensible to rush patients into intensive care at that time or even to keep them there in an alien and anxiety-creating environment, with all its terrifying mechanical and electronic gadgetry. The real usefulness of coronary care units in keeping people alive has never been put to the test. With its sometimes grotesque procedures, the new heroic medicine may turn out to be yet another instance of reflex preference of modern medicine for the highest-tech fix for a problem.

What have perhaps contributed most to the falling coronary death rate, particularly in the United States, are not these costly patch-up management techniques but moves to healthier lifestyles consequent upon better understanding of the causes of much heart disease. Here, the breakthrough has been through chemistry. The dangers of athero-sclerosis, or the laying down of fatty plaques in the walls of the arteries, became clear. The main component of such arterial plaques was found by Michael Brown (b. 1941) and Joseph Goldstein (b. 1940) to be cholesterol, manufactured in the liver and supplemented by fat-rich foodstuffs. This reinforced the findings of statisticians and epidemiolo-gists that the wealthy were more prone to heart disease than the poor: rich people had richer diets. A counter-explanation argued that stress was the chief cause, pointing out that the most vulnerable were ambitious, anxious types, those with a so-called 'type A' personality. The stress theory lost ground, however: Finnish lumberjacks, who led a low-stress life with plenty of exercise, had one of the highest rates of coronary deaths, presumably because their diet was full of animal fats.

Understanding of the role of cholesterol promoted new ideas about diet and drugs in the prevention and treatment of strokes and heart attacks caused by the clogging of arteries. Public understanding of risk factors – smoking, diet, obesity, lack of exercise – improved, and lifestyle shifts made a fundamental contribution to reducing the problem. Sales of butter and other dairy products dropped while purchases of vegetable oils containing polyunsaturated fats rose; jogging became the rage. Partly as a consequence coronary heart disease in the United States dropped by half between 1970 and 1990 – a reduction of around 300,000 deaths a year – there was also a substantial decline in strokes.

Improvements were not uniform; the educated classes changed their habits most. Nor were they so marked in other countries where the strenuous pursuit of personal health and well-being counts for less. In Scotland and Northern Ireland, for example, coronary death rates continued to rise, and in Britain as a whole male deaths from coronary disease remain 50 per cent higher than in the US. Overall, heart disease, like lung cancer, appears to be a problem medicine can palliate at enormous cost, but which is dramatically reduced by simple attention to diet and lifestyle.

GENETICS

The nexus of basic science, clinical research and practical medicine has been notable in two fields in particular in the latter half of the twentieth century. One is genetics.

The idea that particular features may be hereditary ('like begets like') is ancient, but down the centuries, as the battles between 'ovists', 'animalculists' and the like show, there was no agreement about how inheritance operated. Many diseases were believed to be heritable, for instance gout, and some pointed to a hereditary tendency to colour blindness and haemophilia. In 1814 the British physician Joseph Adams (1756–1818) offered a full summary of the extant state of knowledge, drawing distinctions between familial diseases (which he deemed confined to a single generation), and hereditary diseases, passed on from generation to generation.* Coming from a line of physicians, Charles Darwin was fascinated by evidence for disease inheritance, but notoriously unsure about the mechanics of the process.

Modern genetics stems from the hybridization experiments Gregor Mendel (1822–84) conducted with the common garden pea, *Pisum sativum*, at the Augustinian monastery in Brno in Bohemia. He reported his results in 1865, but little attention was paid. In Cambridge William Bateson (1861–1926), an ardent evolutionist, was unable to reconcile his belief in the discontinuous nature of hereditary variation with Darwin's model of evolution through continuous variation, spending years in doubt before reading about Mendel's experiments, where he found the mechanism for discontinuous variation.

* In modern usage, hereditary refers to the passage of a trait from generation to generation (surnames may be hereditary but they are not genetic). An hereditary trait is genetic only when its passage from generation to generation is determined by genes. A congenital trait (one present at birth) is not necessarily genetic.

Though the workings of heredity remained obscure and contro-versial, bedside medicine continued to accumulate data about inherited disease. In 1897 Archibald Garrod became fascinated by alkaptonuria, a disorder which turns the urine dark and often leads to arthritis. The popular theory was that it was due to a bacillus, but Garrod concluded it arose out of an 'error of metabolism', which was congenital. He noted that among four families in which unaffected parents had produced alkaptonuric offspring, three of the parental pairs were first cousins. From this he deduced that the pathology must be discontinuous, all or none, affected or normal. He suspected that other disorders, such as albinism, might share the same hereditary mechanism.

Garrod's incorporation of biochemistry and Mendelian laws into the study of diseases was farsighted, but his theories went largely unnoticed. Proof that many human diseases had a hereditary basis did not come until the mid twentieth century. Two disorders paved the way to this acceptance: sickle-cell anaemia and Down's syndrome.

Sickle-cell anaemia was first reported in 1910 by the Chicago physi-cian, J. B. Herrick (1861–1954), and the first scientific investigation of 'sickling' was described seven years later by another American, V. E. Emmel (1878–1928). Reporting the case of a black woman with severe anaemia and leg ulcers, he found a small proportion of the red cells from the patient's father (who was not anaemic) underwent sickling in cell culture conditions. Emmel did not point to a possible hereditary component – that came in 1923 from J. G. Huck, who explored the family pedigrees in sickle-cell cases. Once sickle-cell anaemia had been accepted as a hereditary disease, its cellular abnormalities came under scrutiny. The Nobel Prize-winning chemist Linus Pauling (1901–1994) showed in 1949 that the haemoglobin molecules in individuals with sickle-cell anaemia were fundamentally different from normal ones. The abnormality would be found, he predicted, in the globin part of the molecule and not in the heme groups; investigations proved him correct.

Soon after, an old medical puzzle was finally solved. A condition called 'furfuraceous idiocy' had been described in 1846 by Eduard Séguin (1812–1880). Its traits included unusual facial features, slow and incomplete growth and mental retardation. In 1867 J. Langdon Down suggested these might be a throwback to the Mongol racial type, though the term 'Mongoloid' was to yield to 'Down's syndrome'. For nearly a century, however, studies failed to produce a viable aetiological hypoth-esis. Then, in the 1950s, improvements in cell-examining techniques provided the solution: in 1959 three French cytologists announced that Down's syndrome children had an extra chromosome (chromosome 21).

Meantime, a still more fundamental breakthrough had been achieved concerning the nature of the genetic material itself. The Swiss biochemist Friedrich Miescher had discovered in 1869 that the same substance occurred in the nucleus of every living tissue cell. This came to be called 'nucleic acid'. By the 1920s, two distinct forms of nucleic acid had been identified: DNA (deoxyribonucleic acid) and RNA (ribonucleic acid). It was believed that the DNA structure was simple and repetitive, and thus could not transmit information. Since chromosomes contained protein as well as DNA, scientists assumed that protein was the transmitter of inheritance, with DNA simply holding the protein together. In one of the most spectacular developments in modern science, however, that view was overturned. In 1953 Francis Crick and James Watson demonstrated the double helical structure of DNA – the twisted-chain ladder – and it was accepted that a complicated code could be contained in DNA. This opened a whole new research field for genetics. Further advances occurred in the 1980s when it became possible chemically to read the genetic code in DNA and to isolate genes and clone (duplicate) them. This had practical pay-offs. Thanks to advances like amniocentesis and biopsies, doctors developed the ability to screen unborn babies for genetic diseases, and an increasing number of inherited and other congenital disorders can now be diagnosed before birth. Moreover, diseases and conditions caused by the absence of a specific gene product or a defective one could now (at least in principle) be treated by isolating the gene which encodes the protein and using it to produce large quantities of the desired protein.

Here lies the background to the launching in the mid 1980s of the international Human Genome Project, designed to clone and sequence all human genes. James Watson, who briefly headed the enterprise, described it as 'the ultimate tool for understanding ourselves at the molecular level'. The understanding of life had moved from organs, to tissues, to cells, to molecules. The project has become the major driving force for the encouragement of large-scale genetic testing for inherited traits, with a view to gene transplantation as a means of rectifying inherited diseases.

By the early 1990s, researchers had labelled and decoded some 2000 genes, and identifed a fair number of those responsible for specific diseases, including Duchenne muscular dystrophy, cystic fibrosis, some cancers, inherited high blood cholesterol levels and inherited forms of Alzheimer's disease. In the age of Bichat, two hundred years ago, more and more was known about diseases doctors could not cure. Now we have the ability to manipulate our own genes – the stuff of life itself.

The expectation is that genetic engineering should tackle genetic disease head-on. But it has become controversial whether, in this climate of hyperbole, there will be undue expectations about 'finding' genetic causes for all 'diseases', from anorexia nervosa to criminality, leading to a new eugenics. The issue of 'copyrighting' genes also raises the relation-ship between big science and private power. Other dilemmas loom. Genetic screening creates ethical dilemmas of the kind thrown up by the development of a test for Huntington's chorea. The degeneration of brain cells which underlies Huntington's disease leads to an irreversible dementia and eventually death, but the first signs of the illness do not normally appear until the second half of adult life. The test for Huntington's means that adults who may be currently healthy would have the option of discovering their fate.

IMMUNOLOGY

The further field of spectacular development during recent decades has been immunology. By 1900 bacteriological investigations were alerting medical scientists to the complexities of the body's immunological defences. The activities of phagocytes, granulocytes, leucocytes and lymphocytes were becoming known, at least in part. Serum defence had been identified, and effective diphtheria and tetanus antitoxins created; vaccination had been introduced against cholera, rabies, bubonic plague and typhoid. The hunt was on for more vaccines and sera.

There was a dawning awareness of the diversity of immunological processes: species or natural immunity, some species not being liable to diseases to which others fall victim; acquired immunity – active when the body makes its own immunity, following some stimulus, passive when the protective substances are applied. It was recognized that infants were commonly immune to many diseases because the baby received certain substances from the mother in the womb (congenital passive immunity). Artificial passive immunity could be created if the blood serum of an individual containing substances protective against diphtheria were injected into a susceptible.

Immunology came in with a bang, with the production of protective vaccines and antisera, alongside quinine the first truly effective medical treatments. The startling success of diphtheria serum created interest in antigen-antibody reactions and the nature of specificity. The earliest lucid formulation came with Ehrlich's side-chain theory. This in its turn drew criticism: it seemed to presuppose that the side-chains bound to their receptors firmly and irreversibly and to require that the body be provided with pre-existing antibodies for every antigen. To many that seemed an implausible supposition. An alternative idea – that the antigen-antibody reaction was not chemical but physical – was taken up by Karl Landsteiner (1868–1943) in Vienna, who advanced a physico-chemical model for antigen-antibody reactions: the precipitation of inorganic colloids. Colloid chemistry, which deals with the behaviour of materials forming particles so large that their reactions depend on physical properties rather than their chemical nature, seemed to hold great promise for explaining the antigen-antibody reaction, because it was thought that only proteins were antigenic.

The central dogma of immunology was the notion that antigens were recognized by the immune response triggered in foreign cell walls, and immunity was conferred by the presence of antibodies after an attack. But initially there was no real conception of an immune *system*; immune reactions were viewed piecemeal, and each individual component had its location: granulocytes and macrophages came from bone marrow; plasma cells produced antibodies; lymphocytes derived from lymph nodes. It was the American researcher Robert A. Good (b. 1922) who played a key part in showing that there was an integrative factor binding the whole together – the lymphocytes. Lymphocytes derived, Good demonstrated, from the primitive cells around the embryonic yolk sac at the beginning of the development of the embryo.

Immunology was transformed from *ad hoc* reactions into sophisticated theory. This transformation owed much to Landsteiner's pioneering studies with blood, which won him the Nobel Prize in 1930. After the unsuccessful seventeenth-century trials, blood transfusions had been abandoned. In 1900, investigating failed transfusions, Landsteiner found that fusing the blood of particular individuals with that of others made the red cells 'clump' together, resulting in death; but this agglutination did not happen with all possible mixtures. He concluded that clumping must depend on the presence or absence of two antigens on the surfaces of the red cells. He labelled these antigen A and antigen B. The red cells from two of his colleagues carried antigen A (group A) while those from two others carried antigen B (group B). When these mingled, clumping occurred. When the blood of other colleagues brought no clumping when mixed with samples from either group, Landsteiner decided that these blood cells carried no antigen and named their blood group O (zero). Shortly afterwards he realized that he had left out another blood group – AB – in which the red cells carry both antigens.

Landsteiner's discovery of blood types received scant recognition, and the possibilities it might have opened up for blood transfusion were little considered for many years. Transfusion did not become a regular hospital procedure until the establishment of blood banks shortly before World War II, in the anticipation of huge civilian casualties. Landsteiner meanwhile emigrated to the United States to continue his work at the Rockefeller Institute for Medical Research in New York.

In 1939, two American scientists, Philip Levine (1900–87) and Rufus Stetson (1886–1967), reported a peculiar case. After a stillbirth, a mother was given a transfusion of her husband's blood which, like hers, was group O. Despite this apparent compatibility, she suffered a severe reaction: red cells from her husband clumped. When Levine and Stetson mixed her serum with red cells from other donors, all group O, clumping occurred in four fifths of the cases. Evidently her red cells had a hitherto unknown antigen: she had developed antibodies after exposure to the antigen from her unborn baby, who must have inherited it from the father. When she received her husband's blood, the antibodies she had developed attacked his red cells, causing them to clump. This finding had the most profound implications concerning the understanding of what the body regarded as an enemy, as self or not self.

In the short term, this case led to a further nuance in the perception of blood groups. Testing transfusions from the rhesus monkey (*Macacus rhesus*) into guineapigs and rabbits, Landsteiner found that the anti-rhesus antibodies produced by the animals caused not only the monkey's red blood cells to clump but those of six out of seven white New Yorkers. Both the monkey and the majority of New Yorkers must, he surmised, have a common antigen, which he called the 'rhesus factor'. He termed the blood of the monkey and of the New Yorkers rhesus positive

(Rh+) while the unaffected blood was called rhesus negative (Rhx).

This discovery had immense implications for the health of unborn babies. Using Landsteiner's findings, Levine and Stetson concluded that the stillbirth woman must have been Rhx, and saw this rhesus incompatibility as the cause of diseases now renamed 'haemolytic diseases of the newborn'. Tests were produced for the antigen, and treatments followed. The significance of this development for immunology was that 'natural antibodies' had been found whose presence in the body was independent of infection.

The complex phenomena of immunized animals and immune cells catalyzed a new theory. During the 1940s, nuggets of crucial evidence accumulated. One was the phenomenon of tolerance. Ray Owen (b. 1915) in California found that twin calves sharing intrauterine circulation before birth each contained some of the other's blood cells; for that reason as adults they made no antibody to them. In 1949 the Australian MacFarlane Burnet (1899–1985) suggested more broadly that an animal body had a mechanism for distinguishing 'self' from 'not-self'. Antigens present before birth were accepted as self, and no antibody was made to them. These ideas had a practical relevance. Treating those burned in the Blitz, Peter Medawar (1915–1987) tried to use grafts of donor skin in the same way as donor blood, but donor skin did not 'take'. He concluded that graft rejection must be a immunogenetic phenomenon: self-tolerance was established in the womb.

With new attention being paid in the early 1950s to tolerance, the 'natural selection' theory advanced by the Dane, Niels Kaj Jerne (1911–94), assumed great importance. This proposed that 'natural' antibodies were continuously being formed, even before any antigen threat. A given antigen would select its match from among the assorted antibodies and would make an antigen-antibody complex. This would then be attacked by a phagocyte, setting off further production of the same antibody specificity. Jerne's theory chimed with Burnet's concept of self-tolerance: the idea of an anti-self antibody made no sense in biological and evolutionary terms.

In the late 1950s Burnet went on to modify Jerne's model, developing a clonal selection theory which eventually won acceptance. He suggested that the natural antibody was not loose in the serum but fixed to the cell surface as a receptor, rather as Ehrlich had conjectured. The antigen then attached itself to the cell bearing the right antibody, and this was the signal for the cell to start multiplying. Burnet's theory neatly accounted for various biological phenomena associated with immunity. It explained tolerance of self as the absence of 'forbidden clones' of cells which would have made anti-self antibody. And it made sense of the tempo of antibody production: the delay following inoculation of the antigen while the initial generations of cells were made, and the exponential rise with each new generation. Cells of the right clones already existed, ready to proliferate. Supporting evidence for the clonal selection theory was produced by Gustav Nossal (b. 1931) and Joshua Lederberg (b. 1925).

The thymus was a mystery organ: it seemed to have no function. Unlike, say, thyroidectomy, thymectomy seemed to have no effect. In 1961 Burnet suggested testing the effect of thymectomy not on adults but on newborns in whom, according to his theory, self-tolerance was still being established. Mice experiments showed an arresting effect. Thymectomized mice got ill, and were hardly able to produce any antibody. The America paediatrician Robert Good comparably found that children with immune deficiencies often had congenital absence of the thymus. Like the mice, they suffered from countless infections and failed to produce antibodies. It seemed that alongside the bone-marrow (or B) cells that produced antibody, thymus (or T) cells were needed as 'helpers'. Investigation showed that T cells were composed of helpers, suppressors and cytotoxic cells.

These discoveries further illuminated an old enigma. In 1890, Koch had announced his notorious tuberculosis cure by means of tuberculin. It produced a striking flare-up of skin lesions, but it was not a cure. Working on the 'serum sickness' which frequently followed injection of diphtheria serum, the Viennese pediatrician Clemens von Pirquet (1874–1929) recognized that the tuberculin reaction had a bearing on his concept of 'allergy', or altered reactivity. In 1939 at the Rockefeller Institute, Landsteiner saw the connection between delayed hypersensitivity and contact hypersensitivity to such things as poison ivy, on the one hand, and – on the other – the artificial antigens on which he had long been working. He deduced that delayed hypersensitivity could assume the form of autoimmune disease.

Immunologists accepted the clonal selection theory, and in the 1970s the phenomenon of immunity assumed a centrality to biomedicine that brought together cell biologists and immunochemists (with their culture techniques) and genetics and molecular biology (with their sequence studies). Immunology research skyrocketed: between 1970 and

1988 no fewer than forty-seven new immunological journals came into being! This had not a little to do with the arrival of AIDS.

In the summer of 1981, the Centers for Disease Control, the US federal monitoring organization in Atlanta, Georgia, revealed details of a baffling outbreak of illness in San Francisco. Five men had been diagnosed as suffering from *Pneumocystis carinii*, a rare and deadly type of pneumonia. The CDC spotted a link: each was homosexual, but was that significant to their illnesses? And, if so, how? Was the connection their lifestyle or their sexual contacts? The CDC's findings were followed by similar reports from physicians in San Francisco, Los Angeles and New York, indicating unusual disorders among homosexual males, each seemingly involving a potentially fatal breakdown in the patient's immune system. Some of the disorders they suffered, such as pneumocystis pneumonia, had heretofore been identified only in people whose immune systems had been damaged or suppressed, for example by drugs used to facilitate transplants.

Though experts at first called it 'Gay-Related Immune Disease', it was soon perceived not to be unique to homosexual men. Cases were diagnosed among intravenous drug users, blood transfusion recipients, haemophiliacs – and others of both sexes, all ages and every sexual preference. The condition was redesignated Acquired Immuno-Deficiency Syndrome (AIDS).

Suspicion grew that AIDS was caused by a virus capable of person-to-person transmission. By early 1984, a French team under Luc Montagnier (b. 1932) had succeeded in establishing that a virus deactivated the immune system by destroying white blood cells. The organism was eventually named the Human Immuno-deficiency Virus (HIV). Unseemly wrangles followed with the American, Robert Gallo (b. 1937), over priority in this discovery, but French and American researchers soon devised a test to indicate its presence before symptoms appeared. Studies indicated that the AIDS virus was transmitted by infected blood or other bodily fluids.

It became clear that HIV could lie dormant for a long time in the body while the carrier seemed healthy or suffered general disorders such as night sweats, which bore no outward relation to AIDS. It was later discovered that AIDS could also penetrate into the central nervous system, leading to meningitis and dementia.

By mid 1986, about 21,000 cases had been diagnosed worldwide, more than half being in the United States, but experts feared the figures were only the tip of an iceberg, estimating that up to 500,000 people could have the lesser disorders that might be a prelude to AIDS (the Aids-Related Complex, ARC) – and that perhaps two million could be carrying HIV, though asymptomatic. The search for a cure was stepped up, but there were overwhelming difficulties. HIV mutates much faster than most influenza viruses (the cliché was that attempts to develop a vaccine were like 'trying to hit a moving target'). Above all, a cure seemed particularly elusive, because treatments for infectious diseases typically rely on support from the body's immune system – the target which the HIV virus attacks. It is ironic indeed that a lethal disease which disables the immune system should have come upon the scene at the moment when the enormity of the fact could at last be understood.

CONCLUSION

Basic research, clinical science and technology working with one another have characterized the cutting edge of modern medicine. Progress has been made. For almost all diseases something can be done; some can be prevented or fully cured.

Nevertheless, a century which has brought the most intense concentration of attention and resources on medical research ends with many of the major killers of western society – particularly heart and vascular disease, cancer, and chronic degenerative illnesses – largely incurable and in many cases increasing in incidence. It can be argued that one reason why there has been relatively little success in eradicating them is because the strategies which earlier worked so well for tackling acute infectious diseases have proved inappropriate for dealing with chronic and degenerative conditions, and it has been hard to discard the successful 'microbe hunters' formula.

In large measure, the progress that has been made in their management can be described, in Sir David Weatherall's (b. 1933) evocative phrase, as 'increasingly expensive symptomatic patch-up procedures'. The causes of many still elude us, as do their prevention and cure. Asking of modern medicine, 'How well are we doing?', Weatherall, Regius professor of medicine at Oxford, has sombrely noted that, after a century of dedicated endeavour, 'we seem to have reached an impasse in our understanding of the major killers of Western society, particularly heart and vascular disease, cancer and the chronic illnesses whose victims fill our hospitals'. Cancer patients can, to some degree, be 'patched up', but only at the price of 'the spiralling cost of health care, which threatens to cripple our economy'. The trouble, Sir David concludes, is that 'although we have learned more and more about the minutiae of how these diseases make patients sick, we have made little headway in determining why they arise in the first place.'

CHAPTER XIX

SURGERY

AFTER LISTER

MEDICINE HABITUALLY EDGES FORWARD with minor improvements; in surgery, new technical know-how brought Plaster of Paris bandages, safer artery clips, flexible rubber tubes, rubber gloves and so forth, all doing their bit in the latter part of the nineteenth century. But blazing changes were also occurring.

'Operating theatres which resembled shambles in 1860', recalled one surgeon fifty years later, 'are replaced by rooms of spotless purity containing cantilevered metal furniture and ingenious electric lights. All concerned in the operation are clothed from nose-tip to toe-tip in sterilised linen gowns, and their hands are covered with sterilised rubber gloves.' Sepsis had ceased to have surgery by the throat. 'In my under-graduate days every surgical case got erysipelas,' Dr George Dock (1860–1951) explained to his students at the University of Michigan in 1904. 'If a man came in with a compound fracture, he got erysipelas. It was considered part of hospital life.' By then that was becoming a thing of the past, and the combination of anaesthesia and asepsis offered the unprecedented prospect of safe and virtually unlimited surgical inter-vention. For thousands of years surgery had been a business of boils and broken bones, hernias, venesection and the occasional amputation; 'an operation on the heart would be a prostitution of surgery,' declared the young Theodor Billroth (1829–94). Yet this high-minded caution rapidly became old-fashioned.

Contrast the operations undertaken by Joseph Lister between 1877 and 1893 with those of his protégé, William Watson Cheyne (1852–1932). About 60 per cent of Lister's practice concerned accident and orthopaedic cases, with tubercular conditions prominent, and his

597

surgical repertoire focused on bones, joints and superficial tumours. Though his results were excellent, his operations were traditional. Up to 1893, Lister attempted no abdominal surgery and Cheyne undertook just one bowel operation. In the new century, this branch of Cheyne's practice rose to around three in ten cases; opening the abdomen became the bread-and-butter of surgery.

Surgeons began attempting operations on organs and lesions hitherto taboo: bowel inflammations, the pancreas, the liver and biliary tracts, peptic ulcers, gallstones, and a range of cancers – and also knife and gunshot wounds in the abdomen. One consequence was that surgery's profile rose. A sign of the times was the Mayo Clinic at Rochester, Minnesota, founded by the brothers William (1861–1939) and Charles Mayo (1865–1939), masters respectively of abdominal and thyroid surgery. Sons of a rugged individualist surgeon who had prided himself on his skill in the removal of ovarian tumours, the Mayos followed in their father's footsteps and turned the local Minnesota hospital, St Mary's, into a surgical powerhouse. In 1800 a big London hospital staged no more than two hundred operations a year; a century later the Mayos and their team were performing over three thousand, while 1924 saw their clinic logging a staggering 23,628 operations, with 60,063 patients on the books. Surgery had developed a scope and achieved a popularity hitherto quite unthinkable; the Mayos became household names and millionaires. The new surgery was accompanied by new procedures and the routinization of systematic testing: blood counts (important for the diagnosis of typhoid fever or the prognosis of pneumonia), urinalysis and, with the discovery of insulin, the measurement of urinary sugar.

The Columbus of the new surgical techniques was Theodor Billroth. Educated in Göttingen, Billroth was a man of many talents; he wrote a book called *Wer ist musikalisch?* (1895) [Who is Musical?] and was a good friend of Brahms, who dedicated two string quartets to him. In 1856 he was appointed assistant to the greatest German surgeon of the day, Berhard von Langenbeck (1810–87) at the Berlin Charité hospital. Four years later he became professor in Zürich, then moved on to Vienna in 1867, where he capitalized on the splendid facilities at the General Hospital, modernized by Rokitansky and Skoda. Talented acolytes gathered around him at the 'second Vienna school'.

The all-round scientific surgeon, Billroth moved easily from the bedside to the microscope in the laboratory and to the operating theatre.

His classic *Die allgemeine chirurgische Pathologie und Chirurgie* (1863) [General Surgical Pathology and Surgery] derived indications of surgery from the underlying pathophysiology of wound-healing, regeneration, inflammation, haemorrhage, etc. The work established his reputation worldwide, running through sixteen editions and being translated into ten languages.

An innovator on many fronts, Billroth refined Listerian antisepsis and pioneered regular temperature measurement for post-operative control, drawing on Wunderlich's works, which taught that temperature rise was a sign of complications. Superb technique and a dauntless temperament ensured him a leading role in developing new operations, and he was the first to have success with some: gastric resections, removal of the whole oesophagus, and the creation of detours around acute or chronic intestinal obstructions through the use of anastomoses (new channels and connexions – replumbing in effect) between parts of the digestive tract. Frankly experimental, his new methods sacrificed many lives but, as his practices became refined and post-operative care improved, mortality rates dipped.

With role-models like Billroth to follow, the ambitious surgeon was beguiled into believing that all manner of diseases could be cured or checked by chloroforming the patient and plying the knife and needle. The potential of surgery became almost a matter of faith: if patients failed to improve after a operation, didn't this show that further lesions remained to be excised, yet more fixing-up to be done? Probing around in the thorax and the abdomen would and did unearth assorted anomalies, which were then deemed pathological and hence indications for further intervention. The body's interior seemed an Africa in microcosm, that dark continent being opened up, mapped and transformed. Fame and fortune awaited the surgical pioneer who first laid the knife to some hitherto untouched part – perhaps he would be immortalized by an eponymous operation.

Some surgeons grew quite cavalier: the dazzling Irish-born William Arbuthnot Lane (1856–1943) viewed the innards as little more than a problem in plumbing. He urged, for instance, colectomies – removal of lengths of the gut – to treat that favourite English malaise, constipation, or even as a prophylactic against 'intestinal stasis' and 'autointoxication' (the self-poisoning which he supposed resulted from the artificialities of modern civilization). In Lane's pathological model, poisons were absorbed from a sluggish colon, producing pelvic pain and other symptoms. An overloaded colon might lead to 'Lane's kinks', which he claimed to iron out. He was, significantly, in great demand; the sick were beginning to look to surgery as the new panacea.

Appendectomy, not only for the acute condition but for so-called 'chronic' appendicitis (the 'grumbling appendix'), enjoyed a vogue in the 1920s and 1930s. The pathology of the condition had long been familiar, described post mortem in the sixteenth century by Berengario da Carpi and Jean Fernel. The condition had been diagnosed in a living patient in 1734 by Wilhelm Ballonius, and in 1812 James Parkinson (1775–1824) described how inflammation of the appendix preceded peritonitis. But though appendicitis thus came to be recognized as dangerous, pre-Lister treatments invariably and inevitably remained, in the time-honoured Hippocratic manner, medical: blood-letting, leeches and enemas.

Various surgeons have been credited with the first appendectomy; in England, Robert Lawson Tait (1845–99) performed the operation in 1880; another pioneer (1886) was Ulrich Rudolf Krönlein (1847–1910). The optimal surgical approach remained contested. On the whole, the British preferred to wait until the inflammation died down before operating and some surgeons, including Frederick Treves (1853–1923), even hesitated to remove the whole organ. He won eminence and a baronetcy when on 24 June 1902 he drained the appendix of the Prince of Wales, who had gone down with appendicitis shortly before he was to be crowned as Edward VII.* Treves was a passionate champion of the new surgery. 'It is less dangerous to leap from the Clifton Suspension Bridge', he declared, 'than to suffer from acute intestinal obstruction and decline operation.'

All manner of new operations were tried; some became established, others disappeared. Procedures were devised to fix abdominal organs found upon X-ray or exploratory operation to be 'misplaced' or 'dropped' (dropped organs were thought to cause neurosis and vague, unlocalized abdominal pains). 'Hitching up the kidneys' was recommended as a fix for back pain; fragments of vertebrae were removed for the same reason. And countless tonsillectomies were performed on small children; it was an easy, relatively safe, and lucrative operation. In 1925

---

* Treves was also famous for his dealings with Joseph Merrick (1860–90), the 'Elephant Man', suffering from hideous deformities, whom he befriended, rescuing him from freak shows and securing permanent accommodation for him at the London Hospital.

a staggering 25.5 per cent of patients admitted to the Pennsylvania Hospital were allegedly suffering from diseases of the tonsils – tonsillectomy became for a while easily the most common hospital procedure.

Tonsils – sometimes viewed as an organ that evolution had rendered functionless – were removed not only because they were ulcerated but because they seemed enlarged, and doctors and parents were convinced that surgical intervention would solve the problem of never-ending childhood infections. A study undertaken in New York in 1934 revealed that of 1000 eleven-year-olds in state schools, 611 had already had their tonsils removed. The other 389 were evaluated by a panel of doctors, and the procedure was recommended for 174 more. Different physicians were brought in to inspect the remaining 215 and they chose to operate on 99 more, leaving 116 from the original 1000 'surgery-free'. These 116 were evaluated by a third panel of doctors, who recommended a further 51 for surgery. In this 'can-do, will-do' atmosphere, surgical operations took on the quality of a cure-all. Since it is now known that tonsils form part of the immune system, removal must have been positively damaging – and over eighty children died annually in England in the 1930s because of post-operative complications following tonsillectomies.

Hysterectomies also had a vogue; removal became popular in the belief that it would deal not only with the assumed physical pathology but with emotional and psychological difficulties. Another fashionable inter-war diagnosis was focal sepsis: the notion that pockets of pus were lurking in the sickly body, causing infections and requiring surgical extraction. It thus became routine to extract teeth, often all the teeth of patients in psychiatric hospitals. Other surgical fads included operations to remove sympathetic nerves, so as to end spasm of the gut or artery.

Recourse to the knife became almost a reflex. Its appeal lay in the fact that it was new, quick and, supposedly, painless and safe; who would refuse a short-cut to end suffering? (Indeed a class of patients emerged suffering from an addiction to surgery: Münchausen's syndrome; no label seems to have been devised, however, for surgeons addicted to surgery.) The myth of the surgeon as hero blossomed; at long last the craft had thrown off its associations with pain, blood and butchery and become linked by the public and the press with science and life-saving. The truth was rather more complicated: up to the 1940s appendectomy, for example, had a one in five mortality, and post-operative complications remain to this day one of the main sources of iatrogenic disorders and hospital-caught infections.

NEW OPERATIONS

Surgery was extended to many familiar grave conditions and to organs hitherto untouched. Cholecystotomy, removing gallstones, was first performed in 1867 by the American John S. Bobbs (1809–70). Removal of the gall bladder (cholecystectomy) also became routine, being first attempted in 1882 by Carl Langenbuch (1846–1901) in Berlin. In 1884, J. Knowsley Thornton (1845–1904) tried something different: finding two big stones inside a patient's duct, he crushed them using a rubber-jawed pincer designed for nose-polyps. Two months later, he opened the duct of another patient and took out gallstones – the first choledocholithotomy. Confidence grew in opening up the gall bladder, and eventually surgery was recommended even for general indications, such as pain in the gall bladder area; biliary disease began to slide from the physicians' hold into the surgeons' grasp. (In a later technological age, gallstones were fragmented by the shock-wave method, a technique also used for kidney stones.)

Kidney operations had been extremely rare and undertaken only *in extremis*. The first known nephrectomy (surgical removal of a kidney) was done in 1861, by E. B. Wolcott (1804–80) of Milwaukee, who removed a large kidney tumour, though his patient died two weeks later. Success dates from 1870 with the German surgeon Gustav Simon (1824–76), though the mortality rate was initially high.

Surgery also became viable for ulcers. An operation for chronic peptic ulcers was described in 1881 by another of Billroth's protégés, Anton Wölfler (1850–1917); it was first performed for duodenal ulcers in 1892 by Eugene Doyen (1859–1916) in Paris. An alternative was to remove much of the stomach (gastric resection), so as to reduce secretion of hydrochloric acid. Billroth attempted this in January 1881 on a woman named Thérèse Heller; the operation took ninety minutes and she recovered well, only to die of liver cancer four months later. Connecting the resected stomach with the duodenum, his method became known as 'Billroth I'.

An acute perforated ulcer spells danger: the hole must be sutured to prevent fatal peritonitis. 'Every doctor, faced with a perforated ulcer of the stomach or intestine', wrote one of Billroth's devotees, 'must consider opening the abdomen, sewing up the hole and averting a possible or actual inflammation by carefully cleansing the abdominal cavity.' This was first done on 19 May 1892. A man with stomach ulcers suddenly went down with peritonitis; Ludwig Heusner (1846–1916) was summoned to his home where he accomplished the operation in two and a half hours; a similar operation was performed the next year in England by Hastings Gilford (1861–1941). By the mid nineties, the suture of perforations of the stomach and duodenum had become part of the repertoire.

Other conditions were being subjected to surgery for the first time, including certain cancers. Breast cancer operations date back to antiquity: Aetius of Amida had emphasized that the knife should cut healthy tissue around a tumour and that a cauterizing-iron should stanch the blood. The Florentine Angelo Nannoni (1715–90) published a book in 1746 on the surgical treatment of breast cancer; in his *Traité des maladies chirurgicales et les opérations qui leur conviennent* (1774–6) [Treatise on Surgical Ailments and Operations], the French surgeon Jean-Louis Petit advocated radical removal of the breast muscle and lymph nodes. The mastectomy Larrey performed on Fanny Burney in 1810 was probably along these lines.

Radical mastectomy was advocated by Sir Astley Cooper. He wrote in his *Lectures on the Principles and Practice of Surgery* (1824–7), 'it will be sometimes necessary to remove the whole breast where much is apparently contaminated, for there is more generally diseased than perceived and it is best not to leave any small portion of it as tubercles reappear in them. If a gland in the axilla [armpit] be enlarged, it should be removed and with it all the intervening cellular substance.' The operation was attempted by Charles Hewitt Moore (1821–70) at the Middlesex Hospital in London, which had a special cancer ward, but without success. In 1879 Billroth reported that out of 143 women who had undergone it, a mere thirty-five survived for any length of time (surgeons may have felt less uncomfortable about practising their techniques on such desperate cases). Billroth did not specialize in breast cancer, but he did envisage surgery as bringing hope for cancer sufferers. He tackled stomach cancer, for instance, with 'Billroth II', closing the top of the duodenum and connecting the resected stomach with the jejunum. Such methods proved popular for stomach cancer, as well as for duodenal ulcers.

Among Billroth's students in Vienna was the American William Stewart Halsted (1852–1922). He quickly became one of the top young surgeons in New York, until, in 1884, he and some colleagues began to experiment with cocaine. He became addicted, his work deteriorated, and his chief, William Welch, arranged for him to go on a detoxifying cruise before taking up a post at the Johns Hopkins Medical School as professor of pathology. Within six months, Halsted was back in the psychiatric hospital, having switched from cocaine to morphine in hopes of beating his addiction.

At Baltimore he enjoyed a remarkable career spanning thirty-three years, training the best surgeons of the next generation, including the neuro-surgeon Harvey Cushing. Halsted ushered in a new 'surgery of safety', aiming not to injure tissues more than was avoidable, but his operations were radical. He evolved striking advances in bile duct, intestine and thyroid gland surgery, and the Halsted II procedure for repairing inguinal hernias. But he was best known for his cancer treatments. Cognizant of how cancer of the breast spread through the lymph system, he advocated radical mastectomy, in which the breast, all the lymph glands in the nearest armpit and the chest wall muscles were removed. Introduced in the 1890s, this was the treatment of choice for breast cancer for over half a century. Its underlying premise was that cancer remained in the breast for some time before spreading, and that the lymphatic system was relatively separate from blood vessels, so removal of lymph nodes would prevent the passage of cancer cells.

In 1937, however, the *British Medical Journal* reported that an identical percentage of women survived after less severe surgery, with Geoffrey Keynes (1887–1982) of St Bartholomew's Hospital claiming equally good results with the simple removal of breast tumours ('lumpectomies'), followed by radiation. By the 1970s it was accepted that tumours could not be cut out by their roots like weeds: by the time breast cancer was diagnosed, most patients had cancer elsewh_re in their bodies. The lymphatic system and bloodstream were found to be utterly integrated, so the removal of lymph nodes to prevent cancer spread was mistaken. Many decades of experience offered little cause for satisfaction. In 1975, a World Health Organization survey showed that, despite the growing sophistication of surgery and other interventions, deaths from breast cancer had failed to decline since 1900. Surgery wasn't the answer.

Operations were also developed for other forms of cancer. Lung resections were begun in 1933 by Evarts Graham (1883–1957) in Washington. Lobectomy (removing a lung lobe), segmental resection (removing only part of a lobe) and pulmectomy (taking out the whole lung) were also tackled, as was prostate cancer. In 1889 a Leeds surgeon, A. F. McGill (1850–90), reported 37 prostatectomies with good results, and in 1890 William Belfield (1856–1929) of Chicago reported eighty cases with a mortality of 14 per cent – considered excellent at the time. Surgeons were thus boldly going into the body, where none had gone before.

SEEING INTO INNER SPACE

Such interventions marched forward in line with other new probes and advances in diagnostic techniques. First had come the stethoscope; Helmholtz had developed the ophthalmoscope (1851), and in 1868 the oesophagoscope was produced by John Bevan, enabling foreign objects in the gullet to be located and removed. That year, too, the first stomach gastroscopy was done by an assistant to Adolf Kussmaul (1822–1902), who engaged a professional sword-swallower to swallow a pipe, nearly half a metre long, equipped with a lamp and lenses. An American surgeon, Howard Kelly (1858–1943), created the equivalent rectoscope in 1895, which was soon adapted by gynaecologists to explore the abdomen (laparoscopy).

Early gastroscopes were stiff, causing soreness and injury, but from the 1930s flexible versions were devised, making use of glass-fibre optics, which directed light though a tube by total internal reflection. Tiny cameras were later incorporated into such endoscopic devices, as well as tongs to take biopsy samples and lasers to stop bleeding.

The most decisive new windows into the body, however, were X-rays. On 8 November 1895, Karl Wilhelm Röntgen (1845–1923), a physics professor at Würzburg interested in cathode rays (the glow radiating from a wire vacuum sealed in a Crookes tube when a high voltage was applied) hit upon a new phenomenon while testing a tube. Having darkened his laboratory and wrapped the tube in black cardboard to screen out the light it emitted, he was surprised to find that, on switching on the current, a fluorescent screen coated with barium platinocyanide glowed a faint green colour. The tube was obviously giving off something else beside the familiar cathode rays; invisible rays were passing through the cardboard cover and bombarding the screen.

If these rays could penetrate card, what else might they pass through? Experimenting with playing-cards, a book, some wood, hard rubber and assorted metal sheets, Röntgen found that only lead barred the rays totally. He held some lead between the tube and the screen; its shadow was visible on the screen and so was the outline of the bones of his hand. Aware that cathode rays darkened photographic plates, he asked his wife to hold one in her hand, while he beamed the new rays onto it; her hand was distinctly outlined, and its bones and rings highlighted against the silhouette of the surrounding flesh.

Röntgen announced his discovery in *Eine neue Art von Strahlen* (1896) [A New Kind of Ray]. News of the rays (which he styled X-rays because their nature was unknown) made headlines, and coverage peaked in 1901 when he received the first Nobel Prize for Physics. Public excitement and anxiety followed: to capitalize on fears of Peeping Toms with 'X-ray eyes' peering through women's underclothes, one enterprising firm advertised X-ray-proof knickers.

The diagnostic possibilities were quickly exploited. As early as 7 January 1896, a radiograph was taken for clinical purposes. Though initially only bones were examined, soon other things, like gallstones, were seen too, and the rays were valuable in diagnosing fractures and locating foreign bodies. In the Spanish-American War, an X-ray machine was used to scan for bullets, though its utility was reduced by the long exposure times (up to thirty-five minutes!). In December 1896, Walter Cannon at Harvard found that if laboratory animals were fed bismuth salts as a diagnostic meal the workings of their intestines could be observed on a fluorescent screen. By 1904 that technique was being applied to humans, with the substitution of the safer barium sulphate. 'Barium swallows' became routine, until largely superseded by endoscopy.

Early chest radiographs were unsatisfactory, since exposure times needed to be long (initially at least twenty minutes) and contrasts were poor – one of the reasons why, despite public fear over the scourge of tuberculosis, mass chest X-ray screening was not developed until the 1920s. What the stethoscope had been to the nineteenth century, the X-ray became for the twentieth: an impressive diagnostic tool and a symbol of medical power.

Not merely diagnostically valuable, X-rays were regarded as therapeutically promising. Röntgen found that prolonged exposure produced skin burns and ulcerations, hair loss and dermatitis, though these effects were turned to therapeutic account by physicians who used them to burn off moles or treat skin conditions ranging from acne to lupus (skin tuberculosis). The properties of other sorts of rays were also being touted. The Danish physician Niels Finsen (1860–1904) suggested that ultraviolet rays were bactericidal, and so could be useful against conditions like lupus. Many early hospital radiology departments provided both radiation and ultraviolet light therapy, and Finsen's researches stimulated high-altitude tuberculosis sanatoria and inspired the unfortunate belief that sun-tans were healthy. The dangers of X-rays were also recognized; a relationship between exposure and skin cancer was reported as early as 1902. Benefits and costs have always been precariously balanced on the radiation research accounts sheet.

A few weeks after Röntgen's discovery, the French scientist Henri Becquerel (1852–1908), in the course of setting up an experiment to investigate the X-ray potential of uranium salts, placed some salts over a photographic plate protected by aluminium; he then developed the plate without carrying out the intended experiment and found, to his surprise, that it had darkened at the point where the salts had been. Hence, uranium emitted rays which, like X-rays, penetrated matter. He published his findings, but then lost interest. In 1897, Marie Curie (1867–1934) chose uranium rays as the topic for her doctoral thesis.

Warsaw-born, Maria Sklodowska had left Poland in 1891 to study at the Sorbonne, and married a fellow-scientist Pierre Curie (1859–1906) in 1895. Studying uranium compounds, she noticed that pitchblende (uranium oxide ore occurring in tarry masses) was four times as active as uranium. Soon she was speculating upon the probable existence of a new radioactive element, which her husband joined her in the race to isolate. Laboriously they refined 100g of pitchblende and in July 1898 announced the discovery of the new element, 'polonium', called after Marie's beloved Poland.

By November it was apparent that the refined pitchblende liquid, left over after the polonium had been removed, was still highly radioactive: it had to contain another undiscovered element. Further refinement produced a substance 900 times more radioactive than uranium: on 26 December 1898, they announced the discovery of radium. Both Mme Curie and Becquerel had burned themselves accidentally when carrying radium phials in their pockets, and in 1901 Pierre did so deliberately by strapping some to his arm. Demonstrations in 1904 that radium rays destroyed diseased cells, led to radiation treatments for cancer and other diseases. When in 1906 Pierre was knocked down and killed by a cart, Marie was offered his chair, becoming the first woman professor at the Sorbonne. In 1911, she was twice rewarded: she received her second Nobel Prize (her first had been in 1904), and the Sorbonne and the Pasteur Institute helped to fund her Radium Institute.

X-rays and radiation provoked immense interest among scientifically minded physicians. Before the First World War, various radium institutes sprang up, there were radiology journals and societies, and the new 'miracle cures' had been tried out for more than a hundred diseases, most notably cancer. Scores of proprietary cures, some sponsored by renowned doctors, traded on the conjectured therapeutic powers of radioactivity. Therapeutic enthusiasm outran caution, and the dangers of radiotherapy were determined at great cost to patients and radiographers alike (many of the latter lost their lives). Little thought was given to the long-term consequences of repeated exposure to heavy radiation – for instance, among technicians involved in handling X-ray machines. Fluoroscopes went on being employed quite casually in shoe-shops and X-rays in ante-natal clinics. As late as the 1940s benign menstrual bleeding was sometimes treated with X-rays and radium – a therapy which caused cervical cancer.

Exposure did not become a subject of deep and lasting public concern until the consequences of the devastation of Hiroshima and Nagasaki by atom bombs at the close of World War II became plain. Modern medicine has sometimes been so engrossed in its healing mission as to be cavalier about evaluating safety, benefits and costs.

Other roles for rays were discovered. Scientists found that electromagnetic waves heated up tissues which absorbed them. In 1917 Albert Einstein (1879–1955) announced the principle of the 'laser' (an acronym for **L**ight **A**mplification by **S**timulated **E**mission of **R**adiation), and in due course lasers were harnessed for medical use. Their high-energy waves could be focused to a microscopic point, were sterile, and caused little bleeding or scarring. Such optical 'knives' became deployed to weld a detached retina, burn through a blocked coronary artery, or even to efface an unwanted tattoo.

Other technical advances of great diagnostic importance followed from breakthroughs in microscopy. Microscopes were first used directly on the body in 1899, when the cornea (the transparent covering on the front of the eye) was investigated with a large-field stereo-microscope. In time this led to microsurgery: in 1921, the Scandinavian ear specialist,

C. O. Nylen (b. 1892), performed an operation using a monocular microscope, and operating under microscopes soon became standard practice. What could be seen was, however, limited: since the wavelength of light is about one-thousandth of a millimetre, viruses would not show up under a light microscope.

In 1925, the London microscopist Joseph Bernard developed the ultraviolet microscope, which achieved magnifications of up to 2500 and allowed the larger viruses to be seen. Meanwhile, it became known that electrons travelled with a wave motion similar to light but 100,000 times shorter. Objects far smaller would thus be visible through an electron microscope. The first was developed by a Belgian, L. L. Marton (1901–79). By 1934, researchers had achieved the same magnification as with the best light microscopes; within three years, objects could be magnified 7000 times; and, by 1946, over 200,000 times with electron microscopes. Many medically significant aspects of cell structure were revealed: macrophages tangled with asbestos fibres, synapses between nerves, histamine-releasing granules, and so forth. In the 1970s scanning electron microscopes also became important.

Another development of immediate diagnostic significance was ultrasound, for assessing foetal progress through pregnancy. Developed in the 1950s by Ian Donald (1910–87), professor of midwifery in Glasgow, this drew on the naval echo-sounding technique known as sonar (**So**und **Na**vigation and **R**anging). When subjected to an electric charge certain crystals emit sound waves at frequencies too high to be heard by the human ear; these ultrasonic waves travel through water, sending back echoes when they encounter a solid object. Distance can be calculated from the time-lapse.

Applying this principle to the body, Donald initially concentrated on showing how different classes of abdominal tumours give off distinct echoes, diagnosing them with a view to surgery; but by 1957 he was using ultrasound to diagnose foetal disorders, later applying it to establish pregnancy itself. Experience allayed fears that ultrasound could prove harmful to the foetus in the manner of X-rays, and foetuses became minutely monitored for abnormalities. A similar diagnostic technique made use of the infra-red radiation found in heat rather than sound waves. Different body parts emit varying heat patterns, measurable by the intensity of the infra-red waves they contain. These may be analysed to identify abnormalities: cancerous tumours, for example, show up as 'hot spots'.

In 1967, Godfrey Hounsfield (b. 1919), an engineer and computer expert working for the British company EMI, had the idea of developing a system to build up a three-dimensional body image. Computerized axial tomography (CAT) transmits fine X-rays through the patient to produce detailed cross-sections, which are computer processed to create a three-dimensional picture whose shading depends on tissue density – more compact tissues absorb more of the X-ray beam. Refinements enabled the computer to colour the scan.

In what came to be called 'imaging', the CAT (or CT) scanner led to the PETT (positron emission transaxial tomography) scanner, used to diagnose and monitor brain disorders. Dispensing with X-rays (and hence the irradiation of the patient), this relies on radioactive emissions and enables doctors to study brain activity. Patients are injected with radioactive glucose, and distinct brain areas soak up different amounts depending on their activity-level. Analysis allows identification of the tell-tale patterns diagnostic of brain disorder in cases of strokes, psychiatric conditions and the like.

A still more advanced technique of making the body transparent is magnetic resonance imaging (MRI), which exploits the fact that hydrogen atoms resonate when bombarded with energy from magnets. Like CAT, MRI displays three-dimensional body images on a screen; its main advantage is that it does not involve radiation. Allowing body chemistry to be studied while physiological events are actually taking place, it can be used to monitor surgery involving organ transplants as well as the course of such diseases as muscular dystrophy. MRI scans are particularly useful for showing soft-tissue injuries within the spine, such as prolapsed disc.

NEW SURGICAL FIELDS

Stimulated by technical innovations and driven by outside pressures, not least the appalling wounds of two world wars, surgery moved stage-centre in the twentieth century. Initially its mission, like that of the Commandos, seemed to be to go in and destroy all threats, mainly with the knife. Surgeons focused on tumours and stenosis (constriction of vessels), especially in the digestive, respiratory and urogenital tracts, removing or relieving these by excision or fissuring, as in tracheotomy for tuberculosis or throat cancer. Abdominal surgery produced herniotomies, treatments for appendicitis and colon disorders, extirpation of cancer of the rectum, and so forth, in what has been called surgery's heroic, even knife-happy, age. And if such invasions were at first frankly experimental and desperately hit-and-miss, in time and at a cost to life routinization brought greater safety and reliability. All the cavities and organs of the body were conquered, and certain departments of surgery were utterly novel, for instance neurosurgery. The operating theatre became the high altar of the hospital, and the white-coated, masked and capped surgeon, so cool in an emergency, became the high priest of medicine in images which pervaded popular culture, TV soap operas and the press.

Encouraged by new techniques and intoxicated by their own rhetoric and even successes, the profession was liable to offer surgical fixes for everything. High on the list of diseases the new surgery was eager to cure was tuberculosis. Though dipping by the closing decades of the nineteenth century, TB mortality remained shockingly high. Certain breakthroughs had been achieved, including the identification of the bacillus, but all therapies had proved failures (including of course Koch's much-fêted tuberculin). No wonder the possibility of a surgical solution was prized. In 1921, Sir James Kingston Fowler (1852–1934) hailed the pneumothorax technique of collapsing and immobilizing the lung – resting it, so as to encourage the lesions to heal – as one of 'two real advances in the treatment of pulmonary tuberculosis' (the other he had in mind was the sanitorium).

In reality, the surgical handling of the disease was far less clear-cut; a multitude of technical problems had first to be surmounted. One obstacle facing this and similar thoracic operations was air pressure. This is normally low in the pleural cavities around the lungs, but opening the body lets in air, which causes the lungs to collapse, and breathing becomes impossible. Great ingenuity was needed to overcome such difficulties.

Convinced the only way to defeat TB was to operate, Carlo Forlanini (1847–1918) of Pavia attempted the first pneumothorax operation in 1888. The 'cavern' area could be made to rest, he believed, if the ribs were mostly removed so that the chest wall and the lung collapsed. Forlanini injected an inert gas between the two layers of the pleura; the result was compression and lung collapse. Initially unsuccessful, this operation was worked upon by Ferdinand Sauerbruch (1875–1951), who had trained in Berlin under Langerhans before becoming professor at Berlin's Charité Hospital. Sauerbruch, whose father had died of the disease, set about solving the problem of lung collapse on the opening of the thorax. He experimented on animals by enclosing the creature's chest in a pressurized cage using gloves built into the cage wall, and developed ways of operating while the animal carried on breathing.

By 1904, a 'negative pressure chamber' had been built to hold a patient, a table and a full operating team. In this, Sauerbruch built up experience in thoracic surgery. By the 1920s, new and improved ways of establishing collapse had been developed; both physicians and surgeons had their part to play. A temporary collapse of the lung could be produced by nitrogen displacement (pneumothorax), which could be performed by physicians. Alternatively, a permanent collapse of the whole lung could be produced by cutting out ribs – the surgeon's turf. Despite all the inventiveness and skill employed, pneumothorax proved of uncertain value, and it was abandoned after the Second World War.*

Brain surgery presented even more daunting problems. For thousands of years, no one had dared to operate on the brain, with the exception of trepanning the head (strictly speaking, *skull* not *brain* surgery). One reason was an almost total ignorance of how the brain worked and where lesions were likely to lie, beyond the guesswork of phrenology. Neurophysiological advances associated with the work of Jackson and Ferrier on epilepsy led to a more confident mapping of brain localization and better-grounded hopes of locating tumours.

Antiseptic techniques allowed surgeons to open up the skull to expose the brain. In 1876 William Macewen (1848–1924), who had studied under Lister, diagnosed and localized a cerebral abscess. His request to operate was refused by the patient's family, but after death he *was* allowed to open the cranium, and the abscess was found as diagnosed. Three years later Macewen successfully removed a fungus-like tumour of the dura (a meningioma). His *Pyogenic Infective Diseases of the Brain and Spinal Cord* (1893) chronicled ten years' work: he had operated on seventy-four patients with intracranial infections, and sixty-three of them had improved.

In 1884, a patient was sent to the Hospital for Epilepsy and Paralysis

---

* Like many top surgeons, Sauerbruch was a driven man, convinced of his sacred mission as a healer. Authoritarian and egotistical, he gave enthusiastic support to the Nazis; after the war his unwillingness to retire, long after his cringing colleagues recognized that his judgment and powers had waned but had done nothing about it, killed many patients.

(Queen Square Hospital) in London with a brain tumour diagnosed between the frontal and parietal lobes. Operated on by Lister's nephew, John Rickman Godlee (1849–1925), a walnut-sized tumour was found exactly as predicted. (The patient, alas, died from complications.) The real trail-blazer in brain surgery was Victor Horsley (1857–1916), at Queen Square, who turned himself into the world's first specialist neurosurgeon, writing about injuries and diseases of the spinal cord and brain. Another was Vilhelm Magnus (1871–1929) in Norway, who first operated on the brain in 1903, removing a tumour from an epileptic. Some twenty years later, he reported more than a hundred brain-tumour operations with a mortality rate of only 8 per cent.*

In the United States the field leader was Harvey Cushing (1869–1939), who learned his technique from Halsted; during the course of his career he removed more than 2000 brain tumours. After studying in England with Sherrington, Cushing returned to Johns Hopkins in 1901, became associate professor of surgery in 1903, and then spent most of his career at Harvard. He pioneered the operation for trigeminal neuralgia (*tic douloureux*).

Cushing favoured the gentle handling of tumours and tissue, using tiny silver clips at bleeding points in the brain to achieve bloodless operations. Brain surgery mortalities had averaged about 40 per cent; by 1915 Cushing had removed 130 tumours with a mortality of just 8 per cent. His work put brain surgery on the map, even if as late as 1932 a textbook was cautioning that no more than 7 per cent of brain tumours could be removed.

THE HEART

The success of the new surgery was chequered. New operations came thick and fast, specialization progressed, the operating theatre became the most prestigious site of medical practice, special clinics were set up for urological, neurological, thoracic, orthopaedic and paediatric conditions. But, as has been seen with cancer and tuberculosis, while giving 'hope', these measures were not always effective. In one high-

---

* Brain surgery for epileptics does not always involve removing tumours; it is possible to remove scarred brain tissue. One of the more common brain operations for epileptics is a temporal lobectomy; temporal lobe epilepsy is the most common form in adults.

profile field, however, a series of spectacular successes in large measure realized surgery's promise, sustaining its impetus into more recent times when various improvements (including new diagnostic technologies and more effective drugs) made surgical intervention generally more effective.

That area was cardiovascular disease, a condition perceived to be dramatically worsening. Like a Himalayan peak, the heart is a great challenge to surgery. Sir Stephen Paget said in 1896 that 'surgery of the heart has probably reached the limits set by Nature to all surgery; no new method, and no new discovery, can overcome the natural difficulties that attend a wound of the heart.' But in the twentieth century, the heart ceased to be a no-go area.

As explored in Chapter 18, clinical knowledge of heart disease was growing, helped by diagnostic technology, notably the electrocardiograph (1903), which became as much a symbol of the modern hospital as the operating theatre. Over the decades other diagnostic improvements brightened prospects for heart surgery. In 1929 a German medical student, Werner Forssmann (1904–79), injected a catheter into his own arm, slid it up a vein and had an X-ray photograph taken of the catheter, whose tip he had pushed (it turned out) into the right atrium of his heart. This caused a sensation. He experimented again on himself in 1931, injecting a radio-opaque substance through a catheter into his heart and then having himself X-rayed (the first angiocardiogram). Building on this, in 1940 the Americans André Cournand (1895–1959) and Dickinson Richards (1895–1973) performed the first catheterization on a patient. Such innovative techniques were to become routine in diagnosis of heart disease.

Catheterization was to prove useful not just diagnostically but therapeutically. It was discovered that the inner lining of coronary arteries (blockage of which is a major cause of heart attacks) can be scoured in a technique known as endarterectomy. In 1964 angioplasty was devised by the Swiss doctor Andreas Grünzig (1939–85): a tiny balloon is inserted into a constricted artery via a catheter and inflated, which clears a path for blood flow. The New York heart surgeon Sol Sobel took this technique a stage further by injecting a powerful carbon dioxide gas jet into an artery via a hypodermic syringe.

As had been understood down the centuries by surgeons faced with aneurysm, the great problem in cardiovascular cases was to find a practical way of reconstructing arteries. This was achieved by a surgeon from

Lyons, Alexis Carrel (1873–1948), a perfectionist who elevated the technical details of his craft into an almost religious mystique. Carrel showed that a piece of the aortal wall could be replaced with a fragment from another artery or vein; above all, having taken lessons from a lacemaker, he developed effective ways of sewing vessels together (anastomosis). In 1910 he described how to transplant an entire vessel, sewing the ends with 'everted' sutures so that the inside was left threadfree, in the belief that the familiar and lethal problem of clotting would thereby be surmounted.

His blood vessel anastomosis operations, joining severed arteries or veins, laid the foundations for later transplant surgery and seemed to presage the realization of the Cartesian model of the body viewed as a machine with replaceable parts. Carrel's early animal experiments from 1902, performed with dog kidneys, ovaries, legs and other organs, attracted such attention that he went to America, working in Chicago and later at the recently founded Rockefeller Institute in New York. In the course of his experiments, he discovered that animals grafted with their own organs thrive, whereas organs sewn on from other animals provoke death; the rejection problem had raised its ugly head.

Traditionally off-limits, the heart and its vessels became the object of intervention thanks to these and related advances. Heart surgery developed by stages, and various operations were tried with improving results. Early efforts to suture stab wounds, for example, resulted in a mortality of 50–60 per cent, due mostly to infection, but by World War II, drawing upon sulfa drugs and antibiotics, surgeons were able to open the heart without undue risk.

Among acquired heart defects, one of the commonest was mitral stenosis, frequently the long-term consequence of childhood rheumatic fever. The valve between the left auricle and ventricle (it supposedly looked like a bishop's mitre) becomes narrowed (stenosis); blood accumulates in the atrium and into the lungs, and the ventricle is not able to supply the body's oxygen needs. The patient is tired and short of breath, and the retardation of blood circulation often results in heart failure. Surgical treatment was envisaged for this constriction in 1902 by Sir Thomas Lauder Brunton (1844–1916), and an operation for mitral stenosis was first attempted in 1923 by Elliott Cutler (1888–1947) in Boston, but without success. In 1925 the English surgeon Henry Souttar (1875–1964) reported operating on a person thought to have mitral stenosis. Though Souttar's diagnosis turned out to be wrong, he discovered that he could stick his finger through the mitral hole, and suggested that might be a way of widening a narrowed valve. Failures in further attempts at mitral valvotomy (out of ten attempts to cure mitral stenosis, eight patients died) led to a pause in this form of surgery.

Nothing happened until a Boston surgeon, Dwight Harken (b. 1910), returned to practice after the Second World War, during which he had come to know the heart through removing bullets. Turning to mitral stenosis, he fitted his finger with a small knife, and on 16 June 1948 treated a valve by dilating it with his finger and cutting its calcified ring. A few months afterwards in London, Sir Russell Brock (1903–1980) did likewise, but using his finger. The operation was progressively refined, leading to the 'open commissurotomy' operation used today. By the early 1980s about 16,000 mitral valve replacements were being performed each year in the USA.

The problem of 'blue babies' – those dying because of inadequate oxygen supply – was recognized from the late nineteenth century. Postmortem indicated that four things could be amiss:

- the pulmonary valve between the heart and the pulmonary artery, through which blood should travel to pick up oxygen in the lungs, might be narrowed;
- the right ventricle, the lower right chamber of the heart, could become swollen from having to pump blood through this constricted aperture;
- the partition (septum) between the two sides of the heart might be incomplete: a 'hole in the heart' allowing oxygenated (arterial) and deoxygenated (veinous) blood to mix;
- the aorta, normally supplying oxygenated blood to the rest of the body, could be misplaced so that it took blood from both the left and right ventricles.

Congenital defects of these kinds meant the baby's body would receive insufficient oxygen and would become cyanosed, giving the skin its blue tinge. 'Blue babies' died young. Could blue baby syndrome be rectified surgically? This was first attempted at Johns Hopkins in November 1944. Denied entry to Harvard because she was a woman, Helen Taussig (1898–1986) had joined Johns Hopkins Medical School in 1921, becoming a specialist in paediatric cardiology. She found that some of her blue baby patients had another congenital heart defect – persistent ductus – yet they paradoxically seemed to do better: evidently the ductus or passage allowed blood to bypass the narrowed pulmonary valve and flow better to the lungs. The answer seemed to be to build an artificial ductus or shunt. She turned to the surgeon Alfred Blalock (1899–1964).

On 29 November 1944, Blalock operated on fifteen-month-old Eileen Saxon, a blue baby close to death. She hovered between life and death, slowly improved, and two months later was discharged from the hospital. By the end of 1950, Blalock and his co-workers had performed over a thousand such operations, and the mortality rate had fallen to 5 per cent. Taussig's *Congenital Malformations of the Heart* (1947) became the Bible of paediatric cardiology.

With mitral stenosis, the surgeon could work on a regularly beating heart, since the procedure could be done in a trice; but more time was needed to correct other inborn heart defects, including a 'hole in the heart'. This takes about six minutes, but the brain can go without blood for only four. How could the available operating time be increased? One idea was to cool the body, as the brain requires less oxygen at lower temperatures. Dog experiments supported this hypothermia approach, and it proved workable on humans.

But hypothermia would be useless for the more serious defects. John Gibbon (1903–73), in Philadelphia, addressed that problem: to devise a machine that would take on the work of the heart and lungs while the patient was under surgery, pumping oxygenated blood around a patient's circulation while bypassing the heart so that it could be operated on at leisure. Having developed a heart-lung machine, in 1950 he began a series of animal experiments to perfect his surgical techniques in correcting heart defects. In 1952 he operated on his first human patient, a fifteen-month-old baby, who died shortly afterwards. His second patient was eighteen-year-old Cecilia Bavolek, who had a hole in the heart. On 6 May 1953 he operated, connecting her to his heart-lung machine for forty-five minutes – for twenty-seven minutes it was her sole source of circulation and respiration.

The operation was a success, and advances thereafter were dramatic. Use of low-temperature techniques with a heart-lung machine initiated open-heart surgery. In 1952, the American surgeon Charles A. Hufnagel (1916–1989) inserted a plastic valve into the descending part of the aorta in the chest, to take over from a diseased aortic heart valve, and, three years later, surgeons began to replace failed valves with ones from human cadavers.

From the 1950s blocked arteries in the limbs were being replaced, and in 1967 coronary arteries were tackled for the first time, when Rene

Favaloro (b. 1923), a cardiovascular surgeon at the Cleveland Clinic, Ohio, 'bypassed' an occluded artery by grafting on a section of healthy vein from the patient's leg above and below the blockage, inaugurating the celebrated coronary bypass. The plumbing involved in coronary artery surgery is quite simple; the aims are to reduce heart pain (angina), improve heart function, and to cut the subsequent incidence of heart attack and sudden death.

By the mid 1980s more than a million Americans had undergone a bypass operation. Over 100,000 are being undertaken every year and technically the operation has become routine. What is in doubt is the long-term value of such arterial surgery. It is effective in relieving angina pains, but it is not clear that, compared with other medical treatments, it improves life expectancy.

TRANSPLANTS

Initially the accent in modern surgery was upon excision. In time, plastic and replacement surgery began to grow in importance and stature. Such reconstructive surgery may take many forms. It can include removing malignant skin tumours and treating birth defects – such as cleft lips and palates – as well as burns and face traumas, urogenital deformities and cancer scars, to say nothing of cosmetic or aesthetic operations like breast implants.

Experience showed that skin and bone tissues could be 'autotransplanted' from one site to another in the same patient. In Paris Félix Jean Casimir Guyon (1831–1920) reported in 1869 that he had got small pieces of skin to heal on a naked wound, while in the same year, noticing that large wounds healed not only from the edges but from 'islands' of skin, Jacques Reverdin (1842–1908), in Geneva, had the idea of aiding the process by strewing slivers of skin on the wound: these extra islands, too, formed new skin. It was also discovered that corneas could be transplanted in a 'keroplastic' operation, originated by Eduard Zirm (1863–1944) in 1906, which saved the sight of many whose corneas had become opaque.

It was the First World War which decisively advanced skin transplants. Confronted by horrific facial injuries, Harold Gillies (1882–1960) set up a plastic surgery unit at Aldershot in the south of England. He was one of the first plastic surgeons to take the patient's appearance into consideration ('a beautiful woman', he believed, 'is worth preserving'). After the Battle of the Somme in 1916, he dealt personally with about 2000 cases of facial damage, and in 1932, he hired as his assistant his cousin, Archibald Hector McIndoe (1900–60), who had gained experience at the Mayo Clinic. Shortly after the outbreak of the Second World War, he founded a unit at Queen Victoria Hospital in East Grinstead, Sussex.

The Battle of Britain in 1940 brought McIndoe some 4000 airmen with terrible new injuries: facial and hand burns from ignited airplane fuel. McIndoe felt that 'plastic surgery' did not truly describe what was required for these, which frequently took years and many operations to rectify, so he coined the term 'reconstructive surgery'. For major facial injuries, he used Gillies's tubed pedicle graft – a large piece of skin from the donor site, which remained attached by a stalk to provide it with a blood supply until a new one established itself. A surgical artist, McIndoe had a gift for cutting complicated shapes from skin freehand.

What about organ transplantation? Thanks to Carrel's new suturing techniques, transplants had become a technical possibility. Using experimental animals, Carrel had begun to transplant kidneys, hearts and the spleen; surgically, his experiments were successes, but rejection was frequent and always led to death: some obscure biological process was at work. There the matter rested, until work undertaken during the 1940s at the National Institute for Medical Research in London by Peter Medawar (1915–1987) clarified the underlying immune reactions. Medawar demonstrated that a transplant's lifespan was much shorter in a host animal which had previously received a graft from the same donor, as it also was in a host injected with white blood cells from the donor. Evidently animals contained or developed antigens which were interfering with the transplanted organ: the host fought the transplant as it would a disease, treating it as an alien invader.

In 1951 Medawar had the idea of drawing on cortisone, a new drug known to be immunosuppressive. In most circumstances immunosuppressiveness would be regarded as a blemish, but here it could be a virtue, undermining the host's resistance. A better immunosuppressor, azathioprine, was developed by Roy Calne (b. 1930) and J. E. Murray (b. 1919) in 1959; but the real breakthrough came in the late 1970s with the application of a new high-powered immunosuppressor, cyclosporine, which became indispensable to further progress in transplanting organs.

The kidney blazed the transplant trail. That was inevitable. The organ was easily tissue-typed and simple to remove; and the fact that everyone has two but needs only one meant that living donors could be used. Should a transplant fail, dialysis was available as a safety-net. Kidneys had long been objects of attention. As early as 1914, a team at Johns Hopkins developed the first artificial kidney (for dogs) designed to perform dialysis – the separation of particles in a liquid according to their capacity to pass through a membrane into another liquid. In the Netherlands, Willem Kolff (b. 1911) constructed the first workable dialysis machine for people thirty years later. At first, they were used only for treating patients dying of acute kidney failure, or from poisoning by drugs which could be removed through dialysis, the idea being to keep them alive long enough for their kidneys to recover. By the early 1960s, however, Belding Scribner (b. 1921), in Seattle, was treating patients with chronic kidney failure with long-term dialysis.

Human kidney transplants were tried in the United States from 1951 – for example on patients with terminal Bright's disease – but the death rate was so awful that only very courageous, reckless, thick-skinned or far-sighted surgeons persevered. Why did they fail? Analysis made it clear that organs had diverse types of tissue, rather as with different blood types, and highlighted questions of compatibility and rejection. Meticulous matching of the tissues of donor and host would give a transplant more of a chance; the ideal case would be that of identical twins, an unlikely event. Nevertheless, the first successful human transplant was indeed performed on identical twins: the donated organ was a kidney transplanted to a twenty-four-year-old man who had two diseased kidneys and was close to death. The healthy kidney came from his identical twin brother, so there was no immunological barrier. The operation was carried out in December 1954 in Boston by J. Hartwell Harrison and Joseph Murray, and its success helped Murray to a Nobel Prize.

Once kidney transplants had been seen to work, the way was open for all other organs. In June 1963, James Hardy (b. 1918) transplanted the lung of a man who had died of a heart attack into a fifty-eight-year-old dying of lung cancer. The new lung functioned immediately and did so for eighteen days until the patient died from kidney failure. In the same year human liver transplantation was first attempted by Thomas Starzl (b. 1926) in Denver.

What of the heart? Transplanting the heart poses problems independent of rejection. Since it deteriorates within minutes of death and is impossible to store, it must be removed and transplanted with great speed, even without full tissue-typing. Nevertheless, it was bound to be the coveted prize for transplant surgeons, for all the obvious emotional, cultural and personal reasons, not least because soaring incidence of heart disease meant this breakthrough could have enormous utility.

The first human heart transplant was attempted on 23 January 1964 at the Mississippi Medical Centre. James Hardy, the pioneer of lung transplants, put a sixty-eight-year-old man with advanced heart disease on a heart-lung machine and prepared for the first transplant between humans. The donor was to be a young man dying from irreversible brain damage, but he was still alive when the potential recipient's heart failed. Hardy stitched in a chimpanzee's heart which was too small to cope, and the patient died.

The world had to wait another four years for the big event: at the Groote Schuur Hospital in Cape Town on 3 December 1967 Christiaan Barnard (b. 1922) transplanted the heart of a young woman, Denise Darvall, certified brain-dead after a car smash. It may be no accident that South Africa got in first; the land of apartheid had fewer ethical rules hedging what doctors could do. While Barnard had contemplated practising on a black man his chief was mindful that 'overseas they will say we are experimenting on non-whites', and this would have tarnished the triumph.

Barnard's patient was fifty-three-year-old Louis Washkansky, who had suffered a series of heart attacks in the previous seven years and had been given only a few weeks to live: he died of pneumonia eighteen days later. Before his demise, publicity seemed to take precedence over the patient's health: the press was admitted to see the recipient within days of the operation (something that would not be permissable today) and Barnard immediately began jetting around the world; he was abroad when Washkansky's condition started to deteriorate.

Barnard was followed in January 1968 by Norman Shumway (b. 1923) at Stanford University in California, and in May that year by Denton Cooley (b. 1920), in Houston. Heart transplants became the rage as media coverage generated funding and fame. In the following year more than a hundred were performed around the world in eighteen different countries; two thirds of the patients were dead within three months. Criticism mounted of such rash human experimentation, especially in view of the lack of attention to tissue-typing (matching compatible tissues).

Initially heart transplants had paltry success; it was not until cyclo-sporin became available over ten years later that the rejection problem was surmounted. Cyclosporin brought to an end the period when kid-ney, liver, heart, heart-and-lung and other interventions were more beneficial to researchers than to the recipients. By the mid 1980s there were 29 centres in the US alone carrying out heart transplants. Approxi-mately 300 were performed in 1984; of the recipients, 75 per cent lived for at. least a year and almost 66 per cent for five years. By 1987 the tally of transplanted hearts had risen to 7000.

By temperament, transplant surgeons were an audacious breed. A colleague of the Texan Denton Cooley commented in the 1990s, 'Twenty-five years ago [Cooley] didn't feel it was worth coming into the hospital unless he had at least ten patients to operate on.' Such men were not fazed by failure: out of seventeen transplants Cooley performed in 1968 only three survived more than six months. So were there limits to what might be achieved? And if so, what were they?

By 1990, Robert White (b. 1926) was beginning to experiment in Chicago on monkeys with 'total-body transplants' – that is, giving heads entirely new bodies. In 1992 the English child Laura Davies suffered, many thought, as a human guineapig at the hands of the Pittsburgh surgeon Andreas Tzakis; she underwent, in the full glare of publicity, to multiple transplants and re-transplants, involving as many as six organs, before she died. The BBC documentary producer, Tony Stark, tells in his book, *Knife to the Heart*, the story of an ex-patient of Tzakis's, Benito Agrelo, a teenager who, experiencing agonizing side-effects from his post-transplant medication, quit his drugs with his family's approval and chose to have a few months of normal life rather than a few years of agony. As a consequence, the medical authorities had him formally taken into care (on the grounds that medical non-compliance was a symptom of personality disorder). He was taken from his home, handcuffed and tied to a stretcher, and ambulanced back to hospital.

The life-and-death excitement of transplants could bring out a ruth-less edge, a belief that 'medical progress' is an end which justifies almost any means. Critics allege that such incidents epitomize the disturbing inability of today's high-tech medicine to accept the autonomy of patients and the reality of death. Barnard's published autobiography portrays the author as a man obsessed by success; he became besotted by his opportuni-ties for fame and sexual conquest. (It is ironic that his surgical career was cut short by a condition so banal as arthritis.)

Other forms of replacement surgery have been less glamorous, costly and controversial – and arguably far more valuable. Hip replacement was developed around 1960 by John Charnley (1911–82) at the Manchester Royal Infirmary. He tackled a widespread problem. When a degenerative disease causes the breakdown of bone tissue, the joint surfaces become rough and irregular, so that when the ball of the femur rubs against the hip socket even the slightest pressure can be extremely painful. Various replacement hips had been designed, including some fashioned from stainless steel. Unsafe and uncomfortable, the metal ball was attached to the femur with a screw, which loosened and eventually became unfastened. In addition, the steel hip squeaked with every step. Charnley tried to overcome these problems. Realizing that the body's fluids could not lubricate the steel sufficiently, he carried out exhaustive studies on lubricants, adhesives and plastics, applying the principles of tribology (the science of wear). He performed the first clinical tests of a prosthetic hip in November 1972. The mechanical success of his hip replacement was remarkable, and within four years his procedure had helped more than 9000 patients to walk without crutches. By the 1990s some of the removal of bone was being done by robotic devices, doubtless heralding a trend towards mechanically driven surgery.

The first successful replantation of a severed limb took place in Boston in 1962. A twelve-year-old boy had his right arm cut off just below the shoulder in an accident. The boy and his arm were taken to Massachusetts General Hospital where the arm was grafted back on. Some months later the nerves were reconnected, and within two years the boy had regained almost full use of the arm and hand, to the point of being able to lift small weights. Replant operations became standard. In 1993 John Bobbitt became headline news when his penis, sliced off by his enraged wife, was sewn back on. Bobbitt blossomed into a porno movie star.

REPRODUCTION

Transplants were just one of many new procedures which radically increased the scope of intervention after 1950. Human reproduction has been spectacularly affected, leading to possibilities and ethical quandaries that transcend technical success or failure in the individual case.

Aware that many women were infertile because of blockage of their

Fallopian tubes, the British gynaecologist Patrick Steptoe (1913–88) saw that if an egg were removed from an ovary, using a laparoscope, and fertilized with sperm, it could be placed in the mother's uterus for normal development. This has become known as 'test-tube' fertilization, though the fertilization takes place not in a test-tube but in petri dishes.

Steptoe went into collaboration with Robert Edwards (b. 1925), a Cambridge University physiologist. In February 1969, they announced that they had for the first time achieved fertilization of thirteen human eggs (out of fifty-six) outside the body. Nine years later, in July 1978, Louise Brown was born at Oldham District Hospital, the first 'test-tube baby'. Despite enthusiastic media coverage, by May 1989 only one in ten of such *in vitro* fertilization (IVF) treatments in Britain produced live babies.

Louise Brown's birth was condemned by voices as diverse as Nobel laureate James Watson, the Vatican, and some feminist philosophers, for the foetus's brief extra-uterine existence raised controversial moral questions: did every extra-uterine embryo have a right to be implanted? must surplus extra-uterine embryos be destroyed or stored and used for later research? if so, was ectogenesis (growth in an artificial environment) permissible? Together with artificial insemination by donor (AID), IVF also raised perplexing questions about the legitimacy of surrogate motherhood.

Efforts were made to resolve these issues. In July 1982 the Warnock Committee, chaired by philosopher Mary Warnock (b. 1924), was convened by the UK Department of Health and Social Security to examine the problems. It recommended that IVF be considered a legitimate medical option for infertile women, while limiting the extra-uterine maintenance of an embryo to fourteen days after fertilization: only then was experimentation admissible. The Committee also advised against the implantation of embryos used as research subjects in humans or in other species. It did not address surrogate motherhood, which is still contentious.

Meanwhile the Vatican came out against IVF; payments to surrogate mothers (receiving eggs and sperm from couples unable to have their own children) were outlawed in some countries; and there was shock when it was revealed, in 1992, that a fifty-nine-year-old Italian woman had been impregnated with a donor egg fertilized by her husband's sperm. At the same time, an American doctor was sentenced to ten years in prison for having used his own sperm when artificially inseminating dozens of his female patients. In 1997, a sixty-three year-old mother gave birth after in vitro fertilization.

Advances in reproduction technology and transplant surgery have thus raised worries that pressures for legalization of the hire of wombs and the sale of organs will become overwhelming. In the United States Dr H. Barry Jacobs (b. 1942) floated the International Kidney Exchange Inc., with a view to importing Third World kidneys for sale to American citizens. Executed criminals in China already have their organs harvested; kidney sales by poor people have become common in various developing countries, and are not unknown in Harley Street. The disquieting parallel between the nineteenth-century Burke and Hare and these modern variants of body-snatching was a theme central to the film *Coma*, directed by Michael Crichton (1977).

Such developments have brought into question the whole status of the body: is it a 'thing', disposable on the market like any other piece of private property? (If so, who owns it after death?) The case for regarding it as a commodity has been advanced by some American utilitarian philosophers: rational choice and market forces, they argue, would create an optimum trade in body commodities such as sperm, embryos, wombs and babies. A 'futures market' in organs has been proposed. Donors (or rather *vendors*) would be paid in advance, on condition that they bequeathed their corpses to be 'harvested' on death. Linked also to the staggering growth of aesthetic surgery – over 800,000 facial procedures are annually performed in the United States alone – the new world of surgery is challenging traditional ideas of the person and the integrity of the individual life.

CONCLUSION

Some pattern may be seen in the development of surgical interventions. In its heroic, Billrothian stage, surgery was principally preoccupied with removal of pathological matter. In due course, thanks to better immunological knowledge and the evolution of anti-bacterial drugs, surgery entered a new phase, more concerned with restoration and replacement. Practitioners acquired a capacity to control and re-establish the functioning of the heart, lungs and kidneys, and also fluid balance. Since the mid twentieth century, one result has been a greater assimilation of surgical intervention into other forms of treatment.

Take angina, first depicted in the eighteenth century by William Heberden. For a time it was expected that surgical intervention would solve this, through the implantation of a bypass or balloon dilatation (coronary angioplasty). Indeed, the Russian president, Boris Yeltsin, who had suffered three heart attacks, underwent a quintuple bypass operation in November 1996. But angina has not only been tackled through surgery – drugs have played their part, notably beta-blockers. In a similar way, most cancers today are handled by a combination of surgery, radiotherapy, chemotherapy and, in some cases, hormone treatment.

Telling also has been the growth of implants as part of a wider strategy of controlling and re-establishing organ functioning. The first implantation of such a prosthesis came in 1959 with the heart pacemaker, developed in Sweden by Rune Elmqvist (b. 1935) and implanted by Ake Sening (b. 1915), designed to adjust beat frequency by electrical impulses in the case of arrhythmic variations. Remedy for many patients suffering from an abnormally slow heartbeat is now offered by an artificial pacemaker. By the early 1990s more than 200,000 were being implanted each year worldwide, approximately half in the United States (about the same number of bypass operations were being performed). Restorative procedures now range from eye lenses to penis implants to facilitate erection. Implanting a prosthesis is traditionally considered part of surgery, but is it so very different from 'implanting' a drug, the work of physic?

This contemporary blurring of the boundaries is evident, too, in changes in urology. Early in the twentieth century, disorders like bladder carcinoma were treated by cutting out malignant tumours. An alternative was provided by radiotherapy, also used for prostate cancer. Bladder cancer was one of the first cancers to be successfully treated with hormones (1941). These days the most frequent form of male cancer, prostate, is rarely dealt with by radical prostatectomy; most treatment is palliative: anti-androgen therapy helps, involving giving the female hormone, oestrogen. In other words, surgery has become increasingly integrated into wider therapeutic strategies, eroding the obsolescent barriers between physic and surgery.

It has thus gone through successive, if overlapping, phases of development. The age of extirpation, involving new ways of dealing with tumours and injuries by surgical excision, gave way to a period of restoration, in which stress fell on physiology and pharmacology, aimed at repairing endangered or impaired function. More recently replacement has come to the fore, with the introduction of biological or artificial organs and tissues. This has implied a more systemic approach to treatment, foreshadowing the ending of old professional identities.

CHAPTER XX

MEDICINE, STATE AND SOCIETY

MEDICINE USED TO BE ATOMIZED, a jumble of patient-doctor trans-actions. Practitioners were mainly self-employed, with at most a tiny back-up team: an apothecary compounding medicines or a surgeon's apprentices pinning down a screaming amputee. Patient-doctor relations typically involved a personal contract, initiated by the sick person calling in a physician or a surgeon.

Other kinds of healing encounters, such as medical charities, made much of the personal touch, the face-to-face relationship believed essential to the office and alchemy of healing. There were of course exceptions: in plague epidemics doctors worked in teams under magistrates within a bureaucratic framework; medics banded together in colleges for *esprit de corps* and pomp and ceremony; and some served in larger social institutions, like the armed forces. But these were anomalous to the normal petty-capitalist occupational patterns. Writing in industrializing Manchester, Dr Thomas Percival presented in his *Medical Ethics* (1803) a picture of a fragmented, divided occupation, in which petty tensions and rivalries between individual doctors (every man for himself) threatened good relations and good practice. Medicine was traditionally small-scale, disaggregated, restricted and piecemeal in its operations.

What could be more different from today? Medicine has now turned into the proverbial Leviathan, comparable to the military machine or the civil service, and is in many cases no less business- and money-oriented than the great oligopolistic corporations. A former chairman of a fast-food chain who quit to head the Hospital Corporation of America (Nashville, Tennessee), explained his move thus; 'The growth potential in hospitals is unlimited: it's even better than Kentucky Fried Chicken.' No wonder he thought that, since astonishing transformations in scale were taking place in what has become known as the industrial–medical complex.

The annual number of hospital admissions in the United States rose from an estimated 146,500 in 1873 to more than 29 million in the late 1960s. While the nation's population was growing five-fold, use of hospitals – the new capital-intensive factories of medicine – rose almost two-hundred-fold. In 1909 there were 400,000 beds in the USA; by 1973 there were 1.5 million. (In Britain, the number of beds per thousand population doubled between 1860 and 1940, and doubled again by 1980.) In the process, medicine became inordinately expensive, claiming a greater share of the gross national product than any other component (in the United States, a staggering 15 per cent by the 1990s). Critics complained that it was out of control, or at least driven more by profit to the supplier than by the needs of the consumer.

The transition from one-man to corporate enterprise is partly the institutional dimension of the developments sketched in the last few chapters: giant strides in basic and clinical research, and the pharmacological and surgical revolutions. In the 1850s Claude Bernard funded his research out of his wife's dowry, while George Sumner Huntington, who discovered the disease named after him, was an obscure country practitioner in New York state; in those days all the tools of the country doctor's trade fitted into a battered pigskin saddle-bag. But even Koch, who started small, ended up the satrap of several palatial research institutions, and since then the iron law has been expansion and amalgamation. These days medicine is practised, at least at its cutting edge, in purpose-built institutions blessed or burdened with complex infrastructures, bureaucracies, funding arrangements and back-up facilities. Orthodox medicine is unthinkable without its research centres and teaching hospitals served by armies of paramedics, technicians, ancillary staff, managers, accountants and fund-raisers, all kept in place by rigorous professional hierarchies and codes of conduct. The medical machine has a programme dedicated to the investigation of all that is objective and measurable and to the pursuit of high-tech, closely monitored practice. It has acquired an extraordinary momentum.

In a medical division of labour that has become elaborate, physicians remain superior in status; however, today they are but the tip of a gigantic health-care iceberg – of the 4.5 million employees involved in health-care in America (5 per cent of the total labour force), only about one in seventeen (300,000) is a practising physician. Perhaps nine out of ten of those employed never directly treat the sick. Time was when medical power lay with clinicians who attended kings and the carriage-trade; in *ancien régime* Denmark it was not odd that Dr Struensee (1737–72) was both royal physician and prime minister (an affair with the queen cost him his head). Today, though one or two transplant surgeons are household names, the real medical power lies in the hands of Nobel Prize-winning researchers, the presidents of the great medical schools, and the boards of multi-billion dollar hospital conglomerates, health maintenance organizations and pharmaceutical companies.

In many nations the largest single employer, medicine's politics have become controverted. Providing life-saving services and priding itself upon being, as Sir William Osler asserted around 1900, distinguished from all other professions 'by its *singular beneficence*', medicine lays claim to a privileged autonomy. Yet that is also the special pleading of an institution dependent upon the market and the state for its financing and anxious to protect its corner.

Modern medicine has been able to root, spread and propagate itself in this way in part because it changed its objectives. Traditionally the physician simply patched up the sick individual; but medicine gradually asserted a more central role in the ordering of society, staking claims for a mission in the home, the office and the factory, in law courts and schools, within what came to be called, by friend and foe alike, a welfare or therapeutic state. The more medicine seemed scientific and effective, the more the public became beguiled by the allure of medical beneficence, regarding the healing arts as a therapeutic cornucopia showering benefits on all, or, like a fairy godmother, potentially granting everybody's wishes. In 1993 the distinguished American writer, Harold Brodkey, who was suffering from AIDS, declared in a magazine, 'I want [President] Clinton to save my life.' Brodkey assumed all that was needed was larger federal grants to AIDS researchers. The previous year, the US government had spent $4.3 billion dollars on AIDS – more than any other disease except cancer.

In western market societies driven by consumption and fashion, medicine was one commodity for which rising demand could not summarily be dismissed by critics of 'I want it now' materialistic individualism. And ever since wily Chancellor Bismarck set up state-run medical insurance in Germany in 1883, politicians have been able to look to health care as a service appealing to virtually the entire electorate. Alongside bread and circuses, there came to be votes in pills and hospital beds. Yet medical politics, of course, never proved simple, and the consequence is that, at the close of the twentieth century, public debates on medical care and its costs have become sources of strife in both America and Britain.

In 1992 one of the campaign issues securing Bill Clinton's election was his undertaking to reform health care. That he dropped the issue once he was president, on meeting opposition from the corporate bodies dominating medicine and their friends in Congress, indicates how medicine has become a political hot potato. In the UK, once Margaret Thatcher became prime minister in 1979, the future of the much-valued National Health Service, threatened by the Conservative government's agenda for privatizing public services, was rarely out of the headlines. Her government felt obliged to reassure voters time and again that, despite the closure of hospital wards and cuts in services, the NHS was safe in its hands. How different from the nineteenth century! Medical issues were then marginal to high politics. Nations did not even possess a ministry of health, hospital beds had no place in election manifestos, and the provision of health care was not considered the state's business.

Of course, the state's role in such matters had been growing during the nineteenth century, but up to 1900 its activities were *ad hoc*. Statutory medical provision tended to be limited to particular problems (e.g., policing of communicable disease) and was viewed by cabinets as a necessary evil rather than the true business of state or a vote-winner. (As noted, faced with cholera in 1848, *The Times* had remonstrated against being 'bullied into health'; its readers probably agreed.) By 1900 medical professionals were generally licensed by law, even in the United States where medical sectarianism was rampant, but nowhere did the state outlaw irregulars. In industrialized nations public-health legislation had entered the statute book in respect of matters like sewage, sanitation and smallpox. But in the USA and elsewhere the management of health was still a tangle of voluntary, religious and charitable initiatives, as was primary care for the needy, while medicine for those who could afford to pay remained essentially a private transaction.

All this was to change, ceaselessly if unevenly, in the twentieth century. It became widely accepted that the smooth and efficient functioning of intricate producer and consumer economies required a population no less healthy than literate, skilled and law-abiding; and in democracies where workers were also voters, the ampler provision of health services became one way of pre-empting discontent. Health also moved centre-stage in propaganda wars – questions of national fitness came to the fore in the great Darwinist panics over racial decline around 1900. Between the wars, fascist Italy, Nazi Germany and the communist USSR each glorified the trinity of health, power and joy, rejoicing in macho workers and fecund mothers while unmasking social pathogens who supposedly endangered national well-being. The Nazis did not merely seek to exterminate what they called the cancer of the Jews; they encouraged cults of physical fitness (through hiking, paramilitary drill, sport and sun-bathing) and launched the first crusade against cigarette smoking. Hitler (unlike Roosevelt, Stalin and Churchill, a non-smoker) supported anti-tobacco campaigns in the name of hygiene, and smoking was banned in the Luftwaffe. The first major medical paper proposing a link between smoking and lung cancer was published by Dr F. H. Müller in Germany in 1939. In any case, whether democratic or fascist, the hands of great powers were often forced when it came to health matters: world wars required massive injections of public money and resources into centralized health services to keep fighting men in the field and sustain civilian morale.

The twentieth-century ship of state thus took health on board, paying lip service to medical thinkers and social scientists who taught that a healthy population required a new compact between the state, society and medicine: unless medicine were in some measure 'nationalized', society was doomed to be sick and dysfunctional.

Medical philosophers equally recognized that medicine had to revise its aims and objectives. Conventional clinical medicine was myopic and hidebound, reformers argued; only so much could be known from corpses, only so much could be done with sedatives, syringes and sticking-plaster. Why wait for people to fall sick? Prevention was better than patching; far better to determine what made people ill in the first place and then – guided by statistics, sociology and epidemiology – take measures to build positive health. In a rational, democratic and progressive society, medicine should not be restricted and reactive; it should assume a universal and positive presence, it should address the totality of pathological tendencies in the community and correct them through farsighted policies, the law, education and specific agencies.

Why not invest in screening, testing, health education, ante-natal care, infant welfare, school health? Why not conduct surveys to discover health hazards and epidemiological variables? Would it not make sense for medicine to step in to prevent citizens becoming decrepit at the workplace, intervene before they became alcoholics or neurotics, or before imbeciles started breeding? Ill-health could not truly be understood at the individual, clinical level, but only as an expression of the health of the social whole; likewise, it could not be combated *ad hoc*, but only through planned interventions. This was the only way to achieve national efficiency, to create a fit, indeed fighting fit, population.

Such views were widely embraced in war-torn Europe and to a lesser degree in North America from the early twentieth century, among the planners, academics and civil servants charged with administering modern society; among social democrats appalled at the human waste caused by inefficient market mechanisms in the Slump and the Depression; among progressive doctors convinced the profession would fulfil its mission only if the state spurred reform; among medical rationalists with visionary leanings and a taste for the social sciences; and not least among far-right propagandists preoccupied with ensuring national mastery in a cut-throat Darwinian arena whose very law was biomedical: thrive or perish.

The call for medicine to adapt was reinforced by the growing recognition that the disease landscape was changing, or was at long last being understood. Twentieth-century epidemiologists stressed that much of the sickness crippling workers, at immense socio-economic cost, was no longer being produced by the classic air-, water- and bug-borne infections. Typhus, diphtheria and other acute infections were being defeated by better living standards, sanitary improvements and interventions like vaccination. In their place, chronic disorders began to assume a new prominence. Medicine began to fix its gaze on a morass of deep-seated and widespread dysfunctions hitherto hardly appreciated: sickly infants, backward children, anaemic mothers, office workers with ulcers, sufferers from arthritis, back pain, strokes, inherited conditions, depression and other neuroses and all the maladies of old age.

To deal with these, the ontological or bacteriological model of disease was no longer sufficient. The health threats facing modern society had more to do with physiological and psychological abnormalities, broad and perhaps congenital tendencies to sickness surfacing among populations rendered dysfunctional and unproductive by poverty, ignorance, inequality, poor diet and housing, unemployment or overwork. To combat all this waste, hardship and suffering, medicine (it was argued) had to become a positive and systematic enterprise, undertaking planned surveillance of apparently healthy, normal people as well as the sick, tracing groups from infancy to old age, logging the incidence of chronic, inherited and constitutional conditions, correlating ill health against variables like income, education, class, diet and housing.

Diverse policy options were then available. One lay primarily in advice and education – helping citizens to adjust to socio-economic reality by instructing them in hygiene, cleanliness, nutrition and domestic science – the old non-naturals revamped. Another lay in specific interventions: providing free school meals, contraception centres, antenatal clinics and the like. In London in the 1930s, the Peckham Health Centre was a showcase experiment in the voluntary provision of health care, together with leisure and educational facilities, for a working-class community. Or there might be yet more ambitious political programmes, building on the model Virchow had perhaps imagined in 1848 for Silesia: health could not be improved without radical socio-political change designed to ensure greater social justice and equality.

Disease became conceptualized after 1900 as a social no less than a biological phenomenon, to be understood statistically, sociologically, psychologically – even politically. Medicine's gaze had to incorporate wider questions of income, lifestyle, diet, habit, employment, education and family structure – in short, the entire psycho-social economy. Only thus could medicine meet the challenges of mass society, supplanting outmoded clinical practice and transcending the shortsightedness of a laboratory medicine preoccupied with minute investigation of lesions but indifferent as to how they got there. It was not only radicals and prophets who appealed to a new holism – understanding the whole person in the whole society; respected figures within the temple of medical science, including Kurt Goldstein (1878–1965) and René Dubos (1901–82), author of *Mirage of Health* (1959), were emphatic that the mechanical model of the body and the sticking-plaster formula would at best palliate disease (too little, too late) but never produce true health.

The twentieth century generated a welter of programmes and policies devoted to the people's health. The underlying ideologies extended from the socialist left (state medicine should aid the underprivileged) to the fascist right (nations must defend themselves against socio-pathogenic tendencies). Either way, the hallowed liberal-individualist Hippocratic model of a sacred private contract between patient and doctor seemed as passé as Smithian political economy in the age of Keynes. As medicine transformed itself after 1900 into a vast edifice, philosophies changed with it, embracing an expansive vision of the socialization of medicine and the medicalization of society. Buoyed up by the indisputable success of Listerian surgery, Pasteurian bacteriology and so forth, confidence was running high about what medicine and health care might achieve. In a world torn by war, violence, class struggle and economic depression, medicine at least would be a force for good! The benefits were clear; the disadvantages would surface only later.

MEDICINE AND THE STATE

Over the centuries medicine had slowly and incompletely become incorporated into the public domain. From medieval times the state began to regulate medical practices, creating a profession; in the early-modern period medicine was ascribed a role within mercantilist strategies for the consolidation of national wealth and manpower; and doctors were always liable to be called upon in time of emergency, particularly plague. In the nineteenth century new medical growth points arose, notably the need to cope with the threat of the sick poor and the environmental hazards caused by industrialization.

Spurred by a familiar mix of altruism and prudence, medical measures were devised to alleviate the afflictions of the masses. The nineteenth century brought philanthropic dispensaries and other forms of out-patient care for the ambulant sick, manned by charitable volunteers or by rank-and-file practitioners working for municipal, religious or philanthropic agencies. Hospitals provided beds for the sick poor, supported by charity (religious or secular) and public subsidy; sometimes they were staffed by elite practitioners using hospital positions as platforms for teaching, research and surgical practice. Centralized or municipal poor law organizations had to handle vast numbers of the sick poor and encountered the need to create immediate hospital facilities for them.

The sanitary movement promised a further approach to the health problems of industrial society, preaching and teaching good drains and housekeeping, physical and moral cleanliness, and in some situations being granted judicial powers. Public health set medicine onto a new official plane with the appointment of experts to compile official statistics, remedy nuisances and do the state's business. A cohort of doctors emerged, beholden not to individual clients but in the guise of guardians of the health of the population generally, and with a brief not curative but preventive. The Victorian administrative state created a variety of appointments for doctors – as medical officers of health, public analysts, factory inspectors, forensic experts, prison doctors and asylum super-intendents, to say nothing of those employed in the army, the navy and imperial enterprises such as the Indian Civil Service.

The ideological identification of medicine with public service was consolidated as more doctors earned part or all of their living in the state sector. Their position was far from comfortable, however, since medicine might need to serve two masters. The prison doctor was implicated in a punitive regime, but ethically his duty lay with the well-being of the individual convict. A similar predicament was involved with workmen's compensation schemes for industrial accidents and ill-ness. Doctors on statutory arbitration boards had to handle situations where the causes of illness and injury were contested between workman, master and state. When a coal-miner developed the eye disease nystag-mus, was this to be diagnosed as due to work conditions or to an inherent constitutional diathesis? The practitioner had to act as society's arbitrator.

Further intractable tensions arose over provision and payments for health care. Sickness costs far exceeded the routine capacity of many to pay, and third-party systems were devised for meeting bills. Initially, these took the form of friendly societies and ethnic associations created by labouring people themselves. Workers in a factory or a coal-pit might club together to pay a fixed weekly sum into a common kitty, to procure the annual services of a general practitioner. Though such arrangements provided junior doctors with some guaranteed income, contract practice was resented, since patient-power posed threats to professional dignity and autonomy: doctors were apprehensive that third-party payers would call the tune, reducing them to mere employees, imperilling their clinical freedom, and creating a Dutch auction.

But if the nineteenth-century medic might not be quite sure where he stood, in Europe at least his (and to a small but growing degree *her*) economic prospects were brightening towards 1900, as specialisms became entrenched and antiseptic surgery blossomed, with the post-Lister menu of operations growing rapidly, first tried out on the poor and later performed upon paying private patients. With surgeons under-taking more ambitious work under strict aseptic routines, there was more scope for the setting up of private hospitals, nursing homes and clinics. Meanwhile public hospitals were turning themselves into high-prestige diagnostic and surgical centres, wooing affluent patients and employing almoners to ensure that even the poor paid something towards costs.

As medical institutions learned how to appeal to the better-off, advances in diagnostics and surgical interventions transformed the political economy of medicine, first and foremost in the United States but also among the elite elsewhere. American medicine was inventive and energetic in promoting new specialties and business arrangements, providing wider services and diagnostic tests, and tapping new sources of custom and income. Medicine seemed good for business and business good for medicine. American doctors were bold in setting up their own hospitals, as did religious, ethnic and other groups. Whether private or charitable, all such institutions found themselves in competition for paying patients who, as the twentieth century progressed, constituted a growing proportion of their clientèle. By 1929 the Mayo Clinic in Rochester, Minnesota was a huge operation with 386 physicians on its books and 895 lab technicians, nurses and other workers. The clinic had 288 examining rooms, 21 laboratories and was housed in a 15-storey building.

In the big cities, American private practitioners discovered the advantages of behaving like lawyers or businessmen, setting up offices in downtown medical buildings, with access to common facilities. Forward-looking in the use of secretaries and technicians, they drew in patients by installing X-ray machines and chemical laboratories, and communicating the self-assurance which the successes of bacteriology and surgery seemed to warrant. At the forefront of innovation, or among those serving wealthy clientèles, medicine developed a powerful momentum and met growing public demand by evolving new forms. Archaic distinctions between private and public, commercial and charitable blurred as hospitals became cathedrals of the new medical science and housed every department of practice. From the 1880s the development of hygienic, well-equipped operating theatres turned hospitals from refuges for the poor into institutions fit for all. From the early 1900s surgery became much more intricate, laboratory tests and other investigations were extended, medical technology became essential, and staff costs leapt. Ambulance services made the hospital the heart of emergency care. All this raised it in the public eye – it also raised costs.

At the same time medical elites were increasingly courted by politicians, called upon to sit on committees and public inquiries to pronounce on social health, housing, diet and national welfare. Dealing with charged issues like the health of children or soldiers, leading doctors hobnobbed with ministers and got a sniff of the benefits that could follow from state welfare programmes and Treasury health investment. Medicine imperceptibly obtained a place at the table of power.

But the situation did not look so rosy for all. With politicians dreaming up schemes for health assurance and state medicine, and with the extension of municipal hospitals, baby centres, venereal disease clinics and the like, ordinary private doctors could feel left out, anxious that public medicine would inexorably encroach upon the private practice which was their bread-and-butter. Every enlargement of state, municipal, contract or charitable medicine meant potential patients lost by private medicine and the family doctor. Worker power in medical friendly societies, schemes for public health, and not least the entry of women into the profession – all these were sources of concern for the self-employed practitioner.

At the grassroots, doctors reacted to these threats by digging in their heels. In the early twentieth century, for instance, British Medical Association branches began to operate remarkably like a trade union, threatening to black-leg colleagues who worked for non-approved friendly societies or 'poachers', who set up practices in 'overstocked' areas. Bitter discord flared between those greeting the extension of organized, large-scale state and municipal medicine, expecting better funding and facilities, and those suspicious that these would be financially ruinous and inimical to 'proper' medicine.

A quandary thus faced British doctors in 1911 when the Liberal politician Lloyd George launched his National Insurance scheme, modelled along Bismarckian lines. In this compulsory scheme, workers earning up to £150 a year (roughly speaking the waged working classes) would be insured; their contribution would be fourpence a week, the employer would pay twopence and the state threepence; the insured workers would in return receive approved medical treatments from a 'panel' doctor of their choice, and for the first thirteen weeks of sickness a benefit of 10s per week for men (7s 6d for women – they earned less). There were restrictions upon benefits: hospital costs were not met, except in the case of TB sanatoria, and the families of insured parties were excluded, though there was a 30s maternity grant (babies were prized as the future of the race). It was a measure devised to be popular with the electorate (it gave 'ninepence for fourpence', boasted Lloyd George), while ameliorating the wretched health of ordinary workers.

This had been critically exposed when a high proportion of Boer War volunteers had been found unfit to serve for medical reasons.

Initially practitioners were up in arms against the National Insurance bill. They would not become cogs in a bureaucratic machine run by the state! Doctors would be reduced to the status of petty civil servants. Some, however, looked to the scheme for deliverance from worse servitude – worker-power in friendly societies – and believed the state would be a more benign and distant master, and certain to pay. In the event, after vocal opposition, most opted to become 'panel doctors' and found that their relationship with the state was secure and remunerative; doctors' income rose steadily.

National Insurance reinforced the divide in Britain between the general practitioner and the hospital doctor, which was to have long-term repercussions for the structure of the profession; but it also helped to cement a lasting and valued relationship between the sick and their GPs, secured by the authority of the state. The family doctor was appreciated because he (increasingly she) was a reassuringly tangible presence. 'We never took weekends off except by special arrangement, which meant we worked six and a half days a week and were on call every night', recalled Kenneth Lane, who began practice as a junior partner in Somerset in 1929; his sense of identity as a country GP and devotion to the job were typical.

War and the threat of war did not merely expose the ill health of people in modern industrial society; they provoked grave anxiety generally about the nation's health. Many who might be indifferent about ailing factory workers and insanitary housing became incensed at the thought of sickly soldiers and enfeebled national stock. The most articulate and coherent response on both sides of the Atlantic was the eugenics movement, which directed the health debate to the problem of fitness, understood in national and racial terms.

Diverse nebulous theories of psycho-biological decline were crystallized by Francis Galton (1822–1911), Darwin's cousin, into a eugenics creed which taught that survival lay in selective breeding. Nature counted for more than nurture; in terms of contributions to national health, breeding stock mattered more than housing stock, wage levels, environmental filth and all the variables which had preoccupied Victorian sanitarians. Unemployment and poverty were the results, not the causes, of social incapacity; malnutrition followed from bad household management, not bad wages. There were in England and Wales, as one eugenist put it in 1931, 'four million persons forming the dregs of the community and thriving upon it as the mycelium of some fungus thrives upon a healthy vigorous plant'. What was the answer? The eugenically sound should breed more, and the dysgenic should be dissuaded from reproduction, or even prevented by sterilization or segregation.

These new degenerationist and hereditarian creeds gained vocal and in some cases large followings in Protestant Europe and in the United States, with race purity eugenists dismissing public health reform not simply as a waste of money and effort but as positively mistaken: rescuing the dregs risked ruining the race. Eugenists like Leonard Darwin (1850–1943), Charles Darwin's son, in England, and Charles Davenport (1866–1944) in the USA advocated measures which included stricter marriage regulation, tax reform to encourage the middle classes to produce more babies, detaining defectives, and the sterilization (voluntary or compulsory) of the unfit. The political right had no monopoly on eugenism: 'the legitimate claims of eugenics', pronounced the impeccably left-wing *New Statesman*, 'are not inherently incompatible with the outlook of the collectivist movement.'

Industrial nations adopted various ingredients of these policies. In Britain the Mental Deficiency Act of 1913 increased powers to place 'defectives' in special 'colonies'. American eugenists championed stricter immigration laws and secured the first compulsory sterilization measures, in due course to be law in forty-four states; 15,000 Americans were sterilized by 1930. Public health advocates and many socialists rebutted these arguments: ill health and other impairments were the products of poverty and poor environment, not inborn defects. And they opposed eugenic policies with ambitious programmes of preventive and sanitary medicine and education. 'Social efficiency', environmentalists claimed, lay in public health management and welfare programmes for mothers, infants, school children, the acute and chronic sick, the tubercular and the aged. Some demanded a comprehensive health system, administered by local health authorities and funded by taxation.

The public health and reformist cases on the one hand and the eugenist on the other shared some common ground. Both could embrace the importance of planning for the future. Healthy mothers produced healthy babies, so state and local agencies and activists invested in mother and baby welfare. In this there were already voluntarist traditions on which to build; so-called 'mothers' ignorance' had been tackled in Victorian times. Founded in 1857, the Ladies' National Association for the Diffusion of Sanitary Knowledge had distributed a million and a half tracts, with titles like *Health of Mothers* (which contained advice on pre-natal care, food, exercise and the evils of tight corsets), *How to Rear Healthy Children, How to Manage a Baby* and *The Evils of Wet-Nursing*, full of baby-care jingles like:

> Remember, he can't chew
> And solid food is bad for him
> Tho' very good for you.

From the 1880s milk depots were founded (though before cows' milk was tuberculin-tested, these were a mixed blessing); ante-natal care programmes were initiated; clinics set up, especially in poor neighbour-hoods, where babies were inspected and weighed, given food, vaccina-tions, and, later, vitamin supplements; women were taught baby care and the benefits of breast-feeding – or alternatively encouraged to use brand-name powdered milk as hygienic artificial feeding; instruction and pressure from big food companies meant that bottle-feeding became the norm for American mothers. Propaganda for 'scientific motherhood' denigrated the traditional mother but idealized the mother of the future. Mothers were persuaded to defer to the expertise of doctors and their clinics, and came under pressure from physicians, women's magazines and particularly the hospitals in which they were increasingly delivered. They became key instruments in the dissemination of new health values.

Doctors, district nurses and health visitors were all asserting their superior knowledge and authority, establishing moral sanctions on grounds of health and the national interest, and running down tra-ditional methods of child care – in particular care by anyone except the mother. Neighbours or grandmothers looking after babies were assumed to be dirty, unfit and remiss. The authority of state over individual, of professional over amateur, of science over tradition, of male over female, of ruling class over working class, were all involved in the 'elevation' of motherhood in this period, and in making sure that the mothers of the race were carefully schooled.

In France the emphasis fell on pro-natalism; after the crushing defeat in the Franco-Prussian War of 1870–1 and with the French population being outstripped by the German, health propaganda encouraged large families. A different tack was taken by supporters of

642 MEDICINE, STATE AND SOCIETY

contraception, including Marie Stopes (1880–1958), a dedicated eugenist (as such, she disapproved of her son marrying a woman who wore glasses). Birth control, claimed Stopes and her followers, would permit the spacing of babies and ensure optimal family size. Planned children would be healthier because adequate resources would be available for them. Quality counted more than quantity.

Sceptics complained that all these gestures were designed primarily to produce fitter cannon-fodder for the battlefield. Die they certainly did in unparalleled numbers between 1914 and 1918 as trench warfare in the First World War set new standards in horror and new peaks in victims. The staggering numbers of casualties, most of whom were not professional soldiers but volunteers and conscripts, and the duration of hostilities, forced governments to construct medical organizations far larger and more centralized than anything conceivable in peacetime. Thousands of buildings were requisitioned as hospitals and convalescent centres; staff were recruited; nursing became a major field of war work; doctors, used to practising in their parlour, discovered the advantages of working in a large, co-ordinated system in which civil servants, specialists, surgeons and women availed themselves of opportunities hitherto denied them.

Though such medical machines were dismantled after the armistice, outlooks were permanently changed. Among the victors, doctors who had specialized in wartime surgery, shellshock or heart medicine returned to civilian life with a passionate vision of a better medical future, partly thanks to contact with American specialists accustomed to well-equipped hospitals and enthusiastic for the new medical technology. Wartime medicine gave doctors a vision and a voice.

The Great War was a watershed, confirming that health was a national concern, but its impact on medicine varied from nation to nation. After Prime Minister Lloyd George's ringing promise to create a land fit for heroes, and his insistence that 'a C–3 population would not do for an A–1 empire', the victorious British were troubled by the accusing contrast of postwar poverty, unemployment, hunger and sickness. Consonant with Lloyd George's belief that 'at no distant date, the state will acknowlege a full responsibility in the matter of provision for sickness, breakdown or unemployment,' a Ministry of Health was established in 1919 and an inquiry set up, leading to the Dawson Report, written by the eminent London physician, Bertrand (later Lord) Dawson (1864–1945).

Insisting that 'the best means for procuring health and curing disease should be available for every citizen by right and not by favour,' Dawson recommended a state-organized rationalization of medical provision based on district hospitals and primary health centres. These would in effect be cottage hospitals, staffed by GPs, who would use them as their surgeries. They would provide operating and treatment rooms, laboratory and X-ray facilities and dentistry, and would also be used by the local authority for maternity and child welfare work and by the school medical service. The Dawson Report aroused much interest before financial crisis led to its being shelved and abandoned.

The conviction among senior civil servants that the state must do something led, if not to better medical provision for the people, at least to better funding for medical scientists. In the 1920s the Medical Research Council was led by a new breed of investigators, scornful of traditional clinicians but on good terms with government. Investment in research was the way, they claimed, to eliminate worthless practices and yield remedies for disease. With the state shouldering the cost of medical care for the labouring classes, it made sense to study prevalent diseases and develop 'social medicine', in line with Virchow's insistence that 'medicine is a social science, and politics nothing else but medicine on a large scale.'

Offering a broad vision of public health which transcended Chadwick's 'sanitary idea', social medicine was pioneered between the wars by medical progressives, typically politically left-wing, impressed by the socialization of medicine in the USSR, and convinced that medical professionals knew best. Influential health policy experts like Sidney (1859–1947) and Beatrice Webb (1858–1943) in Britain, and Henry Sigerist (1891–1957) in the United States, praised the Soviet medical system and urged its emulation. In contrast to socialized medicine in Russia – which prized science, planning and expertise and attempted to create a 'social medicine' incorporating statistics, social science and prevention – the surgeries run by British general practitioners and the dingy hospital outpatient departments were old-fashioned, chaotic, wasteful and trifling with the nation's health.

The leading spokesman for this group was John Ryle (1889–1950), a clinician at Guy's Hospital, later Regius professor of physic in Cambridge and eventually the first professor of social medicine at Oxford. Traditional public health, Ryle reflected, had been concerned with issues such as drainage and water supply. The central object of social medicine, however, should be man and his relation to his environment, which embraced 'the whole of the economic, nutritional, occupational, educational, and psychological opportunity or experience of the individual or the community'. Ryle and his followers were committed to a socialist vision which attributed bad health to social injustice and advocated care for all.

Humble general practitioners, too, chafed at the petty snobberies which continued to dog English medical care. 'There were four distinct classes of patient – private, panel, club and parish – in a peck order as rigid as the social groups of the eighteenth century,' commented Dr Kenneth Lane on his practice in rural Somerset around 1930, and the receptionist

> never allowed anyone to forget which class they belonged to. The private patients had their medicines wrapped in strong white paper and sealed. They were addressed with respect. The panel, club, and parish patients had no wrapping for their medicines and had to provide the bottle or pay tuppence for it. Mean as this sounds it was almost universal practice. As a further distinction between panel and parish patients she would hand the latter their bottles of medicine at arm's length with her head turned away as though she was afraid of catching something. At first this made me laugh then it began to irritate me.

Though inter-war governments did little, medicine continued in piecemeal but significant ways to interact with society. At last gaining the vote in many countries, women carried more weight in the political sphere, and women's groups campaigned for maternity hospitals, better ante-natal and midwifery care, child care services and the like. Fearful over 'degeneration', central government and municipalities were fairly responsive, though in the UK, except for maternity benefits, women and children remained beyond the state insurance system and dependent on medical charities. Responding to public anxieties, governments also built up hospital-centred services for tuberculosis and maternity.

After the abolition of workhouses in 1929, former Poor Law infirmaries were absorbed into municipal government; local authorities assumed responsibility for the bulk of health services: not just drains and notifiable diseases, but clinics, health education, the majority of hospital beds and some special hospitals. Only the ancient, well-endowed charity hospitals retained their splendid isolation, wholly outside a growing local government health remit. State or charity, hospital services were now for all; paupers were no longer segregated and the rich no longer had their surgery at home.

In the inter-war years Mr and Mrs Average and their children were becoming the focus of public medicine and health policies. What developed varied from state to state. The USSR moved in the 1930s from a state insurance system to a salaried medical and hospitalized service which valued science and expertise. Germany continued to operate its Bismarckian state-regulated insurance scheme for workers, administered, as was its mirror in Britain, through friendly societies or employer schemes. Excluded from state benefits, some of the middle classes pre-paid for treatment through private or occupational insurance schemes. In France a state insurance system reimbursed patients rather than physicians, giving free choice of doctor and hospital. Public hospitals, however, were cash-starved and inferior, and the insured flocked to private hospitals, in some cases doctor-owned, which benefited from the system. The ethos of economic liberalism remained strong in France, stressing the freedom of both patients and doctors, and shying away from the 'Germanic' policy of compulsory state medical insurance. A social insurance law was finally enacted in France in 1930.

Everywhere medicine, psychiatry and the social sciences infiltrated everyday life. In England a milestone was the founding in 1920 of the Tavistock Square Clinic by Hugh Crichton-Miller (1877–1959). Chiming with the aims of the 'mental hygiene' movement, which viewed psychiatry's agenda in terms of the mental health problems not just of the insane but of the man and woman in the street, the Tavistock approach became important in raising awareness of family psychodynamics and childhood problems. Its children's department boosted the child guidance movement, which acquired institutional form in the Child Guidance Council (1927), through which emotional lives (buttoned up in the Victorian era) became objects of professional inquiry and expert direction.

The delivery of medical care developed differently in the USA, where the emphasis remained on the market not the state, and on private consumers rather than organized labour or citizens. Beleaguered in the nineteenth century by medical sects and quacks, regulars grew more confident. One of the consequences of the Flexner Report (1910) was the elimination of over half the existing medical schools; this reduced the quantity and improved the quality of medical graduates. Fewer doctors meant higher status and incomes. Economic prosperity from the 'gilded era' up to the 'Crash' (1929) brought a brisk demand for medical services. It became more common to visit a private doctor for a check-up, or for vaccines and routine ailments, rather as people were increasingly opting for elective and not just emergency surgery; this was the golden age for tonsillectomies. American physicians' salaries began their uninterrupted climb, and the formerly weak American Medical Association (AMA) became a force in the land. Championing the causes of maternal and child health, health education, pure food and drug laws, and better vital statistics, the AMA's basic pitch was that what the nation needed to promote all these desiderata was more medicine.

In the United States as well as Europe, health insurance became a major issue. In 1912 the short-lived Progressive Party embraced the concept of compulsory health insurance. The AMA showed interest, keeping its options open, but in the chauvinistic atmosphere during and after the First World War, when everything German or Russian was vilified, attitudes hardened and the association went on record in 1920 as opposing any plan of compulsory health insurance. Morris Fishbein (1889–1976), editor of the *Journal of the American Medical Association*, explained that it boiled down to 'Americanism versus Sovietism for the American people'. 'Compulsory Health Insurance', declared one Brooklyn physician, 'is an Un-American, Unsafe, Uneconomic, Unscientific, Unfair and Unscrupulous type of Legislation supported by ... Misguided Clergymen and Hysterical Women.'

Growing more conservative in the 1920s, the AMA resisted the Sheppard-Towner Act, which provided federal subsidies for states to establish maternal and child health programmes; it also opposed the establishing of veterans' hospitals in 1924. (Both were seen as taking the bread out of the mouth of the private physician.) As group hospitalization plans developed, the AMA at first expressed reservations and by 1930 was denouncing them as socialist. A few doctors demurred, the Medical League for Socialised Medicine of New York City strongly advocating compulsory health insurance under professional control.

President Franklin Roosevelt's New Deal, designed to steer the nation out of the Depression, seemed to be leading America in the direction of a national health programme – many New Deal agencies were involved in health. From June 1933 the Federal Emergency Relief Administration authorized the use of its funds for medical care; the Civil Works Administration promoted rural sanitation and participated in schemes to control malaria and other diseases; and the Public Works Administration built hospitals and contributed to other public health projects. In 1935 the Social Security Act authorized the use of federal funds for crippled children, maternity and child care, and the promotion of state and local public health agencies.

The Depression and the popularity of President Roosevelt – himself a polio victim – forced the AMA to temper its views, although it constantly warned of the danger of the government encroaching upon the domain of medicine. The Association counter-attacked by citing the alleged failure of the British National Insurance system. During the Depression, when many could no longer afford to pay and the hospital sector plunged into crisis, charity hospitals began to introduce voluntary insurance schemes to cushion their users; commercial companies also moved into the hospital insurance market. In 1929 a group of school teachers in Dallas contracted with Baylor University Hospital to provide health benefits at a fixed rate. The idea of group hospitalization was picked up by the American Hospital Association in the early 1930s, leading to the Blue Cross (hospital) and Blue Shield (medical and surgical) pre-paid programmes. Initially suspicious, the AMA had the foresight to recognise that private schemes suited their interests better than compulsory federal ones.

Private health insurance became big and lucrative business. In the twenty years from 1940 to 1960 it experienced explosive growth, encouraged by the medical profession's endorsement; and thereafter dominated the American private medicine market. Middle-class families (or often their employers) paid for primary and hospital care through insurance schemes, and physicians and hospitals competed with each other to attract their custom.

With its stress on specialization and surgery, America enjoyed a hospital boom, and hospitals in turn became the great power-base for the medical elite, the automated factories of the medical production-line. By 1900, the profession had everywhere gained effective control of such institutions and their leadership was reinforced by proclamations that advances in biomedical science were the pledge of progress. Hospital laboratories would generate medical advances, while hospital-based education would disseminate them through a hierarchy of practitioners and institutions. Funds for flagship hospitals and research and teaching facilities were prised out of Washington, state governments, and notably from philanthropic bodies such as the Rockefeller Foundation. Between the wars, the Foundation gave millions to university departments and hospitals in many countries to support the science-based medicine Flexner had envisaged.

The transformation of the hospital from a poorhouse to the nerve centre and headquarters of the new medicine had profound implications. It increased the complexity and costs of medical education. Attached to prestigious universities and hospitals, medical schools had to be subsidized, and support for medical education and training came indirectly from the public, from voluntary bodies which financed capital expenditures, and from payments for poor patients. One consequence was that, by mid century, hospitals were absorbing about two thirds of the resources spent on health care in the United States, and the percentage continued to rise. These hospitals became key centres of medical research, in the conviction that this would generate health improvements. Medical research and medical education grew inseparable, and bigger, costlier and more prestigious hospitals were their status symbols.

Medical politics took an altogether different turn in Germany. In the twenties the Weimar Republic (1918–33) made moves to put medicine on a social footing, with clinics for mothers and children and similar measures. But the desire to avenge defeat in the war fostered the rise of ideologies of national fitness, which in practice meant strengthening the strong and eliminating the weak. Building on a German tradition of racial politics, Hitler, who became chancellor in 1933, demonized Jews, gypsies and other groups as enemies of the Aryan master race in his *Mein Kampf* (1927) [My Struggle], and Nazi medicine in due course defined some non-Aryan races as subhuman. The anti-semitism which culminated in the Holocaust received strong ideological and practical backing from doctors and psychiatrists, natural and social scientists, organized in particular through the Nazi Physicians' League.

Founded in 1908, the *Archiv für Rassenhygiene* [Archive of Race Hygiene], the main organ of the German eugenics movement, had long been urging action to stop what it deplored as the biological and psychological deterioration of the German race. The enthusiasm of German physicians in endorsing ideas of racial degeneracy and implementing race hygiene policies indicated personal opportunism, but it was also the expression of widely held biomedical and anthropological doctrines. Physicians and scientists participated eagerly in the administration of key elements of Nazi policies such as the sterilization of the genetically unfit. Presiding at genetic health courts to adjudicate cases, physicians ordered sterilization of nearly 400,000 mentally handicapped and ill persons, epileptics and alcoholics even before the outbreak of war in September 1939. Thereafter, 'mercy deaths', including 'euthanasia by starvation', became routine at mental hospitals. Between January 1940 and September 1942, 70,723 mental patients were gassed, chosen from lists of those whose 'lives were not worth living', drawn up by nine leading professors of psychiatry and thirty-nine top physicians. To make sure that the programmes were expertly conducted, doctors had the exclusive right to supervise the elimination process by selecting prisoners on arrival at Auschwitz and other extermination camps.

Some of the victims were selected so that German medical scientists could conduct programmes of human experimentation. Camp doctors used inmates to study the effects of mustard gas, gangrene, freezing, and typhus and other fatal diseases. Children were injected with petrol, frozen to death, drowned or simply slain for dissection purposes. The leading Auschwitz physician, Josef Mengele (1911–79), had doctorates in both medicine and anthropology, and won his spurs before the war as assistant to the distinguished professor, Otmar Freiherr von Verschuer (1896–1969), giving expert medical testimony against those accused of committing *Rassenschande* (racial disgrace, i.e., sexual relationships between Jews and Aryans).

Dedicated to human experimentation, as camp doctor at Auschwitz, Mengele selected over one hundred pairs of twins, injecting them with typhoid and tuberculosis bacteria; after their deaths he thoughtfully sent their organs to other scientists. In the name of science, he also investigated the serological reactions of different racial groups to infectious diseases in projects financed by the Deutsche Forschungsgemeinschaft [German Research Foundation] under the auspices of the country's most eminent surgeon, Ferdinand Sauerbruch. After the war, Mengele fled to South America; he was never brought to trial. Twenty doctors were, however, tried at Nuremberg for crimes against humanity and four were hanged; but the vast majority of those involved in the atrocities, including Sauerbruch, were allowed to return to their university posts or medical practices.*

Doctors also played a key role in the pursuit of human experimentation in Japan. In 1936 the 'Epidemic Prevention and Water Supply

---

* Nazi practices seemingly confirmed the fears of nineteenth-century antivivisectionists who had prophesied that vivisection experimentation was bound to proceed from animals to humans. The novelist Ouida wrote, 'Claude Bernard, Schiff and many other physiologists have candidly said that human subjects are absolutely necessary to the perfecting of science: who can doubt that in a few years time, they will be openly and successfully demanded and conceded?'

Unit' was formed as a new Japanese army division (it was also known as Unit 731). Hundreds of doctors, scientists and technicians led by Dr Shiro Ishii were set up in the small town of Pingfan in northern Manchuria, then under Japanese occupation, to pioneer bacterial warfare research, producing enough lethal microbes – anthrax, dysentery, typhoid, cholera and, especially, bubonic plague – to wipe out the world several times over. Disease bombs were tested in raids on China. Dr Ishii also developed facilities for experimenting on human guineapigs or *marutas* (the word means 'logs'). Investigating plague and other lethal diseases, he used some 3000 *marutas* to investigate infection patterns and to ascertain the quantity of lethal bacteria necessary to ensure epidemics. Other experimental victims were shot in ballistic tests, were frozen to death to investigate frostbite, were electrocuted, boiled alive, exposed to lethal radiation or vivisected. Like Dr Mengele, Dr Ishii experimented to determine the differential reactions of various races to disease. Initially, his research had all been on Asians, but he broadened his programme to include American, British and Commonwealth prisoners-of-war.

At the end of the war, surviving Pingfan victims were gassed or poisoned, the facilities destroyed and the plague-ridden rats released. Dr Ishii and his team did a deal with the American authorities, trading their research to avoid prosecution as war criminals. The American government chose to keep these atrocities secret. The United States had been manufacturing anthrax and botulin bombs during the war, largely in the expectation that Germany would resort to biological weapons. Britain undertook anthrax tests on the Scottish island of Gruinard and at the Porton Down research station in Dorset. During and after the war, the American military subjected its troops to secret radiation tests as part of its atomic programme: in the climate of World War and Cold War, it was easy for medical scientists to persuade themselves that their involvement in such un-Hippocratic activities would contribute to medical advance, national survival and the benefit of mankind.

One of the reactions in the postwar years against such perversions has been an international ethical movement for medicine. Though the Nuremberg Code, drawn up after the trials, failed to define genocide as a crime,* it was intended to ensure medical research could never

---

* The International Convention on the Prevention and Punishment of the Crime of Genocide was adopted by the United Nations General Assembly in Paris on 9 December 1948; it was ratified by the USA in 1988.

again be abused. The Code consisted of ten points giving ethical guidance. The first and crucial one read: 'The voluntary consent of the subject is essential.' The other nine principles governing medical research stated:

2 The experiment should be such as to yield fruitful results for the good of society, unprocurable by other methods or means of study, and not random or unnecessary in nature.
3 The experiments should be so designed as to be based on animal experimentation and . . . that the anticipated results will justify the performance of the experiment.
4 The experiment should be so conducted as to avoid all unnecessary physical and mental suffering and injury.
5 No experiment should be conducted where there is an *a priori* reason to believe that death or disabling injury will occur; except, perhaps, where the experimental physicians also serve as subjects.
6 The degree of risk taken should never exceed that determined by the humanitarian importance of the problem . . .
7 [Adequate facilities should be used, and precautions taken] to protect the experimental subject against even remote possibilities of injury, disability or death.
8 [E]xperiments should be conducted only by scientifically qualified persons . . .
9 [The] subject should be at liberty to bring the experiment to an end . . .
10 [The] experiment . . . must be . . . terminate[d] . . . [if] continuation is likely to result in injury, disability, or death to the experimental subject.

These principles were further refined in the Declaration of Helsinki on medical research in 1964, which defined the difference between therapeutic experiments (in which clinical research is combined with professional care) and non-therapeutic experiments (in which the experiments may be of no benefit to the subject concerned but may contribute to knowledge). These guidelines carried no sanctions, and subsequent scandals made it frighteningly clear that it was not only fascist powers who had been engaging in unethical research.

In the postwar years whistle-blowers such as H. K. Beecher (1904–76) in the United States and M. H. Pappworth (1910–94) in Britain were to the fore in exposing the routine performance of unethical experiments, often using the mentally ill or defective as human guineapigs, in leading medical schools and published in prestigious journals. One of the more shocking was the Tuskegee (Alabama) experiment, begun in 1932 by the United States Public Health Service. This involved depriving hundreds of syphilitic blacks of proper medical treatment (while pretending that they were being so treated), to make a study of the long-term degenerative effects of syphilis on the nervous system. The experiment continued until the 1960s, and the study was not ended until 1972. It revealed nothing about syphilis, but much about racism. One hundred men died during the course of the experiment.

The Biological Weapons Convention of 1972 outlawed the development, production and stockpiling of biological and toxic weapons as well as their use. It sets out no means of verification, and it is known that disasters have occurred since then in Soviet plants manufacturing anthrax for biological warfare. The extent of Iraq's stockpiles of biological weapons at the time of the Gulf War in 1991 remains unclear.

War is often good for medicine. It gives the medical profession ample opportunities to develop its skills and hone its practices. It can also create a postwar mood eager to beat swords into scalpels. The astonishing success of antibiotics used upon troops during the Second World War heightened expectations of wider public benefits. Only in Great Britain, however, was it followed by a dramatic reorganization of civilian medical services. The USA had emerged unscathed and increasingly suspicious of anything 'unAmerican', while continental Europe was in collapse and unable to implement far-reaching plans.

The blueprint for reform in the UK was the *Beveridge Report on Social Insurance and Allied Services*, the work of civil servant Sir William Beveridge (1879–1963). Published in 1942, it declared war on the five giants that threatened society: Want, Ignorance, Disease, Squalor and Idleness. To combat sickness, Beveridge proposed that a new health service be available to everyone according to need, free at the point of service, without payment or insurance contributions and irrespective of economic status. All means tests would be abolished.

Whether the National Health Service outlined in the Beveridge Report would have been implemented had the Conservatives won the general election of 1945 is doubtful; the Labour Party enjoyed a landslide and set about implementing it. A bill was introduced, in April 1946; on 6 November it received the royal assent and the appointed day for its inauguration was 5 July 1948.

The hospital services were in urgent need of reform. With war looming in 1939, the Ministry of Health had taken over the nation's hospitals on an *ad hoc* basis, instituting a national Emergency Medical Service which gathered more than a thousand voluntary and over 1500 public hospitals into eleven administrative regions. The scheme coped well with the air raids and extensive civilian casualties. At the war's end, it was recognized that most hospitals were financially too feeble to be returned to the voluntary sector, and that they had functioned more effectively during hostilities under government control and financial backing. Moreover, hospitals had begun to count on government payments, and had become used to cooperation within a state-planned scheme. No major private insurance sector was going to keep them afloat, as it did in the United States.

Aneurin Bevan, minister of health in the postwar Labour administration, nationalized municipal as well as charity hospitals. No friend of local government, he wanted hospitals, recognized as the flagships of medicine, under the control of central government. The nationalization of the hospital service divided the country into regions, each administered by a regional hospital board associated with a university and containing one or more medical schools. The teaching hospitals won for themselves (the price paid for their support) a privileged status. Each was to be given a measure of autonomy under its board of governors.

This reorganization was the most far-reaching administrative action concerning hospitals ever brought about in a western nation; in the process the government became responsible for 1143 voluntary hospitals with over 90,000 beds, together with 1545 municipal hospitals containing 390,000 beds. Thanks to nationalization, hospital doctors could look forward to better facilities and consultants were permitted to retain considerable independence, including the right to private practice within NHS hospitals.

For general practitioners, however, the proposed health service seemed an altogether more dubious prospect. Fears were expressed, as in 1911, about the imposition of a full-time salaried medical service. The BMA fomented hostility to the bill, and a questionnaire it conducted in February 1948 showed that 88 per cent of its members were against accepting service. Bevan, however, boasting that he had 'won over the consultants by choking their mouths with gold', denied that he had any intention of introducing a full-time salaried practitioner service, and guaranteed to GPs the continuation of private practice. Faced with such conciliation, opposition subsided, and on schedule, 5 July 1948, the National Health Service came into operation.

Supporters hoped that reorganization of general practice would follow, anticipating the creation of upwards of 2000 health centres. But progress in this direction proved snail-like; ten years after the Act came into force there was only a handful of health centres in the whole country. Even so, the NHS was enormously popular, bringing about a considerable levelling-up of services, though hopes that good treatment would lead to a need for less medicine and hence a reduction of expenditure were naive. Beveridge had calculated the annual cost of the service at £170 million; by 1951 it was £400 million, and by 1960 £726 million. The White Paper of 1944 predicted that it would be several years before the dental service cost £10 million; the cost in the first year was £28 million. Bevan complained about the 'cascades of medicine pouring down British throats', but resigned over the imposition of prescription charges.

The system was efficient and fairly equitable. The NHS did not revolutionize medicine, indeed it perpetuated the old division between hospital consultants and general practitioners, who chose to remain as small businesses under the state. They were widely regarded as less expert than hospital consultants, but their accessibility made them popular. In the 1960s general practice was renovated when, forty years after the Dawson Report, GPs finally began to band together in group practices large enough to employ nurses and other auxiliary services. By then the NHS seemed well established: hospitals, general practitioners and public health were part of a planned and unified service, based on regions and their medical schools. NHS medicine was powerful, popular, and by international standards exceptionally cheap.

Broadly comparable developments had occurred or were to follow in British-influenced countries. In New Zealand, government health care assistance had begun in late-Victorian times with the creation of a national hospital system. The first Hospitals and Charitable Institutions Act (1885) divided the country into twenty-eight hospital districts, each controlled by a board whose members were appointed annually by local authorities. The hospitals were to be financed by patient fees, by voluntary contributions and local rates. The introduction of hospital benefits under the Social Security Act 1938 relieved patients of the payment of fees.

Canada took the path of socialized medicine, though at a later date. Saskatchewan began its Medical Care Insurance and Hospital Services Plan in 1962, enabling residents to obtain insurance covering many medical services. This government administered programme was funded by an annual tax and by the use of federal funds. Shortly afterwards, British Columbia, Alberta and the other provinces adopted similar schemes. A central Medical Care Act (1967) co-ordinated the system. The medical profession initially resisted what seemed to be the encroachment of state medicine, but (as generally happened) fell into line. As health expenditure rose, the Canadian government launched prevention campaigns for traffic accidents, alcohol abuse and smoking, in the hope of curbing costs.

As western Europe recovered from World War II, and moved during the 1950s into an era of prosperity, various forms of state-supported medical systems took shape. Sweden established medical care and sickness benefit insurance in 1955; it was a compulsory scheme, with costs divided among employer, employee and the government. Doctors were not employed by the state, but the government regulated physician and hospital fees.

In postwar divided Germany, the West (the FRG) continued to use sick funds which reimbursed doctors, and France still relied on state welfare benefits through which patients were refunded for most of their medical outlay. Dependants were included in nationalized social security schemes. Private hospitals multiplied and attracted rapidly rising expenditure, while public hospitals (typically rundown buildings catering for long-stay patients) languished. As the French economy recovered, the shabbiness of the public sector became embarrassing and, to counter this, the Debré Law (1965) encouraged liaisons between public hospitals and medical schools, offering incentives to doctors to combine patient care with research and teaching. New installations were added, often housing research laboratories and pursuing science projects found in other nations in universities or other non-clinical institutions. The French state assumed powers to control hospital development, to secure better distribution of services and reduce duplication.

Climbing from the 1950s, West German health expenditure skyrocketed in the 1970s, hospitals accounting for (as everywhere) the bulk of the budget. A law of 1972 led to state governments assuming responsibility for hospital building, and sick funds were obliged to pay the full daily costs of approved hospitals. Gleaming new hospitals drove up standards and caused costs to spiral, so that by the late 1970s Germany, like other nations, was looking for ways to peg expenditure.

Meanwhile the United States went its own way. From the 1930s those able to afford it took out private health insurance, increasingly through occupational schemes tax-deductible for employers and employees alike. Under a fee-for-service system which rewarded doctors for every procedure undertaken, physicians and hospitals competed to offer superior services: more check-ups, better tests, the latest procedures, a wider range of elective surgery, and so forth; Americans began to see their physicians more often, and to consult a greater diversity of specialists. Living longer, they were beguiled by the possibility that medicine would truly deliver the secret of a healthier and more extended life. In these circumstances, costs inevitably spiralled, on the supposition that everyone wanted, and many could afford, more extensive, more expensive benefits: the sky was the limit, nothing could be too good. While capital expenditures on hospitals were steep, they were often subsidized by federal funds; and rising health costs were masked by insurance and cushioned by affluence. In any event, spending more on health seemed like a good investment.

In the 1930s Franklin Roosevelt had toyed with the possibility of introducing some kind of national health insurance as part of the New Deal, but the postwar mood scotched that. In the Cold War's anti-communist, anti-foreigner atmosphere, any socialized system smacked of Germanism and Stalinism. When Harry Truman mooted a national health programme in 1948, the AMA campaigned vigorously and effectively against it. Government money, insisted the medical apologists, should fund science not socialized medicine. 'We are convinced', maintained Curtis Bok (1897–1962), 'that the only genuine medical insurance for this country lies in making the benefits of science available to all practitioners and to all patients'. In similar vein in the 1950s a Republican congressman maintained that 'medical research is the best kind of health insurance.'

Complementing private insurance schemes like Blue Cross came the Health Maintenance Organizations (HMOs), originating with the Kaiser Foundation Health Plan organized in California in 1942 and the Health Insurance Plan of Greater New York dating from 1947. By 1960 each of these was providing complete medical care to over half a million subscribers, and by 1990 the Kaiser-Permanente programme, based in

Oakland, California, was employing 2500 physicians and operating 58 clinics and 23 hospitals. Subscribers to these and other HMOs paid monthly dues entitling them to comprehensive medical care. Physicians received a salary plus a percentage of profits. The remuneration system was designed to keep the lid on costs, by curbing the multiplication of unnecessary tests and procedures, inessential hospitalization, surgery and other expensive and lucrative practices encouraged by traditional health insurance with its fee-for-service basis. The number of surgical operations and the amount of hospitalization deployed in HMOs was around a third less than in ordinary private practice. By 1990 HMOs were providing medical care for about eight million Americans.

Despite acclaim for private medicine and private medical insurance, the American government became committed to shouldering a growing proportion of health care. Federal government provided direct medical care to millions of individuals through the Armed Services and Veterans Administration. Some thirty million war veterans are currently eligible for inpatient and outpatient services at the Veterans Administration Hospitals and Clinics, and approximately two million personnel in the armed services, to say nothing of their dependants. The Public Health Service, the Indian Health Service, and a wide range of other governmental agencies provide federally funded health services of one sort or another.

Awareness grew of the disparity between the increasingly lavish provision of health care for the affluent and the situation of the poor and the old. This injustice became a source of national embarrassment and a campaigning platform for the Democratic Party. With the election of John F. Kennedy as president in 1960 and the possibility of federal intervention, the AMA once again issued a call to arms and fought a rearguard struggle against rising public support for a programme to provide medical care for the aged. Capitalizing on a wave of idealism following Kennedy's assassination in 1963, his successor Lyndon B. Johnson, offering a unifying and healing vision of a 'great society', was able to amend the social security laws. In 1965 Congress made medical care a benefit through Medicaid, set up alongside Medicare, the parallel health-and-care plan for old people. Federal grants were made to state governments to cover the costs.

The Medicare programme, which became effective in July 1966, provided a federally financed insurance system for paying hospital, doctor, and other medical bills, covering all individuals eligible for social security benefits. Medicaid was to provide federal assistance to state medical programmes which might include a variety of services: family planning, nursing homes, screening and diagnostic programmes, laboratory and X-ray services, and so forth. Medicaid and Medicare – essentially government-subsidized medical insurance for social security recipients – proved inflationary because providers were reimbursed on the standard fee-for-service basis.

Health became one of the major growth industries in America, encompassing the pharmaceutical industry, manufacturers of sophisticated and costly diagnostic apparatus, laboratory instruments and therapeutic devices, quite aside from medical personnel, hospitals and their penumbra of corporate finance, insurers, lawyers, accountants and so forth. Expenditure has continued to rise at a quite disproportionate rate, as the accompanying table shows. The 1996 figure for the United States was touching 15 per cent. Many factors contribute to this. Private medical insurance is a lucrative business, and insurers benefit from boosting costs as high as the market can bear. Physicians' incomes run at seven times the national average, and with the rise of medical litigation through malpractice suits, medicine has become a profitable source of business for lawyers, accountants and other expensive professions parasitical upon medicine. Hospital trustees and administrators traditionally have a stake in making medical care lavish and munificent, so hospitals added costly units – kidney machines, scanners and coronary care centres – as prestige items or to gratify local pride, often duplicating similar facilities in neighbouring institutions. Managing 'non-profit' institutions, hospital boards have typically had little incentive to curb expenses, being able to meet their growing budgets by raising charges, staging appeals and securing public money. Vast inefficiency and duplication have come to characterize health care delivery.

No small factor in spiralling costs has been the ceaseless growth of specialties. Specialty practice is attractive to physicians. Specialists generally earn more money, and achieve greater professional and social recognition than the GP. Specialization has inevitably led to a growing population of practitioners and a proliferation of consultations.

In short, from the 1930s the United States has invested in more, more elaborate, and more expensive health care for the well-off. The number of medical schools jumped from 77 in 1945–6 to about 120 in 1990, the number of graduates doubled, and the uptake of physicians' services increased at an even greater rate as medicine rose in the public

Comparison of health care expenditure as share of Gross Domestic Product in OECD countries, 1970–92

COUNTRY	1970	1975	1980	1985	1990	1991	1992
Australia	5.7	7.5	7.3	7.7	8.2	8.5	8.8
Austria	5.4	5.3	7.9	8.1	8.4	8.6	8.8
Belgium	4.1	5.9	6.6	7.4	7.6	8.1	8.2
Canada	7.1	7.2	7.4	8.5	9.4	10.0	10.3
Denmark	6.1	6.5	6.8	6.3	6.3	6.6	6.5
Finland	5.7	6.4	6.5	7.3	8.0	9.1	9.4
France	5.8	7.0	7.6	8.5	8.9	9.1	9.4
Germany	5.9	8.1	8.4	8.7	8.3	8.4	8.7
Greece	4.0	4.1	4.3	4.8	5.3	5.3	5.4
Iceland	5.2	6.2	6.4	7.0	8.2	8.4	8.5
Ireland	5.6	8.0	9.2	8.2	7.0	7.6	7.1
Italy	5.2	6.1	6.9	7.0	8.1	8.6	8.5
Japan	4.6	5.6	6.6	6.5	6.6	6.7	6.9
Luxembourg	4.1	5.6	6.8	6.8	7.2	7.3	7.4
Netherlands	6.0	7.6	8.0	6.0	8.2	8.4	8.6
New Zealand	5.2	6.7	7.2	6.5	7.3	7.7	7.5
Norway	5.0	6.7	6.6	6.4	7.5	8.0	8.3
Portugal	3.1	6.4	5.8	7.0	5.4	5.9	6.0
Spain	3.7	4.8	5.6	6.7	6.6	6.5	7.0
Sweden	7.2	7.8	9.4	8.9	8.6	8.5	7.9
Switzerland	5.2	7.0	7.3	8.1	8.4	9.0	9.5
Turkey	–	3.5	4.0	2.8	4.0	4.7	4.1
United Kingdom	4.5	5.5	5.8	6.0	6.2	6.6	7.1
United States	7.4	8.4	9.2	10.5	12.4	13.4	14.0

Source: OECD, 1996

estimation. Infectious diseases were, it seemed, being conquered, and doctors were innovation-oriented, as were 'research-based' pharmaceutical companies like Hoffman-La Roche, Merck, Hoechst, Eli Lilly, Upjohn and others, producing a series of new and costly drugs. Requiring elaborate tests, the proliferation of paramedical staff and the provision of sophisticated drugs, new medical procedures dramatically increased medical labour and costs – to say nothing of outlays on services aimed at documenting and justifying clinical procedures, so-called 'defensive medicine' (taking an X-ray in case the obvious sprained ankle turned out to be a fracture).

Such developments – medicine seemingly expanding to consume all the funds available – were bound to draw growing criticism. Some denounced Medicare and Medicaid as a blank cheque, corrupting to consumers and providers alike. Others deplored the channelling of vast resources into a defective, high-tech, high-cost system geared to benefiting suppliers rather than sufferers. Scientific medicine (the fulfilment of Flexner's dreams) came under attack, especially in the 1960s' populist counter-culture backlash when all established institutions were fair game. Critics of vast, impersonal mental hospitals campaigned for 'community care'. Feminists lambasted the evils of 'patriarchal medicine', as evidenced in the hospitalization of normal births, and called for the right to choose home confinement. Other consumer groups mobilized patients and challenged the profession's monopoly. High-tech medicine came under fire as part of a wider critique of the shortcomings of science and technology. Disasters with new drugs, notably the thalidomide tragedy, were seen as proof of technical failure and professional dominance – the interests of medi-business taking precedence over the sick.

Radical criticism eroded confidence, caused questioning, and led many into the paths of alternative medicine. But it produced few structural reforms. What achieved most during the 1980s and 1990s were new pressures towards financial stringency in reaction to the soaring cost of high-tech medicine and the uncontrollable and insatiable demand it had excited. Since then the leading factor in medical policy-making has become the quest for cost restraint. The consequences of budgetary crisis have been most crudely evident in the former USSR and the eastern bloc, where political and economic transformation and restructuring – in some cases this has meant collapse – have led to a permanent health care crisis, with shortages of drugs and medical staff not being paid. But everywhere a new financial stringency is in the driving seat.

Medical policy had for so long been focused on conquering disease; from around 1980 the conquest of costs assumed prime importance. Slogans like 'if it's not hurting, it's not working', used by the Conservative administration in the UK in the 1990s, seemed to symbolize the fact that high taxes and high inflation had become, at least in the government's eyes, more of a threat to national well-being than poor health.

In this cost-cutting atmosphere in various countries, professional autonomy simultaneously became threatened by the economic liberalism of the resurgent New Right, which questioned state-provided services, criticized professional monopoly and deified market mechanisms in the name of efficiency and competitiveness. Aware that (as an earlier health minister, Enoch Powell, had put it) 'there is virtually no limit to the amount of health care an individual is capable of absorbing,' and looking for ways to cap NHS spending, the Conservative administrations of the late 1980s came up with the idea of an 'internal market'.

Larger hospitals were encouraged to become independent trusts and to compete with each other for patients and resources. GPs were encouraged to accept independent budgets in the expectation that this would make them more cost-conscious. Hospital consultants and GPs were given stakes in the provision of patient care at less cost; the 'discipline of the market' was supposed to achieve a more cost-effective and socially responsive service. These measures met stern opposition from large parts of the medical profession, particularly as, in trust hospitals, they tended to subordinate senior medical staff to lavishly paid professional managers brought in from industry and commerce.

Concluding that market mechanisms had *increased* administrative costs and inequalities, the new Labour government, elected in May 1997, pledged itself to abolish the internal market. What is conspicuous is that the UK, with the highest percentage of state-controlled medicine in the western world (in 1991, 89 per cent of health care expenditure came from the public sector, compared with 41 per cent in the US) also spends the smallest percentage of the GNP on health. This can be interpreted as proof, despite right-wing propaganda, of the efficiency of state medicine, or that one of the weaknesses of postwar British health policy has been failure to invest adequately in health.

In the United States, the crisis over out-of-control health costs highlighted the plight of those excluded from the mainstream. As of the 1990s, over 35 million Americans had no medical insurance: almost one in six citizens under the age of sixty-five. Another 20 million had such inadequate insurance that a major illness would lead to bankruptcy. Indeed, almost 17 million Americans who are gainfully employed lack health insurance – 3 million more than in 1982, and each year approximately 200,000 are turned away from hospital emergency rooms for this reason. Half a million American mothers have no form of insurance when they give birth, and 11 million American children are not covered by any medical insurance. The failure of President Clinton's health initiative in 1992–94 makes it unlikely that this question will be tackled in the near future.

Meanwhile, significant changes were occurring within American private medicine, as new managerial business outlooks were applied to hospitals. Humana, one of the largest hospital chains, had ninety-two hospitals and $1.4 billion in revenues by 1980. Its president said it wanted to provide as uniform and reliable a product as a McDonald's hamburger coast to coast. Business attitudes were also extended to HMOs, which realized that their best prospects of high profitability lay not in the proliferation of expensive services but in cost control, cost-cutting, 'down-sizing', rationalization of services and mergers.

Corporate management has taken over HMOs and embarked upon programmes of buying up municipal and non-profit hospitals, closing down others, amalgamating facilities to end duplication, and capping target expenditures for tests, hospital stays and drugs. Staff numbers (including physicians) have been slashed, as has the range of medical choices available to subscribers. Traditional non-profit institutions have been brought into the 'for-profit' sector. To many doctors, it seemed that all rationales in health were being subordinated to the budgetary. A physician who is part of a family medicine unit in a small town in California commented on the medical changes consequent on the financial imperative:

> At first we prided ourselves on keeping our patients healthy and out of the hospital. But the hospital administrators didn't like this. They wanted to keep the hospital full and keep the patients in as long as possible, except for a certain number of indigent patients whom we tried to admit but the administration wanted to keep out. But now the hospital has signed up with a number of HMOs. So it's in the hospital's interests to keep patients out too. This is the crazy logic of health-care financing in the United States.

This new trend underlines how inflationary the physician-driven character of American medicine was during previous generations (the so-called 'golden age' from the 1920s to the 1970s). It is ironic that only when big business moved into medicine was there sufficient incentive to slash costs (and hence often wasteful, futile and unprincipled medicine) in the name of higher profits. It is not clear whether the cutting edge of profitability can produce better medicine in the twenty-first century – and for whom. It is equally unclear whether the increasingly fierce medico-political war being fought, between the traditional medico-industrial complex, the medical profession, the federal government, new managerial finance and the customer, has anything to do with the fulfilment of real health needs in the United States.

POLICING HEALTH

Its spokesmen during the last couple of centuries have liked to emphasize medicine's autonomy and its benevolence as an enabling profession. Notably in the US, the profession has jealously rejected 'encroachments' by the state. In reality, however, medicine and the state have become ever more closely bonded, eating off each other's plates.

The medical profession depends upon government money for institutions, research, education and salaries; and governments have followed and justified various policies on medical grounds. In most respects this growing (if unacknowledged and often disavowed) rapprochement between the state and the medical profession embodied benign logic: who could deny health to the people? Who would doubt that the encouragement of medicine was the best way to supply it? Indeed, the twentieth century brought countless *ad hoc* interventions to create services to reduce health risks and help the helpless. Mothers, babies, children, the elderly, and many other groups, have been objects of interventions benignly intended and often beneficial. But the state and the medical profession have often joined in alliances in which social policing and political goals have counted for more than the promotion of personal health. We shall now survey briefly one such increasingly salient area: narcotics control.

Opium was a commodity traditionally available on the free market. Its chemically produced form, morphia, was introduced in the 1820s, and the hypodermic syringe in the 1850s – 'the greatest boon given to medicine since the discovery of chloroform', it was declared in 1869. 'Nothing did me any good,' Florence Nightingale noted during one of her illnesses, 'but a curious little new fangled operation of putting opium under the skin which relieved one for twenty-four hours.' In 1898, the German company Bayer introduced Heroin (diacetylmorphine), the 'heroic drug' which, they said, had the 'ability of morphine to relieve pain, yet is safer'.

For most of the nineteenth century there was little attempt by governments to regulate the sale of drugs – indeed opium became a bizarre test case in free-trade. Cultivating opium poppies in Bengal, Britain's East India Company exported the drug illegally to China, the trade amounting in 1839 to 400,000 chests of opium. China grew anxious about the threats to health, morale and its silver reserves. The British pushed the drug, China resisted, and war resulted. After the First Opium War (1840–42), China lost Hong Kong; the Second Opium War (1857–60) meant further losses of Chinese sovereignty and an enforced open door for the opium trade.

In Europe, as the hypodermic syringe led to increased morphia use, doctors grew aware of dependency and withdrawal symptoms. In *Die Morphiumsucht* (1878) [The Morbid Craving for Morphia], Eduard Levinstein (1831–82) described morphia addiction. In England, the Society for the Study and Cure of Inebriety, founded in 1884 by Dr Norman Kerr (1834–99), pursued Levinstein's ideas, investigating alcohol abuse, opium, chloral hydrate and cocaine. Morphine and opium usage were soaring, largely due to medical prescribing. In the US, the Ebert Prescription Survey of 1885, covering 15,700 prescriptions dispensed in nine Illinois pharmacies, showed the ingredients most frequently used in medicines were quinine and morphine.

Recognition grew that addiction was mainly iatrogenic. A late nineteenth-century American cartoon features a bartender gazing enviously at a druggist and grumbling, 'The kind of drunkard I make is going out of fashion. I can't begin to compete with this fellow,' while contented customers walk out of the pharmacy carrying opium-based medicines labelled 'Bracer' and 'Soothing Syrup'.

Important in the framing of the 'drugs problem' was the idea developed by doctors and psychiatrists of an 'addict type'. Addiction became defined as a disease. However, after initial hopes, optimism about cures had waned by the 1920s. Concluding in the 1930s that addiction betrayed a psychopathic personality, Dr Lawrence Kolb of the US Public Health Service demanded strict regulation; the drug addict should be considered a potential criminal: predisposition to addiction included a sociopathic tendency.

Restrictive legislation on over-the-counter medicines was first passed in Britain in 1860 in an attempt to control the new substances; prescription-only drugs came into being and the class was subsequently extended. Although patent medicine manufacturers lobbied feverishly, the Pure Food and Drug Act of 1906 ended the availability of narcotics over the counter in the USA and established the first legally enforceable *Pharmacopoeia of the United States of America*. Rather as the Eighteenth Amendment to the Constitution and the Volstead Act (1919) were to prohibit alcohol sale, the comprehensive Harrison Act (1914) criminalized drug addiction, making opiates and other narcotics legally available only on prescription for treating disease. The Supreme Court ruled that supplying addicts through prescriptions was illegal under the act – contraventions led to some 25,000 physicians being arraigned and 3000 of them serving prison terms. The Act made bad worse. In 1925 Robert A. Schless observed that 'most drug addiction today is due directly to the Harrison Anti-Narcotic Act. . . . The Harrison Act made the drug peddler and the drug peddler makes drug addicts.'

Penalization bred panic, drugs were dubbed 'mankind's deadliest foe', and in 1930 the Federal Bureau of Narcotics was formed, many of its officers being laid-off prohibition agents. 'How many murders, suicides, robberies, criminal assaults, hold-ups, burglaries, and deeds of maniacal insanity [smoking marijuana] causes each year, especially among the young, can only be conjectured,' thundered the Bureau's chief commissioner, Harry J. Anslinger (b. 1892). The 'cannabis problem' was created by the passing of the Marijuana Tax Act 1937, which, by imposing huge taxes, bureaucratic restrictions and penalties, put an end to legal use and drove it underground.

The spirit of the 1930s carried over into the 'war on drugs' launched in 1971 by President Nixon, with the allocation of greater federal funds, powers and manpower. 'America's Public Enemy No. 1 is drug abuse,' declared Nixon, who surely knew about public enemies. Soft and hard drugs were demonized together, the consequence being that in the 1980s some 300,000 Americans were being arrested annually on cannabis charges – in 1982 a Virginia man received a forty-year jail sentence for distribution of nine ounces of pot. The war on drugs was hypocrisy; the CIA had long supported Asian and South American drugs barons as props against communism.

As public policy changed, the medical profession changed its tune respecting the dangers of narcotics. Doctors had once thought rather well of cannabis, as of opium. Set up in 1893 by the British government, the Indian Hemp Drugs Commission concluded in a 3000-page report that moderate use had no appreciable medical, psychological or moral effect. Banning it might drive the Indian poor 'to have recourse to alcohol or to stimulants or narcotics which may be more deleterious' and prohibition or even 'repressive measures of a stringent nature' would create 'the army of blackmail'. The commission's findings might have been skewed by the fact that cannabis, like opium, was a key source of revenue to the Raj, but they also reflected sound medical opinion.

With the political drive against cannabis in America from the 1930s, medical thinking shifted. It was in 1934 that 'drug addiction' first appeared in the American Psychiatric Association's diagnostic handbook and, four years after the 1937 Marijuana Act, cannabis disappeared from the US Pharmacopoeia. When a commission of the New York Academy of Medicine set up by Mayor LaGuardia concluded in 1944 that there was little evidence that marijuana harmed health, the American Psychiatric Association advised its members to disregard the commission's findings, because they would do 'great damage to the cause of law enforcement'. The Association knew which side its bread was buttered.

The American medical profession fell into line with the criminalization of narcotics, accepting funds made available for setting up detoxification programmes and developing anti-addiction drugs like methadone. They could easily convince themselves that they were helping addicts and society, while doing their careers a favour. The 1960s brought a shift in Britain too. With the government obliged to be seen to be responding to a growing drugs menace, and sensing that capital was to be made out of scapegoating, new restrictions were imposed. No longer could addicts routinely be supplied by GPs: they had now to be registered at special clinics for treatment. As in America, the upshot of tougher laws and policing was that the traffic went underground, achieved new allure, and became more deeply enmeshed with criminality and corruption.

With respect to narcotics – innumerable other questions from genetic engineering to euthanasia and spare-part surgery could be cited – medicine has bedded down with authority in the modern state. Some of the consequences for sick people of such developments are examined in the final chapter.

CONCLUSION

During the twentieth century medicine became integral to the social and political apparatus of industrialized societies. Its impact is not easy to evaluate. The enormous inequalities of health between rich and poor revealed by nineteenth-century statisticians have certainly not disappeared.

In England the Black Report, published as *Inequalities in Health* in 1980, showed that the affluent continued to live longer than the poor and were far healthier: e.g., in 1971 the death rate for adult males in social class V (unskilled workers) was nearly twice that of adult men in social class I (professional workers). The political upshot of the document was revealing.

Commissioned by a Labour government, the report, written by Sir Douglas Black (b. 1913), was virtually suppressed by the succeeding Conservative government, presumably because it showed how the health of poorer parts of the community still lagged and called for massive public spending to rectify these inequalities:

> Present social inequalities in health in a country with substantial resources like Britain are unacceptable, and deserve to be so declared by every section of public opinion ... we have no doubt that greater equality of health must remain one of our foremost national objectives and that in the last two decades of the twentieth century a new attack upon the forces of inequality has regrettably become necessary.

Patrick Jenkin, then secretary of state for Social Services in Mrs Thatcher's first administration, turned the report's findings to Conservative advantage by contending that they demonstrated that the nature and roots of inequalities of health were such that they *could* not be eradicated by vast injections of public money. The history of the NHS, he said, bore this out: 'We have been spending money in ever-increasing amounts on the NHS for thirty years and it has not actually had much effect on increasing people's health.' Certainly, it is far from clear that the way to end social differentials in health is the provision of more medicine.

CHAPTER XXI

MEDICINE AND THE PEOPLE

MODERN MEDICINE HAS become synonymous with complex infrastructures and towering superstructures: with universities and professional organizations, multi-national pharmaceutical companies and insurance combines, hospitals doubling as medical schools, research sites and lobbies, government departments, international agencies and corporate finance. Medicine in mass society inexorably became inseparable from economics, central and local administration, the law, the social services and the media. At the cutting-edge – bio-technology, genetic engineering and so forth – medicine is the moving frontier, not simply of science and healing but of the future of mankind. With transplant surgery established and human cloning feasible, modern biomedicine is seriously challenging and changing our notions of what a human being is, of what it is to be human. Where has this left people when they fall sick?

Patients, of course, have roles assigned to them within the scripts of the modern medical drama. Depending upon who is doing the analysis or the accountancy, patients appear as demand, costs and benefits, input or output, voters, clients or consumers of services, bearers of rights or pursuers of litigation, the 'tib and fib' in bed 15, frozen sperm in the deep freeze, diseased bodies or clinical material, points on a graph or numbers crunched on a software program.

Above all, perhaps, patients have become the millions to be budgeted for in the now proverbial ageing society. The 'sick man' [sic] is said to have disappeared from the 'medical gaze' with the birth of the clinic around 1800, being reduced to a 'patient', a pathological body studded with lesions. That disappearing act continued during the next two centuries, reducing the patient in due course to an x factor in equations dominated by economics, sociology, diagnostic technology, systems analysis and multitudes of other reference frames.

Yet, aside from the double-entry bookkeeping and flow charts, people went on being ill, suffering, seeing doctors. This chapter tries to sketch modern medicine as bedside encounters and from the publics' viewpoint – obviously a foolhardy undertaking. Over the last two centuries medicine has been astonishingly complex and heterogeneous, a kaleidoscope spangled with contrasts; we are too close to see things in perspective, we are partisan. Current judgments differ wildly. Some medical sociologists cast the twentieth century as an age of medical monopoly and professional dominance, others highlight its diversity, pluralism and populist turn. Some berate physicians for arrogance in wielding the powers of life and death; others see doctors not as white-coated popes but as pawns in a business dominated by the media, the market, the masses and – above all – money.

For its fans, modern medicine, with its microbe-hunters and microchips, has enabled westerners to escape from the valley of the shadow of death, living longer and healthier lives; for critics this is the era of the Holocaust and the Gulags, in whose unspeakable outrages doctors and psychiatrists were hardly reluctant participants. Scientific medicine may be the knight in shining armour or a new body-snatcher. What Shaw called *The Doctor's Dilemma* is humanity's.

THE PATIENT, THE DOCTOR, AND THE BEDSIDE

Modern medicine brought 'primary care', the first port of call for the sick, to everybody for the first time, but has made it problematic. From 1800 primary care became routinely available first to the many, then the majority, and finally to the masses. Successful peasants in Gascony and the petty bourgeoisie in Gloucester would rarely have consulted a professional medic in 1700, but they were routinely seeing the doctor by 1850. Charities, friendly societies and state insurance schemes meant that labouring men were gaining comparable access by the time of the First World War. The provision of primary medical care became a basic service in the modern democratic state.

No less important than its spread has been the power of its ideology. The model personal physician or family doctor looms large in the public imagination, yet has the ring of myth. 'Time was, and not so long ago', wrote the American physician Carl Binger (1889–1976), in 1956, when the family doctor delivered babies and supervised their nursing, their weaning and their teething, when he vaccinated them and saw them through their measles and chicken pox and whooping cough. He told the boy about the facts of life and treated the girl for her menstrual cramps. He advised about diet and rest, gave spring tonics, clipped tonsils, set a broken arm, reassured father who couldn't sleep because of business worries, pulled mother through a case of typhoid or double pneumonia, reprimanded the cook who was found, on her day out, to have a dozen empty whisky bottles in her clothes closet, gave advice about the young man's choice of college and profession, comforted grandma, who was losing her memory and becoming more and more irritable, and closed grandpa's eyes in his final sleep. He went on his endless, mysterious and incessant rounds leaving in his wake a faint odor of carbolic with which he disinfected his beard.

But all that had changed, he concluded: 'This heroic figure is gone from our midst. . . . Who killed Cock Robin?' That is a question to which we will return. This idea of a friendly, familiar doctor 'being there' assumed a key role in deep-rooted ideals of good medical practice – that is, medicine characterized not by perfect health but by a desirable clinical relationship.

Primary care is *prima facie* a simple matter: a sick person treated by a doctor. 'We have been very much at leisure for several days past till Sunday last', wrote old Richard Weekes (1751–1823), a Sussex general practitioner, to his son, Hampton, in 1802. Then the action set in:

I was sent for to Pollards wife at Poynings, who has an Infln of the Plura while I was bleeding her Godly's Wife at Ditchg sent out the man came to Poynings after me when I got to Grainger's Gate met Mrs Bridgers Man with his horse sweating profusely said Mrs lay dead & had been near an hour as he had been to my home when I got there she was recoverd from a strong Convulsion fit has had two before I think them of serious consequence rode home very fast, there was Godley teasing me when I got into the shop there was Dr Dick with Woolven's Son a lad abt 15 or 16 years of age with his hand shatterd all to pieces by the Bursting of a Gun, he had put a Tourniquet on his Arm & layd him flat on his back, just at this instant, one of Chandler's Girls set her clothes on fire & is most terribly burnt while the man & his wife where at Church . . .

If primary care sometimes wore this simple appearance – a pile-up of emergencies attended by a 'fire brigade' physician – it could also be complicated, because the classic reasons for consulting a doctor might be psychological, social, conventional and ritualistic. The open secret of general practice, its strength and weakness, has been that many clients do not actually have a disease; they are sick, sad or solitary; they need solace.

The patient and doctor nexus was challenged by the march of science. Private doctors must, within limits, give patients what they want. 'The doctor who has to live by pleasing his patients in competition with everybody who has walked the hospitals, scraped through the examinations, and bought a brass plate', remarked Shaw,

> soon finds himself prescribing water to teetotallers and brandy or champagne jelly to drunkards; beefsteaks and stout in one house, and 'uric acid free' vegetarian diet over the way; shut windows, big fires, and heavy overcoats to old Colonels, and open air and as much nakedness as is compatible with decency to young faddists, never once daring to say either 'I don't know', or 'I don't agree'.

With the open air or shut windows, the twentieth-century primary-care physician has chosen (indeed has felt obliged) to dispense science, in the guise of expertise, diagnostic equipment, chemical tests and especially as measures of drugs. Tensions were bound to result.

The more the primary physician prescribed science, the more he ran the risk of intimating that it was practitioners other than himself who were the true experts. How could a small-scale operator command the resources of science as effectively as the mighty hospital? Hence advocacy of and allegiance to science proved a double-edged sword for the small man; while boosting him, it threatened to put him out of business. It set up tensions for patients too. They demanded science, because it became associated in the public mind with superior diagnosis and effective treatment. But science demystifies, dehumanizes, creates impersonality, clinical detachment and modes of mechanization, all of which may seem remote and uncaring. Patients may as a consequence criticize modern medicine for reducing them to the status of walking stomachs, blood sugars, heart valves or whatever is the seat of their disease. Beset by such pressures, old-style primary care has had to re-invent itself endlessly in new attire, including coming to terms with alternative therapies and psychotherapy.

*   *   *

The nineteenth-century bourgeois patient would summon a doctor of choice (generally by servant; by 1900, perhaps by telephone); the doctor would then pay a call – on horseback, by pony-and-trap or, latterly, by motor car. Relations between patients and family doctors were face-to-face; personal mettle and social graces counted. It is not easy to say precisely what went on, because much of our picture derives from stray anecdotes about eccentric physicians and insufferable patients.

From the patient's side we hear grumbles about physicians who were officious or brusque: John Abernethy (1764–1831) was apparently in the habit of barking at fat ladies 'Madam, buy a skipping rope', yet he was in demand. Physicians protested against know-all patients and hypochondriacs: the worried well. But such grouses should not be taken at face value. The profession had a stake in cosseting valetudinarians like Mr Woodhouse in Jane Austen's *Emma* (1816) who comprised an eager, if vexatious, clientèle. Cynics suggested that physicians sowed habits of sickness among leisured and lucrative patients, in particular the weaker sex. New diagnostic jargon, fancy prescriptions and regimens, laborious attention to diet and lifestyle – these constituted the ornate rituals of a profession which had to be civil and obsequious to the carriage trade and to snobbish pretenders to gentility. Aspiring doctors set up Alpine sanatoria, rural hydros and seaside clinics where they prescribed rest cures to those with money and time on their hands and a craving to be coddled, or cold baths to the spartan.

The solemn bedside palaver of medical attendance upon the solid bourgeoisie – a grave demeanour, an air of benign and unflappable authority, the art of never leaving without a favourable prognosis – was much prized. A *Punch* cartoon of 1884 featured a conversation between two women:

> First: What sort of doctor is he?
> Second: Oh, well, I don't know very much about his ability; but
>   he's got a very good *bedside manner*!

All this cloaked the fact that disease called the shots; patients of every age and class were liable to be stricken by dangerous infections which in pre-bacteriological days could not even be diagnosed with exactitude, let alone cured. The well-documented medical histories of many eminent Victorians – Charles Darwin, Thomas Carlyle, Alfred Tennyson and all their sickly circles – are tales of woe. From his thirties, Darwin seems to have been poorly, day-in day-out, with headaches, vomiting, palpitations and a devil in his stomach which never went away. 'For 25 years extreme spasmodic daily & nightly flatulence', he related to his physician:

> Age 56–57 – occasional vomiting, on two occasions prolonged during months. Vomiting preceded by shivering, . . . dying sensations . . . & copious very pallid urine. Now vomiting & every passage of flatulence preceded by ringing of ears, treading on air & vision.

Over the years he consulted a gaggle of physicians who gave him diagnoses and remedies galore. Nothing did much good, but he lived well into his seventies, unlike Keats, Chopin, Schubert and other brilliant contemporaries who died tragically young of diseases readily curable today. With Darwin and many others it is a fair assumption that the medicines they took, whether prescribed by doctors or self-administered, did more harm than good and perhaps became the main source of the sickness.

Throughout the nineteenth century, and well into the twentieth, patients were besieged by infections, commonly lethal to old and young alike – diphtheria, chickenpox, scarlet fever, rubella and a multitude of gastro-intestinal and dysenteric troubles claimed millions of infants. Being a family doctor in 1830 and even a century later meant being called out late at night to febrile patients, sweating copiously and hectic in their breathing, suffering from some infant fever or from pneumonia (called 'the old man's friend' because it was often speedily fatal). Measles and the other epidemic diseases of childhood were still killers; tuberculosis, syphilis, diphtheria, meningitis and postpartum sepsis were widely encountered.

Arthur E. Hertzler was born in Iowa in 1870; he took a medical degree at Northwestern University, did graduate work in Berlin in the modern manner, and practised in Kansas before becoming professor of surgery at the University of Kansas in 1909. In his charming autobiography, *The Horse and Buggy Doctor* (1938), he recalled scores of fever cases. One day he was called to a case three hours' drive away. It was empyema, pus in the lungs. The boy in question was 'in deep cyanosis [short of oxygen], with grayish-blue skin and heaving chest, his mouth open and his eyes bulging':

> Grabbing a scalpel I made an incision in his chest wall with one stab – he was too near death to require an anesthetic. As the knife

penetrated his chest, a stream of pus the size of a finger spurted out, striking me under the chin and drenching me. After placing a drain in the opening, I wrapped a blanket about my pus-soaked body and spent another three hours reaching home.

Living amidst a sea of infections and fevers, the old-style doctor had a choice between conservative options (bed-rest, tonics, care and hope), and heroic possibilities, including violent purges (often calomel, the 'blue pill'), or, in Rush's America and Broussais's France, drastic blood-letting (physically dubious if psychologically effective). Often the doctor's decision was made for him; traditional patients had strong views about their illnesses and the treatment they needed. Fortunately, such views usually coincided with age-old medical regimes: blood-letting, sweating, purging, vomiting and other ways of expelling bad humours had a hold upon the popular imagination and reflected medical confidence in such matters.

Blood-letting gradually lost favour, but it was hardly superseded by anything better: the pharmacopoeia was a bag of blanks. As of the late nineteenth century the few medicines that were effective included mercury for syphilis and ringworm, digitalis to strengthen the heart, amyl nitrate to dilate the arteries in angina, quinine for malaria, colchicum for gout – and little else (aspirin was introduced in 1896). Iron was popular as a tonic, and plant-based purgatives such as senna remained prevalent. '120 patients were seen by the physician and dismissed in an hour and ten minutes, or at the rate of 35 seconds each,' wrote an observer of the outpatients' department of London's St Bartholomew's Hospital in 1869. Each patient received 'a doubtful dose of physic, ordered almost at random, and poured out of a huge brown jug'. The medicine dispensed there consisted essentially 'of purgatives; a mixture of iron, sulphate of magnesia, and quassia [both laxatives], and cod-liver oil, fulfilling the two great indications of all therapeutics – elimination, and the supply of some elements to the blood'. The old-time American doctor of the late nineteenth century was said to get by with 'calomel, opium, quinine, buchu [a diuretic], ipecac [an emetic and evacuant], and Dover's powder [used for colds and chills]'.

Nothing was any good against infections, or against other serious conditions such as diabetes, arthritis, asthma or heart attacks. What would a doctor do in a pneumonia case? As late as the 1920s, textbooks were still recommending calomel to open the bowels and an irritant expectorant mixture (perhaps ether-based) to bring up phlegm; digitalis to 'strengthen the heart muscle', morphia, chloral mixtures or bromides as hypnotics to induce sleep and soothe. Brandy and oxygen were employed as stimulants, and, in extreme cases, strychnine. The battle against pneumonia might persist for several days until a 'crisis' was reached, when the fever broke, symptoms subsided and convalescence could begin – were the patient still alive! 'I can scarcely think of a single disease that the doctors actually cured during those early years', Hertzler recalled of the time he put out his shingle; all that doctors could do was 'to relieve suffering, set bones, sew up cuts and open boils on small boys'.

Doctors were thus on the horns of a dilemma, especially because patients remained notoriously self-dosing, drugging themselves with a diet of home-brew kitchen physic, shop-bought nostrums, quacks' mixtures and so forth, all perfectly legal, and they were always sounding out some new doctor in the hope of finding something different. Too many worthless medicines, too few remedies, opinionated patients, insecure doctors and ignorance everywhere made for a dismal situation, somewhat allayed by the fact that in a churchgoing era people were inured to death and did not seriously expect medical miracles. Unlike today, doctors were not likely to be held legally accountable for their failures and mistakes.

The pressures upon doctors to do something explains why the growing availability of strong sedatives, analgesics and narcotics, produced by the new industrial pharmaceutical companies, was a godsend. Many mixtures had a heavy brandy base, and opium was freely dispensed. Thanks to the synthesis of morphine in 1806 and the invention in 1853 of the hypodermic syringe, it became easy to get fast fixes of opiates in strong concentrations to lessen life's troubles. As Edward Shorter has rightly stressed, to the insomniac and the irritable, the depressed and the agitated, the German chemical industry was a fairy-godmother.

In 1869 chloral hydrate came into medical use as a sleeping potion, and chloral addicts became familiar sights in private nervous clinics. In 1888 sulfonal, a more powerful hypnotic (sleeping draught), became available. Bayer also revealed barbitone in 1903, marketed as 'Veronal', phenobarbitone was introduced in 1912 as 'Luminal' and further barbiturates followed, all popular with general practitioners. 'I bought Luminal tablets in five-thousand lots every few months', one Canadian family doctor recalled of the inter-war years. Like so many other drugs introduced at the time, the barbiturates had the drawback of being habit-forming.

If his ability to cure the sick improved only slowly, the GP was nevertheless able to consolidate his position by developing other skills. Diagnostic techniques were being transformed, thanks to new ways of looking at patients – the triumph of the 'medical gaze' promoted by Paris localist patho-anatomy encouraged the slow but steady regularization of physical examinations. At the bedside, the stethoscope and technological aids such as the ophthalmoscope and the laryngoscope imparted a new ritual to diagnosis. How much real difference they made is hard to tell. When Europe's top physicians gathered around the bed of Kaiser Friedrich III in 1890, all their new apparatus and tests couldn't help them decide whether or not he had malignant throat cancer. Against the German laryngologists, the English consultant Morell Mackenzie (1837–92) carried the day, denying it and advising against operating, but the Kaiser died shortly after – of cancer. The unseemly repercussions cast doubt on how far things had advanced since the deathbed of Charles II in 1683. Even if the doctors had got the Kaiser's diagnosis right, there was nothing they could have done to save his life.

Physical examinations became more common and more thorough. 'Doctor Williams called,' wrote Harriet Wynne in 1803, 'and made me undergo a *blushing* examination.' Not all patients were so compliant. Dr Arthur Conan Doyle recorded in 1881 how he had to deal with a 'frightful horror' of a patient. 'She won't let me examine her chest. "Young doctors take such liberties, you know my dear."' Faced with obstinacy and with questions of propriety doctors took refuge in professional protocol: 'There can be no indecency, and no sacrifice of self-respect in making any necessary physical examination whatever,' pronounced the American gynaecologist J. Marion Sims (1813–83), 'if it be done with a proper sense of delicacy, and with a dignified, earnest, and conscientious determination to arrive at the truth.' But doctors knew they had to tread carefully. Keep your eyes fixed on the ceiling while making vaginal examinations, William Goodell (1829–94) of the University of Pennsylvania counselled his students. The vaginal speculum proved especially controversial, and some doctors would have none of it. Another Philadelphia man, Charles D. Meigs (1792–1869), was proud 'that in this country . . . there are women who prefer to suffer the extremity of danger and pain rather than waive those scruples of delicacy which prevent their maladies from being explored'. (Such scruples could be invoked to promote the case for the admission of women to the profession.) Patients might be wary of the new-style examinations using stethoscopes and other apparatus, but so might doctors. Resisting what would today be called de-skilling, some elite physicians remained adamant that the trained finger on the pulse and an experienced eye were surer diagnostic aids than any new-fangled machine.

General practice was nevertheless slowly transformed by a professionalism based upon diagnostic skills, a product of the new medical schools, with their (Parisian) stress upon rigorous diagnosis and (German) emphasis upon laboratory, microscopic, bacteriological routines. The prime purpose was diagnostic. 'What makes a great physician?', asked Dr Jacob Bigelow (1787–1879) in 1852, going on to reply to his own question:

> I would answer that he is a great physician who, above other men, understands diagnosis. It is not he who promises to cure all maladies, who has a remedy ready for every symptom, or one remedy for all symptoms; who boasts that success never fails him, when his daily history gives the lie to such assertion.

This approach developed slowly in America, since most pre-Flexner medical colleges were low grade. Nevertheless, the better medical schools taught science, and the bridge between the doctor's scientific knowledge and the patient's symptoms was the physical examination: percussing the chest, palpating the abdomen, and listening to blood and air movements within the cavities through a stethoscope.

Dr George Dock taught at the University of Michigan around 1900. His clinical classes, recorded by a stenographer, reveal that he imparted painstaking training in the arts of diagnosis, based on drills and skills in interpreting the underlying pathology. The patient in the bed facing the professor and his students had rheumatism. After percussing was performed, this interrogation followed:

> DOCK: Now what is the matter with his heart?
> STUDENT: He has a loud blowing murmur which reflects the first sound at the apex.
> DOCK: But what causes that?
> STUDENT: It is caused by mitral regurgitation.
> DOCK: Has he any other signs of mitral regurgitation?
> STUDENT: The sound is conveyed out to the axilla.
> DOCK: Well, what else? What else do you hear? Where is it loudest?

STUDENT: Just to the left of the sternum.

DOCK: What else is there?

STUDENT: Then there is a diastolic murmur in the right second intercostal space. There is a slight accentuation of the second pulmonic.

DOCK: Well, is there anything else in the aortic area?

STUDENT: There is also a murmur, a systolic murmur. [And so forth, at great length.]

Dock's students would certainly have known their diagnosis (even if they would have been able to do little for such patients).

The twentieth-century physician acquired further aids to help him visualize and identify disease. Thermometers measured body temperature, and the fever charts they constructed demonstrated temperature patterns typical of specific diseases. Sphygmomanometers improved pulse lore by telling of abnormalities in the blood pressure, thus helping a physician to characterize circulatory disorders. If he possessed or had access to some kind of diagnostic laboratory, he might examine body fluids – blood, faeces, vomit, sputum and vaginal discharges – by measuring electrolytes, counting blood cells, searching for microbes, and observing unusual tissues and cell types. Microscopes and staining techniques revealed bacteria and permitted the counting of red blood cells and the various types of white blood cells, useful in differential diagnosis.

The doctor proficient at diagnosis based upon the physical examination ritual might command high esteem. American mid-west physicians, Doc Hertzler noted, had traditionally limited themselves to peering at the tongue, feeling the pulse and studying the face:

> The usual procedure for a doctor when he reached the patient's house was to greet the grandmother and aunts effusively and pat all the kids on the head before approaching the bedside. He greeted the patient with a grave look and a pleasant joke. He felt the pulse and inspected the tongue, and asked where it hurt. This done, he was ready to deliver an opinion and prescribe his pet remedy. More modern men had a thermometer and a stethoscope. The temperature was gravely measured, and the chest listened to – or at.

Fresh back from Berlin, young Hertzler had a mind to change all that:

> I had ideas of my own. I passed the aged female relatives up, ignored the children and proceeded with the matter at hand. This

was not based on bravery on my part, but ignorance. I had not yet learned that most of the things one needs to know in the practice of the art of healing never get into the books. But there were compensating factors. I at least examined my patients as well as I knew how. My puerile attempts at physical examination impressed my patients and annoyed my competitors, which, of course, I accepted as a two-time strike. Word went out that the young doctor 'ain't very civil but he is thorough'. Only yesterday one of my old patients recalled that when I came to see her young son I 'stripped him all off and examined him all over'. Members of that family have been my patients for the intervening forty years, so impressed were they. Incidentally, it may be mentioned that in this case I discovered a pleurisy with effusion which had not been apparent to my tongue-inspecting colleague.

Hertzler felt a new dedication to science-based medicine. His was one of many reruns of George Eliot's Tertius Lydgate, only by 1900 it seemed the public on both sides of the Atlantic was more sold on scientific medicine than in the days of Eliot's hero. Writing in 1924, and oozing a cynicism born of more than fifty years of medical practice in a social milieu intensely sceptical towards doctors, Daniel Cathell (1839–1925) reflected upon the importance of the scientific aura:

> Working with the microscope and making analyses of the urine, sputum, blood, and other fluids as an aid to diagnosis, will not only bring fees and lead to valuable information regarding your patient's condition, but will also give you reputation and professional respect, by investing you, in the eyes of the public, with the benefits of being a very scientific man.

Cathell advised the young physician to blind the patient with scientific jargon: 'By employing the terms ac. phenicum for carbolic acid, secale cornutum for ergot, kalium for potassium, natrum for sodium, chinin for quinine, etc., you will debar the average patient from reading your prescriptions.' Cathell's brash counsel conveys an American weakness for the new-fangled and the scientific; physicians from the Old World were likely to warn that science brought losses as well as gains, and that too much science might distract a physician from the true art of healing. Sir James Mackenzie (1853–1925) asserted in his *The Future of Medicine* (1918) that 'laboratory training *unfits* a man for his work as a physician', since it accustomed him to mechanistic ways of thinking. Too much science, too much specialization, too many hours amid the test-tubes might produce a fragmentation of the mind not conducive to healing – one which saw not patients but walking organs and diseases.

On the whole, however, early twentieth-century patients lapped science up, partly because it was the new thing, but also because it gave them the impression of commanding the doctor's attention when he used his stethoscope or sphygmomanometer, when he rapped and tapped and listened. The rituals of scientific, diagnostic medicine spelt out the message that care was being dispensed, and hence strengthened the bond between physician and patient. The well-respected GPs in 1870 or 1900 or 1930 were those who could impress upon patients that they were skilful, serious, attentive, upright: they knew what they were doing, and could be trusted. In that sense the Hippocratic physician was very much alive.

Curing remained a subordinate consideration. Doctors knew their medicines were largely eyewash, which is one reason why the therapeutic nihilism associated with Paris was an honest option. 'Medicine as a natural science cannot have the task of inventing panaceas and discovering miracle cures that banish death,' pronounced the Viennese Joseph Dietl in 1841; its job was to 'discover the conditions under which people become ill, recover, and perish'. Vienna seems to have gained a notoriety in this respect. *Punch* in the 1880s depicted an American physician turning to an English one and saying, 'Now in Vienna they're first-rate at diagnosis; but, then, you see, they always make a point of confirming it by a post-mortem!'

Therapeutic nihilism might be dressed up in more palatable form as acclaim for 'nature's healing ways' (*vis medicatrix naturae*) and rejection of the classic heroic therapies of bleeding and purging – and all the rest of the worthless mass of the pharmacopoeia. 'Throw out opium', said Oliver Wendell Holmes (1809–94), who did not beat about the bush,

> throw out a few specifics ... throw out wine ... and the vapors which produce the miracle of anaesthesia, and I firmly believe that if the whole materia medica, as now used, could be sunk to the bottom of the sea, it would be all the better for mankind, – and all the worse for the fishes.

– and 'the best proof of it', the Harvard professor added, is that 'no families take so little medicine as those of doctors' (apart from apothecaries, he added, who took even less). In a similar manner Sir

William Osler, writing of scarlet fever around the turn of the century, confessed that 'medicines have little or no control over the duration or course of the disease, which, like other self-limited affections, practically takes its own time to disappear.' The same applied to most other infections. His *Principles and Practice of Medicine* (1892) was, first and foremost, a catalogue of disease.

Yet if nihilism was possible at the Paris pauper hospitals where Holmes had studied, or in lectures at high-minded Harvard, it would have been suicidal for a private practitioner in the bedrooms of Manchester or Milwaukee, being begged to 'do something' by mothers with toddlers dying of diarrhoea or convulsions, or themselves wasting away with tuberculosis. 'In some cases I knew, even in the beginning, that my efforts would be futile in the matter of rendering service to anyone,' Hertzler summed up his dilemma, that of every general practitioner in about 1900: 'Of course, one left some medicine ... this was largely the bunk, but someone had to pay for the axle grease, and just plain advice never was productive of revenue unless fortified by a few pills.' The primitive magic associated with such pills was widely appreciated: 'Some of old Ballard's ways', a young British country doctor, Kenneth Lane, observed of his senior partner in the 1930s,

> were so much a part of the practice that it would have taken a revolution to change them quickly. He kept three large bottles of aspirins coloured green, pink, and yellow. These formed an important part of the dispensing. He also prescribed a mixture the dispenser called Mist Explo. It was a clear yellow liquid made from a few bright yellow crystals dissolved in water. The crystals were apt to ignite if left to dry in the sunlight, hence the name Mist Explosive. I don't remember the exact chemistry of this wonder drug but it was a derivative of picric acid and quite harmless when well diluted and used as a bitter tonic.

The distinguished American physician, Lewis Thomas, who was a medical student in the 1930s, recalled a similar situation. 'We were provided with a thin, pocket-size book called *Useful Drugs*, one hundred pages or so', he remembered,

> and we carried this around in our white coats when we entered the teaching wards and clinics in the third year, but I cannot recall any of our instructors ever referring to this volume. Nor do I remember much talk about treating disease at any time in the four years of medical school except by the surgeons. ... The medicine

we were trained to practice was, essentially, Osler's medicine. Our task for the future was to be diagnoses and explanation. Explanation was the real business of medicine. What the ill patient and his family wanted most was to know the name of the illness, and then, if possible, what had caused it, and finally, most important of all, how it was likely to turn out.

One attempt to resolve this therapeutic quandary was the patient-as-a-person movement, a doctrine influential in primary care in the decades after 1900. Medicines would not help much – though these would still be given – but the psychological support of the doctor would. The physician had to be trained to see the patient as a person and not a disease; a sympathetic, caring manner was therapeutic in itself. 'Medicine', insisted Hermann Nothnagel (1841–1905) in his inaugural lecture in 1882, 'is about treating sick people and not diseases. . . . Never forget that it is not a pneumonia but a pneumonic man who is your patient.' Statements like these turned into a refrain. The Canadian medical humanist William Osler taught that 'the good physician treats the disease but the great physician treats the patient'. He also commented, 'It is much more important to know what sort of patient has the disease than to know what sort of disease the patient has.' One of Osler's students, George Canby Robinson (1878–1966), wrote *The Patient as a Person* (1939) which urged the 'treatment of the patient as a whole'. 'The most important difference between a good and indifferent clinician lies in the amount of attention paid to the story of the patient,' pronounced Sir Farquhar Buzzard (1871–1945), professor of medicine at Oxford.

Such views also won backing from the social medicine movement. In the 1930s Milton Winternitz (1885–1959), head of the Institute of Human Relations at Yale, deplored how medicine had lost sight of the fact that individuals were social beings as well as sick bodies. Medical education should combine sociological, psychological and clinical training to produce social physicians, practising 'clinical sociology'. General practitioners found the patient-as-a-person teachings useful in treating those whose symptoms were 'functional' or 'psychosomatic'– without organic lesion – but believed by the patient to be organic. These patients constituted a huge slab of primary care.

The bedside physician was left in a quandary. The implicit message was that the most highly valued aspects of primary care were simply expedients for papering over its inability to make the sick well. Did not this mean that the more medicine developed and the more effective it became, the more primary care would be devalued? This dilemma was spelt out in the early 1920s by a highly-regarded Boston physician and professor of internal medicine at Harvard University, Francis Weld Peabody (1881–1927). He discerned a great irony: at the very time that medicine was improving, a decline in the physician-patient relationship was taking place. Physicians, he argued, were in danger of forsaking the patient for science. Practitioners might become so concerned with the disease as to lose desire to relate to the individual. Similar observations were made by the Hungarian-born British doctor, Michael Balint (1896–1970), whose *The Doctor, the Patient and the Illness* (1957) extolled the 'apostolic function' of the physician and recommended, by way of remedy, that all primary-care physicians in effect became psycho-therapists, so to speak commandeering the placebo effect (*placebo* is Latin for 'I will please').

By then it was too late, at least in the United States, where the old family doctor was an endangered species, a residual survivor. Why was that? Or, to revert to Carl Binger's question, who actually killed Cock Robin? First in America, but elsewhere later, two major trends were at work. There was a shift from general practitioner to specialist; and there was a migration in medical topography from the patient's home to the doctor's surgery and the hospital.

The rise of specialism – as early as 1861 (Sir) William Gull (1816–90) grumbled against 'the popular prejudice for specialists' – has been explored in earlier chapters. It was fuelled by scientific medicine and public demand; specialists were attractive to a public confident about the benefits of progress. By the 1870s, New York had a dermatological society, an obstetrical society, and a forensic medicine society, while London's Harley Street was becoming studded with consultants. And specialists were seen to do well. Daniel Cathell said of the specialist, 'his fees are always good, *sometimes fat*'.

In respect of the pull of specialization a schism opened between the UK and the US. In Britain, primary care remained and remains firmly in the hands of general family doctors, whereas in the United States they became a vanishing breed. In Britain, panel practice under the National Insurance Act, and its reinforcement within the National Health Service, bolstered the general practitioner. And since he had no right to attend patients in hospital, he was cut off from hospital science and what that implied in terms of innovations, attitudes and professional identities. Yet he could not be dislodged: his letter of referral alone gave access to the hospital. On the eve of the Second World War there were in Britain about 2800 full-time consultants but seven times as many general practitioners; among the 43,000 physicians in the UK in 1980, 65 per cent were still GPs.

In the USA, general practitioners inexorably lost out to specialists and hospital outpatient departments. Around 1900 William Osler noted that many households he knew would, in the course of a year, call upon the services of a gynaecologist, an oculist, a laryngologist, a dermatologist and a surgeon; all that was left for the general practitioner was the health of the children – and that would soon fall to the paediatrician. This development, Osler judged, 'though in many ways to be regretted, is not likely to be changed', since 'the rapid increase of knowledge has made concentration of work a necessity; specialism is here and here to stay.' By 1942 fewer than half of all American doctors were GPs. By 1989, of nearly half a million active American physicians, only one in eight was in general and family practice; specialists had hijacked primary care.

Significant too was the shift in medical practice from the patient's home to the doctor's surgery. House calls came to be seen as wasteful of the doctor's time. The coming of the telephone and the motor car cut down some of that waste, but in the long run, the patient went to visit the physician rather than the other way round, as had traditionally been the case. In America, by 1990, only 2 per cent of all physician contacts took place in the patient's home, 60 per cent in the surgery, and 14 per cent in a hospital outpatient department. In Britain, home visiting remained common for much longer because the NHS buttressed the traditional role of the general practitioner; as late as 1977, 19 per cent of all patient contact took place as home visits.

Meanwhile, in the US, physicians had been tending to relocate in big population centres, leading to an office practice with on-the-spot technology. By the 1930s, half the physicians in Dallas were practising in a single building; by the 1950s, half of American general practitioners had an X-ray machine in their offices (a far higher percentage than in Britain).

And what was happening to the sick themselves? After the First World War the ancient illness patterns persisted. Describing his Leeds (Yorkshire) practice in his *Manual of General Medical Practice* (1927), W. Stanley Sykes (1894–1960) put influenza as the commonest complaint; then came acute bronchitis, tonsillitis, measles and whooping cough, and a tail of other infectious illnesses. He still saw a lot of rheumatic fever and erysipelas, and had more pneumonia than cancer cases – and half his pneumonia cases still died.

This disease picture shifted radically. Partly because of the long-term effects of better living standards, better nutrition and an improved environment, and partly as a result of improved therapy, notably the introduction of the sulpha drugs from the mid thirties, the major infections shrank. 'Tuberculosis, meningitis, polio . . . rheumatic fever, chilblains and lobar pneumonia continue to decline,' one British family doctor wrote in 1963, 'and are disappearing from practice in Western countries.' By then it was said that a general practitioner in the West 'might wait eight years to see a case of rheumatic fever in a child under the age of fifteen' – before the war, that was a disease found in every working-class street. Replacing these acute infectious diseases were modern 'lifestyle' conditions: lung cancer, coronary artery disease, diabetes, strokes, and chronic degenerative diseases, such as senile dementia. The age of acute yielded to the age of chronic disease.

Yet though familiar and fatal diseases were disappearing, the population seemed to be feeling worse. The number of self-reported illnesses rose by one and a half times from 1928–31 to 1981, according to one study. Healthier individuals probably grew more sensitive to bodily symptoms and more inclined to seek help for ailments their grandparents would have dismissed as trivial, inescapable or untreatable; they had also been encouraged to expect and demand more of their doctors. The 'doing better, feeling worse' syndrome emerged.

Medical help-seeking was certainly on the increase. In the USA around 1930, the average person visited the doctor 2.9 times a year; by 1990 this had almost doubled. A similar pattern was seen in the UK. Perhaps to counter this rising demand, physicians developed techniques for keeping patients at bay, including answering services. There is still a longing on the part of much of the clientèle for that old doctor, ever available, avuncular and conveying hope.

Sulpha drugs marked the dawn of modern treatment. From 1935 medicine really could overcome the fevers and bacterial infections of the past; penicillin and other antibiotics were soon to give enormous new therapeutic power. After the Second World War, antibiotics provided protection against serious infections, and drugs were discovered which alleviated arthritis, reduced high blood pressure, dissolved clots in blocked coronary arteries, overcame anxiety and relieved depression. If the half century after 1880 was marked by the doctor's ability to diagnose disease scientifically while remaining therapeutically powerless, the post-World War II era was characterized by the ability to triumph over the classic killers and relieve suffering.

But though doctors became therapeutically more potent, in large measure they ceased to give the patients what they want. With effective weapons against organic disease, they tended to forget the psychological significance and benefits of the doctor-patient relationship. The new generation of physicians was filled with therapeutic self-confidence: a display of humanity had become therapeutically unnecessary and risked being forgotten. Interviewing a British NHS doctor in the 1980s, Jonathan Gathorne Hardy (b. 1933) was informed that prescribing pills was a way of avoiding a more time-consuming analysis and treatment, a technique for cutting short the consultation: 'It's a nice way of getting rid of the patient,' explained the GP, 'you scribble something out and rip the thing off the pad. The ripping off is really the "Fuck off".'

The doctor-patient relationship could thus be seen, on both sides, as a rip-off. That disquieting cynicism was symptomatic of a wider medical malaise, or at least disorientation, which had been growing in the second half of the twentieth century.

MEDICALIZATION AND ITS DISCONTENTS

Wave after wave of protest has arisen against the medical system and the medical establishment in recent decades. Some has come from the inside; much from the outside. Rejection of regular medicine is nothing new; after all, in the nineteenth century religious nonconformity and political radicalism often meant an allegiance to alternative medicine. Such movements were mirrored among supporters of the hippie counter-culture of the 1960s and 1970s.

Western society was sick, they said, because capitalism and material-ism had alienated it from nature and from the soul; and high-tech western medicine merely compounded the problem. Changed lifestyles, spiritual healing, eastern philosophy, mysticism and a pinch of user-friendly psychotherapy or drugs were needed to restore wholeness as well as spiritual and physical health. People had to find themselves and recover their bodies. Feminism and other radical movements reinforced aspects of these ideas.

Drop-outs criticized medicine. So did pundits and intellectuals such as the Austrian-born ex-priest Ivan Illich (b. 1926), who maintained that 'the medical establishment has become a major threat to health.' In laying bare what he styled 'iatrogenesis' (doctor-caused illness), Illich exposed many facets of modern medicine as positively counter-productive: pharmaceutical products made you ill, hospitals were hot-beds of infection, surgery was often bungled, tests were lacking or misleading, or they created maladies of their own. Not least, argued critics of for-profit, free-market, fee-for-service medicine, there were too many unnecessary procedures.

In 1974 a Senate investigation reported that 2.4 million unnecessary operations were performed in the United States *per year*, and that they caused 11,900 deaths and cost about $3.9 billion. More deaths, it was noted, were caused annually by surgery than the yearly toll of military deaths during the Vietnam war. In 1954 the Yale Hospital was per-forming 48,000 lab procedures; by 1964 the figure was 200,000. The fetishism of running tests in an obtuse and inhumane manner was satirized in a TV sketch by Groucho Marx:

GROUCHO: If I were found unconscious on the sidewalk, what would you do?
INTERN: I would work up the patient.
GROUCHO: How would you start?
INTERN: Well, I would do the laboratory work first. I would do a red count and hemoglobin and then a total white and differential count.

Critics in the Illichian mould saw medicine out of control; it was driven not by concern for the patient's health needs but by collective professional ambition, corporate financial pressures, and deluded imperatives – not least an itch to intervene. The 'can-do, will-do' technological imperative came under mounting criticism. It has was shown that many procedures benefit doctors and other medical professionals and technocrats more than patients, while others are positively harmful. Though new drugs have to surmount the hurdle of randomized double-blind trials before they may come onto the market in western nations, strict trials have rarely been conducted for myriad other medical procedures, including surgical interventions and diagnostic tests. Studies seemed to suggest that regular medical check-ups and screenings had at best marginal benefits. The perverse incentives of the fee-for-service system gave physicians financial encouragement for unnecessary interventions, as did the threats of law suits for negligence. Finally the funding system for research encouraged hype and overselling. All in all, a powerful critique held that much modern medicine was, at best, subject to the law of diminishing marginal returns and, at worst, on the wrong track entirely.

Quite independently of nonconformists and radical critics, patients generally registered their dissatisfaction with all or some aspects of modern medicine by voting with their feet. Alternative medicine developed a massive uptake from around 1970 among many with no inclination to drop out. By the time of the establishment of the NHS, fringe medicine had dwindled in the UK; only a small fringe of herbalists, mediums, faith-healers and spiritualists were left, and their clients were regarded as cranky. All that changed from the late 1960s; by 1981 an estimated thirteen million visits were made annually to medical irregulars. It was then reckoned that there were some 2209 medically qualified complementary practitioners, a further 11,184 in professional associations, and 16,980 not in professional associations, making a grand total of 30,373: just *higher* than the total number of general practitioners (30,180).

The range of alternative therapies on offer is now enormous: osteo-pathy, acupuncture, aromatherapy, Alexander technique, homoeo-pathy, massage, shiatsu, iridology, chiropractic, herbalism, meditation, transformational workshops, holistic reflexology, kinesiology, colonics and hypnosis – to name only the most popular. What is even more remarkable is that, in the UK, two in five GPs now refer patients to complementary therapists, while in the Netherlands 7 per cent of the population now visits unorthodox healers each year. In 1990 Americans made 425 million visits to unconventional healers compared with 388 million to primary care physicians.

This astonishing resurgence of alternative and complementary medicine throughout the West, among young and old, rich and poor, people of all ethnic and religious backgrounds and all points on the political compass, shows that regular medicine has ceased to convince the public of its own creed: that it is the only, or the best, means to cure their ills.

There is doubtless a 'proof of the pudding' element in this. Western scientific medicine has not fully delivered the goods it promised. Everyone is aware that scientific medicine has not proved successful against lethal diseases such as cancer, many chronic conditions like arthritis, and other severe syndromes, most recently ME (myalgic encephalomyelitis, 'yuppie flu' or chronic fatigue syndrome). But something more is involved: changing attitudes and outlooks in western societies, a growing unwillingness among the public to accept unquestioningly the role of patient (docile and passive), and a desire to have a greater say, to assert more power and legal rights, through the roles of citizen, client, customer and, if need be, litigator.

This new assertion squares with other roles assumed by the populace in the contemporary West. Affluence, education, leisure and many of the values promoted by corporate capitalism have stoked a culture of individual enhancement and free and active choice. As with cars, careers or sexual partners, it has become the done thing to shop around for healing – whether in desperation, as an exercise of the power of the purse, or as part of an odyssey of life. The rigid, pre-programmed work-oriented lives of the bourgeoisie and labouring classes of earlier generations (one job, one spouse, one house, one family) have been explicitly or implicitly rejected in the latter part of the twentieth century as austere, narrow and rigid. Flexibility, permissiveness, variety, self-discovery have assumed greater status in our culture of self-enhancement or narcissism. There is a new self-assertiveness among the sick, perhaps a survival strategy in the teeth of the extreme depersonalization and bureaucratization of regular medicine.

Initially at least, regular medicine reacted in a negative and authoritarian way towards this urge for new medical freedom and pluralism, sternly warning the public against the evils of rampant quackery. As late as the 1980s, the BMA's medical ethics handbook still threatened that practitioners who had dealings with osteopaths and similar healers could expect to be the subject of disciplinary proceedings; and a report brought out by the Association in 1986 was condescending and antagonistic to other kinds of healing.

But by the 1990s the BMA had become somewhat less uptight – or had decided that discretion was the better part of valour. It produced more conciliatory publicity documents, partly on the urging of its president, the Prince of Wales (the English royal family has always had homoeopathic leanings). Thereafter GPs readily gave their blessing to patients seeing complementary healers, so long as the GPs retained overall clinical control. Indeed, substantial numbers of GPs began to practice therapies like acupuncture and aromatherapy. By 1988 the

Royal Society of Medicine was recommending 'bridge building' between conventional and alternative medicine.

In France recourse to alternative healers became so common that the government established a foundation to study 'soft medicine', with five universities offering certificates. In 1997 the founding was announced by Dr Wah Jun Tze, a professor of paediatrics at the University of British Columbia, of the Tzu Chi Institute for Complementary and Alternative Medicine at Vancouver Hospital, Canada's second largest hospital, thanks to a C\$6m (US\$4.5m) endowment from the Buddhist Tzu Chi Foundation of Taiwan. The aim of the institute would be to sift scientifically the useful from the worthless in the welter of non-conventional therapies, and to integrate what works into conventional practice. One in five Canadians are said to use alternative medicine.

Stirred by wider consumer protection and rights movements, the sick learned to abandon the role of 'child' accepting medicine from a paternalistic doctor; they began to assume the guise of adults. Patients' rights were stressed and the importance of informed consent and other ethical desiderata underlined. The mute deference so characteristic of previous generations – the assumption among doctors that patients did not *really* want to know what was wrong with them (it would only cause needless anxiety), or that they could not possibly understand – was challenged. An English GP interviewed in the 1980s confessed, 'I find the older working classes and generally the lower-middle classes of all ages easier to deal with than my own sort. My own sort ask complicated questions and are often dissatisfied with the answers. And want long discussion in the middle of a busy surgery. The others simply listen and do what you ask'. Even 'the others' are no longer so meek.

These new tensions and uncertainties in the patient-doctor relationship are in many ways a response to the modern medicalization of life – the widening provision of medical explanations, opinions, services and interventions; the infiltration of medicine into many spheres of life, from normal pregnancy and childbirth to alcohol and drugs related behaviour, in line with a philosophy that assumes the more medicine the better. As childhood and old age became subsumed within paediatrics and geriatrics, medicine swarmed over new terrains of life during the twentieth century and laid claim both to expertise and to a capacity for benevolent action. New medical skills and agencies were activated from the early decades of the twentieth century, professing to shield the sick, the disabled and the vulnerable from violence, neglect, accidents, poverty and from negative authority figures such as abusive parents/husbands, the police, magistrates, judges or prison officers. Be it the psychoanalyst's couch, the baby clinic, the family-planning centre, the detox clinic, or the group therapy session, medicine (and its increasingly powerful sibling, psychotherapy), could sell itself as a benevolent and compassionate institution, a branch of society devoted not primarily to wealth or power but to welfare. Today's complex and confused attitudes towards medicine are the cumulative responses to a century of the growth of the therapeutic state and the medicalized society.

The profession regarded and represented this new medical umbrella as benign. But the term 'the medicalization of society', used by critics, has a routinely negative ring. Historically speaking, the conspiratorial reading is inaccurate because medicine never was sufficiently powerful to muscle in and assume the reins of control: the resistance of the state and the inertia of the people were too great. It always had to assume authority more subtly: there was always to-and-fro, give-and-take, a collusive tie in which groups or the population at large stood to gain from the empowerment of medicine.

The entry points of such medicalization are familiar. One has been the family, with mothers and babies being targeted. In former centuries, mothers were expected to be medical carers to their babies and infants; traditional doctors were not keen to treat children because they were difficult and unremunerative; and wives and children were excluded from the original national insurance schemes. All that changed in the twentieth century. Charitable, private and municipal mother and baby centres were set up; ante-natal clinics gave instruction on motherhood (benefits like free food supplements and orange juice were conditional on conforming); and mothers were increasingly encouraged and expected to have their babies delivered in hospital rather than, as traditionally, in their own homes. Hospital was an excellent base for instilling medically sanctioned attitudes towards baby-feeding, baby-rearing and what came to be called 'scientific motherhood'.

All of this made perfect sense. The modernized, multipurpose hospital gained a reputation for being 'safe' because of its new aseptic procedures; the prospect of a hospital birth was appealing for busy mothers with the maternity ward affording a brief haven of peace. The hospital could handle emergencies and would be safer in administering anaesthetics, particularly the new 'twilight sleep' popular in the 1920s. In particular, once the sulpha drugs cut puerperal fever and made childbirth safe for mothers, there was a new accent on the power and expertise of the hospital and its professional staff to make birth completely safe for babies too – a doubly attractive goal because, with birth control, women were choosing to have fewer babies, and the survival of each perhaps became more significant. Many procedures were introduced, including forceps births, the use of drugs and oxygen, techniques of induction, and finally caesarian sections – all designed to ensure safer, faster, easier delivery and the saving of premature babies who would otherwise have died. Did not the figures speak for themselves?

Post-natal care might then be laced with instruction in 'mother-craft'. Clinics distributed free or cheap milk, orange juice or medicines to induce regular attendance and compliance. School medical services inspected pupils, advised on dentistry, eye-glasses, hearing aids and other appliances, investigated tendencies to rickets, tuberculosis and growth disorders, and conducted vaccinations. Paediatrics became influential with its concepts of normal development and the abnormal child, physically or psychologically. Parents were instructed through various channels how their children should be brought up: they might be offered psychiatric advice or family guidance; medical agencies would network with social bodies that dealt with children – the police, juvenile courts, family therapy, schools for children with special needs.

Medical interventions grew in all branches of life. All the time surgery and other procedures associated with hospitals (including, for example, blood transfusions) were saving lives that would otherwise have been lost, not least those of war combatants and the victims of motor accidents and civil violence. Hospital casualty or emergency departments became the normal resort for people in times of crisis. And of course these developments had an enormous impact upon the handling of death, traditionally associated with the home. With new monitoring machinery, quasi-surgical interventions and the growth of respirators and all the other technology associated with the intensive care unit – the hospital became the place, not where the patient came to *die* but where the apparently terminal patient might almost miraculously be *rescued* from death. Doctors thereby assumed control over the rituals of death: what was left of the 'good death' of the religious *ars moriendi* yielded to the priests in white coats. In the nineteenth century it had been the physician's role to minister over or administer a peaceful death; his modern successor seemed to promise to overcome death. Rendered a mark of failure, death became a taboo, something to be deferred. The management of death was subjected to medical protocols.

In these and a thousand other ways, twentieth-century medicine promised services which would keep people alive longer and improve the quality of life from cradle to grave. Cosmetic surgery might be on hand to restore damaged people (notably war and accident victims), or to beautify the affluent (through nose-jobs, breast implants, or tummy-tucks). Medicine might make the infertile fertile, psychotherapy would teach the forlorn to know, like and assert themselves.

Such procedures and beliefs – which may collectively be called the medicalization of life – could never have become entrenched had not the offerings of enthusiastic practitioners, surgeons and psychiatrists been accepted as desirable and beneficial. From the inter-war years until the 1970s, patients were disposed to regard medical staff as benign: the nurse was selfless, humane, generous, warm, motherly; the surgeon was a fearless warrior, the physician was wise and dependable. As depicted in media representations such as Dr Kildare, their image was positive. Medicine was a service or commodity everyone wanted more of; for much of the century most people could not get enough of it: greater supply, fairer, faster, freer access was the call.

Most spectacularly, there emerged from the early decades of the twentieth century new and remarkable alliances between organized medicine and the public, notably in the mobilization of campaigns against lethal diseases such as tuberculosis and polio. Once the bacterial cause of tuberculosis became known in the 1880s, the idea gained currency that the disease could be controlled, even eliminated through a great public effort. Around 1900, in Europe and the USA, local and national associations sprang up, launched by activists, to carry out the fight. Tuberculosis societies acquired social prestige, often being headed by royalty and influential patrons. Mass mobilization publicized the disease, educated the people in preventive techniques (campaigns against spitting, etc.), promoted ways to reduce risks of infection, provided for the segregation and care of tubercular patients, and funded research into treatments and cure.

Organized in 1892, the Pennsylvania Society for the Prevention of Tuberculosis created an action programme which became a model for others. The plan was to publicize the contagiousness of the disease, instruct the public how to avoid it, visit sufferers, supply them with medical assistance, and inform them on hygienic principles.

Tuberculosis societies – bodies dedicated to the eradication of a particular targeted disease, and generating their own income – were a twentieth-century and largely American phenomenon. For funding, the societies appealed to the general public, the key being small regular contributions made by the millions. The idea of selling a special tuberculosis Christmas stamp originated in Denmark; by 1920, the American Lung Association was raising nearly $4 million from Christmas seals alone; by 1950, sales had climbed to $20 million.

A parallel programme followed with polio. Outbreaks of poliomyelitis – crippling and sometimes fatal – increased in many European countries in the last decades of the nineteenth century, but it was in the United States that the summer plague struck with greatest severity; there might be 50,000 victims in a bad year, mainly children. Its cause was disputed and no way was known of hindering its spread.

The campaign against polio gained ground once Franklin Delano Roosevelt became involved. Roosevelt had contracted paralytic polio in 1921. Though crippled, he fought to be elected governor of New York and, in 1932, president of the United States. His political standing and his much-publicized fight against the disease were enlisted for fund-raising purposes. The President's Birthday Ball Commission was set up; the money would be used for polio research, and the first grants were made in 1935. This was the basis for the National Foundation for Infantile Paralysis, which brought massive funding to researchers who previously had only small budgets. (Owned and developed by FDR, Warm Springs, Georgia, became a folksy – if Whites Only – rehabilitation resort, the focus of the nation's sympathies.)

The National Foundation undertook a massive public relations campaign whose focus was the 'March of Dimes', symbolic of the power of countless small donations from the people. Publicity was the essence; every advance scientists announced was exploited to demonstrate the value of the work, and to promote further giving. Polio discoveries were news; there were pronouncements about the great 'breakthrough' just around the corner, and both scientists and administrators were involved in promotion. Researchers became accustomed to using Madison Avenue methods, and an unprecedented rapport was forged between doctors, researchers and the people.

Between 1938 and 1962 the National Foundation's annual income averaged $25 million; its total receipts were $630 million: 59 per cent went to medical care, 8 per cent to education, 11 per cent to research and 13 per cent to administration and fund-raising. The American example was followed, on a smaller scale, elsewhere: in 1948, the European Association against Poliomyelitis and Allied Diseases was founded. After 1952, the World Health Organization took a more active role.

Initially there were setbacks. In 1935, a vaccine virus was tested: about 17,000 children were vaccinated with a very dilute virus but twelve developed polio, and six died. The vaccines were deemed unsafe, and inoculation was stopped. Controversies flared, mainly surrounding Elizabeth Kenny (1886–1952). In 1910, while nursing victims of poliomyelitis in her native Australia, 'Sister Kenny' began to evolve a programme of physical therapy involving applications of moist heat and a system of hot packs, passive exercise and constant physical therapy (together with an emphasis on will power). All this contradicted prevailing approaches, in which rest was prized and paralysed limbs were immobilized in casts, braces and splints. Between 1933 and 1937 Kenny opened the Sister Kenny Institute in Minneapolis and several other clinics where she employed her unconventional methods. Revered by many, but reviled and ridiculed by leading members of the medical establishment, she defended her techniques and her clinics spread across America. There was, in effect, a contest between the medical elite, the maverick Kenny, and the public as to who was to have ultimate say in the authorization of new therapies. It was a political struggle often to be repeated in medicine in the latter half of the twentieth century.

Against the backdrop of a serious new polio epidemic with some 50,000 cases annually in the United States, and growing public unrest, the National Foundation decided in 1950 to go for a vaccine solution. They found a leader in Jonas Salk (1914–95), of the University of Pittsburgh. Favouring a killed virus vaccine, he reported a series of successful preliminary tests on 23 January 1953. Though there was also support for the live oral polio vaccine developed by Albert Sabin (1906–93) (its attraction was lasting immunity – and it could be taken on a sugar lump), the Immunization Committee of the National Foundation decided to move ahead. Public relations played a part in these decisions: Salk reassured the public; Sabin, by contrast, was abrasive; the two were at each other's throats. Moreover, the Salk vaccine (which required multiple shots and a booster) was ready for immediate testing, and time counted in the public management of disease control.

An elaborate double-blind test was established involving nearly two million children. The results were announced on 12 April 1955, unequivocally stating the vaccine was safe. (Salk underscored when pressed, 'What is safer than safe?') Licensing followed. A million jabs were given between 22 April and 7 May. The vaccine worked, and its huge and highly publicized success contributed in no small measure to the wave of emotional optimism about the conquest of disease.

The tuberculosis and polio campaigns were successful and relatively uncontroversial. Here were dangerous diseases which the medical profession and the public seemed to be joining forces to overcome. Such crusades were mirrored and repeated in thousands of other battles against illness – cancer, cystic fibrosis or heart disease – or campaigns to buy hospital equipment, such as scanners.

These movements help to explain a further phenomenon common in the twentieth century: the success of medical pundits in talking directly to the public on key health matters – sometimes over the heads of their professional peers, and contravening conventional social, moral and even medical wisdom. Childbirth has been one classic arena. Though birth was slowly becoming safer, a succession of dissenting voices was raised, protesting against the authorized medical rituals.

In the inter-war years, for instance, Grantly Dick-Read (1890–1959) came to believe that the pain suffered during childbirth was created by doctors and others. A Cambridge-educated orthodox physician, his experiences in his private gynaecology practice in London led him to develop and publicize the 'Read Method of Natural Birth Control', which he described in *Natural Childbirth* (1933). Nine years later he published *Childbirth Without Fear* (1942), which became a bestseller, though (predictably) provoking anger from much of the medical establishment. Translated into ten languages, it was the centre of heated debate for both its medical and its social message.

Modern women had grown frightened of childbirth, Dick-Read claimed, and this fear caused muscular tension that led to labour pain – the 'fear-tension-pain syndrome'. The answer lay in ante-natal education; his books sought to speak directly to mothers, instilling confidence. Though railing against the 'unforgivable custom' of routinely anaesthetizing women during childbirth (this was becoming the norm) he did not reject pain relief. If women were aware of what was happening, they would probably not need any; but if they did, then relief should be at hand.

Recommending courses of psychological and physical exercises, Dick-Read promised expectant mothers that they could give birth safely and painlessly without drugs. His preparatory sessions combined educational lectures and physical techniques for breathing and muscle conditioning in a programme emphasizing relaxation, self-assurance, understanding of the physiological aspects of childbirth, and a basking in the experience. In 1956, the National Childbirth Trust was set up in Britain to take his ideas to a wider audience, and there has since been a succession of attempts to rescue childbirth from the high-tech hospitalized routines increasingly favoured by the medical profession. The virtues of the 'active management of labour' were praised by the obstetrician Kieran O'Driscoll in 1969; no labour should last longer than twelve hours, O'Driscoll maintained; the administration of oxytocin (to induce contractions) should be 'a standard procedure, applied in all circumstances and by every member of staff'. Labour would thus be speeded up by conveyor-belt methods. Allegedly, such births were safer; but critics judged them merely an institutional convenience. They were growing. In 1964 induced births in England stood at 15.8 per cent; they had risen to 40 per cent by 1974.

Dick-Read's passionate campaigns found echoes in the work of other physicians and gynaecologists. In the Soviet Union 'psychoprophylaxis' – learning to ignore pain by concentrating on somatic sensations elsewhere – was adopted in 1951 as the official method of childbirth pain relief. The French gynaecologist Fernand Lamaze (1891–1957) went to the USSR to study the method and brought it back to France. His *Painless Childbirth* (1956) copied the Soviet idea, adding a scheme of rapid, shallow breathing to control contractions. He also developed a method of 'psychoprophylactic' preparation for expectant mothers, based on the Pavlovian system of 'deconditioning' popular in the Soviet Union.

He shared with Dick-Read the belief that the pain experienced during childbirth was psychological, and could be avoided by physical and mental preparation. 'Rather than telling the patient to relax,' he said, 'we enable her to help herself in the various phases of labour so that she is able to relax.' Nevertheless, Lamaze retained medical control: 'It is necessary to destroy prejudices based on ignorance,' he declared, 'to enlighten the woman by instructing her about the phenomena involved in childbirth.' By the 1970s statements like that were unacceptably sexist to feminists protesting against medical paternalism and patriarchy; at the time and in context they had an enlightened and benevolent ring. Parallels may be found in the psychological and sex advice literature of the early part of the twentieth century, in which the expert, usually male, assumed that women were in need of instruction in love-making: 'The wife must be *taught*, not only how to behave in coitus, but above all, how and what to feel in this unique act!' proclaimed Theo Van de Velde (1873–1937) in a popular marital advice book of the 1920s. The condescension of that statement did not stop the book being popular with women; the prospect of being released from ignorance had a compulsive appeal.

Fredrique Leboyer (b. 1918), of the Paris Faculty of Medicine, took to heart earlier suggestions of the Italian educator, Maria Montessori (1870–1952), that the first impressions of a baby after birth were vital. In *Pour une naissance sans violence* (1974) [Birth without Violence], he described how it should be a gentle experience with lights dimmed and the baby placed on the mother's belly, immersed in warm water to mimic the amniotic fluids. He influenced a fellow countryman, Michel Odent (b. 1930), who combined the techniques of Leboyer and Lamaze. Odent encouraged women to adopt any position they pleased to deal with contractions; pain relief would hardly ever be needed.

Initially, activists in the women's movement were quite enthusiastic about the campaigns of male physicians who seemed to regard the preferences of women-as-patients over and above medical protocols and convenience. By the 1980s, 'birth rooms' were being set up, birthing chairs, discarded centuries earlier, had returned, the importance of mother-baby bonding was being stressed, and childbirth 'supporters' (usually fathers) had become common. But herein lurked a target for charges that this was another (albeit masked) mode of medical dominance. Situations like this have led feminists to speak of 'the captive womb', which involves expert and, generally, male domination over women.

Such conflicts, with their jockeying for followers and acceptance, have become a central feature of modern medicalization. Let us briefly examine another instance: baby care. Doctors have been giving paediatric advice from at least the seventeenth century; what they said then had little impact upon the way babies were brought up: children were and remained the business of the mother and the nurse. The twentieth century, by contrast, has brought platoons of doctors, psychologists and other professionals and pundits to the fore, proffering 'expert' advice on rearing babies.

'Scientific' baby and infant rearing, designed to end the tyranny of habit, gained momentum early in the twentieth century. The founder of behaviourism, John B. Watson (1878–1958), devised a rigorous approach in which strict control of the child's environment could be guaranteed to produce 'doctor, lawyer, artist, merchant, child, and yes even beggarman and thief'. Frederic Truby King (1858–1938) taught that regularity was paramount: babies should be fed by the clock and not on demand. Both were influential, but neither as significant as Benjamin Spock (b. 1903). Spock stressed freedom, was more relaxed, and chimed with the aspirations and outlooks of the postwar generation. He spent much of his career as professor of child development at Western Reserve University in Cleveland, Ohio, and his approach to child-rearing in *The Common Sense Book of Baby and Child Care* (1946) was a radical departure from the prevailing attitudes. The book sold over thirty million copies, more than any book published in the United States! Foregoing the more rigid methods generally recommended in the 1940s, Spock took a reasonable, individualized approach, which later drew accusations that he had single-handedly produced the 1960s' youth rebellion.

Spock offers perhaps the most striking instance of a modern medical guru, drawing upon his 'expertise' but selling it to the public as 'common sense'. In later life he became something of a political radical, campaigning against the Vietnam War and nuclear weapons, and running for the presidency of the United States. Despite that prominence, sociological critics have cast him as the one who captured child-rearing for medical authority.

From the 1960s public disquiet also grew over the depersonalization of death within the hospital. Institutional death was viewed in the medical profession as a case of failure; the modern hospital was dedicated to saving lives, not managing death. Medicine strove to develop high-tech machinery and the protocols to accompany it, the aim being prolongation of life at all costs.

In heightening awareness of the degradation of death and devising alternatives to it, two figures stand out. The Swiss-born physician and psychiatrist Elisabeth Kübler-Ross (b. 1926) pioneered theoretical and practical ways of coming to terms with dying. A proponent of the Death Awareness Movement, Kübler-Ross's best-selling *On Death and Dying*

(1969) aimed to overcome society's deep-rooted taboos by encouraging frank discussion of death. Meanwhile, in a practical and direct way, Dr Cicely Saunders (b. 1918) developed the hospice movement in Britain, institutions in which a 'good' death was encouraged. In 1967 she founded St Christopher's Hospice in London, so as to create a new *ars moriendi*: pain relief through ample dosing with morphine would dispel fear and enable the dying to experience death in a positive way.

A contrasting philosophy of dying has recently gained ground, again involving an alliance of vocal and radical doctors on the one hand and concerned members of the public on the other: the voluntary euthanasia movement, intended to avoid the indignity of a living death. Thanks to life-support systems, it is now relatively easy to keep many 'dead' people artificially alive. This happened in a grotesquely public way with the Spanish fascist leader, General Franco, in 1975. 'Doctors treating General Franco are using everything they have in a determined effort to keep him alive,' a United Press Agency report began:

> A late medical bulletin said the 82-year-old Spanish leader showed symptoms of pneumonia and doctors sat him up as part of the treatment. One doctor expressed hope for his recovery. At least four mechanical devices are being used in the battle for General Franco's survival.
>
> A defibulator [sic] attached to his chest shocks his heart back to normal when it slows or fades; a pump-like device helps push his blood through his body when it weakens; a respirator helps him breathe, and a kidney machine cleans his blood. At various times in his 25-day crisis, General Franco has had tubes down his windpipe to provide air, down his nose to provide nourishment, in his abdomen to drain accumulative fluids, in his digestive tract to relieve gastric pressure and in his left thigh to relieve the pressure of blood clots. The effort in itself is remarkable considering he has had three major heart attacks.
>
> He has undergone emergency surgery twice – once to patch a ruptured artery to save him from bleeding to death, the second time to remove most of an ulcerated and bleeding stomach for the same reason. He has taken some 15 litres (4 gallons) of blood transfusions. His lungs are congested . . . his kidneys are giving out and his liver is weak. Paralysis periodically affects his intestines . . . he suffers occasional rectal bleeding. Ascites causes an accumulation of fluid in his abdominal cavity. Blood clots have formed and spread in his left thigh. He has lost 9.9kg (22lbs) from his pre-crisis 49kg (110lbs).

Mucus accumulates uncontrollably in his mouth. Influenza was the first official explanation for his confinement to bed on October 17th.

Repugnance grew for the 'cruelty' of this meaningless prolongation of life, particularly amongst those in a 'persistent vegetative state' who entirely lack consciousness. One response has been an advocacy of euthanasia, and many have tried to devise acceptable procedures for mercy-killing, in accordance with the wish of the dying (and their families). These efforts are promoted by pressure groups such as Exit in the UK.

Difficult ethical issues are involved. Euthanasia may be squared with the professional ethics of the physician and with common morality through the argument that, while it is the doctor's duty to save life, that duty does not run so far as to prolong life through artificial means in all circumstances. The Hippocratic oath merely required that the physician should do no harm.

Changes in opinion, medical practice and public policy have been most remarkable in the Netherlands, where since 1984 the medical colleges have accepted euthanasia under strictly controlled circumstances. By 1995 a survey suggested that active euthanasia (a physician humanely intervening to end a terminally ill patient's life at the request of that patient) was taking place in around 1.8 per cent of all deaths. Public acceptance of such practices had been facilitated by the development of 'living wills'. These have been legally binding in South Australia since the Natural Death Act of 1983, and since 1994 in the Netherlands, physicians have been legally obliged to honour them – a development welcomed by the medical profession because it frees them from legal quandaries.

Such practices have met with a much more divided reception elsewhere. In Britain, where euthanasia remains illegal, the pressure group Exit has been subject to prosecution, as has the controversial American pathologist, Dr Jack Kevorkian, who has pioneered doctor-assisted suicide, involving himself in many courtroom struggles. The legal situation remains contested; in 1997, a Northern Territories (Australia) law permitting medically aided euthanasia was overturned by the Australian federal parliament.

Examples of the politicization of medicine could be multiplied *ad infinitum*. The field that has brought the most unstable tug of forces between the profession, the public, the state and activists is psychiatry.

It is noteworthy that all the leading anti-psychiatry campaigners of the 1960s and 1970s – Franco Basaglia (1924–80) in Italy, Thomas Szasz in the US and Ronald Laing in Britain – were themselves practising psychiatrists, who routinely appealed to the public against their own colleagues and profession.

All these instances demonstrate that what has been styled, particularly by critics, 'the medicalization of life' cannot be understood purely or primarily as some kind of professional ramp. What has occurred is not a conspiracy by medical elites to push professional dominance into domains traditionally outside medicine's province, but rather the destabilization of the boundaries of lay and professional competence in an age of democracy, when medical professionals often feel driven to break out from the iron cages which professional strategies have built for them.

If the distinction of function between practitioner and patient, between medical profession and public, was ever simple and clear, it ceased to be so in modern times. Volcanic controversies have erupted *within* the medical profession upon fundamental issues of living and dying, integrity and power. In these the public, the sick person, the disputed body, is sometimes the football – as the title of Brian Clark's (b. 1938) popular play indicates: *Whose Life Is It Anyway?* (1978). Often, though, the public is a player. Medical experts stake their claim for authority with a public eager for the confirmation which authority may confer. These tangled processes can be exemplified through discussion of fields such as sexuality, addiction and anorexia.

It has become widely accepted that concepts of sexual orientation and disposition are socially and historically special. Our discourses specifying male and female roles, heterosexuality and homosexuality, stem largely from late nineteenth-century medicine and psychiatry. Faced with street-walking, child prostitution, domestic violence, incest, and all those other festering moral scandals of the city of dreadful night which shocked bourgeois sensibilities, the prominent sex experts of the *fin de siècle* such as Richard von Krafft-Ebing (1840–1902) delineated sex roles through disciplines like forensic psychiatry and ethnography.

Sexology provided the classificatory and diagnostic systems required to administer the asylums, hospitals, reformatories and jails which had to cope with the chronic masturbators, simpletons, child molesters, rapists, pregnant teenagers, prostitutes, and other sex offenders.

Facing disorder and delinquency, late Victorian sexual science tabulated the varieties of erotic disposition, demarcating the normal from psychopaths, defectives, recidivists and criminals; in some cases detention or medico-psychological therapies were recommended. Krafft-Ebing's encyclopaedic *Psychopathia Sexualis* (1886) itemized, often for the first time, if occasionally in the decent obscurity of Latin, the bestiary of sexual transgressions, from adultery to zooerasty, by way of bestiality, coprolagnia, exhibitionism, fetishism, sado-masochism, satyriasis, urolagnia, voyeurism and a hundred other perversions.

Slightly later, Havelock Ellis's (1859–1939) *Studies in the Psychology of Sex* (1905–28) extended the terminology of psychosexual types: homosexuals, paedophiles, nymphomaniacs, fetishists, transvestites, zoophiles, and so forth, labellings rare before the twentieth century. Perversions were regarded as psychologically based, though deviant people, Ellis believed, were scarred by some revealing physical trait: effeminacy in the male, dull eyes, thick lips, large labia, preternatural hairiness in the female.

Many others around the turn of the century – not least Freud himself in his *Three Essays on the Theory of Sexuality* (1905) – regarded it as advancing the cause of scientific and moral progress to insist upon the biomedical reality of sexual pathologies. 'Perverts', they wished to claim, were not 'wicked', they merely developed that way, their abnormality was a kind of mental or physical sickness, and they should not be punished or condemned. The founders of modern sexology thus staked their intellectual authority on the conviction that certain people were physically and psychologically predisposed to engage in abnormal, inadmissible, and deleterious sexual activity. Until the Victorian era, 'unnatural' acts were regarded mainly as vices which might be indulged by various immature, profligate, impressionable, foreign, or over-sexed individuals, succumbing to lust, intoxication, libertinism, opportunity or necessity (e.g., in a public school or nunnery). Sodomy, self-abuse, and so on had not been interpreted by doctors or moralists as products of abnormal germ plasms or diseased personalities, or as symptomatic of a hereditary group or a psycho-physically bizarre subset. Modern sexual science shifted attention from practices to bodies, genes, brains and psyches, and systematically pigeon-holed such people as 'deviants', inverts or homosexuals, narcissists, masochists, degenerates and exhibitionists. Modern sexual science invented and popularized all the sexual -ists and -isms. But the validity of such identifications has been contested. In particular, the groups identified have wavered between rejecting such names (viewing them as stigmatizing) and embracing them (seeing them as exonerating and empowering). The medicalization of sexuality may thus be either a threat or a blessing.

Uncertainty as to how far, if at all, questions of sexuality do have, and should have, a biomedical substrate, continues to this day, fuelled in part by the AIDS cataclysm. Simon LeVay, an English-born neuroanatomist formerly attached to the Salk Institute in San Diego, has recently claimed that the size of a certain nucleus in the hypothalamus varies with sexual orientation: the INAH-3 nucleus is biggest in heterosexual males, smaller in homosexual males and smallest of all in females. Adducing other evidence – such as experiments showing that rats turned 'gay' if their hormonal balance was altered – LeVay argues that medical science is at last solving 'the homosexuality question'. Being gay is not a matter of choice or a consequence of upbringing, but is encoded in biological destiny; sexual orientation is in the genes or brain.

Himself gay, and looking back admiringly to the late nine-teenth-century sexologists such as Magnus Hirschfeld (1868–1935), LeVay is convinced that scientific support for the 'born that way' claim offers the best strategy for the gay community. Critics, including those aware of how Nazi eugenists treated homosexuals during the Second World War, have accentuated the dangers in this new medicalization of homosexuality.

A parallel case is offered by medical responses to drunkenness and addiction. Inebriation was once viewed as a sin, vice or character defect. The traditional drunk was a weak and selfish man enslaved to his impulses. From the mid nineteenth century, the condition became medicalized, with the Swedish physician Magnus Huss (1807–90) creating the disease category of 'alcoholism'. Powerful voices among the medical and psychiatric communities were happy to accept such a model; drying-out clinics appeared, precursors of the modern twelve-point plans. Lay activists, notably the Alcoholics Anonymous movement, were often receptive to the medical model. It sloughed off responsibility, and it gave hope: if alcoholism were a disease, why should it not be cured? Discussion assumed new foci: what kind of a disease was alcoholism?

This debate has rumbled on. The 1947 edition of *Osler's Principles and Practice of Medicine* took its cue from psychoanalysis, suggesting that alcoholism originated in 'conflicts and maladjustments developing from the patient's family and marital relationships'; two decades later the seventeenth edition construed alcoholism as a liver disease; by 1980 it had become 'a behavior disorder'. Tugged between different groups and values, the concept of alcoholism was predictably less than stable.

Medicalization of the eating disorders has also come to play a crucial role in the social pathology of our consumer society. Self-starvation has a long history. It was initially encultured within a religious agenda, the aim being mortification of the flesh. All Christians were to renounce the deadly sin of gluttony and to fast as directed by the Church, but desert fathers and hermits pursued food asceticism on a heroic scale. They underwent prolonged fasting or supped on nothing but locusts and grass; some female saints pursued particularly pious food preferences, refusing all food but the Host.

Medieval Catholicism recognized its perils: fasting unto death was tantamount to the ultimate sin of suicide, and such austerities might be not piety but vanity, or the promptings of the Devil. Protestantism was robustly dismissive of such superstitious balderdash and, partly for that reason, the Christian era of spiritual fasting gave way to fascination with starvation as spectacle. The nineteenth century promoted the faster as freak, a curiosity for ghouls to swarm around or for commercial exploitation midgets and bearded ladies. Protégés of P. T. Barnum won celebrity as hunger artists, performing before a voyeuristic public, titillated by feats of self-denial and macabre skeletal displays.

At this stage the involvement of the medical profession became significant. Occasionally, physicians authenticated these exhibitions of emaciation, but most often they intervened as sceptics, serving as fraud-busters. This inescapably led to the third stage. For when these public-spirited exposés failed to end the fasting, the doctors had to pronounce that it was not, after all, a swindle but a sickness. Self-starvers (characteristically female) were not cheats but ill – sick in body but, above all, in mind. The label affixed from early Victorian times was 'hysterical': that portmanteau diagnosis for female perversities and expressions of socio-sexual deviance. From the 1850s, however, specialized psychiatric terms were coined: *anorexie nerveuse, anorexie gastrique* and so on.

A priority dispute erupted around 1870 between (Sir) William Gull (1816–90) and the French neuropsychiatrist, Ernest Lasègue (1816–83), about who had first deployed the term *anorexia nervosa* (from the 1870s the historian can without anachronism speak of the anorexia syndrome). These people were self-starvers recognizably akin to the classic anorectics of the post-World War II period. From the 1960s anorexia became 'epidemic', essentially as a consequence of socio-sexual pressures upon teenage girls and young women. Initially, the medical profession was indifferent and dismissive. As with ME at the close of the century, it was not eager to be involved in what might prove a fad. Next, doctors predictably accentuated the physical aspects: anorexia was a weight or eating disorder to be countered by means devised to restore lost flesh. Psychiatric and psychotherapeutic interventions followed, particularly once anorexia was taken up by the women's movement, due partly to Susie Orbach's (b. 1946) *Fat is a Feminist Issue* (1978).

Feminist readings of anorexia appropriate the stories of sufferers no less than those pursuing medicalization. *Anorexia nervosa* cannot be parcelled in a reductionist way, isolated from the wider social systems and cultural beliefs which provide its roots and afford its meanings: it would be false to posit polar rivalry between the 'disease' and the 'protest' models. Modern anorexia is the biopsychosocial disorder mirroring a society with specific tensions and contradictions: the bourgeois family, supportive yet suffocating, and all the paradoxical hypocrisies of modern attitudes towards youth, food, femininity, beauty and sexuality, are whipped up by the media and by multi-million pound food and style industries.

It is no accident in what remains a man's world, with a medical profession still male-dominated, that it is mainly 'women's complaints' which have become medicalized. What is noteworthy is the variety of the responses adopted and made available for negotiation. Menopause is revealing. Anthropologists have pointed out that in many traditional societies menopause presents no subjective problem to women. It marks their escape from a stage in life which may have been burdensome and dangerous (childbearing) and stigmatizing (menstruation viewed as polluting). In the West, however, it is associated with the negative aspects of ageing and loss of sexual appeal. Many strategies have been developed by experts to help women through the so-called mid-life crisis. One school of physicians, mainly gynaecologists, believes menopause should be regarded as a 'deficiency' disease; Hormone Replacement Therapy (HRT) is the treatment of choice. A second group believes that most of those who seek medical care at menopause are suffering from depression, anxious about ageing, loss of sexuality, and a lack of purpose in their lives; perhaps medication is the answer. A third group (mainly family practitioners) believe that trouble at menopause arises out of role conflict, the 'empty nest', a spouse's retirement, and so on. A fourth group, the 'stiff upper lip school', asserts, as do some feminists, that the fuss about menopause is part of a medical plot to demean and pathologize women. Medicine has many tunes and many may sing them.

As all these examples of the politics of contemporary medicine show, it is misleading to represent modern medicine as a monolith. Nothing illustrates this better than the power-play surrounding the disease with the highest public profile: AIDS.

In the early 1980s, in the absence of scientific consensus about the cause of the new syndrome (it did not even have an agreed name), any pundit or self-appointed homophobic television evangelist could pronounce on the 'gay plague' or the 'wrath of God'. Scientists squabbled over whose baby the new disease should be: epidemiologists, public health specialists, virologists, venereologists – who? That clash subsided after 1983, when AIDS was seemingly traced to a virus, but scientific authority was soon tugged and torn by the feud between the virologists Robert Gallo (b. 1937) and Luc Montagnier (b. 1932). This authority was ripped at the seams as the Berkeley immunologist Peter Duesberg denied the causal role of HIV and became the dean of dissent. Gallo claimed that Duesberg had no business at the AIDS table, being a mere 'chemist', who had improperly 'gone public' (a common insult among medical scientists). Duesberg's supporters pointed out that he was a member of the elite National Academy of Sciences.

In such a situation, lay persons and AIDS activists were able to command a role often denied those beyond the magic laboratory: as participants not just patients and, increasingly, as experts. People-With-AIDS possessed a daring born of desperation; moreover, at least among the New York and San Francisco gay communities, PWAs were middle-class, educated and politically astute, thanks to Gay Liberation and especially Act-Up. PWAs developed an expertise of their own as the establishment expressed its astonishment: 'It's frightening sometimes how much they know,' Gallo commented – a most illuminating remark.

This irruption of lay expertise had a surprising impact in the domain of therapeutics. Initially the activists' complaints were simple: treatment was all too little, too late – get 'drugs into bodies' was the campaign slogan. But users' lobbies delved deeper: was the preferred drug AZT (azidothymidine) effective (as prophylactic or treatment)? Or was AZT, as others claimed, 'AIDS by prescription'? Who was to decide? And who was to determine its distribution? And did the system whereby therapeutic innovation was left to the vagaries of drug-company policies, market forces and Food and Drug Administration validation serve patients' interests? Was this 'good medicine'? Who had the right to judge 'good medicine'?

Users' groups even challenged the design and morality of the classical clinical trial, one of medicine's sacred cows since its designs had been standardized in the 1940s. Why did findings seemingly contradict each other? Was it ethically justifiable to maintain the placebo group during a lengthy ('dinosaur') trial, and so perhaps withhold a promising treatment from those whose life was ebbing away? Gay journalists likened such 'laboratory rats' to Nazi holocaust experiment victims.

With time ticking away, AIDS sufferers voted with their feet, setting up 'buyers' clubs', making bootleg drugs, smuggling untried drugs across the border, or, through drug-sharing, subverting clinical trials conducted along the classical model. So persuasive were their reasons, so strong the moral case, that a sizable minority of doctors, scientists and even government appointees were won over – or bowed to political pressure. Fresh thinking followed about how clinical trial protocols needed to be rewritten, so that patient welfare was respected at least as much as the needs of science. The downside, according to many scientists, is that the protocols for 'pure' clinical trials, painstakingly devised over the course of many years, were wrecked, in effect setting AIDS research back a decade and destroying the very safeguards patients had once demanded.

With AIDS, the quarrel of the experts opened a chink into which users and lay people could insert themselves as new carriers of credit. Partly by consequence, the traditional idea of expertise was challenged, provoking a great debate as to who was entitled to a seat at the table in a paternalistic medical set-up forced to become more democratic, accessible and client friendly.

Thus the twentieth century closes with the ownership of the body and the right to speak on sickness profoundly contested. Many voices are raised for repossessing the body from a 'body-snatching' medicine.

One attempt to do so lies in body culture: keeping fit, working-out, body-building. Yet even here problems and paradoxes may lurk: in their extreme forms, these movements are self-medicalizing, since the creation of a 'designer body' often involves dosing with steroids and other hazardous drugs. Empowering 'health-cults' could imperil health.

A parallel may be found in enthusiasms for alternative medicine, which may be no less 'medicalizing' (and risky) than the orthodox medicine they repudiate. Like everybody else, the health-conscious individual is caught in a web of equivocal influences. Modern health preoccupations have spawned a new health mysticism, spurred by big companies which profit from vitamin sales and public health preoccupation. Not least, new psycho-spiritualism ('sickness is all in the personality') uncannily echoes the victim-blaming doctrines of the moral majority ('sickness is God's punishment').

CHAPTER XXII

THE PAST, THE PRESENT
AND THE FUTURE

AT THE CLOSE of the twentieth century, new horizons are visible, but so are new problems. Westerners are now living longer. But longevity means more time for illness, and implies that greater effort and resources will need to be devoted to keeping well – all the more so as it will increasingly fall to individuals to ensure (and insure) their passage through the longer journey. In a more health- and beauty-conscious culture, keeping up appearances will also become more costly and energy-consuming.

We live in an age of science, but science has not eliminated fantasies about health; the stigmas of sickness, the moral meanings of medicine continue. Previous centuries wove stories around leprosy, plague, tuberculosis, and so on, thereby creating terror, guilt and stigma. But the modern age created similar taboos about cancer ('the big C') as untreatable, fatal, and psychogenic, the product of the so-called 'cancer personality', the self that eats itself away through frustration and repressed anger. Therapy was hindered and suffering multiplied. Mythologies have now grown up around AIDS. In important respects, science itself has been the vehicle for the proliferation of health fantasies.

Moreover, despite all the advances, medical self-confidence has been shaken on several occasions during the past century: in 1918–19, when an influenza pandemic of unprecedented virulence swept the world, killing over twenty-five million people, and in medicine's powerlessness against AIDS. Other deadly viral diseases loom, such as the Marburg virus and Ebola fever. The recent discovery that the cattle disease Bovine Spongiform Encephalopathy (BSE) may, through infected beef, be a source of the Creutzfeldt-Jakob Disease (CJD) has sparked fears respecting other pathogens introduced into the food chain by ignorance, carelessness and greed. Such 'new diseases' are not unlucky accidents but part of the political and economic system the West pursues – relentless growth and often destructive development. They are also what the Darwinian struggle for survival predicts will never cease. Earlier optimism about magic bullets and a pill for every ill now seems symptomatic of a shallow high-tech, quick-fix vision of the world, born of the laboratory and expecting the world to be as controllable as a laboratory.

From the olympian view, how does medicine's historical balance-sheet stand? Hard to assess. Let us take the most tragic medical disaster: women dying in childbirth. Throughout the western world, medicalized childbirth has finally, within the last half century, become safe for mother and child, with a less than one-in-10,000 risk of maternal mortality. In 1930 an Englishwoman going into labour had a one-in-250 chance of not surviving, and a dozen women a day died of childbirth just a century ago (it is now down to one a week). In the worst Victorian maternity hospitals, between 9 and 10 per cent of women entering might leave in a coffin. The graph was even grimmer in the American south. Rank and riches afforded no insurance policy; nor were things unambiguously getting better over the years. Maternal mortality – the outcome of sepsis (puerperal fever), haemorrhage or toxaemia (eclampsia) – maintained its tragic plateau from mid Victorian times until the 1930s, and as Semmelweis found in nineteenth-century Vienna, the peaks were sometimes quite Andean.

Was this carnage inevitable? Of course, some women died because they were famished, and others through septic abortions. Until the drugs revolution (sulpha drugs in the 1930s and antibiotics from the 1940s), there was not much that medicine could do to check lethal infections. But the majority of deaths could have been prevented by better obstetrics. In Britain, home deliveries were performed by low-status midwives who had little training, or by GPs whose obstetrical education had been perfunctory. It was not until 1902 that midwives had to be registered. In the United States, deliveries were increasingly performed in hospitals, by a high-intervention factory system which relied on sedation, forceps and caesarians. In both countries, careless and cavalier practices inflated infection rates, long after the Listerian antiseptic revolution could have made labour far safer. Obstetrics was a Cinderella service; male practitioners did not accord mothers and babies much attention.

Things were different in some countries. Scandinavia and the Netherlands were safer places to have a baby. Why? Because their maternity services hinged upon highly qualified domiciliary midwives.

Training equipped them to deal with all but the most exacting emergency cases; they were less trigger-happy with forceps and drugs; and delivery by midwife avoided the lethal cross-infections picked up in the germ-infested hospital or carried by the jack-of-all-trades family practitioner, rushing from infectious cases to women in labour. In short, the safest form of childbirth was traditionally away from hospital and from the doctors' clutches.

Why didn't all nations follow the Dutch or Danish leads? It wasn't because doctors elsewhere did not know the perils facing pregnant women. Pioneers like Semmelweis had already pointed the accusing finger at the profession and its slapdash habits, and many sincere physicians agonized over the slaughter of the innocents. But gut prejudices and professional *esprit de corps* prevailed. Did not hospitals provide the best that science could offer? And how *could* mere midwives provide safer deliveries than top physicians? – midwives, according to one American physician, were 'filthy and ignorant and not far removed from the jungles'. Medicine likes to think it is the most 'beneficent' profession, but it is deeds not words that count.

We should certainly not hanker after some mythic golden age when women gave birth naturally, painlessly and safely: the most appalling western maternal death rate today is among the Faith Assembly religious sect in Indiana, who reject orthodox medicine and practise home births; their perinatal mortality is 92 times greater than in Indiana as a whole. Ignorance may be as lethal as complacency.

Much light is shed on the enigmatic role played by medicine in the modern world by developments over smoking and health. By 1951, it had been determined, in a large sample of hospital patients, that the great majority of lung cancer sufferers were cigarette smokers. In 1956, the results of a five-year study of the smoking habits of 40,000 medical practitioners were published. Lung cancer deaths among doctors who were heavy cigarette smokers (twenty-five or more a day) were over twenty times higher than among non-smokers. The study unleashed the criticism that it did not identify the cause of lung cancer.

The psychologist Hans Eysenck (1916–97) offered a counter-study exonerating cigarettes and claiming a statistical connection between personality types and proneness to lung cancer. Nevertheless, by 1962 the Royal College of Physicians declared that smoking 'causes' lung cancer and, two years later, the US Surgeon-General's Advisory

Committee took the same line. In 1964 the Surgeon-General found that death from cancer for men who smoked was 70 per cent higher than for non-smokers. In 1979 another report from the Surgeon-General announced that the main risk from smoking was not cancer but heart disease. Doctors took the findings to heart: the numbers of British doctors who smoked fell by 50 per cent between 1951 and 1964, a decline much steeper than in the general population. Further links between smoking and other serious diseases became clear – bronchitis, circulatory and cardiovascular disorders.

But politicians were used to the stupendous tax revenues from cigarette sales, and tobacco companies made large political donations and ran forceful political lobbies. Change came slowly. Britain banned television advertising of cigarettes in 1965 and in 1971 secured an agreement from the industry that all cigarette packets would carry a government health warning; in the US, too, health warnings were introduced on cigarette packs. Restrictions on smoking in public places and at work multiplied, particularly since the appearance of data indicting passive smoking. Yet, in the early 1990s, fifty million Americans (nearly a quarter of the entire population, including children) were still regular smokers, and federal experts put the death rate from smoking-related diseases at one thousand a day. Among certain sectors of the population, notably young women, cigarette smoking was conspicuously increasing (smoking allegedly creates a powerful personal aura and is believed to aid slimming).

We now know that tobacco companies were long aware of the health risks of their products, thanks to experiments conducted by their own medical scientists but kept secret. Documentation shows that they deliberately targeted children and artificially raised the nicotine content of their cigarettes so as to increase addiction. In March 1997 the Liggett Group (the smallest of the five big US tobacco companies and the makers of Chesterfield cigarettes) announced a settlement with twenty-two American states in which it admitted that smoking was addictive, caused heart disease, cancer and lung-related illnesses. The company agreed to provide evidence of meetings between industry lawyers which would prove tobacco firms had long known of the dangers of nicotine and had nevertheless continued to target cigarettes at underage smokers.

What has been the role of medicine in this vast health tragedy, costly in lives, costly in resources? Ironically, tobacco was introduced and promoted, around 1600, as a medicine, and long recommended by doctors for calming the nerves. Clinicians were astonishingly slow to sense the dangers; that was the work of statisticians and epidemiologists, once again revealing the divisions within medicine. Despite changes in the political climate – in the United Kingdom, the new Labour government announced in May 1997 its intention to ban all cigarette advertising – the likelihood is that a product known to cause the deaths of one third of a million people a year in the US alone will remain energetically promoted on the open market – because it is profitable to producers and governments, and popular with sectors of the public. Meanwhile, smoking is increasing in many of the poorer parts of the world – in China, cigarette consumption increased from 500 billion in 1978 to 1,700 billion in 1992. Africa shows a similar picture; much of the global increase is the result of hard-selling campaigns by western multinationals.

Blame for all this can hardly be laid at medicine's door, but the facts indicate how little medicine weighs in the balance of health. With stupendous expense of human skill and money – smoking related diseases cost the NHS £610 million a year – modern medicine has developed the capacity, through late-stage crisis management, to bestow a few extra months or years of life on some smokers who would otherwise have died of cardiovascular or lung conditions. The blessing to the individual may be inestimable (or it may simply mean a bad death), but that hardly registers on the global balance-sheet. The contribution of prolonging some smokers' lives is rather slight: most who have been diagnosed and treated do not live more than five years. Commonsense suggests that the money spent on these forms of cardiology and oncology would be more wisely spent on anti-smoking campaigns, and in research into other diseases.

We have invested disproportionately in a form of medicine ('Band Aid' salvage) whose benefits often come late, which buy a little time, and which are easily nullified by external, countervailing factors. Curative, interventionist medicine has played a modest part in shaping wider morbidity and mortality patterns within the community, but in terms of its professed aims – the greatest health of the greatest number – the olympian verdict must be that much medicine has been off target.

Until the last hundred and fifty years, the role of clinical medicine in the improvement of health was tiny. Whether populations grew or shrank, were robust or suffered 'the thousand natural shocks that flesh is heir to', had little to do with medicine, despite its best efforts. That has changed, though not in simple or predictable ways. In the form of contraceptive pills, medical research is today responsible for capping some populations, while, in the form of rehydration kits and measures against infantile diarrhoea, it raises others. Medicine's role in the future of *homo sapiens* on this planet is unforeseeable, because the Darwinian evolutionary battle between mankind and microbes is itself unpredictable. It is unlikely that medicine will play a role as important as politics, economics, or disease.

Its standing is now highly contested. Never has it achieved so much or attracted such great suspicion. The breakthroughs of the last fifty years have saved more lives than those of any epoch since medicine began. Lewis Thomas (b. 1913) wrote that when he began his career in the 1930s

> the major threats to human life were tuberculosis, tetanus, syphilis, rheumatic fever, pneumonia, meningitis, polio, and septicemia of all sorts. These things worried us then the way cancer, heart disease and stroke worry us today. The big problems of the 1930s and 1940s have literally vanished.

Medicine played a large part in that transformation. In 1940, penicillin was just being tried out on mice; within a decade it had saved millions of lives. The 1950s extended the 'first pharmacological revolution' onto a broad front; it produced, in psychotropics like chlorpromazine, the first effective medications for mental illnesses; other drug breakthroughs, notably steroids such as cortisone, made it feasible to capitalize on the growing understanding of the immune system. Immunosuppressants opened brave new world possibilities for transplant surgery. With bypass operations and heart transplants beginning in 1967, surgery seemed to know no bounds.

Technology and science contributed electron microscopes, endoscopes, key-hole surgery, CAT and PETT scans, Magnetic Resonance Imaging, lasers, tracers, ultrasound. Genetic screening and engineering have made great headway; gene replacement therapy beckons. Such advances have come from the vast investment in and endowment of medicine. In several European Union countries, more than 10 per cent of GNP now goes on health; in the US, the figure is touching 15 per cent.

But if medicine is expanding almost beyond the bounds of imagination, the euphoria of the age of penicillin or the 'pill' has turned to anxiety. Today's headlines are much more likely to be of fears about a new cholera epidemic sweeping South America or plague in India, the cloning of sheep today and maybe humans tomorrow. For all medicine's successes, who would deny a certain malaise? The atmosphere is one of hollow conquest. The age of infectious disease gave way to the age of chronic disorders. Longer life means more time to be ill, and medicine is more open to criticism.

Drugs have sometimes been disasters; iatrogenic illness has grown; research on afflictions like cancer, schizophrenia, diabetes, Alzheimer's and other degenerative diseases creeps at a snail's-pace; doubts remain about the very subject of psychiatry. In Britain, the NHS was allowed to disintegrate in the 1980s and became a political football; in the US, insurance and litigation scandals dog the profession. In rich countries, the needy still get a poor medical deal. In the Third World, malaria and many other tropical diseases continue to spread, while diphtheria and tuberculosis, once believed routed, are resurgent in eastern and central Europe and in other industrialized nations. Not least, the AIDS pandemic has destroyed any naive faith that disease itself was *hors de combat*. The fact that AIDS remains without a cure reminds us that panaceas cannot be made to order.

Misgivings may be variously evaluated: do we call partial progress success or failure? Are shortcomings to be blamed on physicians or on politicians? But they are not the heart of the matter: medicine is arguably going through a far more fundamental crisis, the price of progress and its attendant inflated expectations. It is losing its way, or having to redefine its goals. In the *British Medical Journal* in 1949, Lord Horder (1871–1955) posed the question, 'Whither Medicine?', and returned the answer direct: 'Why, whither else but straight ahead'. Today, no thinking person within or outside medicine knows where 'straight ahead' is.

For centuries, the medical enterprise was too feeble to attract radical critiques. From Cato to Chekhov, medicine had its mockers; yet most who could, called the doctor when sick. People did not have high expectations, and when the doctor typically achieved little, they did not blame him much. Medicine was a profession, but it carried little prestige or power. All bowed before death.

In the present century, medicine grew conquering and commanding. It now costs the earth and, as its publicity has mushroomed, it has provoked a crescendo of criticism. Historians, social scientists, political analysts and the public converge to pose searching questions. From the 1950s, sociology put medicine under the microscope – and sometimes on the couch. One school of sociologists mounted assaults on professional dominance. Another contended that the categories of medicine – the very notions of health and sickness, as well as specific diagnosed disorders, like hysteria – were social labels, often involving stigma, victim-blaming, scape-goating and the designation of deviance with respect to class, race and gender. Nor was this critique the ritual chanting of trendy Lefties. At mid century, the doyen of conservative American sociologists, Talcott Parsons (1902–79), drew attention to what he called 'the sick role', a notion reducing the estate of medicine to social ritual. Sociologists now regularly characterize it as a means of social control, reproducing social norms, exercising social power. Once medicine proved effective, the scourge of pestilence was forgotten, and the physician no longer had to be thanked and could be disparaged as a figure of authority, a tool of patriarchy or a stooge of the state.

In another key respect, medicine has become the prisoner of its success. Having conquered many grave diseases and provided relief from suffering, its mandate has become muddled. What are its aims? Where is it to stop? Is its prime duty to keep people alive as long as possible, willy-nilly, whatever the circumstances? Is its charge to *make* people lead healthy lives? Or is it but a service industry, on tap to fulfil whatever fantasies its clients may frame for their bodies, be they cosmetic surgery and designer bodies or the longing of post-menopausal women to have babies? In *Gulliver's Travels* (1726), Jonathan Swift exposed, through his portrait of the wretched Struldbrugs, the follies of hankering after immortality. It may be that medicine has to learn that lesson all over again.

Many of these quandaries in a particular case can be resolved with common decency, goodwill and a sensible ethics committee. But in the wider world, who can decide the direction medicine should now take? In the rich world, it has accomplished its basic targets as understood by Hippocrates, William Harvey or Lord Horder – who will decide its new missions?

The irony is that the healthier western society becomes, the more medicine it craves – indeed, it regards maximum access as a right and duty. Especially in free market America, immense pressures are created – by the medical profession, by medi-business, the media, by the high-pressure advertising of pharmaceutical companies, and dutiful (or susceptible) individuals – to expand the diagnosis of treatable illnesses. Scares are created. People are bamboozled into lab tests, often of dubious reliability. Thanks to diagnostic creep or leap, ever more disorders are revealed. Extensive and expensive treatments are then urged, and the physician who chooses not to treat may expose himself to malpractice accusations. Anxieties and interventions spiral upwards like a space-shot off course.

The root of the trouble is structural. It is endemic to a system in which an expanding medical establishment, faced with a healthier population, is driven to medicalizing normal events like menopause, converting risks into diseases, and treating trivial complaints with fancy procedures. Doctors and 'consumers' are becoming locked within a fantasy that *everyone* has *something* wrong with them, everyone and everything can be cured.

Medical consumerism – like all sorts of consumerism, but more menacingly – is designed to be unsatisfying. The law of diminishing returns necessarily applies. Extending life becomes feasible, but it may be a life exposed to degrading neglect as resources grow overstretched and politics turn mean. What an ignominious destiny if the future of medicine turns into bestowing meagre increments of unenjoyed life!

The close of my history thus suggests that medicine's finest hour is the dawn of its dilemmas. For centuries medicine was impotent and thus unproblematic. From the Greeks to the First World War, its tasks were simple: to grapple with lethal diseases and gross disabilities, to ensure live births and manage pain. It performed these with meagre success. Today, with 'mission accomplished', its triumphs are dissolving in disorientation. Medicine has led to inflated expectations, which the public eagerly swallowed. Yet as those expectations become unlimited, they are unfulfillable: medicine will have to redefine its limits even as it extends its capacities.

FURTHER READING

Every way of organizing a bibliography has its problems; every approach falls between many stools. I have chosen not to present a discursive essay or an annotated bibliography, for that would have duplicated the writings by Gert Brieger, Jonathon Erlen and others listed below in the Bibliography section. Instead I have gone for a series of lists, internally sub-divided and arranged in alphabetic order; this at least has the virtues of brevity, clarity and ease of reference.

I have divided what follows into two parts; first, works of a broad nature and, second, those relevant mainly to a particular chapter. To keep it within manageable proportions, I have stuck almost wholly to English-language sources and mostly omitted scholarly articles, because they are narrower and less accessible. For mention of such works, the footnotes and bibliographies of the books listed should be consulted, especially in the section on Bibliographies. I have set an asterisk (*) against works upon which I have drawn most heavily or which should be a high priority for all wishing to read further. What follows makes no pretence to comprehensiveness; it indicates works which I have found especially helpful and which contain fuller discussions of the materials all too briefly digested in the text.

Certain works are outstandingly valuable and must be mentioned now. There are articles on hundreds of diseases, their historical epidemiology and treatments in Kenneth F. Kiple (ed.), *The Cambridge World History of Human Disease*; these individual articles are not individually referred to below. Roderick E. McGrew's *Encyclopedia of Medical History* is a superb one-volume introduction, unfortunately out of print; the best single-volume medical work of reference is John Walton, Jeremiah A. Barondess and Stephen Lock (eds), *The Oxford Medical Companion*. Fine biographical articles on many of those discussed in this book can be found in the *Dictionary of Scientific Biography*, 16 vols, ed. C. C. Gillispie (New York: Scribner's, 1970–1980). Regrettably there is no thorough, scholarly, up-to-date dictionary of medical biography in English.

BIBLIOGRAPHIES AND HISTORIOGRAPHY

* Gert H. Brieger, 'History of Medicine', in Paul T. Durbin (ed.), *A Guide to the Culture of Science, Technology and Medicine* (New York: Free Press, 1980), 121–96

* Gert H. Brieger, 'The Historiography of Medicine', in W. F. Bynum and Roy Porter (eds), *Companion Encyclopedia of the History of Medicine* (London: Routledge, 1993), 24–44

Jonathon Erlen, *The History of the Health Care Sciences and Health Care 1700–1980: A Selective Annotated Bibliography* (New York: Garland Press, 1984)

Karl M. Figlio, 'The Historiography of Scientific Medicine: An Invitation to the Human Sciences', *Comparative Studies in Society and History*, xix (1977), 262–86

L. J. Jordanova, 'The Social Sciences and History of Science and Medicine', in P. Corsi and P. Weindling (eds), *Information Sources in the History of Science and Medicine* (London: Butterworth Scientific, 1983), 81–98

Christopher Lawrence, 'Democratic, Divine and Heroic: The History and Historiography of Surgery', in Christopher Lawrence (ed.), *Medical Theory, Surgical Practice: Studies in the History of Surgery* (London and New York: Routledge, 1992), 1–47

Leslie T. Morton, *A Medical Bibliography (Garrison and Morton): An Annotated Checklist of Texts Illustrating the History of Medicine*, 4th ed. (Aldershot, Hants: Gower, 1983)

Leslie T. Morton and Robert J. Moore, *A Bibliography of Medical and Biomedical Biography* (Aldershot: Scolar Press, 1989)

Margaret Pelling, 'Medicine Since 1500', in P. Corsi and P. Weindling (eds), *Information Sources in the History of Science and Medicine* (London: Butterworth Scientific, 1983), 379–407

Charles Webster, 'The Historiography of Medicine', in P. Corsi and P. Weindling (eds), *Information Sources in the History of Science and Medicine* (London: Butterworth Scientific, 1983), 29–43

Contemporary research in the history of medicine is comprehensively listed in: *Bibliography of the History of Medicine*, no. 1–28 (Bethesda, Md.: National Library of Medicine, 1965–1993)

Current Work in the History of Medicine. An International Bibliography, no. 1–173 (London: Wellcome Institute for the History of Medicine, 1954–1997). Quarterly. A cumulation of *Current Work*, plus most secondary literature of the twentieth century until 1977, is listed in Wellcome Institute for the History of Medicine, *Subject Catalogue of the History of Medicine*, 18 vols (subject section, 9 vols, biographical section, 5 vols,

topographical section, 4 vols), (Munich: Krays International, 1980).
The annual bibliographies published in the American history of science journal *Isis* contain generous listings of medical history. These have been collected
together up to the 1960s in Magda Whitrow (ed.), *Isis Cumulative Bibliography:
A Bibliography of the History of Science formed from Isis Critical Bibliographies
1–90, 1913–1965*, 3 vols (London: Mansell, 1971–76)

SURVEY HISTORIES AND TEXTBOOKS

* Erwin H. Ackerknecht, *A Short History of Medicine* (Baltimore: Johns
Hopkins University Press, 1968)

F. F. Cartwright, *A Social History of Medicine* (London: Longman, 1977)

* James H. Cassedy, *Medicine in America: A Short History* (Baltimore: Johns
Hopkins University Press, 1991)

Arturo Castiglioni, *A History of Medicine*, tr. and ed. by E. B. Krumbhaar
(New York: Alfred A. Knopf, 1941)

* Lawrence Conrad, Michael Neve, Vivian Nutton, Roy Porter and Andrew
Wear, *The Western Medical Tradition: 800BC to AD1800* (Cambridge:
Cambridge University Press, 1995)

* Nancy Duin, *A History of Medicine: From Prehistory to the Year 2020* (London
and New York: Simon and Schuster, 1992)

* Fielding H. Garrison, *An Introduction to the History of Medicine* (Philadelphia
and London: Saunders, 1917; and many subsequent editions)

Douglas Guthrie, *A History of Medicine* (London: Nelson, 1960)

Robert P. Hudson, *Disease and its Control: The Shaping of Modern Thought*
(Westport: Greenwood Press, 1983)

Irvine Loudon (ed.), *Western Medicine* (Oxford: Oxford University Press,
1997)

* Lois N. Magner, *A History of Medicine* (New York, Basel, Hong Kong:
Marcel Dekker, Inc., 1992)

Ralph H. Major, *A History of Medicine*, 2 vols (Springfield: Charles C. Thomas,
1954)

Max Neuburger, *History of Medicine*, tr. by Ernest Playfair, 2 vols (London:
H. Frowde, 1910–1925)

Roy Porter (ed.), *The Cambridge Illustrated History of Medicine* (Cambridge:
Cambridge University Press, 1996)

Philip Rhodes, *An Outline History of Medicine* (Sevenoaks: Butterworth, 1985)

Richard H. Shryock, *The Development of Modern Medicine: An Interpretation
of the Social and Scientific Factors* (2nd ed., New York: Alfred A. Knopf,
1947; reprinted, Madison, Wisc.: University of Wisconsin Press, 1980)

Henry E. Sigerist, *Civilization and Disease* (Ithaca: Cornell University Press,
1943; reprinted ed., Phoenix: University of Chicago Press, 1962)

Charles Singer and E. Ashworth Underwood, *A Short History of Medicine* (Oxford: Clarendon Press, 1928; 2nd ed., New York: Oxford University Press, 1962)

Jean-Charles Sournia, *The Illustrated History of Medicine* (London: Harold Starke, 1992)

Jean Starobinski, *A History of Medicine* (London: Prentice Hall, 1964)

Andrew Wear (ed.), *Medicine in Society: Historical Essays* (Cambridge: Cambridge University Press, 1992)

BROAD STUDIES COVERING MANY CENTURIES

E. H. Ackerknecht, *Therapeutics from the Primitives to the 20th Century. With an Appendix: The History of Dietetics* (New York: Hafner, 1973)

Philippe Ariès, *The Hour of Our Death* (London: Allen Lane, 1981)

Robert Baker, 'The History of Medical Ethics', in W. F. Bynum and Roy Porter (eds), *Companion Encyclopedia of the History of Medicine* (London: Routledge, 1993), 848–83

W. F. Bynum and Vivian Nutton (eds), *Theories of Fever from Antiquity to the Enlightenment* (London: *Medical History* Supplement 1, 1981)

W. F. Bynum and Roy Porter (eds), *Medicine and the Five Senses* (Cambridge: Cambridge University Press, 1993)

Johann Ludwig Choulant, *History and Bibliography of Anatomic Illustration*, tr. by Frank Mortimer (New York: Henry Schuman, 1945; revised ed. New York: Hafner, 1962)

J. D. Comrie, *History of Scottish Medicine*, 2nd ed., 2 vols (London: Wellcome Historical Medical Museum, 1932)

Harris L. Coulter, *Divided Legacy: A History of the Schism in Medical Thought*, 3 vols (Washington DC: Wehawken Book Company, 1973–1977)

Elizabeth Fee and Daniel M. Fox (eds), *AIDS: The Burdens of History* (Berkeley, Los Angeles and London: University of California Press, 1988)

Jacques Gélis, *History of Childbirth* (Oxford: Polity Press, 1991)

Sander Gilman, *Sexuality: An Illustrated History* (New York: Wiley, 1989)

Lindsay Granshaw and Roy Porter (eds), *The Hospital in History* (London and New York: Routledge, 1989)

Knut Haeger, *The Illustrated History of Surgery* (New York: Bell, 1988)

D. Hamilton, *The Healers: A History of Medicine in Scotland* (Edinburgh: Canongate, 1981)

John Hinnells and Roy Porter (eds), *Religion, Suffering and Healing* (London: Kegan Paul, 1998)

Norman E. Himes, *Medical History of Contraception* (Baltimore: Williams and Wilkins, 1936; New York: Schocken Books, 1970)

Dick Lawson, *The History of Orthopaedics: An Account of the Study and Practice of Orthopaedics from the Earliest Times to the Modern Era* (New Jersey: Parthenon, 1970)

C. D. Leake, *An Historical Account of Pharmacology to the 20th Century* (Springfield, Ill.: C. C. Thomas, 1975)

E. R. Long, *A History of Pathology* (New York: Dover Publications, 1965)

Angus McLaren, *A History of Contraception: From Antiquity to the Present Day* (Oxford: Blackwell, 1993)

Leslie G. Matthews, *History of Pharmacy in Britain* (Edinburgh & London: E. & S. Livingstone, 1962)

Max Neuberger, *The Doctrine of the Healing Power of Nature Throughout the Course of Time*, tr. by Linn J. Boyd (New York: [s.n.], 1943)

Ronald L. Numbers and D. W. Amundsen (eds), *Caring and Curing: Health and Medicine in the Western Religious Tradition* (New York: Macmillan, 1986)

Michael J. O'Dowd and Elliot E. Philipp, *The History of Obstetrics and Gynaecology* (New York and London: The Parthenon Publishing Group, 1994)

K. Pollak and E. A. Underwood, *The Healers: The Doctor Then and Now* (London: Nelson, 1968)

F. N. L. Poynter (ed.), *The Evolution of Pharmacy in Britain* (London: Pitman, 1965)

F. N. L. Poynter (ed.), *The Evolution of Medical Education in Britain* (London: Pitman, 1966)

Terence Ranger and Paul Slack (eds), *Epidemics and Ideas* (Cambridge: Cambridge University Press, 1992)

Stanley Joel Reiser, *Medicine and the Reign of Technology* (Cambridge: Cambridge University Press, 1981)

Roselyne Rey, *History of Pain*, tr. by Elliott Wallace and J. W. and S. W. Cadden (Paris: Éditions la Découverte, 1993)

K. B. Roberts and J. D. W. Tomlinson, *The Fabric of the Body: European Traditions of Anatomical Illustration* (Oxford and New York: Oxford University Press, 1992)

George Rosen, *A History of Public Health* (New York: MD Publications, 1958; new edition, ed. by Elizabeth Fee, with updated bibliography by Edward T. Morman, Baltimore: Johns Hopkins University Press, 1992)

George Rosen, *From Medical Police to Social Medicine: Essays on the History of Health Care* (New York: Science History Publications, 1974)

Charles E. Rosenberg and Janet Golden (eds), *Framing Disease: Studies in Cultural History* (New Brunswick, NJ; Rutgers University Press, 1992)

Karl E. Rothschuh, *History of Physiology*, tr. by G. B. Risse (Huntington, New York: Robert E. Krieger, 1973)

W. J. Sheils (ed.), *The Church and Healing* (Oxford: Basil Blackwell, 1982)

C. Singer, *A Short History of Anatomy and Physiology from the Greeks to Harvey* (New York: Dover, 1957)

Glenn Sonnedecker, *Kremer's and Urdang's History of Pharmacy* (Philadelphia: J. B. Lippincott Company, 1976)

Owsei Temkin, *The Double Face of Janus and Other Essays in the History of Medicine* (Baltimore & London: Johns Hopkins University Press, 1977)

J. D. Thompson and G. Goldin, *The Hospital: A Social and Architectural History* (New Haven & London: Yale University Press, 1975)

John L. Thornton, *Medical Books, Libraries and Collectors: A Study of Bibliography and the Book Trade in Relation to the Medical Sciences*, 2nd ed. (London: André Deutsch, 1966)

Michel Vovelle, *La mort et l'occident de 1300 à nos jours* (Paris: Gallimard, 1983)

Lise Wilkinson, *Animals and Disease: An Introduction to the History of Comparative Medicine* (Cambridge and New York: Cambridge University Press, 1992)

Maxwell M. Wintrobe (ed.), *Blood, Pure and Eloquent: A Story of Discovery, of People, and of Ideas* (New York: McGraw-Hill, 1980)

Leo M. Zimmerman and Ilza Veith, *Great Ideas in the History of Surgery*, 2nd ed. (New York: Dover, 1967)

WORKS OF REFERENCE

Jessica Bendiner and Elmer Bendiner, *Biographical Dictionary of Medicine* (New York: Facts on File, 1990)

W. F. Bynum and Roy Porter (eds), *Companion Encyclopedia of the History of Medicine* (London: Routledge, 1993)

John G. Howells and M. Livia Osborn, *A Reference Companion to the History of Abnormal Psychology*, 2 vols (London: Greenwood Press, 1984)

Kenneth F. Kiple (ed.), *The Cambridge World History of Human Disease* (Cambridge: Cambridge University Press, 1993)

H. O. Lancaster, *Expectations of Life: A Study in the Demography, Statistics, and History of World Mortality* (Berlin and New York: Springer-Verlag, 1990)

Roderick E. McGrew, *Encyclopedia of Medical History* (New York: McGraw-Hill, 1985)

Leslie T. Morton and Robert J. Moore, *A Chronology of Medicine and Related Sciences* (Aldershot: Scolar Press, 1997)

Alvin Rodin and Jack D. Key, *Medicine, Literature and Eponyms: An Encyclopedia of Medical Eponyms Derived from Literary Characters* (Malabar, Fla.: Robert E. Krieger Publishing, 1989)

John Walton, Jeremiah A. Barondess and Stephen Lock (eds), *The Oxford Medical Companion* (Oxford: Oxford University Press, 1994)

RELATED STUDIES, HISTORIES OF SCIENCE

Peter Bowler, *The Fontana History of the Environmental Sciences* (London: Fontana Press, 1992)

W. H. Brock, *The Fontana History of Chemistry* (London: Fontana Press, 1992)

Thomas S. Hall, *Ideas of Life and Matter: Studies in the History of General Physiology 600 BC to AD 1900*, 2 vols (Chicago: University of Chicago Press, 1969)

Lois N. Magner, *A History of the Life Sciences*, 2nd ed. (New York: M. Dekker, 1994)

Eric Nordenskiöld, *The History of Biology* (New York: Alfred A. Knopf, 1928)

R. C. Olby, G. N. Cantor, J. R. R. Christie and M. J. S. Hodge (eds), *Companion to the History of Modern Science* (London: Routledge, 1989)

Roger Smith, *The Fontana History of the Human Sciences* (London: Fontana, 1997)

CONCEPTS OF DISEASE

David Armstrong, 'Medical Sociology', in W. F. Bynum and Roy Porter (eds), *Companion Encyclopedia of the History of Medicine* (London: Routledge, 1993), 1631–52

W. R. Arney and B. J. Bergen, *Medicine and the Management of Living: Taming the Last Great Beast* (Chicago and London: University of Chicago Press, 1985)

Claude Bernard, *Introduction to the Study of Experimental Medicine*, tr. by Henry Greene (New York: Copley, 1957)

Nick Black *et al.* (eds), *Health and Disease: A Reader* (Milton Keynes: Open University Press, 1984)

A. L. Caplan, 'The Concepts of Health, Illness, and Disease', in W. F. Bynum and Roy Porter (eds), *Companion Encyclopedia of the History of Medicine* (London: Routledge, 1993), 233–48

A. L. Caplan, H. T. Engelhardt, and J. J. MacCartney (eds), *Concepts of Health and Disease* (Reading, Mass.: Addison-Wesley, 1981)

Henry Cohen, 'The Evolution of the Concept of Disease', in B. Lush (ed.), *Concepts of Medicine* (Oxford: Pergamon Press, 1961), 159–69

Caroline Currer and Meg Stacey, *Concepts of Health, Illness and Disease: A Comparative Perspective* (Leamington Spa: Berg, 1986)

Mary Douglas, *Purity and Danger: An Analysis of Concepts of Pollution and Taboo* (Harmondsworth: Penguin, 1966)

René Dubos, *The Mirage of Health* (New York: Harper, 1959).

H. Tristram Engelhardt, Jr, 'The Concepts of Health and Disease', in H. Tristram Engelhardt and Stuart F. Spicker (eds), *Evaluation and Explanation in the Biomedical Sciences* (Dordrecht: Reidel, 1975), 125–141

P. Lain Entralgo, *Doctor and Patient*, tr. by Frances Partridge (London: Weidenfeld & Nicolson, 1969)

Pédro Lain Entralgo, *The Therapy of the Word in Classical Antiquity*, ed. and tr. by L. J. Rather and John M. Sharp (New Haven: Yale University Press, 1970)

Uta Gerhardt, *Ideas about Illness: An Intellectual and Political History of Medical Sociology* (New York: New York University Press, 1989)

Sander L. Gilman, *Difference and Pathology* (Ithaca and London: Cornell University Press, 1985)

Sander L. Gilman, *Disease and Representation. From Madness to AIDS* (Ithaca: Cornell University Press, 1988)

K. Keele, *Anatomies of Pain* (Oxford: Blackwell Scientific Publications, 1957)

David Mechanic, 'The Concept of Illness Behavior', *Journal of Chronic Diseases*, xv (1962), 189–194

Ronald L. Numbers and Darrel W. Amundsen (eds), *Caring and Curing. Health and Medicine in the Western Medical Traditions* (New York: Macmillan, 1986)

Talcott Parsons, 'Definitions of Health and Illness in the Light of American Values and Social Structure', in E. Gartley Jaco (ed.), *Patients, Physician and Illness* (Glencoe, Ill.: Free Press, 1958), 165–187

L. J. Rather, 'Towards a Philosophical Study of the Idea of Disease', in Chandler McC. Brooks and Paul F. Cranefield (eds), *The Historical Development of Physiological Thought* (New York: Hafner, 1959), 351–73

Walther Riese, *The Conception of Disease, its History, its Versions and its Nature* (New York: Philosophical Library, 1953)

G. Risse, 'Health and Disease: History of the Concepts', in W. T. Reich (ed.), *Encyclopedia of Bioethics*, 4 vols (New York: Free Press, 1978), ii, 579–85

Oliver Sacks, *Awakenings* (Harmondsworth: Penguin, 1976)

Oliver Sacks, *Migraine: Evolution of a Common Disorder* (London: Pan Books, 1981)

Oliver Sacks, *A Leg to Stand On* (London: Duckworth, 1984)

Oliver Sacks, *The Man Who Mistook His Wife for a Hat* (London: Duckworth, 1985)

Susan Sontag, *Illness as Metaphor* (New York: Farrar, Straus & Giroux, 1978; London: Allen Lane, 1979)

Susan Sontag, *AIDS as Metaphor* (Harmondsworth: Allen Lane, 1989)

F. Kräupl Taylor, *The Concepts of Illness, Disease and Morbus* (Cambridge: Cambridge University Press, 1979)

Owsei Temkin, 'The Scientific Approach to Disease: Specific Entity and Individual Sickness', in A. C. Crombie (ed.), *Scientific Change* (London: Heinemann, 1961), 629–647

Bryan S. Turner, *Medical Power and Social Knowledge* (London and Beverly Hills: Sage Publications, 1987)

ANTHOLOGIES, LITERATURE AND CULTURE

Ann G. Carmichael and Richard M. Ratzan (eds), *Medicine: A Treasury of Art and Literature* (New York: Beaux Arts, 1991)

D. J. Enright (ed.), *The Faber Book of Fevers and Frets* (London: Faber, 1989)

Richard Gordon, *The Literary Companion to Medicine: An Anthology of Prose and Poetry* (London: Sinclair-Stevenson, 1993)

Joanne Trautmann and Carol Pollard (comp.), *Literature and Medicine: Topics, Titles and Notes* (Philadelphia: Society for Health and Human Values, 1975)

N. Cousins, *The Physician in Literature* (Philadelphia: Saunders Press, 1982)

Michael Neve, 'Medicine and Literature', in W. F. Bynum and Roy Porter (eds), *Companion Encyclopedia of the History of Medicine* (London: Routledge, 1993), 1510–25

G. S. Rousseau, *Enlightenment Crossings: Pre- and Post-Modern Discourses: Anthropological* (Manchester: Manchester University Press, 1991)

G. S. Rousseau, *Perilous Enlightenment: Pre- and Post-Modern Discourses: Sexual, Historical* (Manchester: Manchester University Press, 1991)

G. S. Rousseau, *Enlightenment Borders: Pre- and Post-Modern Discourses: Medical, Scientific* (Manchester: Manchester University Press, 1991)

GENERAL HISTORIES

Wide Surveys

J. M. Roberts, *History of the World* (Oxford: Oxford University Press, 1994)

Norman Davies, *Europe: A History* (Oxford: Oxford University Press 1996)

Intellectual and Cultural Histories of the West

Philippe Ariès and Georges Duby (general eds), *A History of Private Life*, vol. i, *From Pagan Rome to Byzantium*; ed. P. Veyne, trans. Arthur Goldhammer (Cambridge, Mass.: The Belknap Press, 1987); vol. ii, *Revelations of the Medieval World*, ed. George Duby, trans. Arthur Goldhammer (Cambridge, Mass.: The Belknap Press, 1988); vol. iii, *Passions of the Renaissance*, ed. Roger Chartier, trans. Arthur Goldhammer (Cambridge, Mass.: The Belknap Press, 1989); vol. iv, *From the Fires of Revolution to the Great*

War, ed. Michelle Perrot, trans. Arthur Goldhammer (Cambridge, Mass.: The Belknap Press, 1990); vol. v, *Riddles of Identity in Modern Times*, eds. Antoine Prost and Gerard Vincent, trans. Arthur Goldhammer (Cambridge, Mass.: The Belknap Press, 1991)

William Barrett, *Death of the Soul. Philosophical Thought from Descartes to the Computer* (Oxford: Oxford University Press, 1987)

Jacob Burckhardt, *The Civilization of the Renaissance in Italy* (Oxford: Phaidon, 1981; first edition, 1859)

Ian Burkitt, 'The Shifting Concept of the Self', *History of the Human Sciences*, vii, (1994), 7–28

Michael Carrithers, Steven Collins and Steven Lukes (eds), *The Category of the Person* (Cambridge: Cambridge University Press, 1985)

S. D. Cox, *'The Stranger Within Thee': The Concept of the Self in Late Eighteenth Century Literature* (Pittsburgh: Pittsburgh University Press, 1980)

Norbert Elias, *The Civilizing Process*, vol. 1, *The History of Manners* (New York: Pantheon, 1978); vol. 2, *Power and Civility* (New York: Pantheon, 1982); vol. 3, *The Court Society* (New York: Pantheon, 1983)

Michel Foucault, *The Order of Things: An Archaeology of the Human Sciences* (London: Tavistock, 1970)

Michel Foucault, *The Archaeology of Knowledge*, trans. by A. M. Sheridan Smith (London: Tavistock, 1972)

Michel Foucault, *Histoire de la sexualité*: vol. 1, *La volonté de savoir* (Paris: Gallimard, 1976); trans. Robert Hurley, *The History of Sexuality: Introduction* (London: Allen Lane, 1978; New York: Vintage Books, 1985)

Stephen Greenblatt, *Renaissance Self-Fashioning: From More to Shakespeare* (Chicago: University of Chicago Press, 1980)

Christopher Lasch, *The Culture of Narcissism: American Life in an Age of Diminishing Expectations* (New York: Norton, 1979)

Stephen Lukes, *Individualism* (Oxford: Basil Blackwell, 1973)

Lois McNay, *Foucault and Feminism: Power, Gender and the Self* (Cambridge: Polity, 1992)

John N. Morris, *Versions of the Self: Studies in English Autobiography from John Bunyan to John Stuart Mill* (New York: Basic Books, 1966)

Camille Paglia, *Sexual Personae* (London and New Haven: Yale University Press, 1990)

John Passmore, *The Perfectibility of Man* (London: Duckworth, 1968)

Anthony Smith, *Software for the Self: Culture and Technology* (London: Faber, 1996)

Patricia Meyer Spacks, *Imagining a Self: Autobiography and Novel in Eighteenth Century England* (Cambridge, Mass.: Harvard University Press, 1976)

C. Taylor, *Sources of the Self. The Making of Modern Identity* (Cambridge: Cambridge University Press, 1989)

CHAPTER II: THE ROOTS OF MEDICINE

Disease and History

Erwin H. Ackerknecht, *History and Geography of the Most Important Diseases* (New York: Hafner, 1965)

D. R. Brothwell and A. T. Sandison (eds), *Diseases in Antiquity. A Survey of the Diseases, Injuries and Surgery of Ancient Populations* (Springfield, Ill.: Charles C. Thomas, 1967)

Sir Macfarlane Burnet, *Natural History of Infectious Disease*, 3rd ed. (Cambridge: Cambridge University Press, 1962)

Frederick F. Cartwright, *Disease and History* (New York: Thomas Y. Crowell, 1972)

Aidan Cockburn and Eve Cockburn, *Mummies, Disease, and Ancient Cultures* (Cambridge and New York: Cambridge University Press, 1980)

Mark Nathan Cohen, *Health and the Rise of Civilization* (New Haven; London: Yale University Press, 1989)

C. Creighton, *A History of Epidemics in Britain: with Additional Material by D. E. C. Eversley (and others)*, 2nd ed. (London: Cambridge University Press, 1965)

* Alfred W. Crosby, *The Columbian Exchange, Biological and Cultural Consequences of 1492* (Westport, CT: Greenwood Press, 1972)

Jared Diamond, *Guns, Germs and Steel: The Fates of Human Societies* (London: Random House, 1997)

D. Hopkins, *Princes and Peasants: Smallpox in History* (Chicago: University of Chicago Press, 1983)

A. B. Janetta, *Epidemics and Mortality in Early Modern Japan* (Princeton: Princeton University Press, 1987)

Arno Karlen, *Man and Microbes. Diseases and Plagues in History and Modern Times* (New York: Tarcher/Putnam 1995)

* Kenneth F. Kiple (ed.), *The Cambridge World History of Human Disease* (Cambridge: Cambridge University Press, 1993)

* Kenneth F. Kiple, 'The Ecology of Disease', in W. F. Bynum and Roy Porter (eds), *Companion Encyclopedia of the History of Medicine* (London: Routledge, 1993), 357–81

Richard Lee, *The !Kung San: Men, Women and Work in a Foraging Society* (Cambridge: Cambridge University Press, 1979)

Thomas McKeown, *The Origins of Human Disease* (Oxford: Basil Blackwell 1988)

* W. H. McNeill, *Plagues and Peoples* (Oxford: Anchor Press, 1976)

Randolph M. Nesse and George C. Williams, *Evolution and Healing. The New Science of Darwinian Medicine* (London: Weidenfeld and Nicolson, 1995)

Claude Quétel, *History of Syphilis* (Oxford: Polity Press, 1990)

Calvin Wells, *Bones, Bodies, and Disease: Evidence of Disease and Abnormality in Early Man* (New York: Frederick A. Praeger, 1964)

H. Zinsser, *Rats, Lice and History* (Boston, Mass.: Atlantic Monthly Press, Little, Brown & Co, 1935)

Ideas of Illness, Healers and Healing

W. G. Black, *Folk Medicine: A Chapter in the History of Culture* (London: Folklore Society, 1883)

Marcelle Bouteiller, *Médecine populaire d'hier et d'aujourd'hui* (Paris: Ed. G. P. Maisonneuve and Larose, 1966)

E. E. Evans-Pritchard, *Witchcraft, Oracles and Magic Among the Azande* (Oxford: Clarendon Press, 1937)

Wayland D. Hand (ed.), *American Folk Medicine: A Symposium* (Berkeley, CA: University of California Press, 1976)

Wayland D. Hand, *Magical Medicine; The Folkloric Component of Medicine in the Folk Belief, Custom, and Ritual of the Peoples of Europe and America* (Berkeley, CA: University of California Press, 1980)

C. Helman, '"Feed a Cold, Starve a Fever": Folk Models of Infection in an English Suburban Community, and Their Relation to Medical Treatment', *Culture, Medicine and Psychiatry*, ii, (1978), 107–37

* C. Helman, *Culture, Health and Illness* (Bristol: Wright, 1984)

A. Kleinman, *Patients and Healers in the Context of Culture: An Exploration of the Borderline between Anthropology, Medicine, and Psychiatry* (Berkeley, CA: University of California Press, 1980)

* Murray Last, 'Non-Western Concepts of Disease', in W. F. Bynum and Roy Porter (eds), *Companion Encyclopedia of the History of Medicine* (London: Routledge, 1993), 634–60

Françoise Loux, *Sagesse du corps: Santé et maladie dans les proverbes régionaux français* (Paris: Maisonneuve et Larose, 1978)

Françoise Loux, *Pratiques et savoirs populaires: Le corps dans la société traditionnelle* (Paris: Berger-Levrault, 1979)

* Françoise Loux, 'Popular Culture and Knowledge of the Body: Infancy and the Medical Anthropologists', in Roy Porter and Andrew Wear (eds), *Problems and Methods in the History of Medicine* (London: Croom Helm, 1988), 81–97

* Françoise Loux, 'Folk Medicine', in W. F. Bynum and Roy Porter (eds), *Companion Encyclopedia of the History of Medicine* (London: Routledge, 1993), 661–75

Carol MacCormack, 'Medicine and Anthropology', in W. F. Bynum and Roy Porter (eds), *Companion Encyclopedia of the History of Medicine* (London: Routledge, 1993), 1427–39

Ann McElroy and Patricia Townsend, *Medical Anthropology in Ecological Perspective* (North Scituate, Massachusetts: Duxbury, 1979)

Richard P. Steiner (ed.), *Folk Medicine. The Art and the Science* (Washington, DC: American Chemical Society, 1988)

Virgil H. J. Vogel, *American Indian Medicine* (Norman, OK: University of Oklahoma Press, 1970)

CHAPTER III: ANTIQUITY

Before the Greeks

D. R. Brothwell and B. A. Chiarelli (eds), *Population Biology of the Ancient Egyptians* (New York: Academic Press, 1973)

Rosalie David (ed.), *Mysteries of the Mummies. The Story of the Unwrapping of a 2000-Year-Old Mummy by a Team of Experts* (New York: Scribner, 1970)

B. Ebbell, *The Papyrus Ebers: The Greatest Egyptian Medical Document* (Copenhagen: Levin and Munksgaard, 1937)

J. Worth Estes, *The Medical Skills of Ancient Egypt* (Canton, MA: Science History Publications, 1989)

Carole Reeves, *Egyptian Medicine* (Princes Risborough, Bucks: Shire Publications, 1992)

J. B. de C. M. Saunders, *The Transition from Ancient Egyptian to Greek Medicine* (Lawrence, KS: University of Kansas Press, 1963)

Henry E. Sigerist, *A History of Medicine*, vol. I, *Primitive and Archaic Medicine* (New York: Oxford University Press, 1951)

Greek Medicine

J. Barnes, *The Presocratic Philosophers*, 2 vols (London: Routledge, 1979)

E. R. Dodds, *The Greeks and the Irrational* (Berkeley, CA: University of California Press, 1951)

Emma Edelstein and Ludwig Edelstein, *Asclepius: A Collection and Interpretation of the Testimonies* (Baltimore: Johns Hopkins University Press, 1945)

Ludwig Edelstein, *Ancient Medicine*, Owsei Temkin and C. Lilian Temkin (eds) (Baltimore: Johns Hopkins University Press, 1967)

P. Lain Entralgo, *The Therapy of the Word in Classical Antiquity*, ed. and tr. by L. J. Rather and John M. Sharp (New Haven: Yale University Press, 1970)

D. J. Furley and J. S. Wilkie, *Galen on Respiration and the Arteries* (Princeton: Princeton University Press, 1984)

Mirko D. Grmek, *Diseases in the Ancient Greek World* (Baltimore: Johns Hopkins University Press, 1991)

Charles R. S. Harris, *The Heart and the Vascular System in Ancient Greek Medicine from Alcmaeon to Galen* (Oxford: Clarendon Press, 1973)

W. H. S. Jones, *Malaria and Greek History* (London: Manchester University Press, 1909)

W. H. S. Jones, *The Doctor's Oath. An Essay in the History of Medicine* (Cambridge: Cambridge University Press, 1924)

G. S. Kirk, J. E. Raven, M. Schofield, *The Presocratic Philosophers*, 2nd ed. (Cambridge: Cambridge University Press, 1983)

G. E. R. Lloyd (ed.), *Hippocratic Writings* (Harmondsworth: Penguin, 1978)

G. E. R. Lloyd, *Science, Folklore, and Ideology* (Cambridge: Cambridge University Press, 1983)

James N. Longrigg, 'The Plague of Athens', *History of Science*, xviii (1980), 209–225

James N. Longrigg, *Greek Rational Medicine* (London: Routledge, 1993)

Vivian Nutton, 'Beyond the Hippocratic Oath', in R. Parker (ed.), *Miasma: Pollution and Purification in Early Greek Religion* (Oxford: Clarendon Press, 1983)

* V. Nutton, 'Humoralism', in W. F. Bynum and Roy Porter (eds), *Companion Encyclopedia of the History of Medicine* (London: Routledge, 1993), 281–91

* E. D. Phillips, *Greek Medicine* (London: Thames and Hudson, 1973)

P. Potter, *A Short Handbook of Hippocratic Medicine* (Québec: Les Éditions du Sphinx, 1988)

Henry E. Sigerist, *A History of Medicine*, vol. II, *Early Greek, Hindu and Persian Medicine* (New York: Oxford University Press, 1961)

B. Simon, *Mind and Madness in Ancient Greece. The Classical Roots of Modern Psychiatry* (Ithaca and London: Cornell University Press, 1978)

Wesley D. Smith, *The Hippocratic Tradition* (Ithaca, NY: Cornell University Press, 1979)

Heinrich von Staden, *Herophilus: The Art of Medicine in Early Alexandria* (New York: Cambridge University Press, 1989)

Roman Medicine
Clifford Allbutt, *Greek Medicine in Rome* (London: Macmillan, 1921)

Peter Brain, *Galen on Bloodletting* (New York: Cambridge University Press, 1986)

* Ralph Jackson, *Doctors and Disease in the Roman Empire* (Norman, OK: University of Oklahoma Press, 1988)

Fridolf Kudlien and Richard J. Durling (eds), *Galen's Method of Healing*, Proceedings of the 1982 Galen Symposium (New York: E. J. Brill, 1990)

M. T. May, *Galen on the Usefulness of the Parts of the Body* (Ithaca: Cornell University Press, 1968)

Vivian Nutton, *Galen, On Prognosis* (Berlin: Akademie Verlag, 1979)

* Vivian Nutton (ed.), *Galen: Problems and Prospects* (London: Wellcome Institute for the History of Medicine, 1981)

Vivian Nutton, *From Democedes to Harvey* (London: Variorum, 1988)

John M. Riddle, *Dioscorides on Pharmacy and Medicine* (Austin, TX: University of Texas Press, 1985)

A. Rousselle, *Porneia: On Desire and the Body in Antiquity* (Oxford: Basil Blackwell, 1988)

John Scarborough, *Roman Medicine* (Ithaca, NY: Cornell University Press, 1969)

* Owsei Temkin, *Galenism: Rise and Decline of a Medical Philosophy* (Ithaca, NY: Cornell University Press, 1973)

Gilbert Watson, *Theriac and Mithridatium: A Study in Therapeutics* (London: The Wellcome Historical Medical Library, 1966)

CHAPTER IV: MEDICINE AND FAITH

Late Antiquity and Early Medieval

Nigel Allen, 'Hospice to Hospital in the Near East', *Bulletin of the History of Medicine*, lxiv (1990), 446–462

Wilfred Bonser, *The Medical Background of Anglo-Saxon England: A Study in History, Psychology and Folklore* (London: Wellcome Historical Medical Library, 1963)

Peter Brown, *Society and the Holy in Late Antiquity* (Berkeley, CA: University of California Press, 1982)

Peter Brown, *The Body and Society* (New York: Columbia University Press, 1988)

Peter Brown, *The Cult of the Saints. Its Rise and Function in Latin Christianity* (Chicago: Chicago University Press, 1980)

M. I. Cameron, *Anglo-Saxon Medicine* (Cambridge: Cambridge University Press, 1993)

T. O. Cockayne (ed.), *Leechdoms. Wortcunning and Starcraft of Early England: Being a Collection of Documents*, i and ii, (London: Holland Press, 1961; originally published 1864–65)

P. Horden, 'The Byzantine Welfare State: Image and Reality', *Society of the Social History of Medicine Bulletin*, xxxvii (1985), 7–10

R. Lane-Fox, *Pagans and Christians* (Harmondsworth: Viking, 1986)

L. C. MacKinney, *Early Medieval Medicine* (Baltimore: Johns Hopkins University Press, 1937)

T. S. Miller, *The Birth of the Hospital in the Byzantine Empire* (Baltimore: Johns Hopkins University Press, 1985)

Vivian Nutton, *From Democedes to Harvey* (London: Variorum Reprints, 1988)

* K. Park, 'Medicine and Society in Medieval Europe, 500–1500', in Andrew Wear (ed.), *Medicine in Society: Historical Essays* (Cambridge: Cambridge University Press, 1992), 59–90

Julius Preuss, *Biblical and Talmudic Medicine*, tr. by Fred Rosner (New York: Sanhedrin Press, 1978)

J. Scarborough (ed.), *Symposium on Byzantine Medicine, Dumbarton Oaks Papers*, 38 (Washington DC: Dumbarton Oaks Research Library and Collection, 1985)

* O. Temkin, *Hippocrates in a World of Pagans and Christians* (Baltimore: Johns Hopkins University Press, 1992)

Islam

Albucasis on Surgery and Instruments, tr. by M. S. Spink and G. L. Lewis (Berkeley, CA: University of California Press, 1973)

* L. I. Conrad, 'Arab-Islamic Medicine', in W. F. Bynum and Roy Porter (eds), *Companion Encyclopedia of the History of Medicine* (London: Routledge, 1993), 676–727

Michael W. Dols, *The Black Death in the Middle East* (Princeton, NJ: Princeton University Press, 1977)

* Michael W. Dols, 'Diseases of the Islamic World', in Kenneth F. Kiple (ed.), *The Cambridge World History of Human Disease* (Cambridge: Cambridge University Press, 1993), 334–41

* Nancy E. Gallagher, 'Islamic and Indian Medicine', in Kenneth F. Kiple (ed.), *The Cambridge World History of Human Disease* (Cambridge: Cambridge University Press, 1993), 27–34

M. S. Khan, *Islamic Medicine* (London: Routledge & Kegan Paul, 1986)

Martin Levey, *Early Arabic Pharmacology: An Introduction Based on Ancient and Medieval Sources* (Leiden: E. J. Brill, 1973)

Fazlur Rahman, *Health and Medicine in the Islamic Tradition: Change and Identity* (New York: Crossroad, 1987)

M. Ullman, *Islamic Medicine* (Edinburgh: Edinburgh University Press, 1978)

Faith Wallis, 'The Experience of the Book: Manuscripts, Texts, and the Role of Epistemology in the Early Medieval Medicine', in Don Bates (ed.), *Knowledge and the Scholarly Medical Traditions* (Cambridge: Cambridge University Press, 1995), 101–126

W. M. Watt, *The Influence of Islam upon Medieval Europe* (Edinburgh: Edinburgh University Press, 1973)

G. M. Wickens (ed.), *Avicenna: Scientist and Philosopher, A Millenary Symposium* (London: Luzac, 1952)

CHAPTER V: THE MEDIEVAL WEST

Luis Garcia Ballester, Roger French, Jon Arrizabalaga and Andrew Cunningham, *Practical Medicine from Salerno to the Black Death* (New York: Cambridge University Press, 1994)

J.-N. Biraben, *Les hommes et la peste en France et dans les pays européens et méditerranéens*, 2 vols (Paris: Mouton, 1975)

T. S. R. Boase, *Death in the Middle Ages: Mortality, Judgement and Remembrance* (New York: McGraw-Hill, 1972)

Saul Nathaniel Brody, *The Disease of the Soul: Leprosy in Medieval Literature* (Ithaca, NY: Cornell University Press, 1974)

Sabina Flanagan, *Hildegard of Bingen, 1098–1179: A Visionary Life* (New York: Routledge, 1989)

Robert S. Gottfried, *The Black Death: Natural and Human Disaster in Medieval Europe* (New York: Free Press, 1983)

John Henderson, *Piety and Charity in Late Medieval Florence* (Oxford: Oxford University Press, 1994)

Tony Hunt, *Popular Medicine in Thirteenth-Century England* (Cambridge: D. S. Brewer, 1990)

S. Danielle Jacquart and Claude Thomasset, *Sexuality and Medicine in the Middle Ages* (Cambridge: Polity Press, 1989)

Brian Lawn, *The Salernitan Questions: An Introduction to the History of Medieval and Renaissance Problem Literature* (Oxford: Oxford University Press, 1963)

Ghislaine Lawrence, 'Surgery (Traditional)', in W. F. Bynum and Roy Porter (eds), *Companion Encyclopedia of the History of Medicine* (London: Routledge, 1993), 957–79

Michael R. McVaugh, *Medicine Before the Plague: Practitioners and their Patients in the Crown of Aragon, 1285–1345* (Cambridge: Cambridge University Press, 1993)

Julian Obermann (ed.), *The Code of Maimonides: Book Ten, the Book of Cleanness*, tr. by H. Danby (New Haven, CT: Yale University Press, 1954)

Nicholas Orme and Margaret Webster, *The English Hospital, 1070–1570* (New Haven and London: Yale University Press, 1995)

* Katherine Park, *Doctors and Medicine in Early Renaissance Florence* (Princeton, NJ: Princeton University Press, 1985)

Katharine Park, 'Black Death', in Kenneth F. Kiple (ed.), *The Cambridge World History of Human Disease* (Cambridge: Cambridge University Press, 1993), 612–15

Pierre J. Payer, *The Bridling of Desire: Views of Sex in the Later Middle Ages* (Toronto: Toronto University Press, 1993)

Marie-Christine Pouchelle, *The Body and Surgery in the Middle Ages*, tr. by Rosemary Morris (New Brunswick: Rutgers University Press, 1990; Cambridge: Polity Press, 1990)

Peter Richards, *The Medieval Leper and His Northern Heirs* (Cambridge: D. S. Brewer, 1977)

John M. Riddle, *Contraception and Abortion from the Ancient World to the Renaissance* (Cambridge, Mass./London: Harvard University Press, 1992)

Fred Rosner, *Medicine in the Mishneh Torah of Maimonides* (New York: KTAV, 1984)

Beryl Rowland (ed. and trans.), *Medieval Woman's Guide to Health* (London: Croom Helm, 1981)

Elizabeth Sears, *The Ages of Man. Medieval Interpretation of the Life Cycle* (Princeton: Princeton University Press, 1986)

* Nancy G. Siraisi, *Medieval & Early Renaissance Medicine: An Introduction to Knowledge and Practice* (Chicago and London: Chicago University Press, 1990)

* Charles H. Talbot, *Medicine in Medieval England* (London: Oldbourne; New York: American Elsevier, 1967)

Philip Ziegler, *The Black Death* (New York: Harper Torchbooks, 1969)

CHAPTER VI: INDIAN MEDICINE

F. U. Baquai, *Traditional Medicine in Pakistan* (Karachi: Hamdard Foundation, 1977)

S. L. Bhatia, *Medical Science in Ancient India* (Bangalore: Bangalore University, 1972)

Caraka, *Agnivesa's Caraka Samhita*, tr. by Ram Karan Sharma and Vaidya Bhagwan Dash (Varanasi, India: Chowkhamba Sanskrit Series Office, 1976)

* Nancy E. Gallagher, 'Islamic and Indian Medicine', in Kenneth F. Kiple (ed.), *The Cambridge World History of Human Disease* (Cambridge: Cambridge University Press, 1993), 27–34

Girindranath Mukhopadhyaya, *History of Indian Medicine*, 3 vols (Calcutta: University of Calcutta Press, 1923–29)

P. Ray, H. Gupta and Mira Roy, *Susruta Samhita: A Scientific Synopsis* (New Delhi: Indian Science Academy, 1980)

* Dominik Wujastyk, 'Indian Medicine', in W. F. Bynum and Roy Porter (eds), *Companion Encyclopedia of the History of Medicine* (London: Routledge, 1993), 755–78

Kenneth G. Zysk, *Religious Healing in the Vedas* (Philadelphia: The American Philosophical Society, 1985)

CHAPTER VII: CHINESE MEDICINE

John Z. Bowers, *When the Twain Meet: The Rise of Western Medicine in Japan* (Baltimore, MD: Johns Hopkins University Press, 1981)

John Z. Bowers, J. W. Hess and Nathan Sivin (eds), *Science and Medicine in*

Twentieth-Century China (Ann Arbor, MI: University of Michigan Press, 1989)

* Francesca Bray, 'Chinese Medicine', in W. F. Bynum and Roy Porter (eds), *Companion Encyclopedia of the History of Medicine* (London: Routledge, 1993), 728–54

* Lu Gwei-Djen and Joseph Needham, 'Diseases of Antiquity in China', in Kenneth F. Kiple (ed.), *The Cambridge World History of Human Disease* (Cambridge: Cambridge University Press, 1993), 345–53

Lu Gwei-Djen and Joseph Needham, *Celestial Lances. A History and Rationale of Acupuncture and Moxa* (Cambridge: Cambridge University Press, 1980)

* Dominique Hoizey, *A History of Chinese Medicine* (Edinburgh: Edinburgh University Press, 1993)

* A. Kleinman, *Social Origins of Distress and Disease: Depression, Neurasthenia, and Pain in Modern China* (New Haven, Conn.: Yale University Press, 1986)

M. Porkert, *The Theoretical Foundations of Chinese Medicine: System of Correspondence* (Cambridge, Mass.: MIT Press, 1974)

* Manfred Porkert and Christian Ullmann, *Chinese Medicine: Its History, Philosophy and Practice* (New York: William Morrow, 1988)

* Nathan Sivin (ed.), *Traditional Medicine in Contemporary China* (Ann Arbor, MI: University of Michigan Press, 1987)

Nathan Sivin, 'Text and Experience in Classical Chinese Medicine', in Don Bates (ed.), *Knowledge and the Scholarly Medical Traditions* (Cambridge: Cambridge University Press, 1995), 177–204

Margaret Trawick, 'Writing the Body and Ruling the Land: Western Reflections on Chinese and Indian Medicine', in Don Bates (ed.), *Knowledge and the Scholarly Medical Traditions* (Cambridge: Cambridge University Press, 1995), 279–319

* Paul U. Unschuld, 'History of Chinese Medicine', in Kenneth F. Kiple (ed.), *The Cambridge World History of Human Disease* (Cambridge: Cambridge University Press, 1993), 20–26

Paul U. Unschuld, *Medicine in China: A History of Ideas* (Berkeley: University of California Press, 1985)

I. Veith, introduction and translation, *The Yellow Emperor's Classic of Internal Medicine* (Berkeley: University of California Press, 1972)

CHAPTER VIII: RENAISSANCE

Disease and Society

* Jon Arrizabalaga, John Henderson, and Roger French, *The Great Pox: The French Disease in Renaissance Europe* (New Haven: Yale University Press, 1997)

P. M. Ashburn, *The Ranks of Death: A Medical History of the Conquest of America* (New York: Coward-McCann, 1947)

Jane E. Buikstra, 'Diseases of the Pre-Columbian Americas', in Kenneth F. Kiple (ed.), *The Cambridge World History of Human Disease* (Cambridge: Cambridge University Press, 1993), 305–17

* Ann G. Carmichael, *Plague and the Poor in Renaissance Florence* (Cambridge and New York: Cambridge University Press, 1986)

Carlo Cipolla, *Public Health and the Medical Profession in the Renaissance* (Cambridge: Cambridge University Press, 1976)

Carlo Cipolla, *Faith, Reason and the Plague in Seventeenth Century Tuscany* (Ithaca: Cornell University Press, 1979)

* Alfred W. Crosby, *Ecological Imperialism: The Biological Expansion of Europe, 900–1900* (New York: Cambridge University Press, 1986)

Brian Pullan, *Rich and Poor in Renaissance Venice* (Oxford: Blackwell, 1971)

Ann Ramenofsky, 'Diseases of the Americas, 1492–1700', in Kenneth F. Kiple (ed.), *The Cambridge World History of Human Disease* (Cambridge: Cambridge University Press, 1993), 317–27

* Paul Slack, *The Impact of Plague in Tudor and Stuart England* (London: Routledge & Kegan Paul, 1985)

Paul Slack, *Poverty and Policy in Tudor and Stuart England* (London: Longman, 1988)

John Walter and Roger Schofield (eds), *Famine, Disease and the Social Order in Early Modern Society* (Cambridge: Cambridge University Press, 1989)

Medicine

Agnes Arber, *Herbals*, 3rd ed. (Cambridge: Cambridge University Press, 1986)

Allen G. Debus, *Man and Nature in the Renaissance* (New York: Cambridge University Press, 1978)

Clifford Foust, *Rhubarb. The Wondrous Drug* (Princeton: Princeton University Press, 1992)

Roger French, 'The Anatomical Tradition', in W. F. Bynum and Roy Porter (eds), *Companion Encyclopedia of the History of Medicine* (London: Routledge, 1993), 81–101

Ole Grell and Andrew Cunningham (eds), *Medicine and the Reformation* (London: Routledge, 1993)

Martin Kemp, *Leonardo da Vinci, The Marvellous Works of Nature and Man* (London: J. M. Dent, 1981)

* C. D. O'Malley, *Andreas Vesalius of Brussels 1514–1564* (California: University of California Press, 1964)

* C. D. O'Malley and J. B. de C. M. Saunders (eds), *Leonardo da Vinci on the Human Body* (New York: Schuman, 1952)

* Ambroise Paré, *Ten Books of Surgery*, tr. by R. W. Linker and N. Womack (Athens, GA: University of Georgia Press, 1969)

* Jonathan Sawday, *The Body Emblazoned: Dissection and the Human Body in Renaissance Culture* (London: Routledge, 1995)
B. Schultz, *Art and Anatomy in Renaissance Italy* (Ann Arbor: UMI Research Press, 1985)
Andrew Wear, 'Epistemology and Learned Medicine in Early Modern England', in Don Bates (ed.), *Knowledge and the Scholarly Medical Traditions* (Cambridge: Cambridge University Press, 1995), 151–74
* Andrew Wear, Roger French and Iain Lonie (eds), *The Medical Renaissance of the Sixteenth Century* (Cambridge: Cambridge University Press, 1985)
* C. Webster (ed.), *Health, Medicine and Mortality in the Sixteenth Century* (Cambridge: Cambridge University Press, 1979)

CHAPTER IX: THE NEW SCIENCE

Disease and Society
Walter George Bell, *The Great Plague in London in 1665* (London: John Lane, 1924)
Giulia Calvi, *Histories of a Plague Year: The Social and the Imaginary in Baroque Florence*, tr. by Dario Biocca and Bryant T. Ragan Jr, with a Foreword by Randolph Starn (Berkeley/Los Angeles/Oxford: University of California Press, 1989)
* Carlo M. Cipolla, *Cristofano and the Plague: A Study in the History of Public Health in the Age of Galileo* (Berkeley: University of California Press; London: Collins, 1973)
Colin Jones, 'Charity before *c.*1850', in W. F. Bynum and Roy Porter (eds), *Companion Encyclopedia of the History of Medicine* (London: Routledge, 1993), 1460–70

Medicine
Howard B. Adelmann, *Marcello Malpighi and the Evolution of Embryology*, 5 vols (Ithaca, NY: Cornell University Press, 1966)
* Lucinda McCray Beier, *Sufferers and Healers: The Experience of Illness in Seventeenth-Century England* (London: Routledge & Kegan Paul, 1987)
S. Bradbury, *The Evolution of the Microscope* (Oxford: Pergamon Press, 1967)
* Lawrence Brockliss and Colin Jones, *The Medical World of Early Modern France* (Oxford: Clarendon Press, 1997)
R. B. Carter, *Descartes' Medical Philosophy: The Organic Solution to the Mind-Body Problem* (Baltimore: Johns Hopkins University Press, 1983)
* Harold J. Cook, *The Decline of the Old Medical Regime in Stuart London* (Ithaca, NY: Cornell University Press, 1986)
Allen Debus, *The English Paracelsians* (London: Oldbourne, 1965)
* Allen G. Debus, *The Chemical Philosophy: Paracelsian Science and Medicine*

in the Sixteenth and Seventeenth Centuries (New York: Science History Publications, 1977)

Allen Debus, *The French Paracelsians* (Cambridge: Cambridge University Press, 1991)

Kenneth Dewhurst (ed.), *Dr Thomas Sydenham (1624–1689): His Life and Original Writings* (Berkeley, CA: University of California Press, 1966)

Audrey Davis, *Circulation Physiology and Medical Chemistry in England 1650–80* (Lawrence, KA: Coronado Press, 1973)

Valerie Fildes, *Breasts, Bottles and Babies: A History of Infant Feeding* (Edinburgh: Edinburgh University Press, 1985; 1986)

Valerie Fildes, *Wet Nursing: A History from Antiquity to the Present* (Oxford: Basil Blackwell, 1988)

* Robert G. Frank, *Harvey and the Oxford Physiologists: Scientific Ideas and Social Interaction* (Berkeley, CA: University of California Press, 1980)

* Roger French and Andrew Wear (eds), *The Medical Revolution of the Seventeenth-Century* (Cambridge and New York: Cambridge University Press, 1989)

E. B. Gasking, *Investigations into Generation 1651–1828* (London: Hutchinson, 1964)

William Harvey, *An Anatomical Disputation Concerning the Movement of the Heart and Blood in Living Creatures*, tr. by G. Whitteridge (Oxford: Blackwell Scientific, 1976)

Michael Heyd, *'Be Sober and Reasonable': The Critique of Enthusiasm in the Seventeenth and Early Eighteenth Centuries* (Leiden; New York; Köln: E. J. Brill, 1995)

Saul Jarcho, *Quinine's Predecessor: Francesco Torti and the Early History of Cinchona* (Baltimore: Johns Hopkins University Press, 1993)

* Colin Jones, *The Charitable Imperative. Hospitals and Nursing in Ancien Régime and Revolutionary France* (London: Routledge, 1989)

Kenneth Keele, *William Harvey: The Man, the Physician and the Scientist* (London: Nelson, 1965)

Geoffrey Keynes, *The Life of William Harvey* (Oxford: Clarendon Press, 1978)

* Michael MacDonald, *Mystical Bedlam: Madness, Anxiety and Healing in Seventeenth-Century England* (Cambridge: Cambridge University Press, 1981)

Hilary Marland (ed.), *The Art of Midwifery. Early Modern Midwives in Europe* (London: Routledge, 1993)

Walter Pagel, *Paracelsus: An Introduction to Philosophical Medicine in the Era of the Renaisssance* (Basel: Karger, 1958)

Walter Pagel, *William Harvey's Biological Ideas* (Basel: Karger, 1958)

* Walter Pagel, *New Light on William Harvey* (Basel: Karger, 1976)

Walter Pagel, *Jan Baptista Van Helmont: Reformer of Science and Medicine* (Cambridge: Cambridge University Press, 1982)

David Stannard, *The Puritan Way of Death* (New York: Oxford University Press, 1977)

Keith Thomas, *Religion and the Decline of Magic* (London: Weidenfeld & Nicolson, 1971)

* Charles Webster, *The Great Instauration: Science, Medicine and Reform 1626–1660* (London: Duckworth, 1975)

Charles Webster, *From Paracelsus to Newton. Magic and the Making of Modern Science* (Cambridge: Cambridge University Press, 1982)

* Gweneth Whitteridge, *William Harvey and the Circulation of the Blood* (London: Macdonald; New York: American Elsevier, 1971)

CHAPTER X: ENLIGHTENMENT

The Legacy of the Scientific Revolution and the Enlightenment

* W. F. Bynum, 'Health, Disease and Medical Care', in G. S. Rousseau and Roy Porter (eds), *The Ferment of Knowledge* (Cambridge: Cambridge University Press, 1980), 211–54

Andrew Cunningham and Roger French (eds), *The Medical Enlightenment of the Eighteenth Century* (Cambridge: Cambridge University Press, 1990)

Tore Frängsmyr, J. L. Heilbron and Robin E. Rider (eds), *The Quantifying Spirit in the Eighteenth Century* (Berkeley, Los Angeles and Oxford: University of California Press, 1990)

* Thomas Hankins, *Science and the Enlightenment* (Cambridge: Cambridge University Press, 1985)

Lester S. King, *The Medical World of the Eighteenth Century* (Chicago: University of Chicago Press, 1958)

Lester S. King, *The Road to Medical Enlightenment, 1650–1695* (London: Macdonald; New York: American Elsevier, 1970)

Lester S. King, *The Philosophy of Medicine: The Early Eighteenth Century* (Cambridge, Mass.: Harvard University Press, 1978)

Lester S. King, *Transformations in American Medicine: From Benjamin Rush to William Osler* (Baltimore Johns Hopkins University Press, 1990)

Roy Porter (ed.), *Medicine in the Enlightenment* (Amsterdam: Rodopi, 1995)

* Guenter B. Risse, 'Medicine in the Age of Enlightenment', in A. Wear (ed.), *Medicine in Society: Historical Essays* (Cambridge: Cambridge University Press, 1992), 149–95

Shirley A. Roe, *Matter, Life and Generation: Eighteenth-Century Embryology and the Haller-Wolff Debate* (Cambridge: Cambridge University Press, 1981)

J. Roger, *Les sciences de la vie dans la pensée française du XVIIIe siècle* (Paris: A. Colin, 1971)

Anatomy, Physiology and Pathology

Elizabeth Haigh, *Xavier Bichat and the Medical Thought of the Eighteenth Century* (London: Wellcome Institute for the History of Medicine, *Medical History*, Supplement 4, 1984)

Saul Jarcho (trans. and ed.), *The Clinical Consultations of Giambattista Morgagni* (Boston: Countway Library of Medicine, 1984)

G. A. Lindeboom, *Herman Boerhaave: The Man and His Work* (London: Methuen, 1968)

J. Spillane, *The Doctrine of the Nerves* (London: Oxford University Press, 1981)

Clinical Medicine and Disease Theory

W. F. Bynum and Roy Porter (eds), *Brunonianism in Britain and Europe* (London: *Medical History*, Supplement 8, 1989)

Knud Faber, *Nosography: A History of Clinical Medicine* (New York: Hoeber, 1930)

Irvine Loudon, *Medical Care and the General Practitioner 1750–1850* (Oxford: Clarendon Press, 1986)

Thomas H. Broman, *The Transformation of German Academic Medicine 1750–1820* (Cambridge: Cambridge University Press, 1996)

Therapeutics

W. F. Bynum and Roy Porter (eds), *William Hunter and the Eighteenth-Century Medical World* (Cambridge: Cambridge University Press, 1985)

J. Worth Estes, *Dictionary of Protopharmacology: Therapeutic Practices, 1700–1850* (Canton, MA: Science History Publications, USA, 1990)

R. B. Fisher, *Edward Jenner 1749–1823* (London: André Deutsch, 1991)

M. Foucault, *Folie et déraison: Histoire de la folie à l'age classique* (Paris: Olon, abridged ed., 1964), tr. as *Madness and Civilization* (London: Tavistock, 1967)

G. Miller, *The Adoption of Inoculation for Smallpox in England and France* (London: Oxford University Press, 1957)

Roy Porter, *Mind Forg'd Manacles: Madness and Psychiatry in England from Restoration to Regency* (London, Athlone Press, 1987; paperback edition, Penguin, 1990)

J. R. Smith, *The Speckled Monster. Smallpox in England 1670–1970, with Particular Reference to Essex* (Chelmsford: Essex Record Office, 1987)

Adrian Wilson, *The Making of Man-Midwifery: Childbirth in England 1660–1770* (London: University College Press, 1995)

Surgery

Toby Gelfand, *Professionalizing Modern Medicine: Paris Surgeons and Medical Science and Institutions in the Eighteenth Century* (Westport, Conn.: Greenwood Press, 1982)

Popular Medicine: Elite and Plebeian Culture

M. Bloch, *The Royal Touch: Sacred Monarchy and Scrofula in England and France* (London: Routledge & Kegan Paul, 1973)

Barbara Duden, *Geschichte unter der Haut* (Stuttgart: Klett, Cotta, 1987), translated as *The Woman Beneath the Skin. A Doctor's Patients in Eighteenth-Century Germany*, tr. by Thomas Dunlap (Cambridge, Mass.: Harvard University Press, 1991)

J. McManners, *Death and the Enlightenment: Changing Attitudes Towards Death Among Christians and Unbelievers in Eighteenth-Century France* (Oxford: Clarendon Presss, 1981)

Dorothy Porter and Roy Porter, *Patient's Progress: Doctors and Doctoring in Eighteenth-Century England* (Cambridge: Polity Press, 1989)

Roy Porter (ed.), *The Popularization of Medicine, 1650–1850* (London: Routledge, 1992)

Roy Porter and Dorothy Porter, *In Sickness and in Health: The British Experience 1650–1850* (London: Fourth Estate, 1988)

The Profession and Medical Education

Juanita G. L. Burnby, *A Study of the English Apothecary from 1660 to 1760* (London: Wellcome Institute for the History of Medicine, *Medical History*, Supplement 3, 1983)

Susan C. Lawrence, *Charitable Knowledge: Hospital Pupils and Practitioners in Eighteenth-Century London* (Cambridge: Cambridge University Press, 1995)

* Mary Lindemann, *Health and Healing in Eighteenth-Century Germany* (Baltimore: Johns Hopkins University Press, 1996)

Lisa Rosner, *Medical Education in the Age of Improvement: Edinburgh Students and Apprentices 1760–1826* (Edinburgh: Edinburgh University Press, 1991)

Quackery

Eric Jameson, *The Natural History of Quackery* (London: Michael Joseph, 1961)

Roy Porter, *Health for Sale: Quackery in England 1650–1850* (Manchester: Manchester University Press, 1989)

Medicine and the State: Hospitals

Mary E. Fissell, *Patients, Power, and the Poor in Eighteenth-Century Bristol* (Cambridge: Cambridge University Press, 1991)

Colin Jones, *The Charitable Imperative: Hospitals and Nursing in Ancien Régime and Revolutionary France*, Wellcome Institute Series in the History of Medicine (London and New York: Routledge, 1990)

C. Lloyd and J. L. S. Coulter, *Medicine and the Navy 1200–1900*, vol. 3, *1714–1815* (Edinburgh: Livingstone, 1961)

James C. Riley, *The Eighteenth-Century Campaign to Avoid Disease* (Basingstoke: Macmillan, 1987)

Guenter Risse, *Hospital Life in Enlightenment Scotland: Care and Teaching at the Royal Infirmary of Edinburgh* (Cambridge: Cambridge University Press, 1986)

Dora Weiner, *The Citizen-Patient in Revolutionary and Imperial Paris* (Baltimore and London: Johns Hopkins University Press, 1993)

J. Woodward, *To Do The Sick No Harm. A Study of the British Voluntary Hospital System to 1875* (London & Boston: Routledge & Kegan Paul, 1974)

Disease, Medicine and Society

Roderick Floud, Kenneth Wachter and Annabel Gregory, *Height, Health and History: Nutritional Status in the United Kingdom, 1750–1980* (Cambridge: Cambridge University Press, 1990)

John Komlos, *Nutrition and Economic Development in the Eighteenth-Century Habsburg Monarchy: An Anthropometric History* (Princeton: Princeton University Press, 1989)

T. McKeown, *The Modern Rise of Population* (London: Edward Arnold; New York: Academic Press, 1976)

T. McKeown, *The Role of Medicine: Dream, Mirage or Nemesis?* (Princeton: Princeton University Press, 1979)

James C. Riley, *Sickness, Recovery and Death: A History and Forecast of Ill Health* (Iowa City; University of Iowa Press, 1989)

James C. Riley, *Sick, Not Dead: The Health of British Workingmen During the Mortality Decline* (Baltimore: Johns Hopkins University Press, 1997)

CHAPTER XI: SCIENTIFIC MEDICINE IN THE
NINETEENTH CENTURY

* Erwin H. Ackerknecht, *Rudolf Virchow: Doctor, Statesman, Anthropologist* (Madison, WI: University of Wisconsin Press, 1953)

* Erwin H. Ackerknecht, *Medicine at the Paris Hospital, 1794–1848* (Baltimore: Johns Hopkins University Press, 1967)

W. R. Albury, 'Ideas of Life and Death', in W. F. Bynum and Roy Porter (eds), *Companion Encyclopedia of the History of Medicine* (London: Routledge, 1993), 249–80

Thomas N. Bonner, *American Doctors and German Universities: A Chapter in International Intellectual Relations 1870–1914* (Lincoln, Neb.: University of Nebraska Press, 1963)

Byron A. Boyd, *Rudolf Virchow: The Scientist as Citizen* (New York: Garland, 1991)

B. Bracegirdle, *A History of Microtechnique* (London: Heinemann, 1978)

Brian Bracegirdle, 'The Microscopical Tradition', in W. F. Bynum and Roy Porter (eds), *Companion Encyclopedia of the History of Medicine* (London: Routledge, 1993), 102–19

W. Brock, *From Prototyle to Proton: William Prout and the Nature of Matter, 1785–1985* (Bristol: Hilger, 1985)

* W. H. Brock, 'The Biochemical Tradition', in W. F. Bynum and Roy Porter (eds), *Companion Encyclopedia of the History of Medicine* (London: Routledge, 1993), 153–68

* W. Brock, *Justus van Liebig: the chemical gatekeeper* (Cambridge: Cambridge University Press, 1997)

* W. F. Bynum, *Science and the Practice of Medicine in the Nineteenth Century* (New York: Cambridge University Press, 1994)

* William Coleman and Frederic L. Holmes (eds), *The Investigative Enterprise: Experimental Physiology in Nineteenth-Century Medicine* (Berkeley, Los Angeles and London: University of California Press, 1988)

W. D. Foster, *A Short History of Clinical Pathology* (Edinburgh: Livingstone, 1961)

* M. Foucault, *The Birth of the Clinic*, tr. by A. M. Sheridan Smith (London: Tavistock, 1973)

Richard D. French, *Antivivisection and Medical Science in Victorian Society* (Princeton: Princeton University Press, 1975)

T. H. Grainger, *A Guide to the History of Bacteriology* (New York: Ronald Press, 1958)

* Frederic L. Holmes, *Claude Bernard and Animal Chemistry: The Emergence of a Scientist* (Cambridge, Mass.: Harvard University Press, 1974)

N. Jewson, 'The Disappearance of the Sick Man from Medical Cosmology, 1770–1870', *Sociology*, x (1976), 225–44

* John E. Lesch, *Science and Medicine in France: The Emergence of Experimental Physiology 1790–1855* (Cambridge, Mass.: Harvard University Press, 1984)

* Erna Lesky, *The Vienna Medical School of the 19th Century*, tr. from the German by L. Williams and I. S. Levij (Baltimore and London: Johns Hopkins University Press, 1965)

Diana E. Manuel, *Marshall Hall (1790–1857): Science and Medicine in Early Victorian Society* (Amsterdam: Rodopi, 1996)

J. Rosser Matthews, *Quantification and the Quest for Medical Certainty* (Princeton: Princeton University Press, 1995)

* Russell C. Maulitz, *Morbid Appearances: The Anatomy of Pathology in the Early Nineteenth Century* (Cambridge and New York: Cambridge University Press, 1987)

R. C. Maulitz, 'The Pathological Tradition', in W. F. Bynum and Roy Porter (eds), *Companion Encyclopedia of the History of Medicine* (London: Routledge, 1993), 169–91

Charles Newman, *The Evolution of Medical Education in the Nineteenth Century* (London: Oxford University Press, 1957)

Arlene Marcia Tuchman, *Science, Medicine, and the State in Germany: The Case of Baden, 1815–1871* (Oxford: Oxford University Press, 1993)

David Vess, *Medical Revolution in France, 1789–1796* (Gainesville: University Presses of Florida, 1975)

Maxwell M. Wintrobe, *Hematology, The Blossoming of a Science: A Story of Inspiration and Effort* (Philadelphia: Lea & Febiger, 1985)

CHAPTER XII: NINETEENTH-CENTURY MEDICAL CARE

The Medical Profession

* Thomas Neville Bonner, *To the Ends of the Earth: Women's Search for Education in Medicine* (Cambridge, Mass. and London: Harvard University Press, 1992)

* Thomas Neville Bonner, *Becoming a Physician: Medical Education in Britain, France, Germany and the United States, 1750–1945* (New York and Oxford: Oxford University Press, 1995)

Kate Campbell Hurd-Mead, *A History of Women in Medicine from the Earliest Times to the Beginning of the Nineteenth Century* (Haddam, Conn.: Haddam Press, 1938)

Anne Digby, *Making a Medical Living: Doctors and Patients in the English Market for Medicine, 1720–1911* (Cambridge: Cambridge University Press, 1994)

P. Fleming, *'Harley Street' from Early Times to the Present Day* (London: H. K. Lewis & Co., 1939)

* Toby Gelfand, 'The History of the Medical Profession', in W. F. Bynum and Roy Porter (eds), *Companion Encyclopedia of the History of Medicine* (London: Routledge, 1993), 1113–43

* Johanna Geyer-Kordesch, 'Women and Medicine', in W. F. Bynum and Roy Porter (eds), *Companion Encyclopedia of the History of Medicine* (London: Routledge, 1993), 884–910

Gerald Larkin, 'The Emergence of Para-Medical Professions', in W. F. Bynum and Roy Porter (eds), *Companion Encyclopedia of the History of Medicine* (London: Routledge, 1993), 1321–41

* Christopher Lawrence, *Medicine in the Making of Modern Britain, 1700–1920* (London and New York: Routledge, 1994)

Jacques Léonard, *Médecins, malades et société dans la France du XIXe siècle* (Paris: Sciences en Situation, 1992)

Regina Markell Morantz-Sanchez, *Sympathy and Science: Women Physicians in American Medicine* (New York and Oxford: Oxford University Press, 1985)

M. Jeanne Peterson, *The Medical Profession in Mid-Victorian London* (Berkeley, CA: University of California Press, 1978)

* Matthew Ramsey, *Professional and Popular Medicine in France, 1770–1830* (New York: Cambridge University Press, 1988)

Ruth Richardson, *Death, Dissection and the Destitute: A Political History of the Human Corpse* (London: Routledge & Kegan Paul, 1987)

Shirley Roberts, *Sophia Jex-Blake: A Woman Pioneer in Nineteenth-Century Medical Reform* (London and New York: Routledge, 1993)

Ivan Waddington, *The Medical Profession in the Industrial Revolution* (Dublin: Gill & Macmillan, 1984)

* John Harley Warner, *The Therapeutic Perspective: Medical Practice, Knowledge and Identity in America, 1820–1885* (Cambridge, Mass.: Harvard University Press, 1986)

Surgery

F. F. Cartwright, *The English Pioneers of Anaesthesia: Beddoes, Davy, and Hickman* (Bristol: Wright, 1952)

Ann Dally, *Women Under the Knife: A History of Surgery* (London: Hutchinson Radius, 1991)

Ann Dally, *Fantasy Surgery, 1880–1930* (Amsterdam and Atlanta, GA: Rodopi, 1996)

* Richard B. Fisher, *Joseph Lister, 1827–1912* (London: Macdonald and Jane's, 1977)

* Irvine Loudon, *Death in Childbirth: An International Study of Maternal Care and Maternal Mortality 1800–1950* (Oxford: Clarendon Press, 1992)

Ornella Moscucci, *The Science of Woman: Gynaecology and Gender in England, 1800–1929* (Cambridge: Cambridge University Press, 1990)

Martin S. Pernick, *A Calculus of Suffering: Pain, Professionalism, and Anesthesia in Nineteenth-Century America* (New York: Columbia University Press, 1985)

Hospitals and Nursing

Monica E. Baly, *Florence Nightingale and the Nursing Legacy* (London: Routledge, 1988)

Lindsay Granshaw, *St Mark's Hospital, London: A Social History of a Specialist Hospital* (London: King's Fund, 1985)

* Lindsay Granshaw, 'The Hospital', in W. F. Bynum and Roy Porter (eds), *Companion Encyclopedia of the History of Medicine* (London: Routledge, 1993), 1173–95

Christopher Maggs, 'A General History of Nursing: 1800–1900', in W. F. Bynum and Roy Porter (eds), *Companion Encyclopedia of the History of Medicine* (London: Routledge, 1993), 1300–20

Florence Nightingale, *Notes on Hospitals* (London: John W. Parker & Son, 1859)

F. N. L. Poynter (ed.), *The Evolution of Hospitals in Britain* (London: Pitman, 1964)

Susan M. Reverby, *Ordered to Care: The Dilemma of American Nursing 1850–1945* (Cambridge: Cambridge University Press, 1987)

* Charles E. Rosenberg, *The Care of Strangers: The Rise of America's Hospital System* (New York: Basic Books, 1987)

David Rosner, *A Once Charitable Enterprise: Hospitals and Health Care in Brooklyn and New York, 1865–1915* (Cambridge: Cambridge University Press, 1982)

F. B. Smith, *Florence Nightingale – Reputation and Power* (London: Croom Helm, 1982)

Specialization

A. F. Abt and F. H. Garrison, *History of Paediatrics* (Philadelphia: Saunders, 1965)

Elizabeth Lomax, *History of Children's Hospitals* (London: Wellcome Institute, 1996)

* George Rosen, *The Specialization of Medicine with Special Reference to Ophthalmology* (New York: Froben Press, 1944)

A. Sorsby, *A Short History of Ophthalmology* (London: Bale, 1948)

George F. Still, *The History of Paediatrics; the Progress of the Study of Diseases of Children up to the End of the Eighteenth Century* (London: Oxford University Press, 1931; London: Dawsons, 1965)

Irregular Medicine and Quackery

T. Cook, *Samuel Hahnemann* (Wellingborough: Thorson's, 1981)

* Norman Gevitz, *Other Healers: Unorthodox Medicine in America* (Baltimore and London: Johns Hopkins University Press, 1988)

Norman Gevitz, 'Unorthodox Medical Theories', in W. F. Bynum and Roy Porter (eds), *Companion Encyclopedia of the History of Medicine* (London: Routledge, 1993), 603–33

Martin Kaufman, *Homeopathy in America: The Rise and Fall of a Medical Heresy* (Baltimore, MD: Johns Hopkins University Press, 1971)

B. Inglis, *Fringe Medicine* (London: Faber & Faber, 1964)

B. Inglis, *Natural Medicine* (London: Collins, 1979)

Phillip A. Nicholls, *Homoeopathy and the Medical Profession* (London and New York: Croom Helm, 1988)

* Mike Saks (ed.), *Alternative Medicine in Britain* (Oxford: Clarendon Press, 1992)

* J. C. Whorton, *Crusaders for Fitness: The History of American Health Reformers* (Princeton: Princeton University Press, 1982)

* James Harvey Young, *The Toadstool Millionaires: A Social History of Patent Medicines in America before Federal Regulation* (Princeton, NJ: Princeton University Press, 1961)

James Harvey Young, *The Medical Messiahs: A Social History of Health Quackery in Twentieth-Century America* (Princeton, NJ: Princeton University Press, 1997)

James Harvey Young, *American Self-Dosage Medicines: An Historical Perspective* (Lawrence, KA: Coronado, 1974)

CHAPTER XIII: PUBLIC MEDICINE

Public Health

Jeanne L. Brand, *Doctors and the State: The British Medical Profession and Government Action in Public Health, 1870-1912* (Baltimore: Johns Hopkins University Press, 1965)

W. Coleman, *Death is a Social Disease: Public Health and Political Economy in Early Industrial France* (Madison, Wisc.: University of Wisconsin Press, 1982)

Alain Corbin, *The Foul and the Fragrant: Odor and the French Social Imagination* (Cambridge, MA: Harvard University Press, 1986)

John Duffy, *The Sword of Pestilence: The New Orleans Yellow Fever Epidemic of 1853* (Baton Rouge: Louisiana State University Press, 1966)

* John Duffy, *The Sanitarians: A History of American Public Health* (Urbana and Chicago: University of Illinois Press, 1990)

John Duffy, 'History of Public Health and Sanitation in the West since 1700', in Kenneth F. Kiple (ed.), *The Cambridge World History of Human Disease* (Cambridge: Cambridge University Press, 1993), 200-206

M. Durey, *The Return of the Plague: British Society and the Cholera 1831-2* (Dublin: Gill & Macmillan, 1979)

* Richard J. Evans, *Death in Hamburg: Society and Politics in the Cholera Years 1830-1910* (Oxford/New York: Oxford University Press, 1987)

R. J. Evans, 'Epidemics and Revolutions: Cholera in Nineteenth-Century Europe', *Past and Present*, 120 (1988), 123-146

John M. Eyler, *Victorian Social Medicine: The Ideas and Methods of William Farr* (Baltimore and London: Johns Hopkins University Press, 1979)

* S. E. Finer, *The Life and Times of Sir Edwin Chadwick* (London: Methuen, 1952)

W. M. Frazer, *A History of English Public Health 1834-1939* (London: Baillière, Tindall & Cox, 1950)

Christopher Hamlin, *Public Health and Social Justice in the Age of Chadwick* (Cambridge: Cambridge University Press, 1997)

Anne Hardy, *The Epidemic Streets: Infectious Disease and the Rise of Preventive Medicine, 1856-1900* (Oxford and New York: Oxford University Press, 1993)

Alan M. Kraut, *Silent Travellers: Germs, Genes, and the 'Immigrant Menace'* (New York, NY: Basic Books 1994)

S. J. Kunitz, 'Medicine, Mortality and Morbidity', in W. F. Bynum and Roy Porter (eds), *Companion Encyclopedia of the History of Medicine* (London: Routledge, 1993), 1693–1711

* Anne La Berge, *Mission and Method: The Early Nineteenth-Century French Public Health Movement* (Cambridge and New York: Cambridge University Press, 1992)

R. Lambert, *Sir John Simon 1816-1904 and English Social Administration* (London: MacGibbon & Kee, 1963)

R. J. Morris, *Cholera, 1832: The Social Response to an Epidemic* (London: Croom Helm, 1976)

Margaret Pelling, *Cholera, Fever and English Medicine 1825-1865* (Oxford: Oxford University Press, 1978)

* Dorothy Porter, 'Public Health', in W. F. Bynum and Roy Porter (eds), *Companion Encyclopedia of the History of Medicine* (London: Routledge, 1993), 1223–53

* Dorothy Porter (ed.), *The History of Health and the Modern State* (Amsterdam: Rodopi, 1994)

Charles E. Rosenberg, *The Cholera Years: The United States in 1832, 1849 and 1866* (Chicago: University of Chicago Press, 1962)

Richard H. Shryock, *Medicine and Society in America 1660-1860* (New York: New York University Press, 1960)

* F. B. Smith, *The People's Health, 1830-1910* (London: Croom Helm, 1979; New York: Holmes & Meier, 1979)

Frank M. Snowden, *Naples in the Time of Cholera, 1884-1911* (Cambridge: Cambridge University Press, 1995)

Georges Vigarello, *Concepts of Cleanliness: Changing Attitudes in France Since the Middle Ages*, tr. by Jean Birrell (Cambridge: Cambridge University Press, 1988)

Paul Weindling (ed.), *The Social History of Occupational Health* (London: Croom Helm, 1985)

Anthony S. Wohl, *Endangered Lives: Public Health in Victorian Britain* (London: Dent; Cambridge: Harvard University Press, 1983)

Policing Disease

David S. Barnes, *The Making of a Social Disease: Tuberculosis in Nineteenth-Century France* (Berkeley, Los Angeles and London: University of California Press, 1995)

L. Bryder, *Below the Magic Mountain: A Social History of Tuberculosis in Twentieth-Century Britain* (Oxford: Clarendon Press, 1988)

René Dubos and Jean Dubos, *The White Plague: Tuberculosis, Man and Society* (Boston: Boston-Little, 1952)

Judith Walzer Leavitt, *Typhoid Mary: Captive to the Public's Health* (Boston: Beacon Press, 1996)

Barbara Gutmann Rosenkrantz (ed.), *From Consumption to Tuberculosis: A Documentary History* (New York: Garland, 1994)

Sheila M. Rothman, *Living in the Shadow of Death: Tuberculosis and the Social Experience of Illness in American History* (New York: Basic Books, 1994)

F. B. Smith, *The Retreat of Tuberculosis 1850-1950* (London and New York: Croom Helm, 1988)

Venereal Disease

* A. M. Brandt, *No Magic Bullet: A Social History of Venereal Disease in the United States since 1880* (New York: Oxford University Press, 1985)

Allan M. Brandt, 'Sexually-Transmitted Diseases', in W. F. Bynum and Roy Porter (eds), *Companion Encyclopedia of the History of Medicine* (London: Routledge, 1993), 561–83

John C. Fout (ed.), *Forbidden History: The State, Society, and the Regulation of Sexuality in Modern Europe* (Chicago: University of Chicago Press, 1992)

Frank Mort, *Dangerous Sexualities: Medico-Moral Politics in England Since 1830* (London and New York: Routledge & Kegan Paul, 1987)

* Theodore Rosebury, *Microbes and Morals: The Strange Story of Venereal Disease* (New York: Viking, 1971; New York: Ballantine Books, 1973)

CHAPTER XIV: FROM PASTEUR TO PENICILLIN

Microbiology

* Thomas D. Brock, *Robert Koch: A Life in Medicine and Bacteriology* (Madison, Wisc.: Science Tech Publishers, 1988)

John Farley, *The Spontaneous Generation Controversy from Descartes to Oparin* (Baltimore: Johns Hopkins University Press, 1977)

F. Fenner and A. Gibbs (eds), *A History of Virology* (Basel: Karger, 1988)

W. D. Foster, *A History of Medical Bacteriology and Immunology* (London: Heinemann, 1970)

* Gerald L. Geison, *The Private Science of Louis Pasteur* (Princeton: Princeton University Press, 1995)

* Ronald Hare, *The Birth of Penicillin* (London: George Allen and Unwin, 1970)

Gladys L. Hobby, *Penicillin: Meeting the Challenge* (New Haven, CT: Yale University Press, 1984)

Sally Smith Hughes, *The Virus: A History of the Concept* (New York: Science History Publications, 1977)

Bruno Latour, *The Pasteurization of France*, tr. by Alan Sheridan and John Law (Cambridge, MA: Harvard University Press, 1988)

J. Liebenau, *Medical Science and Medical Industry: The Formation of the American Pharmaceutical Industry* (London: Macmillan, 1987)

Gwyn Macfarlane, *Alexander Fleming: The Man and the Myth* (New York: Oxford University Press, 1985)

* Wesley W. Spink, *Infectious Diseases: Prevention and Treatment in the Nineteenth and Twentieth Centuries* (Folkestone: Dawson, 1978; Minneapolis: University of Minneapolis Press, 1978; 1979)

Alfred I. Tauber and Leon Chernyak, *Metchnikoff and the Origins of Immunology* (New York: Oxford University Press, 1991)

A. P. Waterson and Lise Wilkinson, *An Introduction to the History of Virology* (New York: Cambridge University Press, 1978)

Therapeutics
Arabella Melville and Colin Johnson, *Cured to Death: The Effects of Prescription Drugs* (London: Secker and Warburg, 1982)

J. Parascandola, *The Development of American Pharmacology: John J. Abel and the Shaping of a Discipline* (Baltimore and London: Johns Hopkins University Press, 1992)

Walter Sneader, *Drug Discovery: The Evolution of Modern Medicines* (Chichester: Wiley, 1985)

* M. Weatherall, *In Search of a Cure: A History of the Pharmaceutical Industry* (Oxford; New York: Oxford University Press, 1990)

CHAPTER XV: TROPICAL MEDICINE, WORLD DISEASES

Tropical Medicine
* David Arnold, *Colonizing the Body: State Medicine and Epidemic Disease in Nineteenth-Century India* (Berkeley, CA: University of California Press, 1993)

* David Arnold, 'Medicine and Colonialism', in W. F. Bynum and Roy Porter (eds), *Companion Encyclopedia of the History of Medicine* (London: Routledge, 1993), 1385–1405

Philip D. Curtin, *Death by Migration: Europe's Encounter with the Tropical World in the Nineteenth Century* (Cambridge and New York: Cambridge University Press, 1989)

Robert S. Desowitz, *Tropical Diseases: From 50,000 BC to 2,500 AD* (London: HarperCollins, 1997)

John Ettling, *The Germ of Laziness: Rockefeller Philanthropy and Public Health in the New South* (Cambridge: Harvard University Press, 1981)

* John Farley, *Bilharzia: A History of Imperial Tropical Medicine* (Cambridge and New York: Cambridge University Press, 1991)

Elizabeth Fee, *Disease and Discovery: A History of the Johns Hopkins School of Hygiene and Public Health, 1916–1939* (Baltimore: Johns Hopkins University Press, 1987)

W. D. Foster, *A History of Parasitology* (Edinburgh, London: E. & S. Livingstone, 1961)

Gordon A. Harrison, *Mosquitoes, Malaria, and Man* (New York: Dutton, 1978)

* Mark Harrison, *Public Health in British India: Anglo-Indian Preventive Medicine, 1859–1914* (Cambridge and New York: Cambridge University Press, 1994)

Margaret Humphreys, *Yellow Fever and the South* (New Brunswick, NJ: Rutgers University Press, 1992)

Kenneth F. Kiple, *The Caribbean Slave: A Biological History* (Cambridge and New York: Cambridge University Press, 1984)

LaVerne Kuhnke, *Lives at Risk: Public Health in Nineteenth-Century Egypt* (Berkeley: University of California Press, 1991)

* Maryinez Lyons, *The Colonial Disease: A Social History of Sleeping Sickness in Northern Zaire, 1900–1940* (Cambridge and New York: Cambridge University Press, 1992)

Jock McCulloch, *Colonial Psychiatry and the 'African Mind'* (Cambridge and New York: Cambridge University Press, 1995)

Roy MacLeod and Milton Lewis (eds), *Disease, Medicine and Empire: Perspectives on Western Medicine and the Experience of European Expansion* (London and New York: Routledge, 1988)

Terence Ranger and Paul Slack (eds), *Epidemics and Ideas: Essays on the Historical Perception of Pestilence* (Cambridge: Cambridge University Press, 1992)

Richard Rhodes, *Deadly Feasts: Tracking the Secrets of a Terrifying New Plague* (New York: Simon and Schuster, 1997)

R. B. Sheridan, *Doctors and Slaves. A Medical and Demographic History of Slavery in the British West Indies, 1680–1834* (Cambridge: Cambridge University Press, 1985)

David E. Stannard, *Before the Horror: The Population of Hawaii on the Eve of Western Contact* (Honolulu: University of Hawaii Press, 1989)

* Megan Vaughan, *Curing Their Ills: Colonial Power and African Illness* (Stanford, Calif.: Stanford University Press, 1991)

Sheldon Watts, *Epidemics and History: Disease, Power and Imperialism* (New Haven and London: Yale University Press, 1997)

* M. Worboys, 'Tropical Diseases', in W. F. Bynum and Roy Porter (eds), *Companion Encyclopedia of the History of Medicine* (London: Routledge, 1993), 511-60

World Health and Disease

A. W. Crosby Jr, *Epidemic and Peace 1918* (Westport, Conn. and London: Greenwood Press, 1976)

Laurie Garrett, *The Coming Plague* (Harmondsworth: Penguin, 1994)

Mirko D. Grmek, *Histoire du Sida: Début et Origine d'une Pandémie Actuelle* (Paris: Payot, 1992); tr. by Russell C. Maulitz and Jacalyn Duffin as *History of AIDS: Emergence and Origin of a Modern Pandemic* (Princeton: Princeton University Press, 1994)

M. I. Roemer, 'Internationalism in Medicine and Public Health', in W. F. Bynum and Roy Porter (eds), *Companion Encyclopedia of the History of Medicine* (London: Routledge, 1993), 1408-26

Paul Weindling (ed.), *The Rise of Medical Internationalism* (Oxford: Oxford University Press, 1996)

World Health Organization, *The Global Eradication of Smallpox* (Geneva: World Health Organization, 1980)

CHAPTER XVI: PSYCHIATRY

Franz G. Alexander and Sheldon T. Selesnick, *The History of Psychiatry: An Evaluation of Psychiatric Thought and Practice from Prehistoric Times to the Present* (London: George Allen & Unwin, 1967)

Jonathan Andrews, Asa Briggs, Roy Porter, Penny Tucker and Keir Waddington, *The History of Bethlem* (London: Routledge, 1997)

Peter Barham, *Closing the Asylum: The Mental Patient in Modern Society* (Harmondsworth: Penguin, 1992)

G. E. Berrios, *History of Mental Symptoms* (Cambridge: Cambridge University Press, 1996)

* German E. Berrios and Roy Porter (eds), *A History of Clinical Psychiatry. The Origin and History of Psychiatric Disorders* (London: Athlone, 1995)

* W. F. Bynum, Roy Porter and Michael Shepherd (eds), *The Anatomy of Madness*, 3 vols (London: Tavistock, 1985-8)

Henri F. Ellenberger, *The Discovery of the Unconscious: The History and Evolution of Dynamic Psychiatry* (New York: Basic Books, 1970)

Peter Gay, *Freud, A Life for Our Time* (London: Dent, 1988)

* Sander L. Gilman, *Seeing the Insane* (New York: Brunner, Mazel, 1982)

Jan Goldstein, *Console and Classify: The French Psychiatric Profession in the Nineteenth Century* (Cambridge: Cambridge University Press, 1987)

Gerald Grob, *The Mad Among Us: A History of the Care of America's Mentally Ill* (New York: Free Press, 1994)

Richard Hunter and Ida Macalpine, *Three Hundred Years of Psychiatry: 1535– 1860* (London: Oxford University Press, 1963)

Peter D. Kramer, *Listening to Prozac* (London: Fourth Estate, 1994)

R. D. Laing, *The Divided Self* (New York: Random House, 1969)

Mark Micale and Roy Porter (eds), *Discovering the History of Psychiatry* (New York and Oxford: Oxford University Press, 1994)

Richard Noll, *The Jung Cult. Origins of a Charismatic Movement* (Princeton: Princeton University Press, 1995)

Daniel Pick, *Faces of Degeneration: A European Disorder, c.1848–1918* (Cambridge: Cambridge University Press, 1989)

Roy Porter, *A Social History of Madness* (London: Weidenfeld & Nicolson, 1987)

Jack D. Pressman, 'Concepts of Mental Illness in the West', in Kenneth F. Kiple (ed.), *The Cambridge World History of Human Disease* (Cambridge: Cambridge University Press, 1993), 59–84

David Rothman, *The Discovery of the Asylum: Social Order and Disorder in the New Republic* (Boston: Little, Brown, 1971)

* Andrew Scull, *The Most Solitary of Afflictions: Madness and Society in Britain, 1700–1900* (New Haven and London: Yale University Press, 1993)

* Andrew Scull, *Decarceration: Community Treatment and the Deviant – A Radical View*, 2nd ed. (Oxford: Polity Press; New Brunswick: Rutgers University Press, 1984)

Edward Shorter, *From Paralysis to Fatigue. A History of Psychosomatic Illness in the Modern Era* (New York: Free Press, 1992)

* Edward Shorter, *A History of Psychiatry* (New York: Free Press, 1997)

Thomas S. Szasz, *The Myth of Mental Illness: Foundations of a Theory of Personal Conduct* (London: Granada, 1972; revised ed., New York: Harper and Row, 1974)

Thomas Szasz, *The Manufacture of Madness* (New York: Harper & Row, 1970)

CHAPTER XVII: MEDICAL RESEARCH

Research

Joan Austoker and Linda Bryder (eds), *Historical Perspectives on the Role of the MRC: Essays in the History of the Medical Research Council of the United Kingdom and Its Predecessor, the Medical Research Committee, 1913–1953* (Oxford and New York: Oxford University Press, 1989)

Christopher Booth, *Doctors in Science and Society: Essays of a Clinical Scientist* (London: British Medical Journal, 1987)

* Christopher Booth, 'Clinical Research', in W. F. Bynum and Roy Porter (eds), *Companion Encyclopedia of the History of Medicine* (London: Routledge, 1993), 205–29

* W. F. Bynum, 'Medical Philanthropy after 1850', in W. F. Bynum and Roy Porter (eds), *Companion Encyclopedia of the History of Medicine* (London: Routledge, 1993), 1480–1494

Alan M. Chesney, *The Johns Hopkins Hospital and the Johns Hopkins University School of Medicine: A Chronicle*, vol. I, *Early Years, 1867–1893* (Baltimore: Johns Hopkins University Press, 1943)

Harriette Chick, Margaret Hume and Marjorie Macfarlane, *War on Diseases: A History of the Lister Institute* (London: Deutsch, 1971)

* William Coleman and Frederic L. Holmes (eds), *The Investigative Enterprise: Experimental Physiology in Nineteenth-Century Medicine* (Berkeley: University of California Press, 1988)

A. McGehee Harvey, *Science at the Bedside: Clinical Research in American Medicine 1905–1945* (Baltimore: Johns Hopkins University Press, 1981)

John V. Pickstone (ed.), *Medical Innovations in Historical Perspective* (London: Macmillan, 1991)

* David Weatherall, *Science and the Quiet Art: Medical Research and Patient Care* (Oxford: Oxford University Press, 1995)

Neurology

Robert B. Aird, *Foundations of Modern Neurology, A Century of Progress* (New York: Raven Press, 1993)

Christopher G. Goetz, Michel Bonduelle, and Toby Gelfand, *Charcot. Constructing Neurology* (Oxford: Oxford University Press, 1996)

J. Spillane, *The Doctrine of the Nerves* (London: Oxford University Press, 1981)

Owsei Temkin, *The Falling Sickness: A History of Epilepsy from the Greeks to the Beginnings of Modern Neurology* (Baltimore: Johns Hopkins University Press, 1945; 1971; 1974)

Nutrition

W. R. Akroyd, *Conquest of Deficiency Diseases* (Geneva: World Health Organization, 1970)

* K. J. Carpenter, *The History of Scurvy and Vitamin C* (Cambridge: Cambridge University Press, 1986)

K. J. Carpenter, 'Nutritional Diseases', in W. F. Bynum and Roy Porter (eds), *Companion Encyclopedia of the History of Medicine* (London: Routledge, 1993), 463–82

* Kenneth J. Carpenter, *Protein and Energy: A Study of Changing Ideas in Nutrition* (Cambridge: Cambridge University Press, 1994)

Samuel A. Goldblith and M. A. Joslyn, *Milestones in Nutrition: An Anthology of Food Sciences*, 3 vols (Westport, CT: Avi Publishing Co., 1964)

Ralph W. Moss, *Free Radical: Albert Szent-Györgyi and the Battle Over Vitamin C* (New York: Paragon House Publishers, 1987)

Daphne A. Roe, *A Plague of Corn: The Social History of Pellagra* (Ithaca, NY: Cornell University Press, 1973)

CHAPTER XVIII: CLINICAL SCIENCE

Endocrinology

* Michael Bliss, *The Discovery of Insulin* (Edinburgh: Paul Harris, 1983)

* R. B. Welbourn, 'Endocrine Diseases', in W. F. Bynum and Roy Porter (eds), *Companion Encyclopedia of the History of Medicine* (London: Routledge, 1993), 483–511

Cancer

Joan Austoker, *A History of the Imperial Cancer Research Fund 1902–1986* (Oxford: Oxford University Press, 1988)

Thomas G. Benedek and Kenneth F. Kiple, 'Concepts of Cancer', in Kenneth F. Kiple (ed.), *The Cambridge World History of Human Disease* (Cambridge: Cambridge University Press, 1993), 102–10

David Cantor, 'Cancer', in W. F. Bynum and Roy Porter (eds), *Companion Encyclopedia of the History of Medicine* (London: Routledge, 1993), 561–83

Lesley Doyal, *Cancer in Britain. The Politics of Prevention* (London: Pluto Press, 1983)

Sandra Panem, *The Interferon Crusade* (Washington DC: The Brookings Institute, 1984)

* James T. Patterson, *The Dread Disease: Cancer and Modern American Culture* (Cambridge, MA: Harvard University Press, 1987)

* Robert N. Proctor, *Cancer Wars: How Politics Shape What We Know & Don't Know About Cancer* (New York: Basic Books, 1995)

L. J. Rather, *The Genesis of Cancer. A Study in the History of Ideas* (Baltimore and London: Johns Hopkins University Press, 1978)

Richard A. Rettig, *Cancer Crusade: The Story of the National Cancer Act of 1971* (Princeton, NJ: Princeton University Press, 1977)

Evelleen Richards, *Vitamin C and Cancer: Medicine or Politics?* (Basingstoke and London: Macmillan, 1991)

Cardiology

W. F. Bynum, C. J. Lawrence and V. Nutton (eds), *The Emergence of Modern Cardiology* (London: Wellcome Institute, *Medical History* Supplement 5, 1985)

Peter Fleming, *A History of Cardiology* (Amsterdam: Rodopi, 1997)

Joel D. Howell, 'Concepts of Heart-Related Diseases', in Kenneth F. Kiple (ed.), *The Cambridge World History of Human Disease* (Cambridge: Cambridge University Press, 1993), 91–101

F. A. Willus and T. E. Keys (eds), *Classics of Cardiology*, 2 vols (New York: Dover, 1961)

Genetics

Eric J. Devor, 'Genetic Disease', in Kenneth F. Kiple (ed.), *The Cambridge World History of Human Disease* (Cambridge: Cambridge University Press, 1993), 113–25

Stuart J. Edelstein, *The Sickled Cell: From Myths to Molecules* (Cambridge, MA: Harvard University Press, 1986)

Horace Judson, *The Eighth Day of Creation: Makers of the Revolution in Biology* (New York: Simon & Schuster, 1979)

* Daniel J. Kevles and Leroy Hood (eds), *The Code of Codes: Scientific and Social Issues in the Human Genome Project* (Cambridge, Mass. and London: Harvard University Press, 1992)

* Pauline M. H. Mazumdar, *Eugenics, Human Genetics and Human Failings: The Eugenics Society, its Sources and its Critics in Britain* (London and New York: Routledge, 1992)

* Robert Olby, 'Constitutional and Hereditary Disorders', in W. F. Bynum and Roy Porter (eds), *Companion Encyclopedia of the History of Medicine* (London: Routledge, 1993), 412–37

Tom Wilkie, *Perilous Knowledge: The Human Genome Project and its Implications* (Berkeley: University of California Press, 1993)

Immunology

Sir Frank Macfarlane Burnet and David O. White, *The Natural History of Infectious Disease*, 4th ed. (New York: Cambridge University Press, 1972)

Stephen S. Hall, *A Commotion in the Blood: Life, Death and the Immune System* (New York: Henry Holt and Company, 1997)

Pauline M. H. Mazumdar (ed.), *Immunology, 1930–1980: Essays on the History of Immunology* (Toronto: Wall & Thompson, 1989)

* Pauline M. H. Mazumdar, 'Immunology', in Kenneth F. Kiple (ed.), *The Cambridge World History of Human Disease* (Cambridge: Cambridge University Press, 1993), 126–39

* Pauline M. H. Mazumdar, *Species and Specificity: An Interpretation of the History of Immunology* (Cambridge: Cambridge University Press, 1994)

Arthur M. Silverstein, *A History of Immunology* (New York: Academic Press, 1989)

* P. Weindling, 'The Immunological Tradition', in W. F. Bynum and Roy

Porter (eds), *Companion Encyclopedia of the History of Medicine* (London: Routledge, 1993), 192–204

CHAPTER XIX: SURGERY

Robert Bud, *The Uses of Life: A History of Biotechnology* (Cambridge and New York: Cambridge University Press, 1994)

* F. F. Cartwright, *The Development of Modern Surgery* (London: Arthur Barker, 1967)

Roger Cooter, 'War and Modern Medicine', in W. F. Bynum and Roy Porter (eds), *Companion Encyclopedia of the History of Medicine* (London: Routledge, 1993), 1526–63

Roger Cooter, *Surgery and Society in Peace and War: Orthopaedics and the Organization of Modern Medicine, 1880–1948* (Basingstoke: Macmillan Press, 1993)

S. J. Crowe, *Halsted of Johns Hopkins: The Man and His Men* (Springfield, IL: Charles C. Thomas, 1957)

Renée C. Fox and Judith P. Swazey, *The Courage to Fail: A Social View of Organ Transplants and Dialysis*, 2nd ed. (Chicago: University of Chicago Press, 1978)

Eliot Freidson (ed.), *The Hospital in Modern Society* (London: Collier and Macmillan, 1963)

* Joel D. Howell, *Technology in the Hospital: Transforming Patient Care in the Early Twentieth Century* (Baltimore: Johns Hopkins University Press, 1995)

Alfred Hurwitz and George A. Degenshein, *Milestones in Modern Surgery* (New York: Hoeber-Harper, 1958)

Bettann Holtzmann Kevles, *Naked to the Bone: Medical Imaging in the Twentieth Century* (New Brunswick: Rutgers University Press, 1997)

Christopher Lawrence, (ed.), *Medical Theory, Surgical Practice: Studies in the History of Surgery* (London and New York: Routledge, 1992)

Naomi Pfeffer, *The Stork and the Syringe: A Political History of Reproductive Medicine* (Cambridge: Polity Press, 1993)

Mark M. Ravitch, *A Century of Surgery: 1880–1980*, 2 vols (Philadelphia: J. B. Lippincott Co., 1981)

Ada Romaine-David, *John Gibbon and his Heart-Lung Machine* (Philadelphia: University of Pennsylvania Press, 1992)

Ira M. Rutkow, *Surgery: An Illustrated History* (St Louis: Mosby-Year Book Inc., in collaboration with Norman Publishing, 1993)

Tony Stark, *Knife to the Heart* (London: Macmillan, 1996)

Rosemary Stevens, *In Sickness and in Wealth: American Hospitals in the Twentieth Century* (New York: Basic Books, 1989)

* Ulrich Tröhler, 'Surgery (Modern)', in W. F. Bynum and Roy Porter (eds), *Companion Encyclopedia of the History of Medicine* (London: Routledge, 1993), 980–1023

Morris J. Vogel, *The Invention of the Modern Hospital: Boston 1870–1930* (Chicago: Chicago University Press, 1980)

Anthony F. Wallace, *The Progress of Plastic Surgery: An Introductory History* (Oxford: William A. Meeuws, 1982)

* Owen H. Wangensteen and Sarah D. Wangensteen, *The Rise of Surgery: From Empiric Craft to Scientific Discipline* (Minneapolis: University of Minnesota Press, 1978; Folkestone, Kent: Dawson, 1978)

CHAPTER XX: MEDICINE, STATE AND SOCIETY

Medical Politics

B. Abel-Smith, *The Hospitals 1500–1848: A Study in Social Administration in England and Wales* (London: Heinemann, 1964)

* David Armstrong, *Political Anatomy of the Body: Medical Knowledge in Britain in the Twentieth Century* (Cambridge: Cambridge University Press, 1983)

Jeffrey L. Berlant, *Profession and Monopoly: A Study of Medicine in the United States and Great Britain* (Berkeley: University of California Press, 1975)

B. and J. Ehrenreich, *The American Health Empire: Power, Profits and Politics* (New York: Random House, 1970)

Karl M. Figlio, 'How does Illness Mediate Social Relations? Workmen's Compensation and Medico-Legal Practices, 1890–1940', in P. Wright and A. Treacher (eds), *The Problem of Medical Knowledge: Examining the Social Construction of Medicine* (Edinburgh: University of Edinburgh Press, 1982), 174–224

* Daniel M. Fox, *Health Policies, Health Politics: British and American Experience 1911–1965* (Princeton, NJ: Princeton University Press, 1986)

* Daniel M. Fox, *Power and Illness: The Failure and Future of American Health Policy* (Berkeley: University of California Press, 1993)

Daniel M. Fox, 'The Medical Institutions and the State', in W. F. Bynum and Roy Porter (eds), *Companion Encyclopedia of the History of Medicine* (London: Routledge, 1993), 1196–1222

Derek Fraser, *The Evolution of the British Welfare State: The History of Social Policy Since the Industrial Revolution* (London: Macmillan, 1973)

Eliot Freidson, *Profession of Medicine: A Study of the Sociology of Applied Knowledge* (New York: Dodd, Mead, 1970)

Edward S. Golub, *The Limits of Medicine: How Science Shapes Our Hope for the Cure* (New York: Times Books, 1994)

D. Hirshfield, *The Lost Reform: The Campaign for Compulsory Health Insurance in the United States from 1932 to 1943* (Cambridge, Mass.: Harvard University Press, 1970)

* J. Rogers Hollingsworth, *A Political Economy of Medicine: Great Britain and the United States* (Baltimore: Johns Hopkins University Press, 1986)

* J. Rogers Hollingsworth, Jerald Hage and Robert A. Hanneman, *State Intervention in Medical Care: Consequences for Britain, France, Sweden and the United States 1890–1970* (Ithaca, NY and London: Cornell University Press, 1990)

* Helen Jones, *Health and Society in Twentieth-Century Britain* (London and New York: Longman, 1994)

James H. Jones, *Bad Blood: The Tuskegee Syphilis Experiment* (New York: Free Press, 1981)

* Rudolf Klein, *The Politics of the National Health Service*, 2nd edition (London: Longmans, 1989)

Rodney Lowe, *The Welfare State in Britain since 1945* (London: Macmillan, 1993)

Benno Müller-Hill, *Murderous Science* (Oxford: Oxford University Press, 1988)

Ronald Numbers, *Almost Persuaded: American Physicians and Compulsory Health Insurance 1912–1920* (Baltimore: Johns Hopkins University Press, 1978)

John Pickstone, *Medicine and Industrial Society: A History of Hospital Development in Manchester and its Region 1752–1946* (Manchester: Manchester University Press, 1985)

S. G. Solomon and J. F. Hutchinson, *Health and Society in Revolutionary Russia* (Bloomington: Indiana University Press, 1990)

Charles Webster, *The Health Services Since the War: Volume 1: Problems of Health Care. The National Health Service Before 1957* (London: Her Majesty's Stationery Office, 1988)

Charles Webster, *The Health Services Since the War: Volume 2:* (London: Her Majesty's Stationery Office, 1997)

Paul Weindling, *Health, Race and German Politics between National Unification and Nazism, 1870–1945* (Cambridge: Cambridge University Press, 1993)

James Woycke, *Birth Control in Germany 1871–1933* (London and New York: Routledge, 1988)

Drugs

V. Berridge and G. Edwards, *Opium and the People* (London: Allen Lane, 1981)

Lester Grinspoon and James B. Bakalar, *Marihuana, The Forbidden Medicine* (New Haven, CT.: Yale University Press, 1993)

H. Wayn Morgan, *Drugs in America: A Social History 1800–1980* (Syracuse: Syracuse University Press, 1981)

David F. Musto, *The American Disease: Origins of Narcotic Control* (New Haven:

Yale University Press, 1973; New York: Oxford University Press, 1988)
David F. Musto, 'Concepts of Addiction: The US Experience', in Kenneth
F. Kiple (ed.), *The Cambridge World History of Human Disease* (Cambridge:
Cambridge University Press, 1993), 170–75

Eugenics

Mark Haller, *Eugenics: Hereditarian Attitudes in American Thought* (New Brunswick, NJ: Rutgers University Press, 1984)
Daniel Kevles, *In the Name of Eugenics: Genetics and the Uses of Human Heredity*
(New York: Knopf, 1985)
Robert N. Proctor, *Racial Hygiene: Medicine Under the Nazis* (Cambridge, MA
and London: Harvard University Press, 1988)
Philip R. Reilly, *The Surgical Solution: A History of Involuntary Sterilization in
the United States* (Baltimore and London: Johns Hopkins University Press,
1991)

Mothers and Children

Rima D. Apple, *Mothers and Medicine: A Social History of Infant Feeding 1890–
1950* (Madison and London: University of Wisconsin Press, 1987)
Catherine Arnup, *Education for Motherhood: Advice for Mothers in Twentieth-
Century Canada* (Toronto: University of Toronto Press, 1994)
Roger Cooter (ed.), *In the Name of the Child: Health and Welfare* (New York
and London: Routledge, 1992)
Deborah Dwork, *War is Good for Babies and Other Young Children: A History
of the Infant and Child Welfare Movement in England 1898–1919* (London
& New York: Tavistock Publications, 1987)
D. Dwork, 'Childhood', in W. F. Bynum and Roy Porter (eds), *Companion
Encyclopedia of the History of Medicine* (London: Routledge, 1993), 1067–86
Richard A. Meckel, *'Save The Babies': American Public Health Reform And The
Prevention Of Infant Mortality, 1850–1929* (Baltimore: Johns Hopkins
University Press, 1990)

CHAPTER XXI: MEDICINE AND THE PEOPLE

General Practice

M. Balint, *The Doctor, His Patient, and the Illness* (London: Pitman, 1957)
Ann Cartwright and Robert Anderson, *General Practice Revisited: A Second
Study of Patients and Their Doctors* (London: Tavistock, 1981)
John Cule, *A Doctor for the People: 200 Years of General Practice in Britain*
(London: Update, 1980)
Jonathan Gathorne-Hardy, *Doctors: The Lives and Work of GPs* (London:
Weidenfeld and Nicolson, 1984)

* Edward Shorter, *Bedside Manners: The Troubled History of Doctors and Patients* (New York: Simon & Schuster, 1985) [later editions under the title *Doctors and their Patients: A Social History*]
* P. Starr, *The Social Transformation of American Medicine* (New York: Basic Books, 1982)

Medicine in Society
Barbara Brookes, *Abortion in England 1900–1967* (London and New York: Croom Helm, 1988)
J. J. Brumberg, *Fasting Girls: The Emergence of Anorexia Nervosa as a Modern Disease* (Cambridge, Mass.: Harvard University Press, 1988)
Rosalind Coward, *The Whole Truth: The Myth of Alternative Health* (London: Faber & Faber, 1989)
J. Donnison, *Midwives and Medical Men: A History of Interprofessional Rivalries and Women's Rights* (London: Heinemann Educational, 1977)
Elizabeth Fee and Daniel M. Fox (eds), *AIDS: The Making of a Chronic Disease* (Berkeley, Los Angeles and London: University of California Press, 1992)
Tony Gould, *A Summer Plague: Polio and its Survivors* (New Haven: Yale University Press, 1995)
David F. Greenberg, *The Construction of Homosexuality* (Chicago, Ill.: The University of Chicago Press, 1988)
I. Illich, *Limits to Medicine: The Expropriation of Health* (Harmondsworth: Penguin, 1977)
Anne Karpf, *Doctoring the Media: The Reporting of Health and Medicine* (London: Routledge, 1988)
Ian Kennedy, *Treat Me Right* (Oxford: Oxford University Press, 1989)
William L. Kissick, *Medicine's Dilemmas: Infinite Needs versus Finite Resources* (New Haven: Yale University Press, 1994)
Melvin Konner, *The Trouble with Medicine* (London: BBC Books, 1993)
Judith Walzer Leavitt, *Brought to Bed: Childbearing in America 1750–1950* (New York and Oxford: Oxford University Press, 1986)
Simon LeVay, *Queer Science. The Use and Abuse of Research on Homosexuality* (Cambridge, Mass.: MIT Press, 1996)
A. Oakley, *The Captured Womb: A History of Medical Care of Pregnant Women* (Oxford: Basil Blackwell, 1984)
Naomi Rogers, *Dirt and Disease: Polio before FDR* (New Brunswick, NJ: Rutgers University Press, 1992)
Edward Shorter, *A History of Women's Bodies* (London: Allen Lane, 1983)

In the Balance

Diana B. Dutton, *Worse than the Disease. Pitfalls of Medical Progress* (New York: Cambridge University Press, 1988)

Steven Epstein, *Impure Science. AIDS, Activism and the Politics of Knowledge* (Berkeley: University of California Press, 1996)

* I. Illich, *Limits to Medicine: The Expropriation of Health* (Harmondsworth: Penguin, 1977)

* Lynn Payer, *Medicine and Culture: Notions of Health and Sickness in Britain, the US, France and West Germany* (London: Victor Gollancz, 1989)

Lynn Payer, *Disease-Mongers: How Doctors, Drug Companies, and Insurers are Making You Feel Sick* (New York, *et al.*: John Wiley & Sons, 1992)

Mike Saks (ed.), *Alternative Medicine in Britain* (Oxford: Clarendon Press, 1992)

Randy Shilts, *And the Band Played On: People, Politics and the AIDS Epidemic* (New York: St. Martin's Press, 1988)

Elaine Showalter, *Hystories* (London: Picador, 1997)

Owen Tully Stratton, *Medicine Man* (Norman: University of Oklahoma Press, 1989)

Richard Taylor, *Medicine out of Control: The Anatomy of a Malignant Technology* (Melbourne: Sun Books, 1979)

Geoff Watts, *Pleasing the Patient* (London: Faber, 1992)

E. M. Whelan and F. J. Stare, *The 100% Natural, Purely Organic, Cholesterol-Free, Megavitamin, Low-Carbohydrate Nutrition Hoax* (New York: Atheneum, 1983)

Alexandra Wyke, *21st Century Miracle Medicine: RoboSurgery Wonder Cures and the Quest for Immortality* (New York: Plenum, 1997)

Two additional books, just published, should be mentioned.

Alan Macfarlane's *The Savage Wars of Peace* (Oxford: Blackwell, 1997) offers a convincing model of the role of health and public health in the modern demographic transition, especially in respect of Britain and Japan

Robert A. Erickson's *The Language of the Heart 1600–1750* (Philadelphia: University of Pennsylvania Press, 1997) explores the cultural significance of the Harveyan physiology of the heart.

INDEX

Numbers in bold denote main reference to subject.